ANNUAL PROGRESS IN CHILD PSYCHIATRY AND CHILD DEVELOPMENT 1991

ANNUAL PROGRESS IN CHILD PSYCHIATRY AND CHILD DEVELOPMENT 1991

Edited by

STELLA CHESS, M.D.

Professor of Child Psychiatry
New York University Medical Center

and

MARGARET E. HERTZIG, M.D.

Associate Professor of Psychiatry
Cornell University Medical College

BRUNNER/MAZEL, *Publishers* ● **New York**

Library of Congress Card No. 68-23452
ISBN 0-87630-651-2
ISSN 0066-4030

Published by
BRUNNER/MAZEL, Inc.
19 Union Square
New York, New York 10003

Manufactured in the United States of America
10 9 8 7 6 5 4 3 2 1

CONTENTS

I.   DEVELOPMENTAL STUDIES   1

    1. Home Enviroment and Cognitive Ability of Seven-Year-Old Children in the Colorado Adoption Project: Genetic and Environmental Etiologies   5

       Hilary Coon, David W. Fulker, J.C. DeFries, and Robert Plomin

    2. Nonshared Experiences Within the Family: Correlates of Behavioral Problems in Middle Childhood   27

       Judy Dunn, Clare Stocker, and Robert Plomin

    3. Children and Their Fathers After Parental Separation   45

       Joseph M. Healy Jr., Janet E. Malley, and Abigail J. Stewart

    4. A Comparison of Stepfamilies With and Without Child-Focused Problems   62

       Anne Chalfant Brown, Robert Jay Green, and Joan Druckman

    5. Masculinity, Femininity, and Sex Role Attitudes in Early Adolescence: Exploring Gender Intensification   77

       Nancy L. Galambos, David M. Almeida, and Anne C. Petersen

    6. Prediction of Behavior Problems in Four-Year-Olds Born Prematurely   92

       Susan Goldberg, Carl Corter, Mirek Lojkasek, and Klaus Minde

II.   STRESS AND VULNERABILITY   115

    7. Vulnerability in Research: A Developmental Perspective on Research Risk   119

       Ross A. Thompson

    8. Does Brain Dysfunction Increase Children's Vulnerability to Environmental Stress?   144

       Naomi Breslau

    9. Long-Term Effects of Food Supplementation and Psychosocial Intervention on the Physical Growth of Colombian Infants at Risk of Malnutrition   160

       Charles M. Super, M. Guillermo Herrera, and José O. Mora

III.   LANGUAGE STUDIES..   191
        10. Annotation: The Genetics of Dyslexia   193
            Bruce F. Pennington
        11. Very Early Language Deficits in Dyslexic Children   204
            Hollis S. Scarborough
        12. The Effect of Hearing Impairment on the Quality of
            Attachment and Mother-Toddler Interaction   228
            Amy R. Lederberg and Caryl E. Mobley

IV.   TEMPERAMENT STUDIES..   243
        13. Extreme Temperament and Diagnosis: A Study in a
            Psychiatric Sample of Consecutive Children   247
            *Michel Maziade, Chantal Caron, Robert Côté, Pierrette
            Boutin, and Jacques Thivierge*
        14. Psychiatric Correlates of Behavioral Inhibition in Young
            Children of Parents With and Without Psychiatric
            Disorders   269
            *Joseph Biederman, Jerrold F. Rosenbaum, Dina R.
            Hirshfeld, Stephen V. Faraone, Elizabeth A. Bolduc,
            Michelle Gersten, Susan R. Meminger Jerome Kagan,
            Nancy Snidman, and J. Steven Reznick*
        15. Temperament, Stress and Family Factors in Behavioural
            Adjustment of Three-Five-Year-Old Children   285
            Michael Kyrios and Margot Prior
        16. Infant Proneness-to-Distress Temperament, Maternal Person-
            ality, and Mother-Infant Attachment: Associations
            and Goodness of Fit...................................   312
            *Sarah Mangelsdorf, Megan Gunnar, Roberta Kestenbaum,
            Sarah Lang, and Debra Andreas*

V.   CLINICAL SYNDROMES   331
        17. Borderline Disorders of Childhood: An Overview...........   335
            Theodore A. Petti and Ricardo M. Vela
        18. Reliability and Validity of the Structured Interview for
            Personality Disorders in Adolescents................   359
            *David A. Brent, Janice P. Zelenak, Oscar Bukstein, and
            Robert V. Brown*

19. Childhood Obsessive–Compulsive Disorder: A Prospective Follow-up Study... 373

Martine F. Flament, Elisabeth Koby, Judith L. Rapoport, Carol J. Berg, Theodore Zahn, Christine Cox, Martha Denckla, and Marge Lenane

20. Annotation: Child and Adolescent Mania—Diagnostic Considerations 395

Gabrielle A. Carlson

21. Anxiety Disorders in a Pediatric Sample 408

Richardean S. Benjamin, Elizabeth J. Costello, and Marcia Warren

22. Psychological Effects of Chronic Disease 434

Christine Eiser

VI. DIAGNOSIS AND TREATMENT 451

23. Magnetic Resonance Imaging Evidence for a Defect of Cerebral Cortical Development in Autism.......... 455

Joseph Piven, Marcelo L. Berthier, Sergio E. Starkstein, Eileen Nehme, Godfrey Pearlson, and Susan Folstein

24. Neuropsychology of Early-treated Phenylketonuria: Specific Executive Function Deficits.......................... 466

Marilyn C. Welsh, Bruce F. Pennington, Sally Ozonoff, Bobbye Rouse, and Edward R.B. McCabe

25. Treatment of Attentional and Hyperactivity Problems in Children with Sympathomimetic Drugs: A Comprehensive Review...................................... 492

Deborah Jacobvitz, L. Alan Sroufe, Mark Stewart, and Nancy Leffert

26. A Review of the Pharmacotherapy of Aggression in Children and Adolescents 519

Jonathan T. Stewart, Wade C. Myers, Roger C. Burket, and W. Bradford Lyles

VII. PSYCHOSOCIAL ISSUES.. 541

27. Adolescent Drug Use and Psychological Health: A Longitudinal Inquiry 545

Jonathan Shedler and Jack Block

28. Nuclear Freedom and Students' Sense of Efficacy About Prevention of Nuclear War 585

Pam Oliver

29. Are Head Start Effects Sustained? A Longitudinal Follow-up
Comparison of Disadvantaged Children Attending
Head Start, No Preschool, and Other Preschool
Programs 600
Valerie E. Lee, J. Brooks-Gunn, Elizabeth Schnur, and
Fong-Ruey Liaw
30. The Seventh Jack Tizard Memorial Lecture: Aspects of
Adoption... 619
Lionel Hersov

ANNUAL PROGRESS IN CHILD PSYCHIATRY AND CHILD DEVELOPMENT 1991

Part I

DEVELOPMENTAL STUDIES

The nature-nurture controversy has long and honorable roots in religious and philosophical thought as well as in academic psychology. In the first paper in this section, Coon, Fulker, DeFries, and Plomin use the methodology of quantitative behavioral genetics to examine the extent to which associations between various measures of family environment and children's cognitive ability are either genetically or environmentally mediated. The logic of this elegantly conceived and executed study is as follows. Correlations between measures of the family environment and measures of children's cognitive ability may have both genetic and environmental components. In adoptive families, relations between measures of the home environment and children's cognitive development are due solely to environmental influences, because adoptive parents do not share heredity with their adopted children. However, such relations in nonadoptive families can be due to heredity and environment. Consequently, a comparison of environment-development relations in adoptive and nonadoptive families can reveal the extent to which influences traditionally attributed to environment are mediated genetically. Measures of the home environment obtained from infancy to seven years of age and WISC-R full-scale IQ at age seven on a sample of 153 adoptive and 163 nonadoptive families were analyzed. Some aspects of the home environment, most notably activity-recreation orientation measured by the Moos FES scales and organized environment measured by the Caldwell HOME inventory, were found to have significant direct environmental effects on the cognitive ability of seven-year olds. However, within this sample, which is described as representative of a broad cross section of metropolitan white families in the United States, aspects of the family environment as measured by the FES and Caldwell scales were found to have little direct impact on IQ. Rather significant relations between ostensible environmental measures and cognitive development are mediated primarily genetically. A thoughtful discussion clarifies and illuminates the findings for the reader who is unfamiliar with the methods of behavior genetics. The findings are of great theoretical interest; however, their generalizability is limited by both the sensitivity of the measures used and the relatively homogeneous nature of the study sample. As the authors acknowledge, this powerful methodology needs to be extended to samples taken from low SES groups and from different cultures using more sensitive instruments to measure the home environment.

The second paper in this section by Dunn, Stocker, and Plomin also uses data derived from the Colorado Adoption Project to examine the issue of the relation of

1

nonshared experiences of siblings within the family to the emergence of individual psychopathology. The rationale for identifying the salient experiences within the family that differ for two children growing up together—the nonshared environment—is clearly outlined. In sum, although family variables frequently thought to be of importance in the development of adjustment and personality such as parental mental health, the quality of the marital relationship, parental child-rearing style, or the parents' own childhood experiences are apparently shared by siblings, these siblings grow up to be strikingly different from one another. Therefore, experiences that are shared cannot be important in the etiology of individual differences in normal or abnormal development. Only nonshared environmental factors can be responsible for the development of individual differences in psychopathology and personality. In the study reported, Dunn, Stocker, and Plomin sought to identify environmental factors that differ for young siblings and to assess the associations between these nonshared factors and the difference in the older siblings' outcome as measured by the internalizing and externalizing behavior scales of the Achenbach Child Behavior Checklist. Maternal interview and observations of differential maternal and sibling behavior were compared within 67 sibling dyads (younger and older siblings averaged four and seven years respectively). Older siblings showed internalizing problems in families in which mothers were less affectionate to the older sibling than to the younger sibling. Greater maternal control toward the older sibling than the younger sibling predicted both internalizing and externalizing problems. The significance of this approach is far reaching. As the authors suggest, investigating why two children growing up in the same family are so different may well provide a key to understanding the nature of environmental influence on the development of all children, not just siblings. The importance of the theory of nonshared environment is the implication that the specific, and most probably subtle, differences experienced or perceived by siblings are important environmental factors that drive both normal and pathological development.

Increasingly, investigative interest has focused on aspects of the impact of divorce on children and how it may be further effected by the nature of the postdivorce experiences of both parents and children. The paper by Healy, Malley, and Stewart, which examines the interacting effects of child's age and gender, frequency and regularity of visitation, father-child closeness, and parental legal conflict on children's self-esteem and behavioral adjustment at two time points following divorce, is squarely in this tradition. The subjects were a nonclinical sample of 121 six-to-12-year-old children in the custody of their mothers. Although the authors deliberately restricted their attention to a relatively small number of variables, the results of the analysis of data proved to be extraordinarily complex. The child's relationship with a noncustodial father does not have simple direct effects, either positive or negative; rather it has different implications for different kinds of children, depending on age, gender, and situation. The authors conclude that their findings suggest the futility of seeking simple answers to whether ongoing contact with fathers following divorce is beneficial or detrimental to children. Alternatively, they stress the importance of individualizing each postdivorce situation in ways that are respectful of both children and parents.

The paper by Brown, Green, and Druckman addresses yet another consequence of divorce—the stepfamily. Family triads, consisting of a biological parent, stepparent, and child aged 11 to 16 years, were selected from two populations: those in therapy for a child-focused problem (N = 23) and those neither in therapy nor having child-focused problems (N = 27). Families were excluded if the child's problem predated the stepfamily's formation. Presenting problems included resisting authority, depression, temper outbursts, hostility, truancy, academic underachievement, behavioral problems in school, substance abuse, difficulties with peers, sibling conflict, jealousy, bulimia nervosa, and running away. Measures of stepparent role, family environment, management of conflict, continued emotional attachment to the former spouse, and the quality of divorced coparental relationships were made. The pattern of findings indicated that the emotional and behavioral problems of stepchildren are associated most strongly with dysfunctional role and conflict management processes within the custodial stepfamily household. Child problems in these stepfamilies do not seem to be strongly related to unresolved, emotional divorce and coparenting processes between the binuclear households. The two groups of stepfamilies did not differ on the amount of authority-related or nurturing-befriending behavior initiated by the stepparent, but they did differ with regard to how stepchildren reacted to that behavior. Stepchildren in families in treatment for child-focused problems tend to reject stepparent's nurturing-befriending and authority-related parental behavior and to view their biological parents as giving less support to the stepparent in his or her role. The findings extend our understanding of the functioning of both more and less successful stepfamilies. In addition, they have implications for the treatment of behavior disorders as they present in children living in reconstituted families. The authors conclude that family treatments may not be sufficient to clarify a given child's lack of reciprocity, therefore individual exploration may also be required.

The study by Galambos, Almeida, and Petersen utilizes data derived from a longitudinal study of 200 young adolescent girls and boys (mean age 11.6 years in sixth grade) to test the hypothesis that differences between boys and girls regarding sex role (masculine or feminine) and sex-role attitudes would intensify across the sixth, seventh, and eighth grades (between 11 and 13 years) and that pubertal timing (early, on time, late) would play a role in this intensification. The findings were different for boys and for girls. Boys viewed themselves as more masculine than girls viewed themselves as feminine at each grade level, with the magnitude of the difference increasing over time. Pubertal timing did not contribute significantly to the divergence. In contrast, among girls there was no escalation of femininity. From the sixth to the eighth grades, girls increasingly approved of male-female equality, whereas boys approved less. Neither direction of difference was related to pubertal timing. A thoughtful discussion of these findings suggests that the lack of an effect of pubertal timing may be an indication that sex-role socialization by parents and teachers may be a more powerful influence on masculinity, femininity, and sex-role attitudes than are physical characteristics. The most salient aspect of pubertal change for gender intensification may be that a cohort becomes pubertal, not that an individual enters puberty. As students enter successively higher grades, the messages regarding sex roles that they receive and observe may be similar, regardless of outward physical appearance.

In the final paper in this section, Goldberg, Corter, Lojkasek, and Minde used longitudinal follow-up data for 69, very low birth weight, preterm infants to assess the influence of four factors (neonatal medical complications, infant temperament, mother-child relationships, and family environment) on mother and teacher reports of behavior problems of four-year-old children. The rationale for the selection of these measures and the anticipated pattern of findings is clearly presented. Contrary to expectation, neither neonatal medical data nor infant-mother attachment were good predictors of behavior problems at age four. The discussion of these unexpected findings is thoughtful and informative. In particular, the review of recent attachment studies is most valuable in assessing the widely held tenet that disturbances in the mother-child relationship are a source of psychopathology. Alternatively, these authors suggest that it is perhaps more reasonable to consider that although attachment problems may be implicated in some behavior disorders (e.g., oppositional disorder), there may be no reason to suspect poor mother-child relationships as a causal factor for other disorders.

1

Home Environment and Cognitive Ability of Seven-Year-Old Children in the Colorado Adoption Project: Genetic and Environmental Etiologies

Hilary Coon, David W. Fulker, and J. C. DeFries
University of Colorado, Boulder

Robert Plomin
Pennsylvania State University

Family environment may be related to childhood cognitive abilities either directly through environmental transmission or indirectly through correlations with parental genotypes. Using the methodology of quantitative behavioral genetics, the magnitude of such effects can be determined. In the present analysis, these relations were investigated using measures of the home environment obtained from infancy through 7 years of age and WISC–R full scale IQ at age 7 on a sample of 153 adoptive and 136 nonadoptive families. Some aspects of the home environment, including activity–recreation orientation measured by the Moos FES scales and organized environment measured by the Caldwell HOME inventory, were found to have significant direct environmental effects on 7-year-old cognitive ability. However, ostensible environment–development relations for most measures were due to indirect genetic mediation.

Reprinted with permission from *Developmental Psychology*, 1990, Vol. 26, No. 3, 459–468. Copyright © 1990 by the American Psychological Association, Inc.

This research was supported in part by Grants HD-10333 and HD-18426 from the National Institute of Child Health and Human Development (NICHD).

We appreciate the time and effort given by the families participating in the Colorado Adoption Project (CAP) and the adoption agencies, Lutheran Social Services of Colorado and Denver Catholic Community Services, who made the CAP possible. We thank Gregory Carey for his comments on a previous version of this article. In addition, we thank Rebecca G. Miles for her expert editorial assistance.

The impact of family environment on cognitive development has been a focal issue of research in developmental psychology. Unfortunately, most of these studies have used intact nuclear families in which ostensible environmental influences may be correlated with heritable parental characteristics and therefore transmitted genetically to the child (Plomin, Loehlin, & DeFries, 1985). A few studies, however, have used behavioral genetic designs to assess the etiology of environment–development relations (e.g., Plomin, 1986; Scarr & Weinberg, 1978; Willerman, 1979). These analyses, based on the quantitative genetic theory of individual differences (Plomin, DeFries & Fulker, 1988), facilitate an evaluation of the extent to which association between various measures of family environment and children's cognitive ability are either genetically or environmentally mediated.

Although twin data have been used to study these environment–development relations (e.g., Wilson & Matheny, 1983), adoption data provide a more direct test for genetic mediation. Reviewing data from several adoption projects, Plomin et al. (1985) showed that correlations between measures of the family environment and measures of children's cognitive ability may have both genetic and environmental components. In adoptive families, relations between measures of the home environment and children's cognitive development are due solely to environmental influences, because adoptive parents do not share heredity with their adopted children. In contrast, such relations in nonadoptive families can be due to heredity as well as to environment. Therefore, comparison of environment–development relations in adoptive and nonadoptive families can reveal the extent to which ostensible environmental influences are mediated genetically.

Several adoption studies have obtained data pertinent to this issue. Burks (1928), Leahy (1935), Scarr and Weinberg (1978), and Horn, Loehlin, and Willerman (1979) all found higher correlations between measures of the family environment and cognitive development in nonadoptive than in adoptive families, suggesting some genetic mediation. Substantial genetic mediation of the home environment was found in a reanalysis of the Burks and Leahy data (Plomin et al., 1985). Although these differences between correlations in nonadoptive and adoptive families were less pronounced in the two more recent studies, these studies used only socioeconomic status (SES) and parental education as environmental measures, in contrast to the more extensive data obtained in the earlier studies. Considerable variation can occur within SES groups in the quality and amount of parental stimulation potentially capable of affecting cognitive development (Bradley, Caldwell, & Elardo, 1977). Moreover, distal measures such as SES and parental education provide no direct evidence about experiences in the child's environment that may influence cognitive development (Gottfried & Gottfried, 1984; Wachs & Gruen, 1982).

Several analyses of Colorado Adoption Project (CAP) data have been conducted to investigate genetic mediation as well as direct environmental transmission for specific measures of the home environment. DeFries, Plomin, Vandenberg, and Kuse

(1981) found little evidence of genetic mediation of environmental associations with cognitive development during the first year of life. In an investigation of the relation of several environmental measures to several measures of infant development, Plomin et al. (1985) estimated that, on average, about one half of the environment–development relations in nonadoptive families are mediated genetically. The extent to which ostensible environmental influences are genetically mediated may differ as a function of the child's age. Rice (1987), for example, found little evidence for genetic mediation at age 1, increasing genetic mediation at age 2, and considerable genetic mediation at ages 3 and 4. The present study, also using data from the Colorado Adoption Project, is the first investigation of the influence of specific measures of the home environment on cognitive ability at 7 years of age. Assuming that the developmental trend found by Rice continues into middle childhood, we hypothesized that associations between measures of the home environment and children's IQ at 7 years would be mediated genetically to a substantial extent.

METHOD

Subjects

The subjects for this study are participants in the Colorado Adoption Project, a longitudinal adoption study designed to investigate genetic and environmental aspects of behavioral development. Adopted children were separated from their biological mothers a few days after birth and placed in adoptive homes within 1 month, on average. A diverse battery of cognitive and other tests was administered to both biological and adoptive parents of the adopted children. The adopted children were tested annually in their homes within 2 weeks of their birthdays until the age of 4. Further tests were conducted through questionnaires and telephone interviews at ages 5 and 6. The children and their adoptive parents were brought into a laboratory setting for an extensive test session after the child completed first grade, at 7.4 years of age, on average. In addition, the study includes a control group of nonadoptive families that follows this same test schedule. Nonadoptive families were matched to adoptive families on the bases of gender of the child, number of children in the family, age of the father (± 5 years), occupational rating of the father, and total years of education of the father (± 2 years). Educational levels in the nonadoptive and adoptive parents range from 6 to 22 years ($M = 15$ years). Occupations range from floor layer, farm worker, and miner to engineer, bank president, and surgeon. For the present report, data from 153 adoptive and 136 nonadoptive families were analyzed. Further detail concerning the CAP can be found in DeFries et al. (1981), Plomin and DeFries (1985), and Plomin et al. (1988).

Measures

The adult test battery in the CAP includes 13 tests of specific cognitive abilities. The adult measure of cognitive ability used in this analysis was the first unrotated principal component of these 13 tests after they were corrected for age and gender effects (DeFries et al., 1981). Because this measure was obtained from our complete sample, it was used for our analyses in order to maximize sample size. The Wechsler Adult Intelligence Scale-Revised (WAIS–R; Wechsler, 1974) was also given to adults in our study when their children were brought in for testing at age 7, and pre-liminary results show a correlation of .70 between the WAIS–R and our measure of general intelligence measured 7 years earlier. The Wechsler Intelligence Scale for Children–Revised (WISC–R; Wechsler, 1974) full scale IQ was used as the measure of cognitive ability for the children at 7 years of age.

Two measures of the home environment were included: the Home Observation for Measurement of the Environment (HOME; Caldwell & Bradley, 1978) and the Family Environment Scale (FES; Moos, 1986). The Caldwell HOME inventory was developed as a more detailed indicator than SES of the effects of home environment on cognitive development. The HOME consists of both direct observations of the family environment completed by the interviewer and reports given by the parent. Because the HOME was developed predominantly for use in lower class families, the CAP HOME scores show elevated means and reduced variance. Although this indicates that the HOME is probably not a sensitive indicator of the variation in the home environments in this sample, the means and variances are quite similar to those of other middle-class samples (Gottfried & Gottfried, 1984; Hollenbeck, 1978; Ramey, Mills, Campbell, & O'Brien, 1975).

We used the six scales from the HOME—Mother's Responsiveness, Avoidance of Restriction, Organized Environment, Play Facilitation, Maternal Involvement, and Daily Variety—as well as a total of the scale scores. The standard HOME scales were used at 1 and 2 years; however, a nonstandard extension of the HOME was used at 3 and 4 years because the preschool version of the HOME was not available when this testing was begun (see Plomin & DeFries, 1985). Preliminary analyses revealed low longitudinal correlations for the HOME, with average correlations ranging from .12 to .39. In addition, no significant correlations were found between the child's WISC–R score at 7 years and the HOME scales at 3 and 4 years, a find-ing similar to that of Rice, Fulker, DeFries, and Plomin (1988) using IQ from ages 1 to 4. However, significant correlations were found between the 7-year WISC–R scores and the HOME scales for 1 and 2 years. For these reasons, we analyzed the HOME scales only at 1 and 2 years.

The FES is a self-report questionnaire that stresses the quality of social relation-ships within a family. In the CAP, it is completed by parents when the child is 1, 3, 5, and 7 years old; an average of ratings of mothers and fathers is taken if both are available. The CAP uses a 5-point rating scale for the FES, rather than the original true–false format, to provide more variation (see Plomin & DeFries, 1985).

From the FES, we included the 10 scales developed by Moos (1986): Cohesion, Expressivity, Family Conflict, Independence, Achievement Orientation, Intellectual–Cultural Orientation, Active Recreational Orientation, Moral–Religious Orientation, Family Organization, and Control Orientation. High-average longitudinal correlations, ranging from .53 to .85, prompted us to sum the FES scales across years. We also created two factors from the resulting scales, and generated factor scores. The first factor, Personal Growth, has substantial positive loadings on cohesion, expressiveness, independence, intellectual-cultural, and active recreational, and a moderate negative loading on conflict. The second factor, Tradition, has high positive loadings on moral-religious, organization, and control, and a moderate loading on achievement. These factors are similar in structure and interpretation to those developed by Plomin and DeFries (1985) on the CAP sample using FES data from 1 year. They also follow the structure and interpretation of FES factors found in different samples by Boake and Salmon (1983) and by Fowler (1982).

Model

Plomin et al. (1985) proposed a simple path model, depicted in Figure 1, for differentiating genetic and environmental effects of a measure of the home environment (H) on a child's phenotype (P_C), which, in the present context, is child's WISC–R IQ. In adoptive families, the home environment can only affect the child's phenotype through the child's environment, represented by the latent variable E_C. In nonadoptive homes, correlations (r_G) between the home environment and the parents' IQ genotype (G_F and G_M) also provide a passive genetic link between the home environment and the child's phenotype. This link is completed by the genetic transmission of one half from the IQ genotypes of the parents to the IQ genotype of the child, G_C. Mediation in this model is strictly through genetic and environmental variables that determine IQ. The expected correlations between the home environment and the child's phenotype are, therefore, [ef] in adoptive homes and [ef + hr_G] in nonadoptive homes. This is merely a path analytic restatement of the point made earlier: Environment–development associations in adoptive homes are solely environmental in origin, whereas in nonadoptive homes heredity can also contribute to such associations.

Our model is an elaboration of this simple model that (a) provides for parental IQ to influence the child's environment in addition to the home environment and (b) uses the additional information in the adoption design obtained from the biological parents to separate the effects of r_G and h. Our r_G and h have identical meaning to those in the Plomin et al. (1985) model, but by including the effects of parental phenotype on the child's environment, we can obtain more accurate estimates of their values. An introduction to CAP model fitting is available elsewhere (Plomin et al., 1988).

We develop our model in two stages. First, we include the parental phenotypes as shown in Figure 2. For simplicity, this diagram shows only those correlations that link the home environment to the child's phenotype. Two additional symbols are introduced in Figure 2: the path z from parental IQ to children's IQ-relevant environment and the correlation ($r_{H,P}$) between the measure of home environment and parental IQ. Thus, following tracing rules of path analysis, the expected correlations between the home environment and the child's phenotype are [ef + 2ez($r_{H,P}$)] in adoptive families, and [ef + 2ez($r_{H,P}$) + hr_G] in nonadoptive families. These expected correlations include the expectations described previously—[ef] for adoptive families and [ef + hr_G] for nonadoptive families. However, the expectation for phenotypic transmission from parental IQ to children's IQ [2ez($r_{H,P}$)] has been added to the expectations for both adoptive and nonadoptive families. This represents the possibility that parental IQ contributes directly to children's IQ independently of the environmental measure. The difference between the expectations for adoptive and nonadoptive families is sill hr_G as in the simple model in Figure 1.

Figure 3 depicts our final model. Here we have incorporated the biological parent to allow us to estimate h so that the effects of h and r_G can be separated. Also, by including the latent variables for the parent (G_M, G_F, E_M, and E_F, $r_{H,P}$ can be expressed more explicitly as a sum of genetic and nongenetic components [hr_G + er_E], as shown in the expectations of the model presented in Table 1. This extension of the model allows us to estimate er_E once hr_G has been determined. With the power added by the adoption design, h and e can be estimated, allowing the further

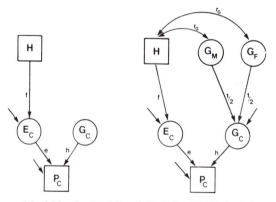

Figure 1. Path model of Plomin, Loehlin, & DeFries (1985) depicting genetic and environmental transmission in adoptive and nonadoptive families. (H is a measure of the home environment. Mother, father, and child are signified by M, F, and C, respectively.)

separation of e and r_E. In addition, the model in Figure 3 allows a more complete description of the effects of assortative mating and genotype-environment correlation. This model is identical to the model presented by Rice et al. (1988), with two minor simplifications. First, previous analyses using CAP data (Fulker, 1988) indicated no differences between maternal and paternal cultural transmission; thus, both are represented by the single path z. Second, no significant differences between maternal and paternal correlations were found for any of our measures of the home; therefore, we constrained r_G and r_E to be equal for mothers and fathers.

Initial tests of selective placement between biological and adoptive parents revealed no significant effects, a result consistent with all previous CAP findings. Therefore, for simplicity, its effects are omitted from the model. In the absence of selective placement, there is no covariance between the genotype and environment of the adopted child of the passive variety (Plomin, DeFries, & Loehlin, 1977). Thus, the phenotypic variance for adopted children is restricted to $V_P = h^2 + e^2$, which may be less than unity if a positive genotype-environment correlation exists in nonadoptive families. Preliminary analyses also yielded no significant differences for assortative mating between wed adoptive and nonadoptive parents and unwed biological parents; therefore, these assortment parameters are represented by p.

This basic model yields the expectations listed in Table 1. In addition to the usual parent-offspring model for estimating heritability of a phenotype, the model facilitates

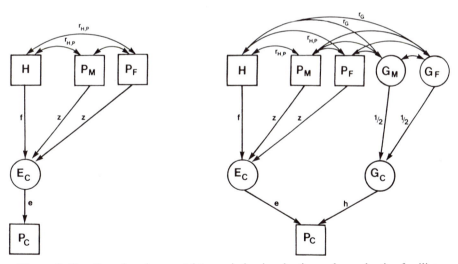

Figure 2. Genetic and environmental transmission in adoptive and nonadoptive families including the effects of the parental phenotype (P_M and P_F). (H is a single measure of the home environment. Mother, father, and child are signified by M, F, and C, respectively. For simplicity, only variables that link H to P_c are shown.)

analyses of ostensible environment–development relations, that is, the comparison between home environment–child phenotype associations in adoptive and nonadoptive families. The difference in expectations between these two correlations is hr_G. The environmental link (er_E between H and parental P is that part of the phenotypic correlation between H and parental P that is not explained by genetic mediation.

These expectations were fitted to three matrices of observed variances and covariances among the variables (see Plomin et al., 1988, for greater detail concerning CAP model fitting). Variables for one matrix included general intelligence scores of nonadoptive mothers and fathers, WISC–R IQ scores of their children, and the home measure under analysis, and it was based on approximately 136 families (sample size depended on missing values for the particular home measure). Two matrices of data were used for adoptive families. The first included data from biological mothers and fathers, adoptive mothers and fathers, the adopted child, and a measure of the home environment. Because relatively few biological fathers were tested, the matrices with data from both biological parents contained only a small number of families (an average of 34). The second matrix included data from families in which the biological fathers were not tested (153 families on average).

The expectations listed in Table 1 were fitted to these observed data using the maximum likelihood estimation procedure. For n observed and expected covariance matrices, the log likelihood ratio chi-square statistic

$$F = \sum_{k=1}^{n} N_K[\ln E(S_K) - \ln S_K + tr(S_K E(S_K)^{-1}) - p_k]$$

was computed, where N_K is the degrees of freedom in the kth matrix, S is the observed covariance matrix, E(S) is the expected covariance matrix, tr is the trace of a matrix, and p_K is the order of the kth matrix. For these analyses, n is 3, and p_K varies from 4 for the matrix of nonadoptive data to 6 for the full matrix of adoptive data.

This function was minimized using the MINUIT optimization software package (CERN, 1977). A difference in the likelihood ratio statistics obtained from the full model and subsequent reduced models allowed a chi-square test for the significance of parameters. Using these techniques, we tested hypotheses concerning the etiology of environment–development relations.

RESULTS

Initial tests for group differences were based on the full sample of adoptive and nonadoptive families. Means and standard deviations are similar to those reported in Plomin et al. (1985). No significant differences between adoptive and nonadoptive families were found for the cognitive measures or for the HOME scales at 1 and 2 years. Consistent with Plomin et al. (1985), significant mean differences were found for several FES scales (Family Conflict, Intellectual–Cultural Orientation, Moral–Religious Orientation, Family Organization, and Control Orientation). However, these differences are all less than .5 *SD*, with the exception of the Moral–Religious Orientation scale, which shows a difference of approximately .66 *SD*. These results suggest an acceptable overlap in range for the two groups, particularly for the purposes of the present study. Because the analyses focus on correlational structures, differences in variance are more important than mean differences. All of the scales show comparable variances, again with the exception of the Moral–Religious Orientation scale, which shows somewhat reduced variance for the adoptive families. These differences for the Moral–Religious Orientation scale are not surprising, given that the adoptive families were recruited through two adoption agencies with religious affiliations.

TABLE 1
Expected Nonadoptive and Adoptive Parent-Offspring Variances and Covariances

Variable	Expectation
Nonadoptive families	
P_M, P_F	$[p]\, V_P$
$P_M, P_H = P_F, P_H$	$[hr_G + er_E]\, V_P^{1/2} V_H^{1/2}$
$P_M, P_C = P_F, P_C$	$[\tfrac{1}{2}h(h + se)(1 + p) + ez(1 + p) +$ $ef(hr_G + er_E)]\, V_P^{1/2} V_{Pc}^{1/2}$
P_H, P_C	$[ef + 2ez(hr_G + er_E) + hr_G] \times$ $V_{Pc}^{1/2} V_H^{1/2}$
$P_M, P_M = P_F, P_F$	$[h^2 + e^2 + 2hse]\, V_P$
P_H, P_H	V_H
P_C, P_C	$[h^2 + e^2 + 2hse]\, V_{Pc}$
Adoptive families	
$P_{BM}, P_{BF} = P_{AM}, P_{AF}$	$[p]\, V_P$
$P_{AM}, P_H = P_{AF}, P_H$	$[hr_G + er_E]\, V_P^{1/2} V_H^{1/2}$
$P_{AM}, P_C = P_{AF}, P_C$	$[ez(1 + p) + ef(hr_G + er_E) \times$ $V_P^{1/2} V_{Pc}^{1/2}$
$P_{BM}, P_C = P_{BF}, P_C$	$[\tfrac{1}{2}h(h + se)(1 + p)]\, V_P^{1/2} V_{Pc}^{1/2}$
P_H, P_C	$[ef + 2ez(hr_G + er_E)]\, V_{Pc}^{1/2} V_H^{1/2}$
$P_{BM}, P_{BM} = P_{BF}, P_{BF} = P_{AM},$ $\quad P_{AM} = P_{AF}, P_{AF}$	$[h^2 + e^2 + 2hse]\, V_P$
P_H, P_H	V_H
P_C, P_C	$[h^2 + e^2]\, V_{Pc}$
Constraints	
r_{GcEc}	$z(h + se)(1 + p) + fr_G$
se	$(zeh(1 + p) + fr_G)/(1 - ze(1 + p))$

Note. P = parental phenotype; M = mother; F = father; H = home environment; C = child; p = assortive mating; h = heritability; e = environmental contribution to phenotype; s = correlation between genotype and environment; z = parent–offspring cultural transmission; G = genotype.

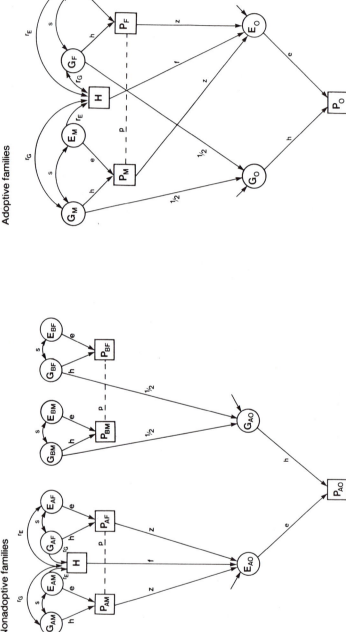

Figure 3. Final model of genetic and environmental transmission in adoptive and control families. (Effects of the biological mother are included. Explicit effects of latent parental variables [G_M, G_F, E_M, and E_F] are included. Mother, father, and child are signified by M, F and C, respectively. Assortative mating occurs through the conditional path p; however, it is assumed that the home environment, H, is present only after the assortment process.)

The results that follow are presented first in terms of simple correlations for the FES and the HOME scales as related to children's IQ and to parents' IQ. Model-fitting results are then presented that confirm the impressions gleaned from the simple correlational results.

FES-IQ Correlations

Table 2 presents correlations of the FES scales and factors with cognitive measures in parents and children. The results in this table show that the FES scales tend to correlate as highly with parent IQ as with children's IQ. Thus, it is reasonable to hypothesize that the correlation between the FES and children's IQ might be mediated to some extent by parental IQ [the 2ez-($r_{H,P}$) paths in Figures 2 and 3].

Correlations of FES measures with parental intelligence were homogeneous

TABLE 2
Correlations Between FES Scales, FES Factors, Parental General Intelligence, and Full Scale WISC–R IQ at Age 7

FES measure	Parental general intelligence ($n = 300$)		Child WISCR full scale IQ ($n = 150$)	
	Mother	Father	Non-adoptive	Adoptive
Scale				
Cohesion	.06	.06	.11	.07
Expressivity	.12*	.10*	.14*	−.03
Conflict	−.02	.00	.06	−.16*
Independence	.12*	.09	.21*	.06
Achievement Orientation	−.13*	−.10*	.06	.04
Intellectual–Cultural Orientation	.19*	.29*	.21*	.01
Active Recreational Orientation	.18*	.08	.00	−.10
Moral-Religious Orientation	−.05	−.16*	−.16*	.05
Family Organization	−.07	−.08	.02	.14*
Control Orientation	−.12*	−.15*	−.14*	−.03
Factor				
Personal Growth	.17*	.16*	.17*	.04
Tradition	−.08	−.15*	−.10	.10

Note. FES = Family Environmental Scale; WISC–R = Wechsler Intelligence Scale for Children–Revised.
* $p = .05$.

across adoptive and nonadoptive parents, and thus were pooled. All of the scales except Cohesion, Family Conflict, and Family Organization show significant correlations with parental intelligence. The Intellectual–Cultural Orientation scale has the highest correlations, whereas significant negative correlations appear for the Achievement, Moral–Religious, and Control Orientation scales. Results similar to these were reported by Garfinkle (1982), Boake and Salmon (1983), and Gottfried and Gottfried (1984). The two factors show different patterns, with positive correlations for Personal Growth and negative correlations for Tradition.

Investigation of the correlations with children's intelligence in adoptive and nonadoptive families provides an initial test of the extent of genetic and environmental mediation of the HOME measures. If the correlations for adopted and nonadopted children are equal, the association between the HOME and IQ is not mediated genetically. Genetic mediation is suggested to the extent that the HOME-IQ correlation is higher for nonadopted children than for adopted children.

Several FES scales are significantly correlated with the child's WISC–R full scale IQ score in nonadoptive families. The Intellectual-Cultural Orientation scale has one of the strongest associations, as has also been found by Harris (1982), Garfinkle (1982), and Wilson and Matheny (1983). Expressivity and independence also correlate positively with child IQ, whereas Moral–Religious and Control Orientation correlate negatively, results consistent with Gottfried and Gottfried (1984). The two factors also follow this trend, with a positive correlation for the Personal Growth and a small negative correlation for Tradition.

As indicated earlier, association between measures of the home environment and children's development found in adoptive families indicates direct environmental influence (Path f in the model). As shown in Table 2, only two correlations are significant for the adopted children: a negative relation with Family Conflict and a positive relationship with Family Organization. Thus, we expect significant estimates for the f parameter for these two scales.

Significant genetic mediation (hr_G) of the association between the FES and offspring IQ is suggested when correlations between FES and offspring IQ are higher in nonadoptive families than in adoptive families. This is the case for Expressivity, Independence, Intellectual–Cultural Orientation, Moral–Religious Orientation, Control Orientation, and Personal Growth. The difference between the FES-offspring IQ correlation in nonadoptive and adoptive families estimates hr_G.

In summary, several of the associations between FES scales and children's IQ in nonadoptive families appear to be mediated genetically because the FES-IQ correlations for nonadopted children exceed those for adopted children. Because these same FES scales also correlate with parental IQ, it is likely that the correlations between FES and children's IQ are mediated to some extent by parental IQ.

TABLE 3
Correlations of HOME Scales for Years 1 and 2 With Parental General Intelligence and Child Full Scale WISC–R IQ at Age 7

| | Year 1 | | | | Year 2 | | | |
| | Parent general intelligence (n = 280) | | Child WISC-R full scale IQ (n = 150) | | Parental general intelligence (n = 260) | | Child WISC-R full scale IQ (n = 145) | |
Caldwell scale	Mother	Father	Nonadoptive	Adoptive	Mother	Father	Nonadoptive	Adoptive
Total	.17*	.15*	.21*	-.08	.16*	.19*	.31*	.08
Mother's Responsiveness	.02	.09	.16*	.02	.08	.16*	.29*	.02
Avoidance of Restriction	.12*	.09	.07	-.08	.14*	.14*	.01	-.06
Organized Environment	.12*	.02	.11	-.09	-.10	-.10	.18*	.20*
Play Facilitation	.15*	.16*	-.01	-.03	.15*	.19*	.16*	-.03
Maternal Involvement	.07	.07	.18*	-.03	.14*	.09	.17*	.00
Daily Variety	.17*	.12*	.08	-.02	.14*	.05	.12	.11

Note. HOME = Home Observation for Measurement of the Environment; WISC–R = Wechsler Intelligence Scale for Children–Revised.
* p = .05.

HOME-IQ Correlations

Results for the HOME scales are presented in Table 3. Similar to the FES, the HOME total score at both 1 and 2 years relates significantly to parental IQ and to nonadopted children's IQ, a result also reported by Wilson and Matheny (1983). However, at both years the HOME-IQ correlation is negligible in adoptive families. Thus, similar to the results for the FES, it appears that the correlations between the HOME total scores at 1 and 2 years and children's IQ at 7 years are primarily genetically mediated. Because the HOME totals at 1 and 2 years also correlate with parental IQ, the correlation between the HOME total and children's IQ is likely to be mediated by parental IQ.

Results for the HOME scales are less clear, perhaps because of reduced reliability of the subscales. Nonetheless, most of the scales correlate with mother's IQ. (Unlike the FES, the HOME focuses on the mother's interaction with her children.) At both 1 and 2 years, Mother's Responsiveness and Maternal Involvement correlate with children's IQ in nonadoptive but not in adoptive families, which suggests genetic mediation of this association. At 2 years, the Play Facilitation scale also shows a significant correlation with children's IQ in nonadoptive families. At 2 years, the Play Facilitation scale also shows a significant correlation with children's IQ in nonadoptive families. At 2 years, the Organized Environment scale correlates with children's IQ in both nonadoptive and adoptive families, suggesting negligible genetic mediation and substantial environmental mediation of this association. This is similar to the finding for the FES organization scale. Daily Variety also appears to have equal effects in both groups, although neither effect is significant, a trend also found by DeFries et al. (1981).

In summary, these HOME correlations suggest significant direct environmental influence (f) for organized environment at 2 years. Differences between adoptive and nonadoptive correlations involving HOME scores and offspring IQ, a measure of hr_G, emerge for the total scores at both 1 and 2 years, for Mother's Responsiveness and Maternal Involvement at 1 and 2 years, and for Play Facilitation at 2 years. The effects of indirect environmental mediation (er_E) appear minimal for all scales, with the exception of the Play Facilitation scale at 1 year, which correlates significantly with parental intelligence, without showing evidence for hr_G.

Model Fitting

In order to test these parameters more rigorously and in the context of the model, matrices of covariances in adoptive and nonadoptive families were fitted to our model using the maximum likelihood estimation procedure described previously. The results of these analyses allowed us to assess the genetic and environmental components of the indirect mediation of the home measures (H) on the child's cognitive ability by comparing the relative magnitudes of hr_G and er_E.

The strengths of r_G and r_E were assessed by first dropping each from the model separately and comparing the fit of these reduced models to the fit of the full model using the likelihood ratio chi-square statistic, or change in chi-square, with 1 *df*. In addition, both r_G and r_E were dropped simultaneously, and again the loss in fit was examined here with 2 *df*. In addition, we assessed the existence of direct effects of the home environment on the child's intelligence by testing the f parameter. The f parameter was dropped from a model containing r_G and r_E if they were found to be significantly different from zero, or from a model omitting them if they could be dropped in the previous test.

Tables 4 and 5 contain parameter estimates of the initial model. Chi-square goodness-of-fit statistics for this initial full model, fit separately for each home measure, ranged from 25.80 for the HOME Play Facilitation scale at 2 years to 38.05 for the FES Moral–Religious Orientation scale. These are all chi-square statistics with 37 *df*, indicating an adequate fit of the data to the full model for all of the home measures. The estimates of the parameters h^2, z, and p in these full models were relatively unaffected by which environmental measure was used, indicating that the underlying model of parent-offspring transmission is independent of the effects of the home measure. Estimates of heritability (h^2), assuming isomorphism of the parental and child intelligence measures, fall between .35 and .40 for all of the home measures tested. Assortative mating (p) was approximately .20, and cultural transmission (z) was effectively zero. These estimates are quite close to those obtained from a similar model, omitting the home measure, which was fitted to parent and 7-year-old cognitive data (Fulker, DeFries, & Plomin, 1988).

Results of the parameter estimates and tests of significance of f, r_G, and r_E for the FES measures given in Table 4 generally confirm the results based on the simple correlations. The greatest estimates of direct environmental transmission (f) involve the four scales with the highest correlations between the FES and adoptee IQ. All of the FES scales that show control-adoptive differences in correlations between FES and offspring IQ yield r_G estimates that were either individually significant or could not be dropped in the 2-*df* test of setting both r_G and r_E to zero.

Earlier examination of the pattern of correlations in Table 2 suggested that the environmental component (er_E) is modest, although some evidence of er_E emerged for control and traditional organization. This is consistent with results of model fitting, which show no significant estimates of the parameter r_E for any of the FES scales, although r_E could not be dropped together with r_G in the 2-*df* test for the Independence, Active Recreational Orientation, and Control Organization scales, and the Personal Growth factor. In comparing models with and without the direct environmental transmission parameter (f), one scale, Active Recreational Orientation, shows a significant loss in fit, with a change in chi-square of 4.60 with

TABLE 4
Parameter Estimates of the Initial Model for the FES Scales and Factors of r_G, r_E, and f

Parameter	Scale										Factor	
	COHSN	EXPR	CONF	INDP	ACH	INTCL	ACTRC	MRELG	ORG	CONT	Growth	Tradition
h^2	.35	.37	.38	.35	.35	.35	.40	.38	.36	.35	.35	.37
z	.02	.04	.02	.02	.03	.02	.04	.03	.04	.02	.03	.04
p	.21	.21	.21	.21	.21	.21	.21	.21	.21	.21	.21	.21
r_G	.15	.41	.31	.33[a]	.02	.37	.25[a]	−.40	.23	−.22[a]	.33[a]	−.37
r_E	−.03	−.14	−.24	−.11[a]	−.14	.06	−.05[a]	.16	.07	−.02[a]	−.01[a]	.12
f	.05	−.09	−.19	.02	.06	.02	−.19	.14	.18	.01	−.01	.17
$\chi^2 (r_E = 0)$	0.03	1.04	3.71	0.74	1.21	0.21	0.15	1.52	0.22	0.04	0.01	0.87
$\chi^2 (r_G = 0)$	0.68	5.57*	3.66	3.30	0.03	4.09*	2.34	5.68*	1.48	1.41	3.25	4.58*
$\chi^2 (r_E = r_G = 0)$	2.78	13.63*	3.85	7.44*	5.87	37.96*	8.53*	11.11*	4.01	11.78*	19.01*	10.76
$\chi^2 (f = 0)$	1.96	0.77	1.12	0.05	1.33	0.11	4.60*	2.08	3.03	0.02	0.01	2.92

Note. Home environment is measured by Family Environment Scales (FES) averaged across 1, 3, 5, and 7 years. Underlined parameters are significantly different from zero. FES subscales are as follows: Cohesion (COHSN), Expressivity (EXPR), Conflict (CONF), Independence (INDP), Achievement orientation (ACH), Intellectual–Cultural Orientation (INTCL), Active Recreational Orientation (ACTRC), Moral–Religious Orientation (MRELG), Family Organization (ORG), Control Orientation (CONT); and Personal Growth and Tradition factors. Parameters estimated are heritability (h^2), parent–offspring cultural transmission (z), assortative mating (p), correlation between parental genotype for IQ and the FES measures (r_G), correlation between parental environment for IQ and the FES measures (r_E), and the direct environmental effect of the FES measures (f).

[a] Parameter is not individually significant; it cannot be dropped on the basis of the 2-*df* test.

* $p = .05$.

TABLE 5
Parameter Estimates of the Initial Model for the HOME Measures and Tests of r_G, r_E, and f

Parameter	Year 1							Year 7						
	Total	RSPNS	RSTRC	ORGNZ	PLAY	INVLV	VRTY	Total	RSPNS	RSTRC	ORGNZ	PLAY	INVLV	VRTY
h^2	.37	.35	.35	.36	.36	.37	.36	.30	.31	.35	.38	.35	.40	.35
z	.05	.03	.04	.03	.04	.03	.03	.01	.01	.01	.04	.01	.01	.03
p	.20	.21	.20	.20	.20	.21	.20	.20	.20	.19	.19	.20	.19	.20
r_G	.50	.29	.23	.32	.12ª	.39	.21ª	.34ª	.41	.02	-.10	.34ª	.26ª	-.02
r_E	-.16	-.14	-.06	-.17	.08ª	-.21	-.01ª	-.03ª	-.16	.10	-.05	-.07ª	-.06ª	.12
f	-.16	-.02	-.11	-.09	-.09	-.11	-.07	.14	-.06	-.07	.31	-.04	.04	.14
$\chi^2(r_E = 0)$	0.85	0.22	1.59	0.40	2.74	0.01	1.72	1.48	0.51	0.19	0.25	0.23	0.83	0.06
$\chi^2(r_G = 0)$	2.48	1.54	3.03	0.39	5.20*	1.37	8.61*	4.72*	0.02	0.28	3.67	2.59	0.02	3.35
$\chi^2(r_E = r_G = 0)$	3.41	4.34	3.88	9.60*	6.35*	8.32*	20.12*	8.50*	4.61	5.15	12.87*	8.22*	3.91	15.36*
$\chi^2(f = 0)$	0.62	0.36	0.08	0.68	1.54	0.38	2.75	0.60	1.15	17.67*	0.16	0.13	2.67	2.35

Note. Home environment is measured by Home Observation for Measurement of the Environment (HOME) scales at years 1 and 2. Underlined parameters are significantly different from zero. HOME scales are as follows: Mother's Responsiveness (RSPNS), Avoidance of Restriction (RSTRC), Organized Environment (ORGNZ), Play Facilitation (PLAY), Maternal Involvement (INVLV), and Daily Variety (VRTY). Parameters estimated are heritability (h^2), parent-offspring cultural transmission (z), assortative mating (p), correlation between parental genotype for IQ and the HOME scales (r_G), correlation between parental environment for IQ and the HOME scales (r_E), and the direct environmental effect of the HOME scales (f).

ª Parameter is not individually significant; it cannot be dropped on the basis of the 2-df test.

* $p = .05$.

1 *df*. This indicates that the Active Recreational Orientation scale has a direct environmental effect on the child's cognitive ability. Using this same model comparison, positive direct environmental effects for the Family Organization scale and the Tradition factor also approached significance, with changes in chi-square of 3.03 and 2.92, respectively. Finally, it is noteworthy that for each of the FES scales, estimates of r_G exceed those of r_E.

The model-fitting results also suggest genetic mediation for the majority of the HOME scales (Table 5). For the HOME total scores at 1 and 2 years, r_G estimates are relatively large; substantial increases in chi-square occurred when this parameter was dropped from the model. In contrast, the increases in chi-square incurred by dropping either r_E or f from the model were negligible.

Findings for the subscales show that the largest r_G parameter estimates occur for those seven HOME scores that show the greatest adoptive-nonadoptive difference in HOME-child-IQ correlations. The only scale with a significant correlation between the Caldwell and adoptee IQ, Family Organization at 2 years, is also the only scale to yield a significant f estimate. This finding is particularly interesting because at this age, Organized Environment has nonsignificant correlations with parental intelligence; this is an environmental measure, uncorrelated with parental intelligence, that has a direct impact on the child. In addition, model-fitting results suggest significant r_G and r_E in the 2-*df* test for play at one year and for variety at 1 year. For each case showing significant correlations with the parental phenotype, the genetic component (r_G) is consistently greater in magnitude than the environmental component (r_E).

DISCUSSION

The model used in this analysis has several advantages for the investigation of relations between measures of the home environment and cognitive development. The model uses quantitative genetic theory to separate the relative importance of direct environmental effects from the indirect effects that operate through genotype and cultural transmission. In addition, the part of the model involving parent-offspring transmission of intelligence is unaffected by the specific home measure being tested.

On the basis of the comparisons of the genetic and nongenetic models proposed, the results indicate that correlations between measures of the home environment and children's IQ at 7 years are often mediated genetically. Correlations are generally lower in adoptive families than in nonadoptive families; in the model-fitting results, estimates of r_G substantially exceed estimates of r_E. Moreover, only one scale, HOME Organized Environment at 2 years, correlated significantly with 7-year IQ in both adoptive and nonadoptive families. In the model-fitting analyses, this scale and one other, FES Active Recreational Orientation, were the only environmental measures to show a direct environmental effect on IQ at 7 years.

To illustrate the finding that environment–development associations are primarily mediated genetically, consider the correlation between the HOME total score at 2 years and 7-year IQ. In nonadoptive families, this correlation is .31, which is remarkable given the 5-year interval between the two assessments. Even though this is a longitudinal correlation, it cannot be assumed that the factors assessed by the HOME measure affect 7-year IQ for environmental reasons. The most telling result is that the correlation in adoptive families is only .08, giving a rough estimate of .31 $-.08 = .23$ for the genetic mediation (hr_G) of the HOME effects on children's IQ. This quantity can also be computed directly from the model-fitting results. As shown in Table 5, h^2 is .30 (which means that h is .55) and r_G is .34; thus, hr_G is .19. These estimates indicate that more than half of the correlation of .31 between the HOME and children's IQ is mediated genetically. The direct environmental path between this HOME measure and 7-year IQ is nonsignificant and modest (.14).

The direct environmental effects of the FES Active Recreational Orientation and the HOME Organized Environment scales on 7-year IQ deserve further comment. The Active Recreational Orientation scale has a significant direct negative impact on the child's cognitive ability. The positive correlation with the parental phenotype indicates that higher parental intelligence corresponds with more family activity. However, the significant negative estimate of direct environmental transmission (f) for this scale suggests that family activity has a negative effect on the child's intelligence. Gottfried and Gottfried (1984) found a significant negative relation between this scale and intelligence at age 3, in addition to negative relations with other measures that could be thought of as distractions, such as noise level in the home and number of siblings. Thus, it is possible that high levels of family activity may detract from time that could be spent in more intellectually stimulating pursuits.

Although results from the HOME may be less robust because of the reduction in variance in the CAP sample, the effect of HOME Organized Environment at 2 years on 7-year IQ is particularly interesting because this scale correlates only slightly (and negatively) with parental IQ. That is, parental intelligence has little association with parental skills of organizing the family environment, but organization has a direct positive influence on the cognitive abilities of the child. Furthermore, a similar result was reported by Bradley and Caldwell (1976), who found that cognitive functioning decreased when the family environment was inadequately organized. Bradley and Caldwell have speculated that children from disorganized families cannot fully concentrate on the cognitive test because of the distractions in their environment when the test is administered in the home. However, our 7-year-old subjects are given the WISC–R in a controlled laboratory setting. In addition, this aspect of the environment was measured when the child was 2 years old. Our results suggest that the effect of Organized Environment on IQ scores is not confined to effects of home testing and that it may have a more lasting impact on the child's cognitive abilities.

Although results of our study indicate that FES Active Recreational Orientation and HOME Organized Environment have significant direct effects, this was the exception rather than the rule. Both the simple correlations and the parameter estimates from fitting our model suggest the prevalence of indirect genetic mediation of the measures of home environment that we tested. Several possibilities could explain this finding. As Plomin et al. (1985) have pointed out, "Although the HOME and the FES were the best environmental measures available when we began the CAP in 1975 and have subsequently become widely used, they represent the first wave of systematic attempts to assess the home environment" (p. 400). They have suggested that more sensitive instruments may reveal other environment–development relationships that are not mediated through the genotypes of the parents.

Another possibility is that direct effects of the environment can only be detected for extreme home environments (Willerman, 1979). Although it will be important to explore these issues in other samples taken from low SES groups and from different cultures, it should be emphasized that the CAP sample is representative of a broad cross-section of metropolitan White families in the United States (Plomin & DeFries, 1985). Within this sample, aspects of the family environment as measured by the FES and Caldwell scales have little direct impact on the cognitive abilities of 7-year-old children. For the broad range of family environments seen in the CAP sample, significant relations between ostensible environmental measures and cognitive development are mediated primarily genetically.

REFERENCES

Boake, C., & Salmon, P. G. (1983). Demographic correlates and factor structure of the Family Environment Scale. *Journal of Clinical Psychology, 39*, 95–100.

Bradley, R. H., & Caldwell, B. M. (1976). Early home environment and changes in mental test performance in children from 6 to 36 months. *Developmental Psychology, 12*, 93–97.

Bradley, R. H., Caldwell, B. M., & Elardo, R. (1977). Home environment, social status, and mental test performance. *Journal of Educational Psychology, 69*, 697–701.

Burks, B. S. (1928). The relative influence of nature and nurture upon mental development. A comparative study of foster-parent-foster-child resemblance and true-parent-true-child resemblance. *27th Yearbook of the National Society for the Study of Education, 27*, 219–316.

Caldwell, B. M., & Bradley, R. H. (1978). *Home Observation for Measurement of the Environment*. Little Rock: University of Arkansas Press.

CERN. (1977). *MINUIT: A system of function minimization and analysis of parameter errors and correlations* [Computer program]. Geneva, Switzerland: Author.

DeFries, J. C., Plomin, R., Vandenberg, S. G., & Kuse, A. R. (1981). Parent-offspring resemblance for cognitive abilities in the Colorado Adoption Project: Biological, adoptive, and control parents and one-year-old children. *Intelligence, 5*, 245–277.

Fowler, P. C. (1982). Factor structure of the Family Environment Scale: Effects of social desirability. *Journal of Clinical Psychology, 38*, 285–292.

Fulker, D. W. (1988). Path analysis of genetic and cultural transmission in human behavior. In B. S. Weir, E. J. Eisen, M. M. Goodman, & G. Namkoong (Eds.), *Proceedings of the Second International Conference on Quantitative Genetics* (pp. 318–340). Sunderland, MA: Sinauer.

Fulker, D. W., DeFries, J. C., & Plomin, R. (1988). Genetic influence on general mental ability increases between infancy and middle childhood. *Nature, 336*, 767–769.

Garfinkle, A. S. (1982). Genetic and environmental influences on the development of Piagetian logico-mathematical concepts and other specific cognitive abilities: A twin study. *Acta Geneticae Medicae et Gemellologiae, 31*, 10–61.

Gottfried, A. E., & Gottfried, A. W. (1984). Home environment and mental development in middle-class children in the first three years. In A. W. Gottfried (Ed.), *Home environment and early cognitive development: Longitudinal research* (pp. 57–115). New York: Academic Press.

Harris, E. L. (1982). Genetic and environmental influences on reading achievement: A study on first- and second-grade twin children. *Acta Geneticae Medicae et Gemellologiae, 31*, 64–116.

Hollenbeck, A. R. (1978). Early infant home environments: Validation of the Home Observation for Measurement of the Environment inventory. *Developmental Psychology, 14*, 416–418.

Horn, J. M., Loehlin, J. C., & Willerman, L. (1979). Intellectual resemblance among adoptive and biological relatives: The Texas Adoption Project. *Behavior Genetics, 9*, 177–208.

Leahy, A. M. (1935). Nature-nurture and intelligence. *Genetic Psychology Monographs, 17*, 235–305.

Moos, R. H. (1986). *Family Environment Scale manual*. Palo Alto, CA: Consulting Psychologists Press.

Plomin, R. (1986). *Development, genetics, and psychology*. Hillsdale, NJ: Erlbaum.

Plomin, R., & DeFries, J. C. (1985). *Origins of individual differences in infancy: The Colorado Adoption Project*. Orlando, FL: Academic Press.

Plomin, R., DeFries, J. C., & Fulker, D. W. (1988). *Nature and nurture during infancy and early childhood*. Cambridge, England: Cambridge University Press.

Plomin, R., DeFries, J. C., & Loehlin, J. C. (1977). Genotype-environment interaction and correlation in the analysis of human behavior. *Psychological Bulletin, 84*, 309–332.

Plomin, R., Loehlin, J. C., & DeFries, J. C. (1985). Genetic and environmental components of "environmental" influences. *Developmental Psychology, 21*, 391–402.

Ramey, C. R., Mills, P., Campbell, F. A., & O'Brien, C. (1975). Infants' home environments: A comparison of high-risk families and families from the general population. *American Journal of Mental Deficiency, 80*, 40–42.

Rice, T. (1987). *Multivariate path analysis of cognitive and environmental measures in the*

Colorado Adoption Project. Unpublished doctoral dissertation, University of Colorado, Boulder.

Rice, T., Fulker, D. W., DeFries, J. C., & Plomin, R. (1988). Path analysis of IQ during infancy and early childhood and an index of the home environment in the Colorado Adoption Project. *Intelligence, 12*, 27–45.

Scarr, S., & Weinberg, R. A. (1978). The influence of "family background" on intellectual attainment. *American Sociological Review, 43*, 674–692.

Wachs, T. D., & Gruen, G. E. (1982). *Early experience and human development*. New York: Plenum Press.

Wechsler, D. (1974). *Examiner's manual: Wechsler Intelligence Scale for Children–Revised*. New York: Psychological Corporation.

Willerman, L. (1979). Effects of families on intellectual development. *American Psychologist, 34*, 923–929.

Wilson, R. S., & Matheny, A. P. (1983). Mental development: Family environment and genetic influences. *Intelligence, 7*, 195–215.

2

Nonshared Experiences Within the Family: Correlates of Behavioral Problems in Middle Childhood

Judy Dunn, Clare Stocker, and Robert Plomin

Pennsylvania State University, University Park

One of the most dramatic findings from quantitative genetic research is that environmental influences shared by siblings in a family do not make the siblings similar in terms of psychopathology. Sibling resemblance for psychopathology appears to be genetic rather than environmental in origin; environmental influences that affect the development of psychopathology must be nonshared and make children in the same family different rather than similar. This study sets out to identify environmental factors that differ for young siblings and to assess associations between such nonshared factors and differences in the older siblings' outcome in two domains: internalizing and externalizing behavior problems. Maternal interview and observations of differential maternal and sibling behavior were compared within 67 sibling dyads (younger and older siblings aged 4 and 7 years, respectively, on average), and differential experiences were related to the adjustment of the older sibling, as assessed by mother and teacher. Differential maternal behavior appeared to be particularly important as a predictor of adjustment problems. Older siblings showed internalizing problems in families in which mothers were less affectionate to the older than to the younger sibling. Greater maternal control toward the older than the younger sibling predicted both internalizing and externalizing problems. Differential maternal behavior explained 34% of the variance of internalizing behavior and 27% of the variance of externalizing behavior

Reprinted with permission from *Development and Psychopathology*, 1990, 113–126. Copyright © 1990 by Cambridge University Press.

This study is supported by the National Science Foundation (BNS-8806589).

problems, independent of variance explained by family structure vari-
ables. Although the sample was unselected for psychopathology and was
too small to permit analyses of the diagnosable extremes of internaliz-
ing and externalizing dimensions, these results are encouraging in rela-
tion to the goal of identifying systematic sources of nonshared
environment that affect the development of psychopathology.

A major challenge to those studying family influence on individual differences in
both normal and abnormal development has recently been put forward by behavioral
geneticists. First, evidence from a wide range of studies has accumulated showing
that siblings, who share 50% of their segregating genes and grow up within the same
family, nevertheless differ markedly from one another in nearly all areas of psychopathology and personality with the possible exceptions of aggressiveness and adolescent delinquency (Daniels, 1986; Plomin & Daniels, 1987; Scarr & Grajek,
1982). The family variables frequently thought to be of prime importance in the
development of adjustment and personality—such as parental mental health, the
quality of the marital relationship, parental childrearing style, or the parents' own
childhood experiences—are apparently shared by siblings. Yet siblings grow up to
be strikingly different from one another. Second, studies of adoptive siblings and of
twins have shown that heredity accounts for sibling resemblance and that the important sources of environmental influence are not shared by siblings (Dunn & Plomin,
1990).

The challenge for those studying family influence then is to answer the question
that these findings pose: What are the salient experiences within the family that *dif-*
fer for two children growing up together, and yet influence their adjustment? That is,
the startling implication of these findings is that experiences shared by siblings in a
family cannot be important in the etiology of individual differences in normal and
abnormal development. Only by specifying such nonshared experiences can we
begin to understand those experiences within the family that are important in development. In contrast to the vast majority of studies that compare single children on a
family-by-family basis, studies of siblings provide a powerful tool to identify environmental factors that differ among children in a family and to assess associations
between such nonshared environmental factors and differences in children's outcomes. Again, the reason for identifying differential experiences of siblings is that
only nonshared environmental factors can be responsible for the development of
individual differences in psychopathology and personality.

Although it has been acknowledged that family-by-family comparisons have
failed to explain more than a small portion of the variance in individual development
(Maccoby & Martin, 1983), we have as yet little evidence that delineates the relative
importance of the various possible sources of nonshared experiences within the family for different outcome domains. A number of potential nonshared influences have

been identified, such as differential parent-child relationships, differences within the sibling relationship itself, and differences in children's experiences with peer groups outside the family (Plomin & Daniels, 1987; Rowe & Plomin, 1981). In addition to such systematic psychosocial sources of nonshared environment, it is possible that chance—nonsystematic, stochastic, epigenetic processes—plays an important role in the divergence of siblings' developmental paths. However, it seems reasonable to begin our exploration of nonshared environment with an examination of potential systematic sources of differential experiences within the family.

Research has begun to document the considerable extent to which children experience different lives within the family (Dunn & Plomin, 1990). In addition to several questionnaire and interview studies, some observational data also suggest that mothers treat their several children differently. Much less is known, however, about associations between siblings' differential experiences and their developmental outcomes. In the first such study, differences in adolescent siblings' outcomes were shown to relate to differential parental behavior as reported by parents as well as by the siblings themselves (Daniels, Dunn, Furstenburg, & Plomin, 1985). Other studies have shown that differences in adolescent siblings' self-reported experiences relate to differences in personality between siblings (Anderson, 1989; Baker & Daniels, in press; Daniels, 1986).

This strategy of relating differences in siblings' experiences to differences in their outcomes provides a sharp scalpel for detecting nonshared environmental effects on outcomes. However, the fundamental issue is the extent to which nonshared environmental factors relate to individual differences in outcome, not just to sibling differences. That is, the phenomenon to be explained is that variance among individuals in adjustment and personality is largely due to nonshared environment. If a nonshared environmental factor were associated with sibling differences in outcome but not with individual differences in outcome, it would not be an important source of nonshared environmental variance.

This article reports the first analyses of this kind. Maternal interviews and observations of maternal and sibling behavior were compared with sibling pairs to determine the extent to which these shared experiences are nonshared. Nonshared experiences were then related to the older sibling's adjustment in two major domains—internalizing and externalizing behavior—as rated by both mothers and teachers. We will also be interested in relating nonshared experience to the adjustment of the younger siblings when they have reached an age when they can be assessed using the same measures of adjustment.

We expected to find that differential experiences in the family, in the context of the mother-child and the sibling-child relationships, would relate to problem behavior in the family as rated by the mother. However, given the lack of concordance between behavioral problems at home and at school, both in terms of observations (Stevenson-Hinde & Hinde, 1986) and as described by parents and by teachers

(Achenbach, McConaughey, & Howell, 1978; Goyette, Conners, & Ulrich, 1978; McGee, Williams, & Silva, 1985; Rutter, Tizard, & Whitmore, 1970; Verhulst & Akkerhuis, 1989), we were not optimistic that differential experiences in the family would carry over to adjustment problems in the school as rated by the teacher. We also expected to find that internalizing problems and externalizing problems would show different patterns of association with nonshared experiences within the family.

METHOD

Sample

The siblings are participating in a subproject of the Colorado Adoption Project (Plomin & DeFries, 1985; Plomin, DeFries, & Fulker, 1988) in which adopted children in adoptive families and nonadopted children in families matched to the adoptive families are studied as individuals when each child is 1, 2, 3, 4, and 7 years of age. Details of the adoption design are not relevant here because the present study employs only the nonadoptive families.

The subproject (the Colorado Sibling Study) involves an additional visit to families with siblings to observe them interacting with each other and with their mother, with the expectation that this would sharpen the search for differential experiences of siblings (Stocker, Dunn, & Plomin, 1989). In this article we report analyses on the 67 sibling dyads of the nonadoptive families. There were 25 boy-boy, 12 boy-girl, 14 girl-boy, and 16 girl-girl pairs. The younger and older siblings were 4 and 7 years old, respectively, on average, at this visit. The mean age spacing between siblings was 31.8 months ($SD = 11.3$ months). Differential sibling experiences are related in the analyses that follow to the adjustment of the older siblings (38 boys, 29 girls), assessed on a different occasion from the home visit, after the first grade of elementary school, usually at 7 years of age.

The nonadoptive families in the present analyses were Caucasian. Mothers and fathers had an average of 15.6 and 16.1 years of education, respectively. The average occupational status of the fathers, rated using the revised National Opinion Research Corporation rating (Hauser & Featherman, 1977), is 52.5. Although this is somewhat above the national norms for the U.S. white labor force, the sample is nearly representative in terms of variance.

Procedure

Each family was visited in their home for approximately 2 hours by a single examiner. Mothers and siblings were videotaped for 30 minutes while they participated in six play settings (see Stocker, Dunn, & Plomin, 1989). Mothers also participated in a 45-minute open-ended interview developed for the project that included questions on differential treatment, as well as the sibling relationship and the siblings' temperaments.

Mothers completed the parent form of the Child Behavior Checklist (CBC; Achenbach & Edelbrock, 1983) in relation to their older child during the summer following the child's first year of elementary school. The child's first-grade teacher received the teacher form of the CBC (TRF) and was asked to rate the target child in April, toward the end of the first grade. Teachers were asked to mail the form directly to the researchers and received an honorarium for their participation. With follow-up reminders, over 90% of the teachers responded.

Measures

Outcome measures were two second-order scales from the CBC as completed by the mothers, and by the children's teachers: *Internalizing* and *Externalizing* behavior. The CBC consists of 118 behavioral problem items that are scored on a 3-point scale, ranging from (0) *not true* of the child, (1) *somewhat or sometimes true*, and (2) *very true or often true*. The items can be scored on eight primary scales and on two second-order dimensions that assess internalizing and externalizing behavior. The Internalizing dimension includes scales that assess depression, social withdrawal, and somatic complaints, and the Externalizing dimension assesses aggressiveness, delinquency, and hyperactivity. The Internalizing and Externalizing scales yield 1-week test-retest reliabilities of .88 and .95, respectively. As in other studies, the correlation between mother and teacher ratings is low (.02) for Internalizing and modest (.34) for Externalizing. Measures of differential maternal and sibling behavior were as follows.

Maternal behavior. From the videotaped observations conducted on the mother with both siblings (Stocker, Dunn, & Plomin, 1989), differences in mothers' behavior to the siblings on two dimensions, *Affection* and *Control*, were considered. Behavior on each dimension was assessed with a 5-point scale, rated for each minute the triad spent in each of the different settings. The scale for Affection ranged from (1) *negative or discouraging remarks, no positive remarks, no physical affection*; (3) *some praise, positive comments, some smiles, laughs*; and (5) *many positive comments, many smiles, positive physical contact*. The scale for Control ranged from (1) *no intruding or directive remarks, does not handle game pieces or take on child's role*; (3) *some helpful comments, a few directive comments not in question form, or several suggestions including questions, suggestions for play*; and (5) *many directive comments, controls child physically, takes child's part in game, organizes child's play*. Two coders independently rated maternal behavior of 10 videotapes. The interrater correlations for maternal affection and control were .83 and .80 for older siblings and .93 and .96 for younger siblings. Test-retest reliabilities for all measures were assessed for a separate sample of 30 families. The families were visited twice at a 2-week interval and participated in identical procedures in both sessions. The test-retest reliabilities for the videotape assessments were .65 and .72 for Affection to the older and younger sibling, respectively, and .83 and .80 for Control. The index of differential maternal behavior was the signed difference between behavior to older and to younger (i.e., behavior to older minus behavior to younger).

The interview with the mothers provides a second source of information concerning differential behavior. In this interview, mothers are asked about relative differences in their affection and control shown toward their two children; these scores served as an index of nonshared environment. The interview was open-ended; mothers were encouraged to talk at length about affection and control issues. For example, the interviewer probed whether mothers found it easier to be more affectionate with one of their children than the other, whether they found one child more "cuddly," and whether they enjoyed physical contact with one more than the other. For control, the interviewer probed whether one child was easier to handle than the other, and whether mothers attempted to control and discipline one child more than the other. From the mothers' extensive comments, the interviewer derived a rating on a 5-point scale representing differences in the frequency of maternal behavior: (1) *younger child much more often*, (2) *younger child a bit more often*, (3) *both children about the same*, (4) *older child a bit more often*, (5) *older child much more often*. Because one interviewer rated each mother's responses during the interview conducted at home, it was not possible to calculate rater agreement. The 2-week test-retest reliabilities are .55 for differential affection and .54 for differential control.

Sibling behavior. From the videotaped observations, coders who had not rated maternal behavior rated each child's behavior to the sibling. Differences in the siblings' behavior to each other on two dimensions, *Conflict* and *Cooperation*, were considered. Behavior on each dimension was rated on a 5-point scale for each minute spent in each of the six settings: For Conflict the scale ranged from (1) *no physical aggression or teasing, no verbal hostility, no protests or disputes*; (3) *mild disputes, arguments, protests, occasional teasing, extended disagreements*; and (5) *intense aggression, physical aggression, frequent criticism of other's actions*. For Cooperation the scale ranged from (1) *no attempts to cooperate, refusal to cooperate or follow suggestions*; (3) *follows suggestions, occasional attempts at cooperation, shares or helps if requested, responds to comments on most occasions, brief sustained conversation*; and (5) *frequent attempts to cooperate with sibling, responds promptly to suggestions or questions, frequent sustained conversation*. Two coders independently rated the siblings' behavior on 10 videotapes. The coders and videotapes were different from those used to assess rater agreement for the measures of maternal behavior. Correlations between the raters were .95 for Conflict and .91 for Cooperation. The 2-week test-retest reliabilities were .58 for Control and .48 for Cooperation. The index of differential sibling behavior employed was the signed difference on each dimension: behavior of older to younger minus behavior of younger to older.

In parallel to the assessments of maternal behavior, maternal interviews were used as well to assess differential sibling behavior. As on the items for differential maternal behavior, mothers were encouraged to discuss at length the siblings' behavior toward each other; sixteen particular aspects of their behavior were discussed. The items comprised frequency of companionship during the week and on the weekend, time spent playing together, desire to play, pretend play, affection, nurturance following distress caused by the sibling or not caused by the sibling, teaching/helping, caretaking, quarrels, physical fights, sharing, competition, jealousy/rivalry focused on the mother and on the father. From the maternal interview, mothers' responses to six open-ended questions concerning each child's behavior to the sibling were rated on 6-point scales ranging for example from (2) *almost never/less than 5%*, (3) *sometimes/about a third of the time together*, (5) *regularly/75-100% of time*. Mothers' responses were included in a principal components analysis from which a positive factor (reflecting joint play, desire to be with the sibling, and affection) and a negative factor (including jealousy of the sibling, physical aggression, competition, and frequency of fights) were derived (for details, see Stocker, Dunn, & Plomin, 1989). A *Positive* and a *Negative* scale were created from these factors, using standardized z scores of the items loading on the factors. The 2-week test-retest reliabilities were .64 for the Positive scale and .79 for the Negative scale. As with the sibling observation measures, the index of differential sibling behavior employed was the signed difference on the positive and the negative scales: behavior of older minus behavior of younger.

Difference Scores

Sibling differences in maternal treatment define our model of nonshared environment because mothers' differences in treatment toward two children provide a within-family measure of differential treatment that is independent of level of treatment and does not depend on any assumptions about the linearity of the regression of scores for one sibling on the other. That is, the extent of mothers' differences in affection toward their two children indicates mothers' relative affection independent of the mothers' absolute level of affection. One could evaluate more complicated models of differential treatment—for example, to assess whether the effect of differential treatment interacts with the absolute level of treatment (Humphreys, in press; Plomin, in press). However, for initial research in this area, it seems reasonable to begin with the more basic model of differential sibling treatment.

Three issues concerning difference scores should be mentioned. First, a difference score is less reliable than its constituent scores to the extent that the constituent scores are correlated. That is, if the constituent scores (e.g., mothers' behavior to each sibling) are correlated, less of the variance of the constituent scores is transferred to the difference score, yet the difference score contains all of the error of measurement because error does not correlate across the constituent scores. Methods to alleviate this problem involve between-family rather than within-family "corrections." For example, partial correlation assesses the association between one sibling's environmental scores and that sibling's outcome score using the other sibling's environmental score as a covariate, "correcting" for the mean linear effect of the other siblings' environmental scores (Cohen & Cohen, 1975). Although these methods can yield more reliable scores than difference scores, they achieve their greater reliability in essence by subtracting a mean linear effect based on a regression for the entire sample, rather than providing a within-family comparison. For this reason, difference scores are preferable for our purposes despite their lower reliability caused by sibling correlations for maternal treatment. It should be borne in mind that the reliability of the difference scores is less than the average reliability of the constituent scores only to the extent that the constituent scores are correlated.

Second, difference scores can correlate with their constituent scores. This is a notorious problem when, for example, a change score is correlated with a pretest score from which the change score was derived. However, our goal does not involve correlating a sibling difference score with the constituent sibling scores. Nonetheless, given that such correlations might exist, one might ask if the between-family variance of the constituent scores (e.g., mother's affection toward each child) should be removed before examining the association between sibling difference scores and their outcomes in order to obtain a "purer" measure of nonshared environment? We suggest that the answer is no, because between-family variance for an environmental measure is not necessarily shared even though within-family variance is nonshared. That is, a measure of mother's affection to a specific child could be shared or nonshared, depending on the extent to which the measure is correlated for siblings. Thus, if variance because of mother's affection to each child is removed before examining the association between differential affection and outcome, some nonshared environmental influence may be eliminated.

The third issue concerns the use of relative or absolute differences. Relative differences are signed differences (in our case older sibling minus younger sibling scores), whereas absolute differences refer to the unsigned differences between siblings. We prefer to use relative differences because they convey information about the direction of the difference, in addition to the magnitude of the difference.

Relating Nonshared Environment to Adjustment

Sibling difference scores for maternal treatment and sibling interactions were related in the analyses that follow to adjustment (internalizing and externalizing problem behavior) of the older sibling, as rated by the mother and by the teacher.

Although many variables could be examined in relation to the association between nonshared environment and adjustment, we chose to control statistically for as many of these variables as possible so that we could focus on associations between non-shared environment and adjustment independent of these complicating factors. Thus, the major form of analysis employed is a multiple regression of older sibling's adjustment on a nonshared measure in a second step after variance in adjustment because these other variables had been removed. These variables include age of older sibling, age spacing of siblings, gender of older sibling, gender status of pair (same sex vs. opposite sex).

RESULTS

Sibling Differences in Maternal Treatment and Sibling Behavior

First, the nature and extent of differential experiences of the siblings should be noted. In Figures 1 and 2, the distribution of scores for the relative differences in the maternal and sibling measures is shown.

As shown in Figure 1, mothers were quite differential in their affection and control toward their two children, as rated by observers and as reported by the mothers. The maternal interview questions on differential control and affection showed that the majority of mothers described differences in their treatment of their children: 30% reported some difference, and a further 35% reported marked difference in affection. For control, 32% reported some difference and 29% much difference.

For the sibling interaction measures (Figure 2), the distribution of sibling differences shows that relative differences were less frequent. During the videotaped observations, the extent of conflict shown by the two siblings was quite similar, but in many pairs the siblings differed in the extent of cooperative behavior shown. According to their mothers' interview accounts, 53% and 31% siblings were rated as showing some differences for the positive and negative scales, respectively. Differences in conflict behavior between the siblings were less common.

An analysis of the magnitude of these differential experiences employing a model that takes into account family constellation variables shows that although these variables contain substantial shared environmental variance, they also assay nonshared environment independent of family constellation variables (Slomkowski, Rende, Stocker, Dunn, & Plomin, 1990). Independent of family constellation variables, non-shared environment accounts for 22% and 26% for observations of maternal affection and control, respectively; 35% and 28% for maternal interviews of sibling positive and negative behavior, respectively; and 42% and 18% for observations of sibling cooperation and conflict, respectively.

*Correlations Between Differential Maternal and Sibling Behavior and
the Adjustment Variables*

As an initial step in the analyses, the children's scores on the maternal CBC and
the teachers' CBC scales of externalizing and internalizing behavior were correlated
with each of the differential maternal and sibling behavior measures. Table 1 shows
the correlations for the maternal CBC scales. None of the correlations with teacher
CBC were significant; in the analyses that follow the focus is therefore on the maternal CBC.

Table 1 shows that differences in maternal affection (interview) were negatively
correlated with children's internalizing scores. Since the sibling difference score represents older sibling minus younger sibling's scores, this negative correlation means
that in families in which the mother was more affectionate to older than to younger,
the older sibling was less likely to show internalizing problems than the older siblings in families in which mothers were less differentially affectionate. In contrast,
the positive correlations between differences in control and both internalizing and
externalizing scores means that older siblings whose mothers were more controlling
to them than to their younger sibling scored relatively high on both scales.

Differences in the siblings' behavior to one another also showed associations with
the adjustment scales, although these only approached statistical significance. Older
siblings who were less positive to their siblings than their younger siblings were to
them were likely to score high on both internalizing and externalizing scales. Those
who were more negative to their siblings than their siblings were to them were likely
to score high on internalizing behavior. Correlations were also conducted between

TABLE 1
Correlations Between Measures of Relative Differences in Maternal and Sibling Behavior
Versus Internalizing and Externalizing CBC Scales

	Internalizing	Externalizing
Maternal measures		
Differential affection (interview)	−.43*	−.13
Differential control (interview)	.48*	.37*
Differential affection (observation)	.21	.00
Differential control (observation)	−.01	−.05
Sibling measures		
Differential positive (interview)	−.29	−.21
Differential negative (interview)	.30	.17
Differential cooperation (observation)	−.01	.12
Differential conflict (observation)	.07	−.26

*$p < .05$.

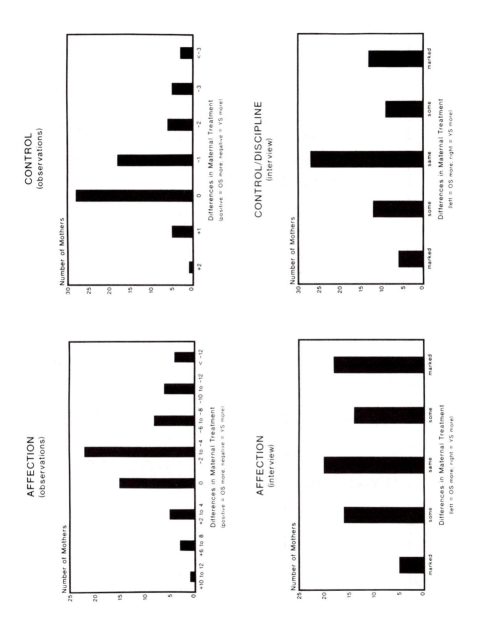

Figure 1. Relative differences in maternal behavior toward siblings

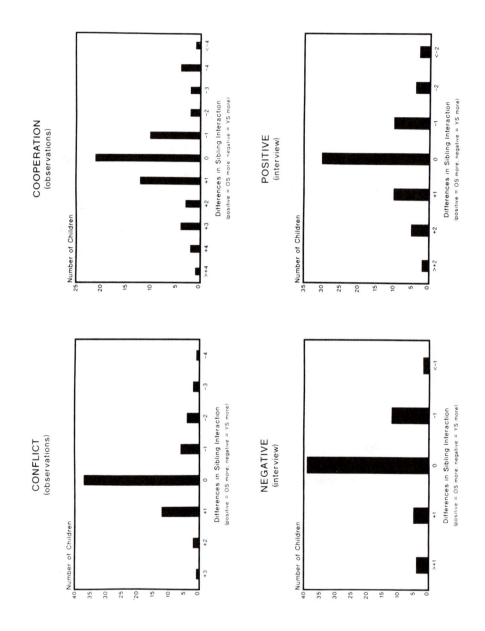

Figure 2. Relative differences in siblings' behavior toward each other

the adjustment scales and the following family structure variables: sex of child, gender composition of sibling dyad, age of older sibling, and age difference between the siblings. None of these correlations were significant.

Multivariate Analyses of the Nonshared Correlates of Internalizing and Externalizing Behavior

The extent to which differential experiences within the family explain variance in internalizing and externalizing problems, independent of family structure variables, was further explored with multiple regression analyses. The family structure variables were entered in the first step of the multiple regression analysis, and then the differential measures were added in a second step. In this way the variance in adjustment related to the effects of differential maternal and sibling experiences can be estimated independent of the variance caused by the family structure variables.

Table 2 shows the variance in adjustment variables explained by family structure and differences in maternal behavior. The family structure variables explained 1% of the variance, and the differential maternal behavior variables independently added 34% to the prediction of the variance in internalizing behavior. For externalizing behavior, the differential maternal behavior measures explained 27% of the variance after the family structure variables had been entered into the analysis.

Table 3 shows the variance in the two adjustment variables explained by family structure and differential sibling behavior variables. After variance due to family structure variables is taken into account, 17% of internalizing variance and 13% of externalizing variance are explained independently by the sibling behavior mea-

TABLE 2

Variance in Internalizing and Externalizing Behavior Problems Explained by Family Structure Variables and by Relative Differences in Maternal Behavior

CBC Scale	Model	r^2 Change	r^2	F	(df)
Internalizing	Family structure[a]	.01		0.12	(4, 26)
	Maternal differential[b]	.34*		4.11	(4, 26)
	Family structure + maternal differential		.46*	2.84	(8, 27)
Externalizing	Family structure[a]	.05		0.45	(4, 25)
	Maternal differential[b]	.27		2.45	(4, 25)
	Family structure + maternal differential		.31	1.45	(8, 26)

[a]Family structure variables included age of older sibling, age spacing of siblings, gender of older sibling, and gender status of pair (same sex vs. opposite sex).
[b]Differential maternal variables included affection (video), control (video), affection (interview), and control (interview).
*$p < .05$.

sures, although neither of these is statistically significant with the current sample size.

DISCUSSION

The first exploration of the relation of differential experience within the family to the development of problem behavior of individual children suggests that there may be systematic associations between differences in sibling experiences within the family and children's adjustment. The results are far from definitive and may be best regarded as preliminary, but promising, for continued investigation of nonshared environment.

Three important points concerning the interpretation of the associations should be noted. First, the sample was unselected for psychopathology, and dimensional measures of behavior problem syndromes were used rather than clinically referred children and psychiatric diagnoses. Thus, these results apply only to the normal range of behavioral problems, and their generalizability to the clinical extremes of these dimensions remains to be investigated. However, sibling concordance for developmental disorders is modest at best, and, on the basis of these results, we speculate that behavioral problems above a diagnosable threshold will also be predicted by differential maternal affection and control. It is possible that there will be even stronger associations with nonshared environmental factors for children at the extremes of the dimensions of behavior problems.

Second, we have examined here only the contemporary association between nonshared experience and adjustment, and thus we can make no inferences about the direction of effects. For example, it could be that mothers differentiate more

TABLE 3

Variance in Internalizing and Externalizing Behavior Problems Explained by Family Structure Variables and by Relative Differences in Sibling Behavior

CBC Scale	Model	r^2 Change	r^2	F	(df)
Internalizing	Family structure[a]	.17		1.50	(4, 25)
	Sibling differential[b]	.17		1.50	(4, 25)
	Family structure + sibling differential		.29	1.36	(8, 26)
Externalizing	Family structure[a]	.01		0.07	(4, 25)
	Sibling differential[b]	.13		0.92	(4, 24)
	Family structure + sibling differential		.17	0.64	(8, 25)

[a]Family structure variables included age of older sibling, age spacing of siblings, gender of older sibling, and gender status of pair (same sex vs. opposite sex).
[b]Differential sibling variables included conflict (video), cooperation (video), positive (interview), and negative (interview).

between their children in their affectionate behavior if one of the siblings is depressive in mood, showing less affection to the depressed child. That is, it may be less easy to express affection equally to two siblings if one is depressed. Indeed, it is possible that the contrast between the siblings in depressive behavior itself makes differentiation between the children by the mothers more likely. Similarly, it could be that mothers show greater differentiation in controlling behavior to their various children if one of the siblings is frequently aggressive, delinquent, or hyperactive. Longitudinal analyses will help in the examination of direction of effects. We are in the process of conducting a 3-year follow-up study of these families using a similar design that will provide the first longitudinal analyses of both differential sibling experiences and outcomes. Meanwhile, analyses of contemporaneous data provide a reasonable first step in identifying associations between nonshared environment and children's outcome.

Third, it should be noted that the significant results come from maternal reports of their own differential behavior and of the children's adjustment. It remains possible, therefore, that the pattern of findings reflects primarily the perception (possibly biased) of a single family member, rather than a more general pattern. However, it may be premature to conclude from these analyses that observational measures of differential treatment and differential sibling behavior are unimportant in the development of adjustment for two reasons. First, other analyses have shown moderate-to-good agreement between the maternal interview data and observational data (Dunn, Stocker, & Plomin, in press; Stocker, Dunn, & Plomin, 1989). Second, the current sample size is relatively small.

While these lines of evidence lead us to infer that the associations in the present study do not solely reflect the perception of the mothers, the lack of association between teachers' accounts of adjustment and differential experiences within the family deserves comment. As with other studies examining both teacher and parent reports of behavioral problems (e.g., Verhulst & Akkerhuis, 1989), the degree to which differences in the description of children's behavior are related to the situational specificity of the children's behavior, or to informant variance, cannot be estimated. As Verhulst and Akkerhuis noted, parents do have more opportunity to give a broad-based assessment of their children in a range of settings, while teachers may be better placed to compare a child's functioning with that of his peers. In general the studies comparing parent and teacher assessment of behavior problems report low to moderate agreement, especially on internalizing problems (Achenbach, McConaughey, & Howell, 1987; Goyette, Conners, & Ulrich, 1978; Rutter, Tizard, & Whitmore, 1970; Verhulst & Akkerhuis, 1989). It is clearly important that the significance of both disagreement and agreement between different informants' judgment should be investigated.

Although interpreting the findings from this study presents these problems, the associations we found are certainly compatible with evidence from a variety of different research approaches that children are sensitive to maternal differential behavior. First, observational studies of children's immediate response to maternal affection and interest in their siblings show that children rarely ignore such interactions, react promptly, and are frequently upset (Dunn & Kendrick, 1982; Dunn & Munn, 1985; Kendrick & Dunn, 1982). Second, studies employing interviews with children show that firstborn children frequently perceive such differences in parental behavior and are upset by it (Koch, 1960). Together these lines of research make it very plausible that perceptions of differences in maternal affection contribute to anxious or depressive feelings in young children, for those who feel themselves to be the less-loved sibling. More generally, evidence is accumulating that children not only monitor their parents' behavior with the other children in the family with considerable sensitivity (see, e.g., Dunn & Shatz, 1989), but also begin to make social comparisons extremely early within the family (Dunn, 1988). To clarify the processes influencing individual differences in children's adjustment and well being, research strategies that are attuned to children's sensitivity to and perceptions of differential experience will be needed.

This research represents but a first step toward identifying nonshared environmental factors that relate to individual differences in adjustment. It seems clear that this is an important research direction if we are to answer the question. Why are children in the same family so different? So often we have assumed—whether we as parents, therapists, or researchers—that the key environmental influences on children's development are shared. Yet to the extent that siblings' experiences are shared, they cannot explain individual differences in children's outcomes. Investigating why two children growing up in the same family are so different from one another is the key for unlocking the secrets of environmental influence on the development of all children, not just siblings.

This new "nonshared" orientation toward understanding why individuals develop the way they do does not involve the dismissal of traditional approaches to family process. Rather, it gives these notions a radically new slant, one that focuses on differences within families rather than family-by-family differences. That is, the importance of the theory of nonshared environment is that it implies that the specific and probably subtle differences experienced or perceived by children growing up in the same family are the key environmental factors that drive normal and abnormal development.

REFERENCES

Achenbach, T. M., & Edelbrock, C. S. (1983). *Manual for the Child Behavior Checklist and Revised Child Behavior Profile.* Burlington: University of Vermont, Department of Psychiatry.

Achenbach, T. M., McConaughey, S. H., & Howell, C. T. (1987). Child/adolescent behavioral/

emotional problems: Implications of cross-informant correlations for situational specificity. *Psychological Bulletin, 101*, 213–232.

Anderson, S. L. (1989). Differential within-family experiences as predictors of adolescent personality and attachment style differences. Unpublished honors thesis, Harvard University, Cambridge, MA.

Baker, L. A., & Daniels, D. (in press). Nonshared environmental influences and personality differences in adult twins. *Journal of Personality and Social Psychology.*

Cohen, J., & Cohen, P. (1975). *Applied multiple regression/correlation analysis for the behavioral sciences.* New York: Halstead.

Daniels, D. (1986). Differential experiences of siblings in the same family as predictors of adolescent sibling personality differences. *Journal of Personality and Social Psychology, 51*, 339–346.

Daniels, D., Dunn, J., Furstenburg, F., & Plomin, R. (1985). Environmental differences within the family and adjustment differences within pairs of adolescent siblings. *Child Development, 56*, 764–774.

Dunn, J. (1988) *The beginnings of social understanding.* Cambridge, MA: Harvard University Press.

Dunn, J., & Kendrick, C. (1982). *Siblings: Love, envy and understanding.* Cambridge, MA: Harvard University Press.

Dunn, J., & Munn, P. (1985). Becoming a family member: Family conflict and the development of social understanding in the second year. *Child Development, 56*, 480–492.

Dunn, J., & Plomin, R. (1990). *Separate lives.* New York: Basic Books.

Dunn, J., & Shatz, M. (1989). Becoming a conversationalist despite (or because of) having an older sibling. *Child Development, 60*, 399–410.

Dunn, J., Stocker, C., & Plomin, R. (in press). Assessing the sibling relationship. *Journal of Child Psychology and Psychiatry.*

Goyette, C. H., Conners, C. K., & Ulrich, R. F. (1978). Normative data on revised Conners parent and Teacher Rating Scales. *Journal of Abnormal Child Psychology, 6*, 221–236.

Hauser, R. M., & Featherman, D. L. (1977). *The process of stratification: Trends and analysis.* New York: Academic.

Humphreys, L. D. (in press). The obvious method of analysis of data is sometimes inadequate. *Behavioral and Brain Sciences.*

Kendrick, C., & Dunn, J. (1982). Protest or pleasure? The reaction of firstborn children to interaction between their mothers and siblings. *Journal of Child Psychology and Psychiatry.*

Koch, H. L. (1960). The relation of certain formal attributes of siblings to attitudes held toward each other and toward their parents. *Monographs of the Society for Research in Child Development, 25* (Serial No. 4).

Maccoby, E. E., & Martin, J. A. (1983). Socialization in the context of the family: Parent-child interaction. In P. H. Mussen (Ed.), *Handbook of child psychology*, Volume IV: *Socialization, personality and social development* (pp. 1–101). New York: Wiley.

McGee, R., Williams, S., & Silva, P. A. (1985). Factor structure and correlates of ratings of inattention, hyperactivity and antisocial behavior in a large sample of 9-year-old children from the general population. *Journal of Consulting and Clinical Psychology, 53*, 480–490.

Plomin, R. (in press). Why are children in the same family so different? Response to commentary by Humphreys. *Behavioral and Brain Sciences.*

Plomin, R., & Daniels, D. (1987). Why are children within the family so different from one another? *Behavioral and Brain Sciences, 10*, 1–16.

Plomin, R., & DeFries, J. C. (1985). *Origins of individual differences in infancy.* New York: Academic.

Plomin, R., DeFries, J. C., & Fulker, D. W. (1988). *Nature and nurture in infancy and early childhood.* New York: Cambridge University Press.

Rowe, D. C., & Plomin, R. (1981). The importance of nonshared (E1) environmental influences in behavioral development. *Developmental Psychology, 17*, 517–531.

Rutter, M., Tizard, J., & Whitmore, K. (1970). *Education, health and behavior.* New York: Wiley.

Scarr, S., & Grajek, S. (1982). Similarities and differences among siblings. In M. E. Lamb & B. Sutton-Smith (Eds.), *Sibling relationships: Their nature and significance across the lifespan* (pp. 357–381). Hillsdale, NJ: Erlbaum.

Slomkowski, C. L., Rende, R. D., Stocker, C., Dunn, J., & Plomin, R. (1990). *Nonshared environmental influences and siblings: A multiple model.* Submitted.

Stevenson-Hinde, J., & Hinde, R. A. (1986). Changes in associations between characteristics and interactions. In R. Plomin & J. Dunn (Eds.), *The study of temperament: Changes, continuities and challenges* (pp. 115–129). Hillsdale, NJ: Erlbaum.

Stocker, C., Dunn, J., & Plomin, R. (1989). Sibling relationships: Links with child temperament, maternal behavior, and family structure. *Child Development, 60*, 715–727.

Verhulst, F. C., & Akkerhuis, G. W. (1989). Agreement between parents' and teachers' ratings of behavioral/emotional problems of children aged 4-12. *Journal of Child Psychology and Psychiatry, 30*, 123–136.

3

Children and Their Fathers After Parental Separation

Joseph M. Healy, Jr.

Rhode Island College, Providence

Janet E. Malley and Abigail J. Stewart

University of Michigan, Ann Arbor

This two-year longitudinal study of 121 6-12-year-old children in the custody of their mothers following parental separation examined main and interacting effects of child's age and gender, frequency and regularity of visitation, father-child closeness, and parental legal conflict on children's self-esteem and behavioral adjustment at two time points. Predictors were found to have different implications for different groups of children and for children in different situations. Findings suggest the futility of seeking simple answers to whether ongoing contact with fathers following divorce is beneficial or detrimental for children.

It has been argued that, after parental separation, children's ties with the non-custodial parent (usually the father) should be severed completely, in the interest of minimizing their continuing pain over the loss of the parent as well as their sense of being torn between two loved parents (*Goldstein, Freud, & Solnit, 1973*). It has also—perhaps more often—been argued that, after parental separation, every effort should be made to maintain close, positive ties between the noncustodial parent and his or her children for the sake of the children's long-term psychological health (*Hess & Camara, 1979; Wallerstein, 1987*). This paper will present data suggesting that, in fact, no blanket recommendation about fathers' relationships with their children after separation can be offered; different children, and different situations, demand different remedies.

Reprinted with permission from *American Journal of Orthopsychiatry,* 1990, Vol. 60, No. 4, 531–543. Copyright © 1990 by the American Orthopsychiatric Association, Inc.

Research was supported by grants to the third author from the Spencer Foundation of Chicago and from the National Institute of Mental Health (RO1-MH38801).

AGE AND GENDER IN DIVORCE ADJUSTMENT

Some previous research has indicated that characteristics of children may moderate the impact of noncustodial parent visitation and involvement. For example, many studies point to the relevance of age at separation for children's divorce adjustment. Specifically, loss of a parent at an early age has been found to have long-term consequences for both boys and girls (*Biller, 1974; Bowlby, 1973; Hetherington, 1972*). Similarly, older children have been found to exhibit better long-term postdivorce adjustment than younger children; on the basis of data from a longitudinal study of eight 17-year-olds, Kurdek, Blisk, and Siesky (*1982*) suggested that the better adjustment of older children might be related to their increased cognitive abilities, such as interpersonal reasoning and locus of control. Others, however, have suggested no quantitative age differences in overall adjustment to divorce but, rather, qualitatively different responses related to specific developmental levels (*Kalter & Rembar, 1971; Wallerstein & Kelly, 1980*).

The findings for gender differences in children's responses to divorce have been equally contradictory. Considerable empirical evidence points to more adjustment problems for boys in divorcing families than for girls (*Emery, 1982; Hetherington, 1979; Hetherington, Cox & Cox, 1982; Kurdek, 1981; Wallerstein & Kelly, 1980*). Guidubaldi and Perry (*1985*) found boys in divorcing families to exhibit more maladaptive symptoms and behavior problems than boys in intact families while girls with divorced parents scored higher in locus of control than their counterparts. Hess and Camara (*1979*) found marital conflict in the divorce situation to be related to problems of undercontrol for boys only. However, Emery (*1982*) and others pointed to evidence for problems of overcontrol or internalizing behavior for girls in conflicted families (*Emery, Hetherington, & DiLalla, 1985; Block, Block, & Morrison, 1981*); Emery suggested that many of the findings of more adjustment problems for boys in divorcing families may reflect the overuse of clinical samples in these studies. He argued that the undercontrolled behavior of boys is more readily observed and more likely to lead to clinical referral. Similarly, Zaslow's (*1988*) review suggests that evidence for sex differences is much more consistent in clinical samples than in nonclinical samples. Others have suggested that psychological distress in response to parental separation is not only expressed differently by girls but may also arise much later for them, especially during adolescence and adulthood (*Hetherington, 1972; Kalter, Riemer, Brickman, & Chen, 1985*). In contrast, Kurdek et al. (*1981*) found no difference between boys and girls in long-term adjustments to their parents' divorce. This finding concurs with Wallerstein and Kelly's (*1980*) view that sex differences in response to parental divorce are minimized over time.

The heightened divorce adjustment problems for boys found in some research may be less related to gender per se than to characteristics of the postdivorce household arrangements. Santrock and Warshak (*1979*) found that both boys and girls in divorcing families exhibited more behavior problems with opposite-sex custodial parents. Since most mothers retain physical custody of their children when divorce occurs (*Weitzman, 1985*), boys' greater adjustment difficulties may be a function of their postseparation household situation. This interpretation is consistent with Zaslow's (*1988*) summary of evidence for sex differences in children's responses to parental divorce. She concluded that boys appear to be more adversely affected by divorce than girls, principally in mother-custody families in which the mother remains unmarried. Similarly, Peterson and Zill (*1986*) found adolescent children to be more likely to exhibit behavior problems if living with the opposite-sex parents. However, Lowenstein and Koopman (*1978*), in their study of 9–14-year-old boys, found no difference in levels of self-esteem for boys living with single mothers and boys living with single fathers. Moreover, as mentioned above, Kurdek et al. (*1981*) found no relationship between long-term negative adjustment and opposite-sex custodial parent, suggesting that any differences between boys and girls may disappear over time.

PARENTAL RELATIONSHIPS

Other studies have suggested that both custodial and noncustodial parents' relationships with their children have important implications for children's postdivorce adjustment (*Hetherington, Cox & Cox, 1978; Wallerstein & Kelly, 1980*). For example, some evidence suggests that the frequency of noncustodial fathers' visitation is important. Lowenstein and Koopman (*1978*) found that boys living with single mothers who saw their fathers more than once a month exhibited higher levels of self-esteem than did those who saw their fathers less frequently. Similarly, Kurdek (*1988*) found that in the first year after parental separation, noncustodial parent involvement was generally associated positively with adjustment in children in divorcing families (especially for children whose parents were experiencing high levels of conflict). However, other studies indicate that the quality of the parent-child relationship may be more consequential than the amount of time spent together. In fact, a negative relationship has been shown between frequency of the noncustodial visitations and the child's more long-term adjustment (*Kurdek et al., 1981*). In contrast, Hess and Camara (*1979*) argued that a good relationship with either parent is related to postdivorce adjustment in children (*Emery, 1982*).

The quality of the relationship between the parents has also been considered an important variable affecting the parent-child relationship, as well as contributing to the child's postdivorce adjustment (*Demo & Acock, 1988; Hetherington, 1979; Koch & Lowery, 1984*). A positive relationship with the ex-spouse has been associated with higher levels of noncustodial father contact with his children (*Ahrons, 1983; Koch & Lowery, 1984*). Similarly, Emery (*1982*) drew a connection between interparent conflict and behavior problems in children. On the other hand, Furstenberg, Morgan, and

Allison (*1987*) suggested that more frequent contact between the child and noncustodial parent may have the effect of increasing both contact and the level of conflict between parents, to the detriment of the child. However, Kurdek (*1988*) found that the advantages of noncustodial parent involvement were greater for children whose parents' interactions were highly conflictual than for those whose parents experienced lower levels of conflict. This finding supports Hess and Camara's (*1979*) conclusion that a good relationship with at least one parent can have a buffering effect for the child, regardless of level of conflict between the parents.

HYPOTHESES

This review of the literature suggests that the implications of the noncustodial father-child relationship for children's divorce adjustment are not clear-cut or straightforward. Some of the conflicting evidence found across studies is the result of methodological differences such as measurement strategy and sample selection. Findings of differences between boys and girls, for example, may reflect the fact that boys express more negative external behavior than do girls, especially in single-parent households (*Zaslow, 1989*). Thus, studies that focus on behavioral outcomes of the child are more likely to find gender differences. However, some evidence suggests that girls who live with stepfathers actually exhibit increased levels of antisocial behavior (*Hetherington, Cox, & Cox, 1985; Zaslow, 1989*). Thus, the study sample characteristics are also an important consideration in assessing discrepant findings. Similarly, conflicting evidence may result from who is reporting on the child's adjustment. Parents' perceptions of children's adjustment may be affected by their own psychological state (*Wallerstein & Kelly, 1980*). In fact, Kurdek et al. (*1981*) found that children's reports of their adjustment were not equivalent to parents' assessment of children's adjustment.

Other discrepancies in empirical findings appear to be related to contextual factors in the divorcing situation which have implications for the child's well-being. Thus, although the child's age and gender appear, generally, to be relevant in assessing post-separation adjustment, length of time since the parents separated appears to diminish these differences. Similarly, other contextual factors, including the child's relationship with the noncustodial parent as well as the custodial and noncustodial parents' relationship, should have implications for the relationship between age and gender and the child's adjustment to divorce.

This study considered the direct and interacting effects of age and gender of the child, several variables assessing the father-child relationship, and parental legal conflict. It should be noted that many potentially important features of the child's situation (socioeconomic status, maternal adjustment, etc.) are not included in these analyses. In addition, not all aspects of the noncustodial parent-child relationship are explored. Instead, our focus is on assessing the simple and complex effects of several specific aspects of the child's relationship with the noncustodial parent. Future analyses may permit a more comprehensive picture of the child's situation.

In order to identify the separate roles of frequency of father contact, regularity of father contact, and father-child closeness, we kept these indicators distinct. Based upon previous research, we expected younger children in our study to show poorer adjustment to divorce than older children. Moreover, we expected boys to exhibit more negative behavior than girls. In terms of the noncustodial parent-child relationship, although more frequent and regular visits may have positive implications for the children, we anticipated that the quality of the parent-child relationship would be a more important predictor of child adjustment. However, overall, we expected that there would be few direct, general relationships between the variables assessing the child's relationship with the noncustodial parent and the child's adjustment. Instead, we expected that individual and situational characteristics would serve as important moderators of those relationships.

METHODS

Subjects

Participants in this study were 121 children from mother-custody families in which the parents had recently separated. These families were participants in a larger, two-year longitudinal study. Excluded from this report are those families in which fathers had physical custody ($N = 17$), in which the parents were reconciled ($N = 6$) or remarried to each other ($N = 1$) by the second year, or in which data from the children are available for only one year ($N = 28$). Families all included at least one child age 6 to 12 years, who was arbitrarily designated the target child by the project staff. Being a "target" child simply permitted parents to answer questionnaire and interview items in terms of that particular child. The parents had all filed for legal separation and had been physically separated for no more than eight months prior to the first-year interview. Families were contacted through a search of court records, and thus represent a nonclinically recruited sample. Moreover, in comparison with other families who did not participate but on whom information was available from the same set of court records, participants did not differ in geographic area of residence, marital and separation history, or number of legal motions accompanying the filing.

Data were collected from all family members (including noncustodial fathers) willing to participate. However, by far the most complete data involve questionnaires and interviews with custodial mothers and target children. All of the data reported in this paper are drawn from these two sources. Wherever possible, measures were obtained from both, under the assumption that mothers and children have validly different perspectives on the family. Follow-up data were collected one year after initial contact (about 18 months after the initial parental separation). At that time about half of the couples were legally divorced.

The mean age of the target children in this study was 8.61 (SD = 1.99); there were 63 boys and 58 girls in the 121 families, and each family had an average of 2.41 (SD = 1.69) children. Based on the socioeconomic status (SES) of the mothers' occupations, the SES of the postseparation households ranged widely. On a seven-point scale used to code the SES of occupations (1 = unskilled labor such as waitress or janitor, 7 = major professions such as doctor or lawyer; adapted from Hollingshead and Redlich [*1958*], the mean SES of mothers' occupations was 3.61 (SD = 1.56) and ranged from unskilled labor to minor professions (e.g., engineers, registered nurses, CPAs, secondary school teachers, etc.). Fathers' occupations ranged even more widely, since they included a few upper-level administrators and major professions. Overall, fathers' mean SES was 4.11 (SD = 1.45). At both data collection points, over 50% of the mothers worked full time and fewer than 25% were not employed for pay outside the home.

Analyses are reported using gender and age as factors. The younger group included the 5–8-year-old children (boys $N = 29$; girls $N = 30$); the older group included the 9–12-year-olds (boys $N = 34$; girls $N = 28$).

Assessing the Father-Child Relationship

We assessed three different aspects of the father-child relationship: *frequency* and *regularity of visits*, and the *closeness of the father and child* from the child's perspective. To measure visits, both mothers and children were asked to describe the father-child visitation schedule. Since half of the children were between six and eight years old, and even some older children were rather vague about the schedule, indicators of the frequency and regularity of father-child visits were taken from mother reports at Time 1. In discussing the child's daily life and schedule of activities, mothers were asked to describe whether or not and how often the children saw their fathers. Frequency of visits was coded into four categories: *1*) never or only once since the separation; *2*) rarely (less than twice a month); *3*) often (two or three times each month); and *4*) frequently (at least once a week). The regularity of visits was divided into two categories: families with a relatively consistent and predictable visitation schedule were considered regular, those with no established visitation routine were considered irregular. Overall, father-child visits were quite frequent at this point; more than two-thirds of the father-child pairs visited at least every other week. About two-thirds of the mothers described the visitation schedule as "regular," and about one-third as "irregular." Interrater reliability for coding of frequency and regularity of visits was greater than .85. Neither of these variables fully captures a third dimension, *duration of visits* (thus, frequent and regular visits may be a few hours or a whole weekend; similarly, even infrequent visits may last a long time). In our data, though, there was a high level of variability in visit lengths *within* a given family, perhaps in part because both fathers and children were experimenting with alternative lengths, trying to arrange their new lives to maximize good outcomes. In any case, reporting in this study was not clear or consistent enough to permit reliable coding of duration of visits.

Children were asked to describe their fathers in general, and their visits with them, and to specify the things they liked and did not like about them, as well as the visits. On the basis of children's descriptions, father-child dyads at Time 1 were coded on a three-point scale, in terms of closeness. Dyads were considered "close" if they shared time together, disclosed feelings to each other, and generally had positive (and, sometimes, negative) feelings toward each other (e.g., "He does a lot with me, he cares a lot, he understands what you mean . . . sometimes he doesn't understand me as well as he thinks he does, but I'm not afraid to talk anything over with him"). Dyads were considered "neutral" if they were described as sharing some activities and as having cordial or civil interactions, but not as sharing intimacy or strong feelings toward each other (e.g., "Sometimes he's nice . . . he lets me do a lot of things . . . Friday nights we go out somewhere and Sunday mornings we go out for donuts"). "Distant" dyads were identified by a general lack of relationship, either because they shared virtually no time together and had no emotional involvement with each other (e.g., "We don't do a lot, we don't dislike each other, really") or because one person wanted contact but the other appeared detached (e.g., "He used to take me roller skating and everyplace . . . I just worry because he hasn't been calling me and he's supposed to call me"). Interrater reliability of this coding was above .90.

Visitation regularity and frequency were correlated .48/<.001; $r = .30$, $p<.05$).

It is important to note here that all of the variables assessing the child's relationship with the noncustodial father were based on reports from the child or the mother, and not the father. This was an unfortunate necessity, given the very low response rate from noncustodial fathers (less than 20%). It is worth noting, though, that for the 21 mother-father pairs in which both a custodial and noncustodial parent reported on visits, the correlations for reports of frequency and regularity were .63 ($p<.01$) and .46 ($p<.05$).

Assessing Children's Adjustment

Measures assessed aspects of the children's adjustment and adaptation from the point of view of both the mother and child.

Children's self-reports of adjustment: Perceived Competence Scale, total score. This measure was used as an estimate of children's overall self-esteem (see Harter, [*1982*] for validity data). Children were read statements that dichotomized feelings of general self-worth and cognitive and social competence (e.g., "Some kids are pretty sure of themselves but other kids are not very sure of themselves") and were asked to say which child they resembled more, then to rate whether they resembled that child "a lot" or "a little." Overall self-esteem scores at Time 1 (based on sums of standardized scale scores) ranged from 28 to 66, with a mean of 51.33 and a SD of 8.98. At Time 2 they ranged from 28 to 68, with a mean of 52.8,5 and a SD of 8.50.

Average raw subscale scores for cognitive and social competence and for general self-worth ranged from 2.8 to 3.2 for our four age-gender groups at both times, as did scores for those three scales for the four normative samples reported by Harter (*1982*). Standard deviations (averaging .50 to .70) were also equivalent.

Mother reports of children's adjustment: Child Behavior Checklist, Parent Form (CBCL-Parent). Individual subscales (e.g., Hyperactive, Depressive) from this widely used, well-validated mother-report checklist of 113 behavior problems (*Achenbach, 1987; Achenbach & Edelbrock, 1983*) were highly intercorrelated in this sample, so only the total score for all kinds of behavior problems (misbehaving, social withdrawal, acting out, depression, etc.) was used in these analyses. Mean scores for the total number of problems (37 for Time 1 and 32 for Time 2, with SDs around 20) were above those reported for Achenbach's (*1987*) sample of 600 children between 6 and 11, in which the mean was about 20 problems. Our *means* were below the cutoff points Achenbach and Edelbrock (*1981*) recommended as useful for diagnostic purposes (37 for girls of this age, 40 for boys). These cutoff points were assigned as identifying the point below which 90% of children from "normal" samples score and above which 80%–90% of children from "clinical" samples score. At Time 1, 45% of the boys and 67% of the girls in our sample scored below the Achenbach and Edelbrock cutoff; at Time 2, it was 67% and 75%.

Overall, then, our sample scored within the "normal" range in self-esteem, but mother reports of behavior problems were elevated above the levels reported for non-clinical samples. Although self-esteem and behavior problems were significantly correlated at Time 1 ($r = -.32$, $p.01$) and at Time 2 ($r = -.25$, $p.05$), the correlations were low enough to suggest that the two indicators are independent.

Moderator Variables

In addition to age and gender, and the three father-child relationship variables, parental legal conflict was included and expected to act both as a predictor and a moderator variable. We chose to use legal conflict as a moderator (rather than parental or child report of parental conflict) because it allows us to rely on a criterion external to any of the family members. However, as is noted below, legal conflict was related to maternal report of tension or conflict in the parental dyad. Legal conflict was defined as dispute over major aspects of the settlement (e.g., custody), and filing of motions and countermotions. The motions and countermotions focused on issues ranging from restraining orders to motions about alimony, child support, visitation, health and life insurance, property, and other financial matters. In order to determine the amount of legal conflict, the motions filed by either parent at three different junctures in the divorce process were counted by trained coders who had achieved interrater reliability greater than .85. The three time periods that were coded were *1*) the initial complaint and the defendant's answer; *2*) the period from the filing of the initial complaint to the Time 1 interview; and *3*) the period from the Time 1 interview to the Time 2 interview. In order to arrive at legal conflict scores for Time 1, we summed the motions for the initial complaint and answer with motions filed up to the Time 1 interview. A total legal conflict score for Time 2 was calculated by adding to the Time 1 legal conflict indicator the number of additional motions filed between the Time 1 and Time 2 interviews. These two indicators were correlated with the mothers' subjective reports of the degree of tension and conflict in the parental relationship both at Time 1 ($r = .37, p<.001$) and at Time 2 ($r = 27$, $p.01$). Moreover, our legal conflict indicators in some sense assess the contributions of both parents to the conflict (at least at the legal level).

Analyses

In keeping with our interest in identifying the unique contributions of our six Time 1 "predictor variables" (the child-focused variables of age and gender, the father-child relationship variables of closeness, visit frequency, and visit regularity, and the family context variable of legal conflict), we performed multiple regressions on the child adjustment indicators at Time 1 and Time 2. In addition, in order to examine the combined effects of the predictors, we created the 15 two-way interaction terms from the six predictors and added them individually to the regression with the six main predictors in order to assess the individual contribution of each interaction term to the adjustment outcomes. For example, in order to assess the effects of legal conflict in combination with visit frequency on child adjustment, we conducted regressions including the six main predictors and the legal conflict by visit frequency interaction term on each of the child adjustment indicators. In this way, the role of all six variables as main effects, and in interaction with the other five variables, was systematically evaluated. Significant interactions were interpreted by calculating and comparing adjustment scores predicted by the regression equation for each cell in the interaction term.

This analysis strategy allowed us to determine whether, as we predicted, there were few main effects on child adjustment outcomes. We could assess directly whether there were main effects for age or gender (we predicted younger children and boys would show poorer adjustment) or the quality and amount of father-child contact. More importantly, by focusing our analyses on the combined effects of our predictors (i.e., the interaction terms), we could assess whether the effect of the father-child relationship on the child's adjustment is moderated by the contextual aspects of the post-separation situation.

RESULTS

Results of the multiple regression analyses are presented in TABLES 1 and 2, separately for each adjustment indicator at each time. As may be seen in these tables, none of the overall regressions of the six "predictors," taken together as main effects, was significant. However, legal conflict was significantly related to behavior problems in both the short and the longer term, and visitation regularity at Time 1 was related to overall self-esteem at Time 2. As predicted, then, there were few overall relationships among these variables and children's adjustment. Also as predicted, though, there proved to be a number of significant interactions, and these in turn often produced significant overall regressions.

TABLE 1
Multiple Regressions on Self-esteem

PREDICTOR VARIABLES[a]	TIME 1		TIME 2	
Main effects	r	β	r	β
Age	$-.10$	$-.12$	$-.09$	$-.12$
Sex (boy = 1, girl = 2)	$-.09$	$-.13$ $R=.21$	$-.08$	$-.11$ $R=.32$
Visit frequency	$-.07$	$-.06$ $df=6,112$	$-.01$	$-.13$ $df=6,83$
Visit regularity	$-.03$	.04 $p=$ NS	.21	.32* $p=$ NS
Father-child closeness	.07	$-.04$	.03	.05
Parental legal conflict	$-.11$	$-.14$	$-.09$	$-.15$
Interactions[b]	p[c]	R[d]	p	R
Sex × Age				
Age × frequency	<.001	.48***		
Age × regularity	<.01	.33†		
Age × closeness				
Age × legal conflict				
Sex × frequency	<.001	.54***	<.01	.45**
Sex × regularity	<.001	.48***	<.01	.44**
Sex × closeness				
Sex × legal conflict				
Frequency × regularity				
Frequency × closeness	<.01	.34*	<.001	.63***
Frequency × legal conflict	<.001	.53***		
Regularity × closeness	<.05	.28		
Regularity × legal conflict	<.05	.29		
Closeness × legal conflict	<.05	.28	<.05	.39†

† $p<.10$; * $p<.05$; ** $p<.01$; *** $p<.001$.
[a] Predictor variables were assessed at Time 1, except that legal conflict was assessed at Time 1 in Time 1 analyses and at Time 2 in Time 2 analyses.
[b] With all main effects and only this interaction entered.
[c] Significance of beta weight associated with interaction term.
[d] Multiple correlation with all main effects and this interaction entered.

The Child's Perspective: Effects on Self-Esteem

As may be seen in TABLE 1, children's age and gender interacted significantly with both frequency and regularity of visits in predicting children's self-esteem at Time 1. Both younger children and boys benefited from more frequent and more regular contact with fathers, while both older children and girls actually had lower self-esteem when father visits were regular. Girls' self-esteem was also lower when father visits were frequent.

Father-child closeness and legal conflict also moderated the effects of frequency and regularity at Time 1. Visit frequency and regularity were both associated with higher self-esteem for children reporting closer relationships with their fathers. Finally, visit regularity was related to high self-esteem when legal conflict was low, but to low self-esteem when legal conflict was high. Father-child closeness also interacted with legal conflict, with closeness associated with high self-esteem only for children without parental conflict.

Only some of these relationships held up over the longer term. Gender and father-child closeness continued to moderate the relationships between self-esteem and frequency and regularity, while father-child closeness moderated the relationship between self-esteem and regularity. In addition, legal conflict continued to moderate the relationship between closeness and self esteem.

The Mother's Perspective: Effects on Behavior

Visit frequency and regularity were associated with children's adjustment as indicated by mother-reported behavior problems at Time 1 for some groups. As may be seen in TABLE 2, gender was an important moderator of both frequency and regularity at Time 1. Girls whose fathers visited frequently and/or regularly were reported as having fewer behavior problems. Boys whose fathers visited regularly were actually reported as having more behavior problems. In addition, frequency and regularity interacted with each other; children with frequent and regular visits showed the fewest behavior problems. Finally, legal conflict interacted with both frequency and regularity. Children showed the most behavior problems if their parents were in legal conflict and the visitation was *not* frequent and/or *not* regular. Thus, reduced visitation in high-conflict divorce situations had detrimental effects.

The pattern of relationships with Time 2 behavior problems was somewhat different. Visit frequency was associated with fewer problems for older children and for children with closer relationships with their fathers. Regularity was unrelated to behavior problems for any group of children, but father-child closeness was associated with fewer behavior problems for children whose parents were not experiencing high levels of legal conflict.

DISCUSSION

Overall, the results of this research suggest that the aspects of the relationships between noncustodial fathers and their children explored here have many implications for children's adjustment. It is important to note that many other factors in children's lives (such as their mothers' adjustment) both directly affect their adjustment and may moderate the impact of their relationship with their noncustodial parents. Moreover, although this study includes attention to frequency and regularity of visits, and quality of the father-child relationship, there are many other aspects of that relationship that may also be important, such as duration of visits or amount of time spent alone with the child.

The analyses presented here show that, even in terms of the variables assessed in this study, the child's relationship with a noncustodial father does not have simple, direct effects; rather, it has different implications for different kinds of children and for children in different situations. In addition, at least in this sample, children's

TABLE 2
Multiple Regressions on Behavior Problems

PREDICTOR VARIABLES[a]	TIME 1		TIME 2	
Main effects	r	β	r	β
Age	.03	.04	.03	.04
Sex (boy = 1, girl = 2)	−.19	−.14 $R = .27$	−.17	−.14 $R = .30$
Visit frequency	.06	.06 $df = 6,97$	.06	.06 $df = 6,89$
Visit regularity	.02	−.04 $p = $ NS	−.06	−.16 $p = $ NS
Father-child closeness	.04	.07	−.06	−.07
Parental legal conflict	.21*	−.19[†]	.22*	.21*
Interactions:[b]	p[c]	R[d]	p	R
Sex × Age				
Age × frequency			<.001	.49***
Age × regularity				
Age × closeness				
Age × legal conflict				
Sex × frequency	<.001	.55***	<.10	.35[†]
Sex × regularity	<.05	.34[†]		
Sex × closeness				
Sex × legal conflict				
Frequency × regularity	<.05	.34[†]		
Frequency × closeness			<.01	.41*
Frequency × legal conflict	<.001	.58***	<.01	.42*
Regularity × closeness				
Regularity × legal conflict				
Closeness × legal conflict	<.05	.36*	<.05	.37[†]

[†] $p < .10$; * $p < .05$; ** $p < .01$; *** $p < .001$.
[a] Predictor variables were assessed at Time 1, except that legal conflict was assessed at Time 1 in Time 1 analyses, and at Time 2 in Time 2 analyses.
[b] With all main effects and only this interaction entered.
[c] Significance of beta weight associated with interaction term.
[d] Multiple correlation with all main effects and this interaction entered.

reports of their self-esteem are not predicted by the same variables as mothers' reports of children's behavior. In fact, in many cases, predictors of high self-esteem were also predictors of more (not fewer) behavior problems. Thus, children's post-separation "adjustment" seems not to be monolithic or unidimensional. It is not clear, though, whether it is the difference in observer (self vs mother) or domain (internal state vs behavior) or both that is salient here. Future research might well be directed to a clarification of this issue.

In the immediate postseparation period, frequent visits by the father were beneficial to children's self-esteem if the children were male, six to eight years old, or especially close to their fathers. It may be that these three groups were most vulnerable to experiencing the separation as a pure *loss* of the father and of the preseparation family. Among children for whom the separation situation is unambiguously a situation of loss, contact with the noncustodial parent should be most comforting. However, every contact also brings a new loss. Thus, at least for boys, high frequency and regularity of contact may be associated with both high self-esteem and with higher mother reports of behavior problems because contact maintained a strong sense of loss. These results provide some confirmation of Wallerstein and Kelly's (*1980*) finding that a good father-child relationship was related to high self-esteem, especially for boys. However, as previously reported, Kurdek et al. (*1981*) found infrequent visitations from the noncustodial parent to be related to better adjustment in children. They suggested that diminished contact with the noncustodial parent may help to reconcile the child to the parents' divorce. Our findings of a relationship with behavior problems only for boys is consistent with general findings that boys are more likely than girls to respond to the divorce with negative behavior.

However, frequent and/or regular visits were actually associated with *low* self-esteem for females, during this period. It is hard to be sure what accounts for this finding, but perhaps frequent contact with the father was more likely to generate or intensify conflict for girls living with their same-sex parent. Perhaps girls, more often than boys, bring to interactions with their fathers a sense of repudiation borrowed from their mothers, or derived from identification with them. If so, more frequent or regular interactions might be experienced *in part* as increased contact with someone who is both loved and missed *and* is an "enemy," or at least an enemy of their mother. The fact that during this period frequent and regular visits were also associated with fewer behavior problems in girls, as reported by their mothers, seems to fit this interpretation as well. Girls visiting often with their fathers during this early period may have been less likely to act up around their mothers for the same reason they showed lower self-esteem: that is, they felt guilty or anxious about the time they spent with their father, but felt relatively more comfortable in the postseparation household. Girls who experience frequent contact with the noncustodial father may be similar to girls living with remarried mothers. Generally, these girls tend to exhibit more negative internalizing behavior than girls living with single mothers (who may be more similar to the girls in our sample with infrequent father contact) (*Peterson & Zill, 1986; Zaslow, 1989*). Similarly, Schwarz and Getter (*cited in Peterson & Zill*) hypothesized that children who are stably allied with the same-sex parent become alienated from their opposite-sex parent. Thus, the girls in our study, living with their mothers, may feel conflict about frequent contact with their noncustodial father, thus contributing to their lower levels of self-esteem. However, our finding of fewer behavior problems for these girls is not consistent with previous findings of increased antisocial behavior for girls whose mothers remarried (*Hetherington, Cox, & Cox, 1985; Zaslow, 1989*). The difference in findings may reflect differences in the samples. The girls in our study were not living with an opposite-sex parent, perhaps resulting in a more comfortable home environment for them than for those girls adjusting to a stepparent in the home.

Across gender, frequent visits were associated with fewer behavior problems when visits were also regular, and with more behavior problems when they were irregular. Infrequent visits were associated with more behavior problems when parental conflict was high, but not when it was low. Similarly, father-child closeness was related to higher self-esteem only when there was lower parental conflict. These findings point up the importance of context in determining the impact of the father-child relationship on children's adjustment. Frequent visits were actually problematic if they were not also regular. Moreover, infrequent visits were only associated with behavior problems when parental legal conflict was high. This evidence confirms Kurdek's (*1988*) finding that the noncustodial father's frequent involvement with his child was most beneficial to the child in cases where interparental conflict was also high.

During this early period, *regular* visits were generally beneficial to children's self-esteem under the same conditions: if children were young, male, and close to their fathers; they were also beneficial if there was little legal conflict. Regular visits were actually problematic for self-esteem, though, for older children, females, and children whose parents were in conflict. Again, predictable contact was probably maximally comforting for those children experiencing a relatively unambivalent and strong sense of loss as a result of parental separation. In contrast, children with age-related needs for autonomy and separation from the family, or experiencing the separation in other ways (as posing internal conflict or as initiating or prolonging parental conflict), may have experienced regularity as a kind of rigidity or inflexibility. For these children, less regular contact, more responsive to their fluctuating feelings, might be more comfortable.

Over time, many of these relationships were attenuated. However, early visitation frequency was still associated with higher self-esteem and high behavior problems for boys, for older children, and for children close to their fathers; it was still associated, as well, with lower self-esteem and fewer behavior problems for girls. Early visitation regularity was still associated with higher self-esteem for boys one year later, as was father-child closeness in the context of low parental conflict. Similarly, low frequency was associated with more behavior problems for children whose parents were in legal conflict. There is, then, some evidence for persistent effects of the early post-separation relationship between fathers and children.

In addition, some new relationships surfaced in predicting Time 2 behavior problems. Although early visitation frequency was not associated with behavior problems for either age group at Time 1, by Time 2 it was associated with fewer such problems for older children. Similarly, although father-child closeness did not affect this relationship at Time 1, early visitation frequency was related to fewer behavior problems at Time 2 for children who were close to their fathers. Finally, early father-child closeness was associated with fewer later behavior problems for children with frequent father-child visits, and parents with low legal conflict. These emergent relationships suggest that father-child closeness, in particular, tends to have relatively longer-term effects on children's behavior, while frequency and regularity tend to have immediate effects, only some of which persist. These results are consistent with those of Hess and Camara (*1979*), who found that the quality of the father-child relationship, but not the amount of contact, was related to positive adjustment in the child.

CONCLUSION

Taken together, our findings point to the importance of children's age and gender as factors influencing the meaning of the regularity and frequency of fathers' visits. Both frequency and regularity seem to enhance self-esteem, and to be associated with behavior problems, for younger children and especially for boys. These results suggest that for children with a relatively uncomplicated sense of loss associated with parental separation, regular or frequent contact with the noncustodial parent is associated with feeling better about the self and openly displaying distress about their loss to the mother (more behavior problems). In contrast, regular or frequent contact has different consequences, because it has a different meaning, for girls and older children. Especially for girls living in mother-custody households, frequent or regular contact with a noncustodial father may arouse or intensify loyalty conflicts, guilt, or anxiety, which in turn lower self-esteem but increase their sense of comfort (fewer behavior problems) in the postseparation custodial household.

Alternatively, it must be noted that both boys and girls seem to be showing sex-role-typical patterns of distress—high self-esteem and high behavior problems for boys, low self-esteem and low behavior problems for girls—when they see their father more—and more regularly. It could be that increased contact with the father has, for both sexes, the effect of strengthening or maintaining traditional sex roles.

Two important aspects of children's family situation also affect the significance of father contact. Both parental legal conflict and father-child closeness make a difference, in ways we might expect and consistent with the literature. Perhaps the most surprising aspect of our findings is the suggestion that it may be especially detrimental to the child to prohibit frequent visits when parents are negated in a protracted legal battle. Generally, though, all of our findings highlight the importance of attention to the psychological meaning *for the child* of each parent, and of the particular postseparation situation. It is clear that children's views of their parents and their families deserve further attention as factors mediating the impact of parents' actions.

REFERENCES

Achenbach, T.M. (1987). Epidemiological comparisons of American and Dutch children:I. Behavioral/emotional problems and competencies reported by parents for ages 4 to 16. *Journal of the American Academy of Child and Adolescent Psychiatry, 26*, 317–325.

Achenbach, T.M., & Edelbrock, C.S. (1981). Behavioral problems and competencies reported by parents of normal and disturbed children aged four to sixteen. *Monograph of the Society for Research in Child Development, 46* (No. 1, Serial No. 188).

Achenbach, T.M., & Edelbrock, C.S. (1983). *Manual for the Child Behavior Checklist and Revised Child Behavior Profile*. Burlington: University of Vermont.

Ahrons, C.R. (1983). Predictors of parental involvement post divorce. *Journal of Divorce, 6*, 55–69.

Biller, H.B. (1974). *Paternal deprivation*. New York: Lexington Books.

Block, J.H., Block, J., & Morrison, A. (1981). Parental agreement-disagreement on child-rearing orientations and gender-related personality correlates in children. *Child Development, 52*, 965–974.

Bowlby, J. (1973). *Attachment and loss: Vol. 2, Separation*. New York: Basic Books.

Demo, D.H., & Acock, A.C. (1988). The impact of divorce on children. *Journal of Marriage and the Family, 50*, 619–648.

Emery, R.E. (1982). Interparent conflict and the children of discord and divorce. *Psychological Bulletin, 92*, 310–330.

Emery, R.E., Hetherington, E.M., & DiLalla, L.F. (1984). Divorce, children, and social policy. In H.W. Stevenson & A.E. Sigel (Eds.), *Child development research and social policy* (pp. 189–266). Chicago: University of Chicago Press.

Furstenberg, F.F., Jr., Morgan, S.P., & Allison, P.D. (1987). Paternal participation and children's well-being after marital dissolution. *American Sociological Review, 52*, 695–701.

Goldstein, J., Freud, A., & Solnit, A.J. (1973). *Beyond the best interests of the child*. New York: Free Press.

Guidubaldi, J., & Perry, J.D. (1985). Divorce and mental health sequelae for children: A two-year follow-up of a nationwide sample. *Journal of the American Academy of Child Psychiatry, 24*, 531–537.

Harter, S. (1982). The perceived competence scale for children. *Child Development, 53*, 87–97.

Hess, R.D., & Camara, K.A. (1979). Post-divorce family relationships as mediating factors in the consequences of divorce for children. *Journal of Social Issues, 35*, 79–96.

Hetherington, E.M., Cox, M., & Cox, R. (1985). Long term effects of divorce and remarriage on the adjustment of children. *Journal of the American Academy of Child Psychiatry, 24*, 518–530.

Hollingshead, A.V., & Redlich, R.C. (1958). *Social class and mental illness: A community study.* New York: John Wiley.

Kalter, N., & Rembar, J. (1981). The significance of a child's age at the time of parental divorce. *American Journal of Orthopsychiatry, 51*, 85–100.

Kalter, N., Riemer, B., Brickman, A., & Chen, J.W. (1985). Implications of parental divorce for female development. *Journal of the American Academy of Child Psychiatry, 24*, 538–544.

Koch, M.P., & Lowery, C.R. (1984). Visitation and the noncustodial father. *Journal of Divorce, 8*, 47–65.

Kurdek, L. (1981). An integrated perspective on children's divorce adjustment. *American Psychologist, 36*, 856–866.

Kurdek, L. (1988). Custodial mothers' perceptions of visitation and payment of child support by noncustodial fathers in families with low and high levels of pre-separation interparent conflict. *Journal of Applied Developmental Psychology, 9*, 315–328.

Kurdek, L.A., Blisk, D., & Siesky, A.E., Jr. (1981). Correlates of children's long-term adjustment to their parents' divorce. *Developmental Psychology, 17*, 565–579.

Lowenstein, J.S., & Koopman, E.J. (1978). A comparison of the self-esteem between boys living with single-parent mothers and single-parent fathers. *Journal of Divorce, 2*, 195–208.

Peterson, J.R., & Zill, N. (1986). Marital disruption, parent-child relationship, and behavior problems in children. *Journal of Marriage and the Family, 48*, 295–307.

Santrock, J.W., & Warshak, R.A. (1979). Father custody and social development in boys and girls. *Social Issues, 35*, 112–125.

Wallerstein, J.S. (1987). Children of divorce: Report of a ten-year follow-up of early latency-age children. *American Journal of Orthopsychiatry, 57*, 199–211.

Wallerstein, J.S., & Kelly, J. (1980). *Surviving the breakup.* New York: Basic Books.

Weitzman, L.J. (1985). *The divorce revolution.* New York: Free Press.

Werner, E.E., & Smith, R.S. (1982). *Vulnerable but not invincible: A study of resilient children.* New York: McGraw-Hill.

Zaslow, M.J. (1988). Sex differences in children's response to parental divorce: 1. Research methodology and postdivorce family forms. *American Journal of Orthopsychiatry, 58*, 355–378.

Zaslow, M.J. (1989). Sex differences in children's response to parental divorce: 2. Samples, variables, ages, and sources. *American Journal of Orthopsychiatry, 59*, 118–141.

4

A Comparison of Stepfamilies With and Without Child-Focused Problems

Anne Chalfant Brown

California Graduate School of Family Psychology, San Rafael

Robert Jay Green

California School of Professional Psychology, Berkeley/Alameda

Joan Druckman

California Graduate School of Family Psychology, San Rafael

Stepfamilies in therapy for a child-focused problem were compared to those without such a problem and not in therapy. Differences were found in reciprocity within the stepparent-stepchild relationship, satisfaction with the stepparent's role, level of stepfamily conflict, and degree of stepfamily expressiveness. Results are discussed in terms of current research and clinical implications.

Given that an estimated one-third of the children living in the United States today will be part of a stepfamily before reaching adulthood (*Glick, 1984*), it is imperative to have accurate data regarding the impact of stepfamily functioning on children. In comparative studies, no overall differences have been found between children growing up in biological families and those in stepfamilies on a range of variables that include academic achievement, social behavior, family relationships, personality characteristics, and self-esteem (*Bohannan & Erickson, 1978; Ganong & Coleman, 1984, 1987; Marotz-Baden, Adams, Bueche, Munro, & Munro, 1979; Wilson, Zurcher, McAdams, & Curtis, 1975*).

These results suggest that family processes other than family constellation are the determining factors in the socialization of stepchildren. There have been, however, no empirical studies comparing stepfamilies in which a child is symptomatic to stepfamilies whose children are not showing problems. One controlled study (*Anderson*

Reprinted with permission from *American Journal of Orthopsychiatry*, 1990, Vol. 60, No. 4, 556–566. Copyright ©1990 by the American Orthopsychiatric Association, Inc.

& *White, 1986*) compared functional and dysfunctional stepfamilies (functional Stepfamilies had no members in therapy, and their Family Adjustment score on the Family Concept Test was in the range for well-functioning families). It was found that functional stepfamily members reported better marital adjustment, more reciprocal positive involvement of stepchild with stepfather, weaker parent-child coalitions, and fewer statements designed to exclude a step-relative from the family. Other clinical studies of dysfunctional stepfamilies (some with problem children) used qualitative methodologies only (*Fast & Cain, 1966; Goldstein, 1974; Kleinman, Rosenberg, & Whiteside, 1979; Ransom, Schlesinger, & Derdeyn, 1979*). Our search of the literature revealed five variables associated with stepfamily stress and possible dysfunction: clarity of the stepparent's role in the stepfamily, management of conflict among members of the stepfamily, management of conflict between the remarried couple, resolution of feelings about the loss of the original family, and quality of the coparental relationship between the divorced couple.

The role of stepparent is ambiguous because no norm exist for sharing parenthood with the biological parent. Problems arise in stepfamilies when the stepparent, biological parent, and stepchild have differing expectations about the role of the stepparent (*Bohannan & Erickson, 1978; Fast & Cain, 1966; Visher & Visher, 1978a, 1978b*). Dysfunctional interactional patterns, such as triangulation, often develop around issues of discipline and nurturance. Frequently in these triangles, the stepparent's authority is not recognized and nurturant behavior not reciprocated by the child, while the natural parent supports the child, thereby undermining the stepparent's parental role (*Messinger, Walker, & Freeman, 1978; Stern, 1978; Visher & Visher, 1978a*).

Higher levels of family conflict have been identified as one of the factors associated with poorer developmental outcomes for children across all family forms (*Marotz-Baden et al., 1979*). For example, in the normative testing of the Family Environment Scale (*Moos, 1974*), normal families consistently score lower on Conflict and higher on Expressiveness than do distressed families (*Moos & Moos, 1981*). Similarly, a study comparing functional and dysfunctional remarriage and first-marriage couples, using the Family Environment Scale, found that functional couples scored lower on Conflict and higher on Expressiveness than did dysfunctional couples (*Medeiros, 1977*).

However, based on clinical studies, another problematic type of conflict management has been identified as associated with stepfamilies. It is characterized as avoidance of conflict, or pseudomutuality, and is thought to arise from the fear of another failure (*Goldstein, 1974; Kleinman et al., 1979*). Thus, a pattern of either too much or too little overt conflict may be characteristic of dysfunctional stepfamilies.

Resolution of feelings about the loss of the original family (i.e., "emotional divorce") is viewed in the stepfamily literature as an integrative developmental task (*Ransom et al., 1979; Visher & Visher, 1979*). Incomplete resolution has been associated with clinical dysfunction in children (*Kleinman et al., 1979; Sager, et al., 1983*). Other postdivorce literature, however, indicates that by the time of stepfamily formation, emotional divorce (at least on the part of the parent) is complete (*Goldsmith, 1980; Hetherington, Cox, & Cox, 1977; Kitson, 1982*).

It is not yet clear in the stepfamily literature whether there is a consistent connection between conflictual divorced coparenting and symptomatology in a child. However, adolescents have reported that conflict between their biological parents is a primary stressor in stepfamily living (*Lutz, 1983*). Also, a two-year study of family response to divorce (in mother-custody families with nursery school children) found two variables associated with the mother's effectiveness in dealing with the child— support in child-rearing from her former husband, and agreement with him on discipline (*Hetherington et al., 1977*).

The purpose of the present study was to assess processes in stepfamilies in which a child is a symptomatic, identified patient. Based on the literature reviewed, and particularly on those variables associated with stepfamily stress, it was hypothesized that nonproblem stepfamilies would show: *1*) greater stepfamily role clarity, *2*) better stepfamily conflict management, *3*) better stepfamily couple conflict management, *4*) less unresolved emotional divorce, and *5*) a better relationship between the divorced coparents. An additional general research question was whether self-report scores on these dependent variables would vary as a function of family role (parent, stepparent, child) regardless of the existence of child problems. Lastly, we looked at whether family role and problem status have interactive effects in terms of the five dependent variables reviewed above.

METHOD

Subjects

Family triads, consisting of a biological parent, stepparent, and child aged 11 through 16 years, were selected from two populations: those in therapy for a child-focused problem (T group) and those neither in therapy nor having child-focused problems (NP group). There were 23 T-group and 27 NP-group stepfamilies in this study. The majority were from the San Francisco Bay Area. The rest were from other urban or suburban settings in California, Michigan, upstate New York, and Pennsylvania.

All the couples had been living together or married for at least six months. Both simple stepfamilies (in which the stepparent had no children from a previous relationship) and complex stepfamilies (in which the stepparent had children from a previous relationship) were included. All the children had lived in the stepfamily at least half-time for at least six months. In addition, all of these children had had face-to-face contact with the other biological parent for at least 10 days during the past year.

The T group was made up of 23 stepfamilies currently in family therapy, or with the child individually in therapy, because of perceived problems with the child. Families were excluded if the child's problem predated the stepfamily's formation. Presenting problems included resisting parental authority, depression, angry flare-ups and hostility, truancy, academic underachievement, acting-out at school, substance abuse, difficulties with peers, conflict with siblings, jealousy in the stepfamily, bulimia, running away, and felonious trespassing.

The NP group was made up of 27 stepfamilies that had not been in therapy for at least two years prior to the date of the study. The parents reported no major problems with the children, and there had been no complaints from the school or other authorities during the previous 12 months.

The two groups did not differ significantly on any demographic, family background, or family composition variables, including sex of child and biological parent, age of child at separation, length of time since divorce, length of the new relationship, whether or not the couple were married, the presence of other children in the household (including a mutual child of the new couple), or whether the stepfamily was simple or complex.

Demographic characteristics. Of the stepchildren, 25 were female and 25 male. In 65% of the stepfamilies, the biological parent was the mother. The mean age for the biological parents was 40.7, for the stepparents 40.3, and for the children 13.9 years (children's subgroup $SD = 1.66$).

Over 90% of the parents and stepparents were Caucasian, and all were middle-class. In 90% of the stepfamilies, the couple was married, with a mean of 5.4 years together. Fifty-four percent of the stepfamilies were complex. The mean number of years since separation from the child's other parent was 7.6. The mean age of the children at the time their parents separated was 5.5 years.

The children's frequency of contact with the other biological parent ranged from "living half-time with him or her" (8%) to "seeing him or her less than one time per month, but at least 10 times in the past year" (36%), with the majority falling between these two extremes.

Instruments

In addition to a Demographic Data Questionnaire, five instruments were used in this study, as follows.

Stepparent Role Scale (SRS) *(Brown, Green, & Druckman, 1988)*. This questionnaire was constructed for the present study. It has three forms, one for each family member, with four subscales and 25 items. The Initiation subscale measures the amount of authority-related and nurturant and befriending behavior initiated by the stepparent; Reciprocity measures the degree of reciprocation by the stepchild of the stepparent's initiatives. Support measures the amount of support by the biological parent for the nurturant and befriending behavior of the stepparent; Satisfaction measures the amount of family satisfaction with the stepparent's role.

The items were developed from behavioral equivalents to concepts described in the literature as being connected with role clarity. Family interaction in the areas of discipline, giving directives, giving and receiving affection, communicating on a personal level, and jointly participating in pleasurable activities were all included. Responses to items were on a five-point Likert scale. Alpha reliability scores were obtained from a sample of 223 respondents and ranged from .70 to .90 on the various subscales of role clarity.

Family Environment Scale–Form R (FES)(Moos, 1974). The FES is a 90-item, true-false instrument that measures the social-environmental characteristics of all types of families. It was used here to measure stepfamily conflict. Normative data on the Form R subscales were collected for 1,125 normal and 500 distressed families. The instrument has good test-retest and internal consistency reliability (with *r*s ranging from .69 to .85 on the various subscales) and has been validated over time in numerous studies (*Moos & Moos, 1981*).

Although the FES was administered to the three family members in its entirety, only data from the Expressiveness and Conflict subscales were used: Expressiveness measures "the extent to which family members are encouraged to act openly and to express their feelings directly;" Conflict measures "the amount of openly expressed anger, aggression and conflict among family members" (*Moos & Moos, 1981, p. 2*). Higher scores on Expressiveness and lower scores on Conflict were assumed to indicate better stepfamily conflict management.

ENRICH (Olson, Fournier, & Druckman, 1982). ENRICH, used here to measure management of conflict between the stepfamily couple, is a 12-scale, 125-item instrument, measuring marital dynamics around personal, interpersonal, and external issues. Responses to the first 115 items are on a Likert scale ranging from 1 = Strongly Agree to 5 = Strongly Disagree. Responses on the last ten items are on four-point Likert scales with varying choices. The instrument has good test-retest and internal consistency reliability, with *r*s ranging from .68 to .92 on the various subscales.

Although the instrument was administered in its entirety, data from only three of the subscales were used: Communication measured the feelings and attitudes of each partner toward the openness of marital communication; Conflict Resolution assessed each partner's feelings and attitudes about the existence of conflict and the couple's ability to handle it in the relationship; Idealistic Distortion (in ENRICH, a modified version of Edmond's Marital Conventionalization Scale) correlates highly with other scales that measure the tendency of individuals to give socially desirable answers to personal questions. It was used in this study as an approximate measure of couple pseudomutality—the presentation of an idyllic, harmonious image of the marriage. Higher scores on Communication and Conflict Resolution and lower scores on Idealistic Distortion were assumed to indicate better couple conflict management.

Attachment Scale (AS) (Kitson, 1982). This scale measures continuing emotional attachment to the former spouse during and after divorce. It is made up of 19 statements, with possible responses on a five-point Likert scale. Items were developed from a model of bereavement by Parkes (*1972*). A factor analysis ensured that attachment and bereavement were on a single dimension. The alpha reliability of the scale was .80. The scale was administered to the biological parent and modified to make the language appropriate for remarried persons, e.g., "husband/wife" became "former husband/wife."

Quality of Divorced Coparental Relationship Scale (QDCR) (Goldsmith, 1980). This instrument measures the amount of cooperation and mutual support between divorced coparents, the amount of hostility and conflict in the coparenting relationship, and the degree of satisfaction with that relationship. Twelve items request responses on five-point Likert scales. The overall reliability coefficient for the scale was .87. A validity study yielded excellent results (*Goldsmith, 1982*). The scale was administered to the biological parent. The instrument was also modified to be appropriate for the child respondent, expanding it by three items in order to include both biological parents in some of the questions. Its internal consistency reliability was .85.

Data Collection

Subjects were volunteers obtained through referrals and advertising. An initial screening interview was conducted by telephone to determine whether the respondent fit the criteria for participation. Questionnaires and instructions were mailed to the participants with return envelopes enclosed.

Data Analysis

Data for stepfamily role clarity and stepfamily conflict management were analyzed using a 2 (T group versus NP group) by 3 (family role: biological parent, stepparent, child) analysis of variance (ANOVA) with the second factor treated as a repeated measure. (The repeated measure was used to allow for possible correlations among the scores by members of the same family.) Thus, main effects for group (T versus NP) represent differences between T group family triad scores (the sum of bioparent plus stepparent plus child scores on a variable) and NP group family triad scores. The main effects for family role represent differences between bioparents, stepparents, and children, regardless of group identify. Finally, interaction effects analyses for group (T versus NP) by family role (biological parent versus stepparent versus child) are presented. Post-hoc Bonferroni analyses, which protect against a Type 1 error rate when there are multiple tests, controlled *alpha* at $\leq.05$ and were conducted, when necessary, to determine which of the subgroups differed significantly from one another when the family role main effects and interaction effects analyses of the ANOVA were significant.

Data for stepfamily couples' conflict management and quality of the divorced coparental relationship were analyzed using a 2 by 2 ANOVA with the second factor treated as a repeated measure, followed by post-hoc Bonferroni analyses, as discussed above. The data for emotional divorce were analyzed using *t*-tests with separate variance estimates.

RESULTS

Results have been organized in terms of each dependent variable, reporting only those tests that were significant at the $p\leq.05$ level. The results comparing the two groups of stepfamilies (NP and T) and two family roles (biological and child) for emotional divorce and quality of the divorced coparental relationship were not significant. Therefore, those dependent variables are not listed below.

Stepfamily Role Clarity (SRC)

Initiation. In the main effect for family role, the stepparents in both groups viewed themselves as initiating authority and nurturing and befriending behavior significantly more often than the stepchildren viewed them as doing ($F = 3.8$, $p\eta.05$). (See TABLE 2.)

Reciprocity. Members of NP-Group stepfamilies reported significantly more role reciprocity by the stepchild in response to the stepparent's initiatives than did members of T-group stepfamilies ($F = 10.34$, $p\leq.01$). (See TABLE 1.)

Support. In the analysis of main effect for family member, the biological parents in both groups viewed themselves as significantly more supportive than either the

TABLE 1
Perceptions by NP and T Family Triads

DEPENDENT VARIABLES	NP PERCEPTIONS			T PERCEPTIONS			
	M	SD	N	M	SD	N	F
Stepchild reciprocity (SRS)	26.9	5.66	78	22.1	6.27	66	10.34*
Stepfamily satisfaction (SRS)	25.5	6.87	81	21.3	6.49	69	6.88*
Stepfamily conflict (FES)	48.9	10.00	81	57.9	8.70	66	22.99**
Stepfamily expressiveness (FES)	48.3	14.85	81	40.4	13.47	66	6.94*

* $p \leq .01$; ** $p \leq .001$.

stepparents or the children viewed them as being ($F = 10.53$, $p \leq .001$). (See TABLE 2.) In the analysis of family member interaction by group, scores for the family members differed between the NP and T groups ($F = 3.88$, $p \leq).05$). Post hoc analyses revealed that, in the T group, the biological parents and stepparents both perceived the biological parent as being significantly more supportive of the stepparent than did the children (Bonferroni t-test, $pp \leq .05$). (See TABLE 3.)

Satisfaction. Members of NP-group stepfamilies expressed significantly more satisfaction about the stepparent's role than did members of T-group stepfamilies ($F = 6.88$, $p \leq .01$). (See TABLE 1).

Stepfamily Conflict Management (FES)

The NP-group stepfamilies reported significantly higher Expressiveness ($F = 6.94$, $p \leq .01$) and lower Conflict ($F = 22.99$, $p \leq -.001$) than did the T-group stepfamilies. (See TABLE 1.) In the analysis of main effect for family member, the biological parents and stepparents both viewed the family as significantly more expressive than did the children ($F = 18.79$, $p \leq .001$). (See TABLE 2.)

Couples' Conflict Management (ENRICH)

Idealistic distortion. In the analysis of family member interaction by group, scores for stepparents and biological parents differed between the NP and T groups ($F = 3.79$, $p \leq .10$). post hoc analyses revealed that, in the T group only, stepparents scored significantly higher than biological parents on this measure (Bonferroni t-test, $p \leq .05$). (See TABLE 3).

In an additional analysis, a comparison was made between the ENRICH normative scores and the scores of stepfamily couples in our sample. Both NP-group and T-group couples scored higher on Communication, Conflict Resolution, and

TABLE 2
Perceptions by Family Members (Combined Groups)

DEPENDENT VARIABLES	BIOLOGICAL PARENTS (B)			STEPPARENTS (S)			CHILDREN (C)				DIFFERING SUBGROUPS[a]
	M	*SD*	*N*	*M*	*SD*	*N*	*M*	*SD*	*N*	*F*	
S initiation (SRS)	22.2	6.11	50	22.3	4.90	50	20.8	5.37	50	3.8*	S>C
B support of S (SRS)	31.2	4.00	49	28.7	5.84	49	26.6	6.71	49	10.53**	B>S, C
Family expressiveness (FES)	46.4	13.42	49	50.1	14.42	49	37.8	13.87	49	18.79**	C<B, S

[a] Results of post hoc analyses to determine which family members differed significantly from one another at $p \leq .05$.
* $p \leq .05$; $p \leq .001$.

Idealistic Distortion than did the couples in the normative sample. This implies that remarried couples function better than the normative sample of married couples.*

DISCUSSION

The findings for NP-group and T-group stepfamilies did not differ on the amount of authority-related or nurturing and befriending behavior initiated by the stepparent; they did, however, differ on the reaction of the stepchildren to that behavior. This suggests that the parental role behavior initiated by the stepparent is less important to stepfamily functioning than is the receptivity of the stepchild to that behavior. Similarly, Anderson and White (*1986*) found no difference between functional and dysfunctional stepfamilies in the stepparent's positive involvement with the child. However, they found that functional stepfamilies were distinguished from dysfunctional ones by a more reciprocal positive involvement of the stepchild with the stepparent.

Explanations of why there were no significant differences for stepparent's initiatives, but were for stepchild responsiveness, are not provided by our data. However, anecdotal data collected by Anderson and White *(1986)* revealed that stepchildren from dysfunctional families react negatively to moves toward premature bonding on the part of the stepparent.

Other unanswered questions arise from the mixed results regarding the biological

TABLE 3
Significant Interaction Effects by Family Role Analyses of Perceptions

	DEPENDENT VARIABLES					
	SUPPORT OF S BY B (SRS)[a]			IDEALISTIC DISTORTION (ENRICH)[b]		
PERCEPTION BY	M	SD	N	M	SD	N
NP Group						
B	31.1	3.93	26	71.0	27.07	27
S	28.1	5.66	26	69.9	26.39	27
C	28.5	5.89	26	—	—	—
T Group						
B	31.2	4.16	23	55.7	22.74	23
S	29.3	6.10	23	66.1	20.89	23
C	24.5	7.06	23	—	—	—

Note. NP = Nonproblem family subjects; T = Therapy family subjects. B = Biological parents; S = Stepparents; C = Children.
[a] Scores for all family members differed between groups: $F = 3.88$, $p \leq .05$. Significant differences at $p \leq .05$ in post hoc analyses: T(C)<T(B) and T(C)< T(S).
[b] Scores for S and B family members differed between groups: $F = 3.79$, $p \leq .10$. Significant differences at $p \leq .05$ in post hoc analyses: T(S)>T(B).

*A table of results for these analyses can be obtained from the first author.

parent's support of the stepparent in the parenting role. There were no significant differences between NP-group and T-group stepfamily triads on this variable. In the T-group stepfamilies, only the stepchildren perceived the biological parents as being less supportive of the stepparents. This latter finding supports the clinical literature, which suggests that when a stepchild rejects the stepparent's initiatives, the biological parent often sides with the child (*Messinger, Walker, & Freeman, 1978; Stern, 1978; Visher & Visher, 1978a*). Along the same lines, Anderson & White (*1986*) found that dysfunctional stepfamilies had a stronger biological parent-child coalition than did functional stepfamilies.

Why only the stepchildren in the T group perceived the biological parents as less supportive is not clear. One explanation is that, in order to create cognitive consistency and justification for their rejection of the stepparent's parenting initiatives, the T-group stepchildren perceived the biological parent as less supportive of the stepparent than was actually so. In this sense, they may be engaging in wishful thinking. Another possible explanation is that the T-group stepchildren were, in fact, correctly observing a lack of support that was being denied by the biological parent and stepparent.

Our finding that NP-group families, as predicted, reported significantly more satisfaction with the stepparent's role highlights the importance of the role clarity as a factor in positive stepfamily functioning. Similarly, recent studies have revealed the centrality of the stepparent-stepchild relationship to the success of the stepfamily. The quality of that relationship has been found to be a better predictor of stepfamily happiness than the quality of the marital relationship (*Crosbie-Burnett, 1984*).

Earlier theory and clinical research considered pseudomutuality to be a typical dysfunctional form of conflict management in stepfamilies (*Goldstein, 1974; Kleinman et al., 1979*). However, in our study, T-group stepfamilies were similar to other distressed families—showing higher levels of overt conflict and less expressiveness than NP-group stepfamilies (*Marotz-Baden et al., 1979; Moos & Moos, 1981*). This suggests that overt conflict, rather than pseudomutual avoidance of conflict, is characteristic of stepfamilies with symptomatic children in our sample's age group.

Although both groups of stepfamily couples showed greater idealistic distortion on ENRICH than a more general population, the NP-group and T-group stepfamilies did not differ on this variable. Therefore, our couple data also fail to support the idea that idealistic distortion (an aspect of pseudomutuality) is related to dysfunction in stepfamilies.

There was no significant difference between the groups in the reported ability of the couples to communicate and resolve conflict, and both groups of couples scored higher than the ENRICH normative sample. One explanation is that the couple relationship tends to be strong and functional, even in dysfunctional stepfamilies. Earlier research found that stepfamily couples in both functional and dysfunctional stepfamilies scored higher on marital adjustment than did couples in functional or dys-functional biological families (*Anderson & White, 1986*). Another possibility, how-ever, is that marital conflict in the T-group stepfamilies is being "detoured" onto the stepchild, contributing to the T-group families' higher scores on the Family Conflict subscale of the Family Environment Scale.

Incomplete emotional divorce did not seem to be an issue for either T-group of NP-group biological parents in our sample. Ninety-two percent reported either low or no attachment to the former spouse. These findings support previous research showing that emotional divorce is usually completed within two years post-separation, and certainly by the time of recoupling (*Goldsmith, 1980; Hetherington et al., 1977; Kitson, 1982*), rather than the prevailing view of incomplete emotional divorce in the stepfamily clinical literature (*Kleinman et al., 1979; Sager et al., 1983*). Our findings thus show that T-group biological parents do not differ from NP-group biological parents on the variable of completed emotional divorce.

However, this particular sample does not provide a test of emotional divorce as an issue for all stepfamilies. The mean number of years since separation for our two groups was 7.6. In a sample drawn from a population that was within two years of separation, unresolved emotional divorce between biological parents might be more pronounced or more associated with dysfunction. In addition, our study did not examine completion of emotional divorce by the stepchildren (i.e., whether stepchil-dren have adequately reached an emotional divorce from the original family-as-a-unit, while still retaining an emotional attachment to each member of that unit.)

The familiar pattern associated with dysfunction in nuclear families, in which a child is triangulated between conflicting biological parents, does not seem to be the case for our study's stepfamilies. However, in our sample, 43% of the T-group bio-logical parents had either joint custody, or sole physical and joint legal custody. Thus, almost half of the biological parents proved to be legally committed to dealing cooperatively with the other biological parent. Our subject selection criterion that the child see the other biological parent at least ten days out of the year may also have skewed the sample in the direction of coparental cooperation.

Other recent research supports our findings that some degree of coparental coop-eration is the norm. Two studies (*Ahrons, 1981; Goldsmith, 1980*) of mother-custody families within one year postdivorce indicated that continued coparenting was common. The majority of those relationships were largely cordial and support-ive, although at times stressful and conflictual. While data collected again at three and five years postdivorce indicated a deterioration in the supportiveness of the coparental relationship, especially following the remarriage of the husband alone, there was no information on how this affected the children (*Ahrons & Wallisch, 1987*). Another study found parallel parenting to be the rule, an arrangement in which communication and joint decision-making was rare, though few reported seri-ous overt undermining or conflict (*Furstenberg & Nord, 1985*). It may be that the binuclear household structure, which allows for less intense contact between the former spouses, dilutes negativity for the children.

Empirical stepfamily research—comparing groups of stepfamilies with differing characteristics—is relatively recent. This study, therefore, can be considered only a beginning. Given the complexity of stepfamilies, future researchers could profitably explore similar dependent variables but select groups for differences between simple and complex stepfamilies, length of time since the initial separation and of the new marriage, age of the index patient, and the amount of contact between the child and the other biological parent.

Furthermore, future studies should include the other biological parent and members of his or her household as respondents. The stepfamily household can be thought of as one component in a binuclear or linked family system (*Ahrons, 1981; Goldsmith, 1980, 1982*). The present study focused primarily on the stepfamily household and touched on the binuclear suprasystem only through the perceptions of the biological parent. Both the significant and the nonsignificant results of this study seem to indicate that the emotional and behavioral problems of stepchildren are associated most strongly with dysfunctional role and conflict management processes within the custodial stepfamily household. Child problems in these stepfamilies do not seem to be strongly related to unresolved emotional divorce and coparenting processes between the binuclear households. However, this conclusion (and the resulting implications for whom to include in the therapeutic system) should be viewed as tentative, because the other part of the binuclear system was investigated in this study only through the perceptions of the focal household stepfamily members.

The major unanswered questions arising from the current study are: why do stepfamilies with child problems have lower levels of expressiveness and higher levels of conflict, and why do stepchildren in these families reject their stepparents' initiatives more? Such rejection does not seem to stem from unresolved attachments or ongoing conflicts between the divorced biological parents. Nor do our data indicate that stepparents in NP-group and T-group families differ in types of initiatives made toward the stepchild. Thus, we believe that the next step in this line of inquiry is to use both in-depth interviews of all family members (especially identified adolescent patients) and observational ratings of family interaction in NP-group and T-group stepfamilies (especially focusing on the biological parent's degree of support for the stepparent's authoritative and nurturing parental behavior).

Clinical Implications

This study reinforced earlier findings that the couple relationship in a stepfamily can be satisfactory even when the stepparent-stepchild subsystem is dysfunctional, and that the quality of the stepparent-stepchild relationship is a more important predictor of good stepfamily functioning than is the marital relationship (*Anderson & White, 1986; Crosbie-Burnett, 1984*). The family therapy axiom that there is marital distress in families with child-focused problems does not seem to hold true for these problem stepfamilies. To the extent that difficulties exist between the new spouses, they may be confined to the parent-stepparent coparenting sphere and not extend into other aspects of the new marriage.

Based on our findings in stepfamilies with an identified child patient between ages 11 and 16 years, therapists can expect to find certain types of interaction patterns in the stepparent-stepchild relationship: overt and hostile (rather than suppressed) family conflict, and a lack of open, direct expression of opinions and feelings. Furthermore, the stepchildren in such problem families tend to reject stepparents' nurturing-befriending and authority-related parental behavior and to view their biological parents as giving less support to the stepparent in his or her role. It is this sequence of stepparent initiatives and child rejections (along with the child's belief that the biological parent is not supportive of the stepparent's initiatives) that may be more problematic. From a therapeutic standpoint, the biological parent may need to clarify to the child the fact that he or she supports the stepparent's role behavior. Other reasons for a given child's lack of reciprocity may need to be explored in individual, systems-oriented therapy sessions with the stepchild, in addition to ongoing conjoint family sessions.

REFERENCES

Ahrons, C. (1981). The continuing coparental relationship between divorced spouses. *American Journal of Orthopsychiatry, 51*, 415–428.

Ahrons, C. & Wallisch, L. (1987). Parenting in the binuclear family: Relationships between biological and stepparents. In K. Pasley & M. Ihinger-Tallman (Eds.), *Remarriage and stepparenting* (pp. 225–257). New York: Guilford Press.

Anderson, J., & White, G. (1986). Dysfunctional intact families and stepfamilies. *Family Process, 25*, 407–422.

Bohannan, P., & Erickson, R. (1978). Stepping in. *Psychology Today, 11*, 53–59.

Brown, A., Green, R.J., & Druckman, J. (1988). *A family measure of stepparent role clarity.* Unpublished manuscript.

Crosbie-Burnett, M. (1984). The centrality of the steprelationship: A challenge to family theory and practice. *Family Relations, 33*, 459–463.

Fast, I., & Cain, A. (1966). The stepparent role: Potential for disturbances in family function. *American Journal of Orthopsychiatry, 36*, 485–491.

Furstenberg, F., & Nord, C. (1985). Parenting apart: Patterns of child-rearing after marital disruption. *Journal of Marriage and the Family, 47*, 893–904.

Ganong, L., & Coleman, M. (1984). The effects of remarriage on children: A review of the empirical literature. *Family Relations, 33*, 389-406.

Ganong, L., & Coleman, M. (1987). Effects of parental remarriage on children: An updated comparison of theories, methods, and findings from clinical and empirical research. In K. Pasley & M. Ihinger-Tallman, (eds.), *Remarriage and stepparenting* (pp. 94–140). New York: Guilford Press.

Glick, P. (1984). Marriage, divorce and living arrangements: Prospective changes. *Journal of Family Issues, 5*, 7–26.

Goldsmith, J. (1980). The relationship between former spouses: Descriptive findings. *Journal of Divorce, 4*, 1–20.

Goldsmith, J. (1982). The post-divorce family system. In F. Walsh (Ed.), *Normal family processes* (pp. 297–330). New York: Guilford Press.

Goldstein, H. (1974). Reconstituted families: The second marriage and its children. *Psychiatric Quarterly, 48*, 433–440.

Hetherington, E.M., Cox, M., & Cox, R. (1977). The aftermath of divorce. In J.H. Stevens, Jr. & Marilyn Matthews (Eds.), *Mother-child, father-child relations*. Washington, DC: National Association for the Education of Young Children.

Kitson, G. (1982). Attachment to the spouse in divorce: A scale and its application, *Journal of Marriage and the Family, 44*, 379–393.

Kleinman, J., Rosenberg, E., & Whiteside, M. (1979). Common developmental tasks in forming reconstituted families. *Journal of Marital and Family Therapy, 5*, 79–86.

Lutz, P. (1983). The stepfamily: An adolescent perspective. *Family Relations, 32*, 367–375.

Marotz-Baden, R., Adams, G., Bueche, N., Munro, B., & Munro, G. (1979). Family form or family process? Reconsidering the deficit family model approach. *The Family Coordinator, 28*, 5–14.

Medeiros, J. (1977). Relationship styles and family environment of stepfamilies. (Doctoral dissertation, California School of Professional Psychology, 1977). *Dissertation Abstracts International, 38*, 4472B.

Messinger, L., Walker, K., & Freeman, S. (1978). Preparation for remarriage following divorce: The use of group techniques. *American Journal of Orthopsychiatry, 48*, 263–272.

Moos, R. (1974). *Family environment scale, Form R*. Palo Alto, CA: Consulting Psychologists Press.

Moos, R., & Moos, B. (1981). *Family environment scale manual*. Palo Alto, CA: Consulting Psychologists Press.

Olson, D., Fournier, D., & Druckman, J. (1982). ENRICH. In D. Olson, H. McCubbin, H. Barnes, A. Larsen, M. Muxen, & M. Wilson (Eds.), *Family inventories* (pp. 49–67). St. Paul: Dept. of Family Social Science, University of Minnesota.

Parkes, C. (1972). *Bereavement: Studies of grief in adult life*. New York: International Universities Press.

Ransom, J., Schlesinger, S., & Derdeyn, A. (1979). A stepfamily in formation. *American Journal of Orthopsychiatry, 49*, 36–43.

Sager, C., Brown, H., Crohn, H., Engel, T., Rodstein, E., & Walker, L. (1983). *Treating the remarried family*. New York: Brunner/Mazel.

Stern, P. (1978). Stepfather families: Integration around child discipline. *Issues in Mental Health Nursing, 1*, 50–56.

Visher, E., & Visher, J. (1978a). Common problems of stepparents and their spouses. *American Journal of Orthopsychiatry, 48*, 252–262.

Visher, E., & Visher, J. (1978b). Major areas of difficulty for stepparent couples. *International Journal of Family Counseling, 6*, 70–80.

Visher, E., & Visher, J. (1979). *Stepfamilies: A guide to working with stepparents and stepchildren.* New York: Brunner/Mazel.

Wilson, K., Zurcher, L., McAdams, D., & Curtis, R. (1975). Stepfathers and stepchildren: An exploratory analysis from two national surveys. *Journal of Marriage and the Family, 37*, 526–536.

5

Masculinity, Femininity, and Sex Role Attitudes in Early Adolescence: Exploring Gender Intensification

Nancy L. Galambos and David M. Almeida
University of Victoria, British Columbia
Anne C. Petersen
Pennsylvania State University

This longitudinal study of 200 young adolescent girls and boys (mean age 11.6 years in sixth grade) investigated the hypothesis that differences in masculinity, femininity, and sex role attitudes would intensify across the sixth, seventh, and eighth grades (between 11 and 13 years of age) and that pubertal timing (early, on time, late) would play a role in this intensification. Analyses revealed that sex differences in masculinity and sex role attitudes increased across grades, but not sex differences in femininity. Pubertal timing was not associated with this gender divergence, although the evidence is equivocal for boys. The results provide support for gender intensification, but the role of pubertal timing may not be as strong as previously supposed.

Considering sex differences in adolescence, Hill and Lynch (1983) argued that, with the onset of puberty, boys and girls experience an intensification of gender-related expectations. This "gender intensification hypothesis" posits that behavioral, attitudinal, and psychological differences between adolescent boys and girls increase with age and are the result of increased socialization pressures to conform to traditional masculine and feminine sex roles. Sex roles denote shared expectations for

Reprinted with permission from *Child Development*, 1990, Vol. 61, 1905–1914. Copyright ©1990 by the Society for Research in Child Development, Inc.

This research was supported by a grant from the National Institute of Mental Health (MH 30252/38142) to A. Petersen. The authors thank three anonymous reviewers for their helpful comments on an earlier version of this paper.

gender-specific sets of behaviors (Worell, 1981), with the masculine role emphasizing instrumental behaviors (e.g., independence) and the feminine role emphasizing expressive behaviors (e.g., nurturance) (Bakan, 1966; Block, 1973). The role that puberty plays in the differentiation of masculine and feminine characteristics may be that it serves as a signal to socializing others (parents, teachers, peers) that the adolescent is beginning the approach to adulthood and should begin to act accordingly, that is, in ways that resemble the stereotypical male or female adult (Hill & Lynch, 1983).

What kind of data constitute evidence for gender intensification in adolescence? First, variables selected for consideration must be gender-salient characteristics on which sex differences already exist before early adolescence. Second, a pattern of increasing differentiation between boys and girls across adolescence must be shown on relevant characteristics. Third, intensification of gender-related attributes should be greatest for those adolescents who have entered puberty, although it is difficult to predict at what point in the pubertal process social pressures and male-female differences will reach their maximum. Will gender-related attributes be most pronounced for those just entering puberty, in the middle of puberty, or when the adolescent clearly resembles an adult (a question of pubertal status)? Furthermore, will increased levels of a given gender-related attribute be greatest for adolescents who are physically on time, early, or late relative to their peers (a question of pubertal timing)?

Gender intensification is evident in the results of several studies, although the role that puberty plays has been considered rarely. Linn and Petersen (1986), for example, reported that during adolescence males gain an advantage over females in certain domains of mathematics achievement. Research on self-image shows that, in early adolescence, girls are more self-conscious and hold themselves in lower esteem than do males (Rosenberg & Simmons, 1975; Simmons & Rosenberg, 1975). Indeed, Simmons, Blyth, Van Cleave, and Bush (1979) found a significant decrease in self-esteem from the sixth to seventh grades among girls who experienced multiple changes, including pubertal development. In a similar vein, two studies found that depression in girls increases during early adolescence (Hirsch & Rapkin, 1987; Petersen, Sarigiani, & Kennedy, in press). Finally, in a study of adolescents followed from the sixth through tenth grades, the rated importance of not acting like the opposite sex peaked in seventh grade for girls and in ninth grade for boys; differences between the sexes in four body-image variables peaked in ninth grade (Simmons & Blyth, 1987).

Guided by the gender intensification hypothesis, Roberts, Sarigiani, Newman, and Petersen (in press) reasoned that if social pressure to behave according to sex stereotypes increases in early adolescence, then the relation between school achievement and a positive self-image should increase among boys and decrease among girls. This would occur because boys are presumed to be pressured to excel academically whereas girls are presumed to be pressured to excel socially. Indeed, from sixth to seventh grade, the relation between school achievement and a positive self-image increased for boys and decreased for girls. At eighth grade, however, less divergence was evident.

Although these studies offer support for the gender intensification hypothesis, others do not. Hirsch and Rapkin (1987) and Petersen and Ebata (1987), for example, did not find that girls' self-image and self-esteem became less positive as they passed through early adolescence. And, based on a meta-analysis, Linn and Petersen (1985) concluded that where sex differences in spatial ability are detected, they are not more prominent in adolescence than earlier or later in the life span. In the domain of vocational development, adult men and women, on average, experience different career trajectories, making it reasonable to assume that sex differences in educational plans and achievement might be seen in adolescence. Simmons and Blyth (1987), however, did not observe a pattern of increasing divergence between boys and girls across adolescence in future work and educational plans, academic performance, and school problem behavior.

Although some progress has been made in examining gender intensification, there are two major shortcomings in the previous research. First, whether adolescents see themselves in an increasingly sex-typed manner as they pass through early adolescence is unknown—a central assumption of gender intensification. Second, as mentioned previously, little is known about the role of puberty in gender intensification.

The present investigation addresses these concerns by using longitudinal data from a study of adolescents to determine whether gender intensification characterizes the development of self-reported masculinity, femininity, and sex role attitudes in early adolescence. Masculinity and femininity are socially desirable attributes that are stereotypically considered to differentiate males and females (Spence & Helmreich, 1978). As such, measurement of these attributes in the adolescent would indicate to what extent the adolescent adheres to sex roles. We considered sex role attitudes because males, relative to females, typically have higher approval of the division of labor, responsibilities, and behaviors based on gender (Galambos, Petersen, Richards, & Gitelson, 1985), and it is important to determine whether this sex difference increases in early adolescence. At the same time, we considered the relation between pubertal timing (early, on time, late) and the above sex-typed attributes. Pubertal timing rather than pubertal status is assessed because timing in particular has been associated with perceptions that others hold of the adolescent (Savin-Williams & Small, 1986) and as such may be influential in shaping self-perceptions. The following predictions were made:

1. Sex differences in masculinity, femininity, and sex role attitudes will become larger during early adolescence (or, in analysis of variance terminology, there will be a sex $\times$ grade interaction).

2. Early-maturing boys will reach higher levels of masculinity sooner than later-developing boys (a pubertal timing × grade interaction); early-maturing girls will reach their height in femininity sooner than later-developing girls. No prediction was made on the relation between pubertal timing and sex role attitudes.

METHODS

Sample

The subjects ($n = 200$; 85 boys, 115 girls) were a subset from a longitudinal study of early adolescence—the Early Adolescence Study (EAS). The design and sample have been described elsewhere (Petersen, 1984; Richardson, Galambos, Schulenberg, & Petersen, 1984). The EAS ($N = 335$; 182 girls and 153 boys) consists of two successive cohorts of students (birth years; 1967 and 1968) who experienced early adolescence in the late 1970s. They were drawn randomly from the sixth-grade class of two primarily white middle- to upper-middle-class Midwestern suburban school districts. About 80% of targeted students participated, and comparisons revealed that those who did participate were not different on any variable studied (e.g., self-image) from students who did not participate.

The adolescents' average age on January 1 of sixth grade was 11.6 years (SD = .34), with no difference in age between boys and girls. Through interviews and group assessments, that were gathered from subjects twice annually in the sixth, seventh, and eighth grades. A longitudinal sample was defined ($n = 253$), present for at least four of six interviews and four of six group testing sessions) for purposes of longitudinal data analyses. It did not differ significantly from the full sample on any measure. Only 6% of the original sample dropped out by the eighth grade; none of these are included in the longitudinal sample. Given the few consistent cohort differences, the two cohorts were combined.

Attempts were made to complete two interviews annually, yielding relatively high completion rates (an average of 88% completion across all interviews), but no attempt was made to gather data from those who missed any of the twice-annual group testing sessions (yielding a still-respectable average of 84% completion across all sessions). Despite the limited amount of incomplete data, the longitudinal pattern for any individual is likely to include some missing data. Since these results are missing at random (i.e., there was no systematic pattern of nonresponse), it was appropriate to estimate scores (see Little & Rubin, 1987). Thus, within the longitudinal sample, estimated scores were generated for those subjects missing masculinity, femininity, or sex role attitudes scores on only one occasion; this involved 33 boys and 54 girls, with a nearly equal proportion of boys and girls having nonresponses within each grade. This resulted in a total of 200 subjects with data required for use in this study.

The score for the missing data point was estimated by weighting the group mean within sex on that occasion by the subject's average deviation from the group mean at the other two data points. This estimation procedure might increase cross-year stability but, because the estimates were generated separately by sex, it may decrease the likelihood of divergence, thus providing a conservative test of gender intensification. The means and standard deviations for this subsample of 200 and all those subjects present on any given occasion were nearly identical. The analyses to be reported using the sample of 200 were conducted also with those subjects present on all three occasions; the results were identical, thereby suggesting that the estimation procedure did not bias the findings.

Measures

Pubertal timing. We measured pubertal timing by using annual height data to assess age at peak height velocity (Bock et al., 1973; Thissen, Bock, Wainer, & Roche, 1976). This maximum-likelihood estimation procedure begins with Bayesian priors based on data from the major growth studies in the United States. Analysis of longitudinal data from these studies has verified the validity of a triple logistic function representing growth in stature from birth (actually conception) to maturity. Although nine parameters are estimated, only one—age at peak height velocity during the adolescent growth spurt—is of interest in the present analysis. Because the estimation begins with Bayesian priors, this measure is useful even for those who do not reach peak growth during the years studied.

The estimates of age at peak height velocity (i.e., age at which growth is fastest) were based on repeated measures of height over the 3 years of the study. However, the nature of the height data differed for the two school districts involved. In one school district, height was measured annually from kindergarten through eighth grade by the school nurse; these data on height obtained directly from school records, were used to estimate age at peak height velocity. In the other district, objective data on height were not available; therefore, we used the adolescents' self-reports of height to make the estimates. The self-reports were obtained from the adolescents in both school districts as part of the semiannual interviews. Thus, reported and objective values could be compared directly in one of the districts, and these comparisons indicated that the self-report data are valid (median $r = 0.94$) (Crockett, Schulenberg, & Petersen, 1987). Moreover, the estimates based on objective data and those based on self-report data were virtually identical. Finally, when estimates from the two districts were compared (one set based on objective data, the other on self-reports), no significant differences emerged. Given these findings, we combined the estimates from both districts in the analyses.

To derive pubertal timing categories, the distribution of scores representing estimated age at peak height velocity was trichotomized, with the lower third being classified as "early," the middle third as "on time," and the upper third as "late" maturers. This procedure was carried out separately for boys and girls in order to take into account the sex differences in the age at which puberty begins. (In other samples, the age at peak height velocity is 11 years for girls and 13 years for boys, with the standard deviation usually around 1 year; Bock et al., 1973.)

The mean ages at peak height velocity for the early, on-time, and late-maturing boys were 12.74 (SD = .50), 13.83 (SD = .19), and 14.76 (SD = .51), respectively; these average ages correspond roughly to mid-seventh, -eighth, and -ninth grades, respectively. The mean ages at peak height velocity for the early, on-time, and late-maturing girls were 10.93 (SD = .51), 11.80 (SD = .51), and 12.64 (SD = .54), respectively; these average ages correspond roughly to mid-fifth, -sixth, and -seventh grades, respectively. This measure has been shown to be predictably related to age at menarche in girls, pubertal status scores in boys and girls, and voice change in boys (Petersen & Crockett, 1985; Petersen, Tobin-Richards, & Boxer, 1983). Early-maturing subjects in the present sample, for example, were more advanced physically (as determined by scores on the Pubertal Development Scale, a measure of pubertal status) than on-time adolescents, and on-time adolescents were more advanced than late maturers; these differences were evident in the sixth, seventh, and eighth grades among both girls and boys (see Petersen & Crockett, 1985). Age at peak height velocity is an appropriate measure of pubertal timing because it is *not* dependent on a single event (e.g., menarche) or on the attainment of the full set of secondary sex characteristics, and is relevant for both boys and girls. Age at peak height velocity occurs at about the middle of the pubertal process for girls and close to the end for boys (Marshall & Tanner, 1969, 1970). Thus, from grades 6 through 8, early-maturing girls move from mid- to postpubertal status, on-time girls from early- to late-pubertal status, and late-maturing girls, from pre- to mid-pubertal status. Similarly, early-maturing boys move from early- to late-pubertal status, on-time boys from pre- to mid-pubertal status, and late-maturing boys enter early puberty by eighth grade.

Masculinity and femininity. Items on the short form of the Bem Sex Role Inventory (BSRI) were used to assess the adolescent's view of himself or herself as masculine and feminine (Bem, 1974, 1981). The short form consists of 10 socially desirable adjectives each to measure masculinity (e.g., "self-reliant") and femininity (e.g., "yielding"). Subjects respond to each item, describing themselves on a scale ranging from *never or almost never true* (1) to *always or almost always true* (7). The mean of the items is computed, with higher scores indicating higher masculinity or femininity. Although the BSRI has been used mostly with young adults, Lamke (1982) found it to be useful for research on adolescents. Alpha coefficients for these scales in our sample range in the .70s and .80s for girls and boys across grades. Sixth-, seventh-, and eighth-grade scores were used.

Although Bem (1977) recommended combining the separate masculinity and femininity scores to place individuals in a fourfold classification scheme (resulting in masculine, feminine, androgynous, and undifferentiated categories), the predictive utility of these combinations has been called into question (Deaux, 1984; Taylor & Hall, 1982). More specifically a comprehensive review of research on psychological androgyny revealed that combinations of masculinity/femininity failed to predict to indices of psychological adjustment above and beyond that predicted by the separate masculinity and femininity scores (Taylor & Hall, 1982). Moreover, Lamke (1982) argued for the importance of using continuous masculinity and femininity scores in research with adolescents. Therefore, masculinity and femininity are treated as independent measures.

Sex role attitudes. The Attitudes toward Women Scale for Adolescents (AWSA) (Galambos et al., 1985) was used to measure sex role attitudes, or the extent to which the adolescent approves of the gender-based division of roles. The AWSA consists of 12 items (e.g., "Girls should have the same freedoms as boys") to which the subject responds on a four-point scale ranging from *agree strongly* to *disagree strongly*. A total scale score consisting of the mean of the responses is computed, with a higher score indicating less approval of gender differences in roles. Galambos et al. (1985) provided evidence for the scale's psychometric adequacy in several samples, including the present (EAS) one. We use sixth-, seventh-, and eighth-grade scores.

Plan of Analysis

Three 2 × 3 × 3 (sex × pubertal timing × grade) repeated-measures analyses of variance (ANOVAs), with grade as the repeated factor, examined the dependent variables of masculinity, femininity, and sex role attitudes. Linear and quadratic polynomial contrasts were used to test hypotheses about change over time (grade). Although the boys and girls in a given pubertal timing category (e.g., early or on time) were not similar in terms of pubertal status (i.e., *absolute* standing on physical maturation) or average age at peak height velocity, within their same-sex peer group they had the same *relative* standing. Therefore, it seemed reasonable to conduct the above ANOVAs. The confound between sex and pubertal timing, however, is addressed in additional analyses following presentation of the main results.

RESULTS

Intercorrelations among Sex Role Measures

Table 1 presents intercorrelations among the masculinity, femininity, and sex role attitudes measures by sex and grade. The significant autocorrelations indicate that, for both boys and girls, there was stability in masculinity, femininity, and sex role attitudes across grade. The pattern of relations also indicates that, both within and across grade, higher masculinity is associated with higher femininity in boys and girls. Young adolescents who describe themselves as having masculine characteristics are likely to describe themselves as having feminine characteristics as well (with the exception of the girls' sixth/eighth-grade comparisons).

One other pattern is noteworthy. Among boys, most correlations between femininity and sex role attitudes are significant both within and across grades. Boys who described themselves as more feminine had more egalitarian sex role attitudes; that is, they were less likely to approve of the division of roles based on sex. In girls, there was no general relation between sex role attitudes and masculinity or femininity.

Masculinity

The first analysis was a $2 \times 3 \times 3$ (sex $\times$ pubertal timing $\times$ grade) repeated-measures ANOVA with grade as the within-subjects factor and masculinity as the dependent variable. Table 2 presents the masculinity scores as a function of sex, grade, and pubertal timing. The results showed a significant main effect of sex, $F(1,194) = 23.04, p < .001$, with boys more masculine than girls. There was also a significant grade effect, $F(2,388) = 18.91, p < .001$, and quadratic, $F(1,194) = 7.97, p < .01$, components. These results indicate that masculinity increased across grade, and that the largest increase was between seventh and eighth grade. There was no significant main effect of pubertal timing. There also was a significant sex

TABLE 1

Intercorrelations Among Masculinity (MASC), Femininity (FEM), and Sex Role Attitudes
(AWSA) by Grade and Sex

Measure	1	2	3	4	5	6	7	8	9
Grade 6:									
1. MASC ...		.49	.11[a]	.65	.44	.16[a]	.61	.49	.14[a]
2. FEM	.28		.33	.29	.64	.42	.30	.66	.33
3. AWSA	.05[a]	.01[a]		−.08[a]	.20	.71	−.01[a]	.13[a]	.67
Grade 7:									
4. MASC ...	.51	.22	.17		.43	−.02[a]	.39	.38	.05[a]
5. FEM	.27	.61	.02[a]	.42		.20	.18	.54	.21
6. AWSA	.06[a]	.07[a]	.66	.15[a]	.12[a]		−.04[a]	.16[a]	.60
Grade 8:									
7. MASC ...	.56	.10[a]	.10[a]	.52	.21	.12[a]		.39	.08[a]
8. FEM	.13[a]	.37	.12[a]	.20	.40	.15[a]	.45		.15[a]
9. AWSA	−.08[a]	.06[a]	.68	.05[a]	−.01[a]	.57	.09[a]	.11[a]	

NOTE.—Correlations for boys ($n = 85$) are above the diagonal; girls ($n = 115$) are below. Higher scores on MASC, FEM, and AWSA indicate higher masculinity, higher femininity, and more egalitarian sex role attitudes, respectively. Cross-time stabilities are in bold.

[a] Correlation not significant.

TABLE 2
Means and Standard Deviations for Masculinity by Sex, Grade, and Pubertal Timing

SEX AND PUBERTAL TIMING	N	GRADE					
		6		7		8	
		M	SD	M	SD	M	SD
Boys:							
Early	28	5.05	.67	5.23	.79	5.51	.80
On time	30	5.07	.89	5.05	.81	5.50	.90
Late	27	5.14	.80	5.08	.77	5.57	.89
Total	85	5.09	.79	5.12	.78	5.53	.85
Girls:							
Early	40	4.85	.62	4.79	.74	4.96	.77
On time	35	4.81	.78	4.76	.74	4.89	.79
Late	40	4.59	.78	4.66	.64	4.85	1.02
Total	115	4.74	.73	4.74	.70	4.90	.86

NOTE.—Higher scores indicate higher masculinity. Possible range: 1–7.

× grade interaction, $F(2,388) = 3.96$, $p < .05$. Although boys were more masculine at all grade levels than were girls, they were most different in the eighth grade. No other interactions were significant.

Femininity

In order to examine evidence for gender intensification in femininity, a 2 × 3 × 3 (sex × pubertal timing × grade) repeated-measures ANOVA was conducted with grade as the within-subjects factor. The means and standard deviations for feminin-

TABLE 3
Means and Standard Deviations for Femininity by Grade, Sex, and Pubertal Timing

SEX AND PUBERTAL TIMING	N	GRADE					
		6		7		8	
		M	SD	M	SD	M	SD
Boys:							
Early	28	4.75	.83	5.07	.67	5.12	.84
On time	30	4.88	1.00	5.14	.75	5.26	.96
Late	27	4.83	.98	4.97	1.00	5.35	.97
Total	85	4.83	.93	5.06	.81	5.24	.92
Girls:							
Early	40	5.48	.77	5.57	.83	5.64	.78
On time	35	5.30	.71	5.28	.78	5.51	.62
Late	40	5.37	.68	5.64	.77	5.61	1.05
Total	115	5.39	.72	5.50	.80	5.59	.84

NOTE.—Higher scores indicate higher femininity. Possible range: 1–7.

ity by sex, grade, and pubertal timing are presented in Table 3. There was a significant main effect of grade, $F(2,388) = 18.91$, $p < .001$, with a significant linear trend, $F(1,194) = 26.70$, $p < .001$. These results indicated an increase in femininity from sixth to eighth grade. There was also a significant main effect of sex, $(1,194) = 20.36$, $p < .001$, indicating that girls were more feminine than boys. No other effects were significant.

Sex Role Attitudes

A $2 \times 3 \times 3$ (sex $\times$ pubertal timing $\times$ grade) repeated-measures ANOVA was conducted to explore whether there was gender intensification of sex role attitudes (AWSA scores). The means and standard deviations on the AWSA by sex, grade, and pubertal timing are seen in Table 4. There was a significant main effect of sex, $F(1,194) = 108.53$, $p < .001$. Girls approved more than boys did of equality between males and females, and given the high means relative to the highest possible score, may be reaching a ceiling effect. There was also a significant sex $\times$ grade interaction, $F(2,388) = 12.70$, $p < .001$. From the sixth to the eighth grades, girls increasingly approved of male-female equality, whereas boys became less approving. There were no main or interaction effects involving pubertal timing.

Additional Analyses

In order to examine whether combining the boys and girls obscured any effects related to pubertal timing (an important issue, given that within the same pubertal

TABLE 4
Means and Standard Deviations for Sex Role Attitudes by Sex, Grade, and Pubertal Timing

SEX AND PUBERTAL TIMING	N	GRADE					
		6		7		8	
		M	SD	M	SD	M	SD
Boys:							
Early	28	2.79	.50	2.79	.56	2.74	.43
On time	30	2.71	.54	2.71	.47	2.59	.62
Late	27	2.96	.51	2.82	.50	2.74	.47
Total	85	2.82	.52	2.77	.51	2.69	.52
Girls:							
Early	40	3.26	.37	3.38	.32	3.37	.34
On time	35	3.23	.34	3.28	.39	3.38	.35
Late	40	3.25	.35	3.34	.30	3.35	.32
Total	115	3.24	.35	3.34	.34	3.37	.34

NOTE.—Higher scores indicate more egalitarian sex role attitudes. Possible range: 1–4.

timing category, girls were ahead of the boys with respect to average age at peak height velocity), three 3×3 (pubertal timing $\times$ grade) repeated-measures ANOVAs were conducted separately within sex. These analyses yielded no new information, that is, pubertal timing did not have an effect on the dependent variables when boys and girls were considered separately.

We also performed a set of 2×3 (sex $\times$ grade) repeated-measures ANOVAs on masculinity, femininity, and sex role attitudes, using only those boys and girls who were *comparable* with respect to age at peak height velocity (early-maturing boys and late-maturing girls; $n = 68$). The results for femininity and sex role attitudes were the same as those found with the larger sample, except that the sex $\times$ grade interaction for sex role attitudes failed to reach significance. In this case, failure to reach significance is probably due to the loss in power associated with smaller sample size.

With respect to masculinity, the main effects of sex and grade were significant (as was the case with the total sample). In contrast to the earlier results, however, there was not a significant sex $\times$ grade interaction. The pattern of results for this smaller sample was different in that late-maturing girls were less masculine in general than other girls, and early-maturing boys were more masculine in the seventh grade than were other boys.

DISCUSSION

The results provide some support for the gender intensification hypothesis. In particular, across early adolescence, sex differences in masculinity and sex role attitudes increased. Pubertal timing, however, did not play an obvious role in the stimulation of this divergence. Why did initial sex differences in masculinity increase over time? Previous research suggests that masculinity is a critical aspect of self among boys, bearing positive relations to self-esteem and peer acceptance (Lamke, 1982; Massad, 1981). In fact, Massad (1981) argued that there is more social pressure placed on early adolescent boys to conform to the masculine sex role than there is for girls to conform to the feminine sex role. Because masculine behaviors, preferences, and interests are socially valued, it is not surprising that there is an escalation of masculinity among boys as they move toward adulthood. Adolescents see sex roles as flexible, to some extent (Carter & Patterson, 1982), but they still have sex-typed interests, activities, and preferences (Erb, 1983; Huston, 1983; Urberg, 1979). And, despite considerable social change over the last 25 years, there has been little evidence of change since then in attitudes, preferences, and interests among adolescent boys and girls (Lewin & Tragos, 1987; Lueptow, 1984).

Contrary to prediction, there was no escalation of femininity in girls relative to boys (i.e., no sex $\times$ grade interaction); rather, the femininity of boys and girls increased in a parallel fashion. Why? One possible explanation derives from longitudinal research showing that boys' and girls' conceptions of femininity become broader across early adolescence, incorporating traditionally masculine attributes along with traditionally feminine attributes (Crockett, Camarena, & Petersen, 1989). With less narrow and rigid definitions of what it means to be feminine, boys might become more comfortable in describing themselves as possessing feminine attributes. Positive correlations between masculinity and femininity among boys and girls in our sample suggest that adolescents have little difficulty in seeing themselves as having both masculine and feminine characteristics. Yet, they still maintain higher levels of sex-typed attributes; that is, girls are more feminine than masculine, and boys are more masculine than feminine.

At the same time, girls may not show dramatic rises in femininity because femininity does not carry with it attributes that are particularly valued or powerful in society (Leahy & Eiter, 1980; Massad; 1981). The disadvantages associated with being female are recognized by adolescent girls—they are more likely than boys to believe that it is hard to be a member of their own sex (Lewin & Tragos, 1987). And girls' recognition of females' relatively inferior position in society may also be seen in the results for sex role attitudes; from the sixth through eighth grades, girls became increasingly egalitarian, and boys became less so. These trends suggest that girls become aware of the personal implications of restrictions placed on them by the feminine sex role, whereas adolescent boys, having limited experience with what it means to be female, may find it easier to adopt less egalitarian attitudes present in society. This is not true for all boys, however; boys who reported having higher levels of feminine attributes were also likely to report more egalitarian sex role attitudes.

Contrary to the gender intensification hypothesis, pubertal timing was unrelated to masculinity, femininity, or sex role attitudes. The possibility remains that pubertal timing may contribute to gender intensification for subjects, especially boys, who are studied beyond the eighth grade. By the end of eighth grade, in contrast to girls, few boys have reached the end of the pubertal process. There might be an effect of pubertal timing among boys, however, once a larger proportion of them experience more of the visible pubertal changes. Indeed, the results of the comparison between early-maturing boys and late-maturing girls on masculinity lead us to suggest that early-maturing boys may be more masculine sooner than later-maturing boys. A fuller test of the gender intensification hypothesis, then, requires an assessment of the effect of pubertal timing as the subjects move through middle adolescence. In this regard, twelfth-grade follow-up data collected on subjects in this study will be useful (Petersen & Ebata, 1987).

Another possible reason for the lack of an effect of pubertal timing is that dimensions of sex typing are shaped by a multiplicity of influences, and despite the prominence of physical characteristics and changes during adolescence, the nature of these other influences on masculinity, femininity, and sex role attitudes may be more powerful. Among the strongest influences are sex role socialization by parents and teachers, messages regarding appropriate behavior as portrayed in the media, and variation in family structure (Huston, 1983). Petersen et al. (1983) argued that behavioral expectations for young adolescents are very much organized around grade in school, and that the experience of puberty is shaped by grade-based experiences. In fact, the most salient aspect of pubertal change for gender intensification may be, not that an individual per se enters puberty, but that a cohort becomes pubertal (Petersen, 1985). With the transition to junior high school for most students, and with successively higher grade levels, the messages regarding sex roles that adolescents receive, observe, and incorporate into their self-concepts may be similar regardless of their outward physical appearance.

Of course, these conclusions should be considered in light of the limitations of the data. The sample is largely middle class and white and consists of adolescents who participated in the study over the course of 3 years. One way in which future investigations could extend the present research is to broaden the age range studied. The present investigation was restricted to early adolescence. Will gender intensification extend into middle adolescence or beyond, or is it limited to early adolescence (see e.g., Petersen & Ebata, 1987)? Could pubertal timing have a more noticeable effect in middle or late adolescence? Another future direction for research is to look at multiple indices of conformity to one's sex role. Huston (1983), for example, discusses many sex-related dimensions that exist, including but not limited to concepts or beliefs about gender, self-perceptions, preferences, and observable behaviors. Through investigation of these issues, we will arrive at a greater understanding of the relation between sex roles and adolescent development.

REFERENCES

Bakan, D. (1966). *The duality of human existence.* Chicago: Rand McNally.

Bem, S.L. (1974). The measurement of psychological androgyny. *Journal of Consulting and Clinical Psychology, 42,* 155–162.

Bem, S.L. (1977). On the utility of alternative procedures for assessing psychological androgyny. *Journal of Consulting and Clinical Psychology, 45,* 196–205.

Bem, S.L. (1981). *Bem Sex-Role Inventory professional manual.* Palo Alto, CA: Consulting Psychologists.

Block, J.H. (1973). Conceptions of sex role: Some cross-cultural and longitudinal perspectives. *American Psychologist, 28,* 512–526.

Bock, R.D., Wainer, H., Petersen, A., Thissen, D., Murray, J., & Roche, A.F. (1973). A parameterization for individual human growth curves. *Human Biology, 45,* 63–80.

Carter, D.B., & Patterson, C.J. (1982). Sex roles as social conventions: The development of children's conceptions of sex-role stereotypes. *Developmental Psychology, 18,* 812–824.

Crockett, L.J., Camarena, P.M., & Petersen, A.C. (1989). *Masculinity and femininity in early adolescence: Developmental change in self-perceptions.* Unpublished manuscript, The Pennsylvania State University.

Crockett, L.J., Schulenberg, J.S., & Petersen, A.C. (1987). Congruence between objective and self-report data in a sample of young adolescents. *Journal of Adolescent Research*, **2**, 383–392.

Deaux, K. (1984). From individual differences to social categories: Analysis of a decade's research on gender. *American Psychologist*, **39**, 105–116.

Erb, T.O. (1983). Career preferences of early adolescents: Age and sex differences. *Journal of Early Adolescence*, **3**, 349–359.

Galambos, N.L., Petersen, A.C., Richards, M., & Gitelson, I.B. (1985). The Attitudes toward Women Scale for Adolescents (AWSA): A study of reliability and validity. *Sex Roles*, **13**, 343–356.

Hill, J.P., & Lynch, M.E. (1983). The intensification of gender-related role expectations during early adolescence. In J. Brooks-Gunn & A.C. Petersen (Eds.), *Girls at puberty: Biological and psychosocial perspectives* (pp. 201–228). New York: Plenum.

Hirsch, B.J., & Rapkin, B.D. (1987). The transition to junior high school: A longitudinal study of self-esteem, school life, and social support. *Child Development*, **58**, 1235–1243.

Huston, A.C. (1983). Sex-typing. In E.M. Hetherington (Ed.), P.H. Mussen (Series Ed.), *Handbook of child psychology: Vol. **4**. Socialization, personality, and social development* (pp. 387–467). New York: Wiley.

Lamke, L.K. (1982). The impact of sex-role orientation on self-esteem in early adolescence. *Child Development*, **53**, 1530–1535.

Leahy, R.L., & Eiter, M. (1980). Moral judgment and the development of real and androgynous self-image during adolescence. *Developmental Psychology*, **16**, 362–370.

Lewin, M., & Tragos, L.M. (1987). Has the feminist movement influenced adolescent sex role attitudes? A reassessment after a quarter century, *Sex Roles*, **16**, 125–135.

Linn, M.C., & Petersen, A.C. (1985). Emergence and characterization of sex differences in spatial ability: A meta-analysis. *Child Development*, **56**, 1479–1498.

Linn, M.C. & Petersen, A.C. (1986). A meta-analysis of gender differences in spatial ability: Implications for math and science achievement. In J.S. Hyde & M.C. Linn (Eds.), *The psychology of gender: Advances through meta-analysis* (pp. 67–101). Baltimore, MD: Johns Hopkins University Press.

Little, R.J.A., & Rubin, O.B. (1987). *Statistical analysis with missing data.* New York: Wiley.

Lueptow, L.B. (1984). *Adolescent sex roles and social change.* New York: Columbia University Press.

Marshall, W.A., & Tanner, J.M. (1969). Variations in the pattern of pubertal changes in girls. *Archives of Disease in Childhood*, **44**, 291–303.

Marshall, W.A., & Tanner, J.M. (1970). Variations in the pattern of pubertal changes in boys. *Archives of Disease in Childhood*, **45**, 13–23.

Massad, C.M. (1981). Sex role identity and adjustment during adolescence. *Child Development*, **52**, 1290–1298.

Petersen, A.C. (1984). The early adolescence study: An overview. *Journal of Early Adolescence*, **4**, 103–106.

Petersen, A.C. (1985). Pubertal development as a cause of disturbance: Myths, realities, and unanswered questions. *Genetic, Social, and General Psychology Monographs*, **111**, 205–232.

Petersen, A.C, & Crockett, L.C. (1985). Pubertal timing and grade effects on adjustment. *Journal of Youth and Adolescence*, **14**, 191–206.

Petersen, A.C., & Ebata, A.T. (1987, July). *Gender-related change in self-image during adolescence.* Paper presented at the biennial meeting of the International Society for the Study of Behavioral Development, Tokyo.

Petersen, A.C., Sarigiani, P.A., & Kennedy, R.E. (in press). Adolescent depression: Why more girls? *Journal of Youth and Adolescence.*

Petersen, A.C., Tobin-Richards, M., & Boxer, A. (1983). Puberty: Its measurement and its meaning. *Journal of Youth and Adolescence*, **3**, 47–62.

Richardson, R.A. Galambos, N.L., Schulenberg, J.E., & Petersen, A.C. (1984). Young adolescents' perceptions of the family environment. *Journal of Early Adolescence*, **4**, 131–153.

Roberts, L.R., Sarigiani, P.A., Newman, J.L., & Petersen, A.C. (in press). Gender differential developmental change over early adolescence in the relationship between school achievement and self-image. *Journal of Early Adolescence.*

Rosenberg, F.R., & Simmons, R.G. (1975). Sex differences in the self-concept in adolescence. *Sex Roles*, **1**, 147–159.

Savin-Williams, R.C., & Small, S.A. (1986). The timing of puberty and its relationship to adolescent and parent perceptions of family interactions. *Developmental Psychology*, **22**, 342–347.

Simmons, R.G., & Blyth, D.A. (1987). *Moving into adolescence: The impact of pubertal change and school context.* New York: Aldine de Gruyter.

Simmons, R.G., Blyth, D.A., Van Cleave, E.F., & Bush, D.M. (1979). Entry into early adolescence: The impact of school structure, puberty, and early dating on self-esteem. *American Sociological Review*, **44**, 948–967.

Simmons, R.G., & Rosenberg, F. (1975). Sex, sex roles, and self-image. *Journal of Youth and Adolescence*, **4**, 229–258.

Spence, J.T., & Helmreich, R.L. (1978). *Masculinity and femininity: Their psychological dimensions, correlates, and antecedents.* Austin: University of Texas Press.

Taylor, M.C., & Hall, J.A. (1982). Psychological androgyny: Theories, methods, and conclusions. *Psychological Bulletin*, **92**, 347–366.

Thissen, D., Bock, R.D., Wainer, H., & Roche, A.F. (1976). Individual growth in stature: A comparison of four growth studies in the USA. *Annals of Human Biology*, **3**, 529n542.

Urberg, K.A. (1979). Sex role conceptualizations in adolescents and adults. *Developmental Psychology*, **15**, 90–92.

Worell, J. (1981). Life-span sex roles: Development, continuity, and change. In R.M. Lerner & N.A. Busch-Rossnagel (Eds.), *Individuals as producers of their development: A life-span perspective* (pp. 313–347). New York: Academic Press.

6

Prediction of Behavior Problems in Four-Year-Olds Born Prematurely

Susan Goldberg and Carl Corter
University of Toronto
Mirek Lojkasek
York University
Klaus Minde
Queen's University

Longitudinal follow-up data for 69 very low birthweight preterm infants were used to assess the influence of four factors (neonatal medical complications, infant temperament, mother-child relationships, and family environment) on mother and teacher reports of behavior problems at 4 years. The proposed model of such influences being tested assumed that (1) the effects of neonatal medical factors would be indirect, and (2) each of the other three factors would show high stability from 1 to 4 years and would have a direct influence on behavior problem outcomes. Neither neonatal medical data nor infant-mother attachment were good predictors of behavior problems at age 4. With these exceptions, teacher report of behavior problems was predicted in a fashion consistent with the preliminary model. However, mother reports of behavior problems was predicted only by prior mother reports of child temperament. Discussion focuses on reasons for discrepancies in these pathways of influence.

Reprinted with permission of *Development and Psychopathology*, Vol. 2, 1990, 15–130. Copyright © 1990 by Cambridge University Press.

The work described here was initiated by Klaus Minde with the support of the Laidlaw Foundation and Ontario Mental Health Foundation. Data collection and analyses were completed under Ontario Mental Health Foundation Grant No. 891–84/86 awarded to Susan Goldberg and Carl Corter. The authors appreciate the cooperation of the neonatal ward and neonatal follow-up clinic of the Hospital for Sick Children and of the families who contributed their time, energy, and enthusiasm to this project.

It is often assumed that preterm birth and its sequelae constitute a risk factor for subsequent behavior disorders. Minde (1984) argued that this assumption is plausible on two grounds: (1) brain damage is known to increase the risk of behavior problems in the population at large, and preterm infants are frequently exposed to damaging perinatal events; and (2) disruptions of normal parental care and high levels of family stress may predispose families toward less optimal caregiving of the preterm infant. However, the empirical evidence to support this assumption is minimal.

Very early articles on outcome of preterm births indicated that at school age, these children were more restless, irritable, and distractible than fullterm peers (Benton, 1940; Mohr & Barthelme, 1934). These reports were largely descriptive and anecdotal. More systematic appraisals were made of later cohorts, followed by Lilienfeld, Pasamanick, and Rogers (1955), Knobloch, Rider, Harper, and Pasamanick (1956), Douglas (1960), and Drillien (1964). While Drillien (1964) found that her low birthweight group was more vulnerable to behavior problems at age 5 than appropriate weight peers, influences of social class and maternal attitudes and behavior were important contributors to behavioral outcome.

From the late 1960s, neonatal care changed dramatically in the direction of more aggressive treatment and large numbers of very young and very small ($\leq 1,500$ grams) preterm infants entered the survival statistics. Therefore, earlier studies provide a poor basis for forming expectations about current cohorts. More current follow-up data have been confined primarily to neurological and cognitive outcomes (Breslau, Klein, & Allen, 1985; Klein, Hach, & Breslau, 1985), and until fairly recently it appeared that altered neonatal treatment had reduced incidence of the previously noted behavior problems (Minde, 1984).

However, there has now been new evidence of increased rates of behavior problems among preterm infants (Escalona, 1984; Field, Dempsey, & Shuman, 1983; see Hoy, Bill, & Sykes, 1988, for a review). In our own most recent follow-up, we found a high rate of behavior problems in a low birthweight preterm group (46% above the cutoff point on the Richman-Graham Behavior Checklist, compared to 6% in a normative survey in the same city) (Minde et al., 1989). While this represents a high rate of behavior problems and confirms that preterm birth is indeed a risk factor in the development of psychopathology, the majority of children in this sample are indistinguishable from fullterm peers in their adjustment. This suggests that some protective factors are operating to the benefit of the majority of this sample. Longitudinal study of this high-risk group provides an opportunity to evaluate the contributions of risk and protective factors for both normal and abnormal outcomes.

The present report is based on a longitudinal study of infants born prematurely at birthweights under 1,500 grams. These children were followed to age 4, at which time both mother and teacher reports of behavior problems were collected. These mother and teacher reports constitute the outcome measures for the present longitudinal analyses. Scores above screening cutoffs on mother and teacher report instruments do not necessarily indicate a psychiatric diagnosis. Therefore, in further discussion, we use the term "behavior problem" to indicate high scores on such screening instruments and "behavior disorder" to indicate psychiatric diagnoses. Four factors traditionally implicated in the etiology of behavior problems for which we had prior information were considered as possible risk and protective factors: medical complications, infant temperament, mother-child relationships, and family environment.

Medical Complications

Although it has been repeatedly shown that medical parameters alone do not account for subsequent developmental outcomes among preterm infants, there is evidence that in the population at large, psychiatric disorders occur more frequently among children with known brain damage (Rutter, Tizard, & Whitmore, 1970; Seidel, Chadwick, & Rutter, 1975). Since it is now known that many very small preterm infants have experienced intraventricular hemorrhages or exposure to potentially damaging perinatal events (e.g., placenta previa, eclampsia), one might predict that those experiencing these events would be more vulnerable to subsequent behavior problems. Medical complications may also contribute to behavior problems by affecting each of the other three predictor variables. The necessity of keeping low birthweight preterm infants with multiple medical problems in hospital, the accompanying stress on parents, and general disruption of family life may threaten to establish poor conditions of care after discharge. Therefore, we felt it necessary to enter medical parameters as a possible predictor and to assume that medical complications can have both direct and indirect influences on subsequent behavior problems. However, on the basis of previous reviews of the literature (e.g., Sameroff & Chandler, 1975) we expected the indirect effects to be more influential than direct effects.

Infant Temperament

Thomas, Chess, and Birch (1968) emphasized the role that difficult temperament and parental ability to adjust to it play in the etiology of behavior problems. Recent studies by Bates and his colleagues (Bates & Bayles, 1988; Bates, Maslin, & Frankel, 1985) and Earls and Jung (1987) indicate a strong association between parent reports of difficult temperament and parent reports of behavior problems in the population of healthy children born at term. In our prior report on the present sample (Minde et al., 1989), we, too, reported that difficult temperament in the first year was associated with a high ($\geqslant 10$) score on the Richman-Graham Behavior Checklist. Conversely, easy temperament may be a protective factor. In the present analyses, we estimate the relative contribution of early temperament as well as the stability of temperament from 1 to 4 years as contributors to 4-year outcomes.

Mother-Child Relationships

The childs' primary relationship with a caregiver (usually the mother) has long been considered an essential foundation of development, and the belief that psychopathology can be traced to "poor mothering" has been a strong one (see Chess & Thomas, 1982, for a refutation of this view). Implicit in this attitude is the assumption that a "good" parent-child relationship can protect the child from subsequent behavior problems. In recent years, with the development of Ainsworth's "Strange Situation" as a standardized paradigm for assessing the quality of the parent-child relationship, a large number of studies have documented the relation between early infant-mother attachment and subsequent child competence in many domains (see Bretherton & Waters, 1985, for recent examples). Data on the relation between attachment and behavior problems are more equivocal with two studies (Erickson, Sroufe, & Egeland, 1985; Lewis, Feiring, McGuffog, & Jaskir, 1984) showing some association between insecure attachment and behavior disorders and two (one of them our own) showing no such association (Bates, Maslin, & Frankel, 1985; Minde et al., 1989). In a prior longitudinal analysis based on data from the present sample (Goldberg, Lojkasek, Gartner, & Corter, 1989), ratings of mother-child interaction in the home were consistently related to 4-year outcomes, although attachment per se was not found to be a strong predictor of behavior problem reports at age 4. In the present analyses, both types of measure were initially considered as predictors of 4-year behavior problem reports. In addition, observations of mother-child interaction at home and in the laboratory at age 4 enabled us to assess stability in the quality of the mother-child relationship and its contribution as a risk or protector in etiology of behavior problems.

Family Environment

There is consistent evidence that competency of young children is strongly related to family mental health and social situations (Broman, Nichols, & Kennedy, 1975; Golden & Birns, 1976; Rutter, 1979; Werner & Smith, 1982). A variety of family factors have been included in such studies. For example, in a recent study of 4-year-olds, Sameroff and his colleagues included ten environmental risk factors: maternal mental health, maternal anxiety, parent attitudes and beliefs about development, quality of mother-infant interaction in prior home observations, occupation of head of household, maternal education, minority status, family support, stressful life events, and family size (Sameroff, Seifer, Barocas, Zax, & Greenspan, 1987). The number of factors on which a child and family was scored nonoptimally was the major determinant of outcomes: the more risk conditions were present, the poorer the outcome in both cognitive and socioemotional domains. Rutter (1987) documented similar findings with behavior disorder as the outcome variable. In the present study, interview, questionnaire, and observational data about each family were collected, and our preliminary analyses indicated that family factors were indeed related to both mother and teacher reports of behavior problems (Minde et al., 1989).

In the present analyses, we estimated the relative contributions of medical status, temperament, mother-child relationships, and family environment to behavior problems at 4 years of age. Figure 1 shows our preliminary model (under each major heading, the label for the operational measure of each factor is indicated). The most important assumption that we made in deriving this model was that with the exception of medical factors (expected to have minimal direct effects), each of the three remaining factors would show reasonably high stability, and this stability would be the route of major influence in all three domains. Furthermore, we considered two types of behavior problem reports: those of mothers and those of teachers. Since parents and teachers see children in different contexts, they may have different views of the same child.

METHOD

Subjects

Participants were recruited from consecutive admissions to a tertiary care neonatal unit in a large pediatric hospital between January 1979 and December 1981. In order to be eligible for the study, infants had to weigh less than 1,500 grams at birth, survive the first 72 hours, and have no known congenital abnormalities. Parents had to live within commuting distance of the hospital, be fluent in English, and agree to participate. The study was initially designed to compare offspring of twin and singleton births. Enrolled were 28 pairs of twins and 26 singletons. In five families, one twin subsequently died leaving 23 intact pairs and 5 single survivors. Comparison of twins and singletons are detailed elsewhere (Goldberg, Perrotta, Minde, & Corter, 1986; Minde et al., 1989). Table 1 shows the characteristics of the group seen at 1 year along with those of the families that returned for follow-up at age 4. At 1 year, 71 infants were observed in the Strange Situation, but 7 could not be scored because of handicaps. At 4 years, we were able to see all single survivors, 21 twin pairs, and 22 singletons. Reasons for subject loss at 4 years were: leaving the province, not locatable, and declining to participate (one family). In addition, we excluded data from nine children with IQ scores below 80 who were not able to participate in all aspects of the follow-up assessment. Because families also had specific missing data the number of subjects differed for various parts of the analysis from 29 to 69. Teacher reports were available for 54 children.

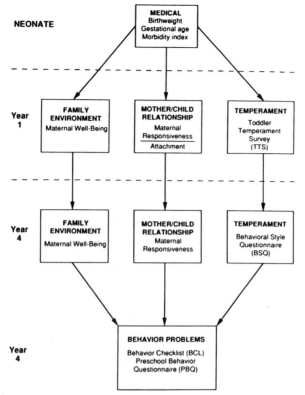

Figure 1. Preliminary model

TABLE 1
Background data (1- and 4-Year Follow-up Samples)

	Year 1 ($N=71$)	Year 4 ($N=69$)
Infants		
$\overline{X}$ birthweight (grams)	1027.7	1071.8
$\overline{X}$ gestational age (weeks)	29.0	29.4
$\overline{X}$ illness score	83.1	77.4
male (%)	57	58
female (%)	43	42
Parents		
Percent married	88	79
Socioeconomic status		
Class		
1, 2 (low)	36	30
3 (middle)	26	33
4, 5 (high)	38	37
$\overline{X}$ age of mother	27.5	30.4

PROCEDURES

Detailed descriptions of the full study are provided in previous papers (Goldberg et al., 1986; Minde et al., 1989). Table 2 provides an overview of the measures collected at each age. In this section, we focus only on those measures entered into the present analyses.

Predictors

Medical status in the neonatal period. In addition to gestational age and birthweight, the Neonatal Morbidity Index (Minde, Whitelaw, Brown, & Fitzhardinge, 1983) was used. This score was obtained from the medical records. Each infant was given a daily score of (0) *not present* to (2) *present and life threatening* for each of 19 possible neonatal complications. A daily summary score was computed, and daily scores were summed for the entire hospital stay to give an overall index that represented both duration and severity of illness. In order to reduce the three measures (gestational age, birthweight, and morbidity score) to a single medical risk indicator, they were entered into a "principal components" analysis (Dillon & Goldstein, 1984). All three measures entered into a single factor with the use of a minimal weight contribution of .5 as a cutoff. For each measure, factor weights were multiplied by the z scores of that measure, and then a sum of the three measures was obtained to give the medical risk score (Cronbach's alpha $= .66$). While now we would wish to examine data on intraventricular hemorrhage, ultrasound was not yet being used routinely for this purpose in 1979–1981 when these children were neonates.

Child Temperament. At 1 year, mothers completed a modification of the Toddler Temperament Survey (TTS; Fullard, McDevitt, & Carey, 1978). This survey consisted of 97 items rated for frequency on a 6-point scale. Although the original instrument contained items related to nine dimensions of temperament, our modification included only items from the five dimensions required to score temperamental difficulty: rhythmicity, approach/withdrawal, adaptability, intensity, and mood. A classification into one of five types of temperament (easy, intermediate low, intermediate high, slow to warm up, and difficult) was derived using a standard algorithm. The score used for the present analyses was this classification from (1) *easy* to (5) *difficult.*

At 4 years, mothers completed the Behavioral Style Questionnaire (BSQ; McDevitt & Carey, 1978), an analogous instrument for 3- to 7-year olds. The full questionnaire was used in this case. The five dimensions relevant to difficult temperament were again used to obtain a classification of temperamental difficulty.

Mother-child relationship. In the first year, extensive observations were made in the home at 6 weeks and 3, 6, and 9 months postterm. After each visit, mother

TABLE 2
Assessment Procedures

	Neonatal Period	6 weeks	3 months	6 months	9 months	12 months	48 months
Psychiatric interview	X					X	X
Mother–child observation							
hospital	X						
home		X	X	X			
laboratory					X	X (Strange Situation)	X (puzzle task)
Temperament						TTS	BSQ
Child developmental status					Bayley Scales		Stanford–Binet
Social skills							Peer Interpersonal Problem Solving Test
Behavior problems							Richman–Graham BCL (mother) Behar PBQ (teacher)

and infant were rated on a series of scales developed by Ainsworth and her colleagues (1971) and subsequently amplified by Egeland, Taraldson, and Brunquell (1977). These yielded a total of 28 ratings at each of four ages. For the purpose of this study, we focused on Ainsworth's four "summary" scores for sensitivity, acceptance, accessibility, and cooperation that have been most widely used to characterize maternal responsiveness. In order to reduce these to a single score for the present analyses, we omitted the 6-week scores that had already been shown to have a different relationship to subsequent outcomes than those at 3, 6, and 9 months (Goldberg, Perrotta, Minde, & Corter, 1986). Since these four ratings are consistently found to be highly correlated, they were summed and averaged over the three age periods to yield a single "maternal responsiveness" score for the first year.

At 12 months corrected age, each child-mother pair participated in Ainsworth's Strange Situation to assess the quality of infant-mother attachment. Classifications of attachment were made using the traditional scheme described by Ainsworth and her colleagues (Ainsworth, Blehar, Waters, & Wall, 1978), which includes three major types: Secure (B), Avoidant (A), and Ambivalent (C). Within major types, there are subgroups: Secure (4 groups), Avoidant (2), and Ambivalent (2). For the purposes of computation, these eight groups were ordered on a scale devised by Crittenden (1985) ranging from (6-B_3) *most secure* to (1-C_2) *least secure*.[1]

At 4 years, children were observed interacting with their mothers both in the laboratory and at home. Since prior analysis had established that measures in the home were highly correlated with both earlier home data and behavior problem outcomes (Goldberg, Lojkasek, Gartner, & Corter, 1989), we included only the home observation for the present analyses. For the purpose of the present analysis, the measure we used was the proportion of total maternal behaviors to the child that were positively responsive.

Family environment. At 1 and 4 years, the parents were interviewed by a child psychiatrist (K.M.), who obtained information on child and family medical, psychological, and social functioning. On the basis of this information, each family was rated on six dimensions: adequacy of housing, financial status, marital relationship, mother's perceived social support, mother's emotional health, and mother's satisfaction with the maternal role. Each was rated on a Likert scale, which varied in range from 3 (e.g., type of housing) to 5 (e.g., marital relationship) with a possible total score of 20. Two raters scored these retrospectively, approximately 1 year after the 4-year data collection. Since both raters had known the families, they were rated without identifying information, and the two protocols for a given

---

[1] In our previous analyses of attachment data, we divided infants into three groups representing a security continuum: (B_2B_3) *secure*, (B_1,B_4) *marginally secure*, (A,C) *insecure*. Crittenden's scale represents an extension of this procedure that we used in correlational analyses because it allowed for greater variability in scores.

family were not rated in sequence. Interrater reliability, based on a subset of 20 protocols, ranged from .84 (mother's emotional health) to .95 (housing) with a mean of .89.

To reduce these scores to a smaller set of measures, a *principal components analysis* was conducted using the same criteria as for the medical risk index. Two factors emerged at both 1 and 4 years, although their components differed somewhat. In general, the first factor was loaded with social class measures. The second factor was loaded with maternal psychosocial measures and was labeled *maternal well-being*. Only this second factor was of interest in these analyses because social class measures were examined separately. At year 1, the maternal well-being factor consisted of mother's emotional health, role satisfaction, and marital relationship (Cronbach's $\alpha = .70$). At year 4, the same three measures entered into the factor in addition to mother's perceived social support (Cronbach's $\alpha = .85$).

Status variables. Gender and twinship status as well as a rating of family socioeconomic status based on father's occupation were considered as possible moderating variables.

Outcomes

Mothers completed the Richman-Graham Behavior Checklist (Richman & Graham, 1971), in which the child is rated on a 3-point scale (0–2) in 12 potential problem areas (e.g., eating, sleeping, activity level). This checklist was chosen because recent local norms for 4-year-olds were available (Minde & Minde, 1977). For children in preschool, teachers completed the Preschool Behavior Questionnaire (Behar, 1977). This instrument includes 36 items rated on a 3-point scale (0–2). On both of these instruments, higher scores represent more serious problems.

ANALYSIS AND RESULTS

Three sets of analyses will be described here: (1) preliminary correlations to select variables for subsequent analysis; (2) regression analyses to determine how well the measures in our four domains predicted the two outcomes (parent and teacher reports of behavior problems), and (3) analyses concerned with testing the model in Figure 1.

On most measures, twins were treated as individuals, since we did, in fact, have independent measures on each member of the pair. However, family measures that contributed to the maternal well-being score could not be independent. Therefore, we first randomly chose one member of each pair to enter into the analysis in the first step. A "replication" analysis was then conducted using the data for the remaining twins. The correlations in the two "replications" were not significantly different.

Therefore, we reported these for the full group and included both twins in the subsequent phases of analysis.

Correlations

Table 3 summarizes the intercorrelations among the measures. First, it is of interest that the two outcome measures—mother-reported problems (BCL) and teacher-reported problems (PBQ)—are not correlated, which indicates that the strategy of treating them as independent outcomes is an appropriate one. Second, *medical risk* was not related to the other measures, except for its relation with attachment assessments at 1 year already noted in a prior publication (Goldberg et al., 1986). Third, attachment status at 1 year was not related to other measures with the exception of its relation with prior maternal responsiveness (also discussed at length by Goldberg et al., 1986). Finally, social class (SES) was not related to the other variables. On this basis, these three measures were excluded from further analyses. The remaining measures, which had modest to high intercorrelations, were retained in subsequent analyses.

Prediction of Outcomes

Regression analyses. For both mother and teacher reports of behavior problems, a series of similar but independent regression analyses were conducted, to answer several questions. First, to rule out the possible confounding effects of gender and twinship, these were entered into a stepwise regression analysis as dummy variables. Neither of these significantly entered the equation for mother or teacher report of behavior problems. As a result, they were excluded from further analyses. We then proceeded to separate but identical series of analyses for mother and teacher reports. To avoid repetition and enhance clarity, we describe the procedures in detail as we consider the maternal reports and only minimally in the subsequent section on teacher reports.

Mother report of behavior problems. (See Table 4.) First, we asked what measures were the best predictions from each age period? Here, we examined whether the predictors entered the stepwise regression equation significantly ($p \leqslant .05$) and the amount of variance accounted for. Temperament was the only significant predictor to enter the regression equation for both years 1 and 4, accounting respectively for 10%, $\Delta F(1, 34) = 4.81, p < .04$, and 30%, $\Delta F)1, 27) = 13.10, p.001$, of the variance.

Second, at each age, how well do the combined measures predict the outcomes? In this step, we forced in predictors that did not significantly contribute to the equation in step 1 and calculated the significance of the overall equation as well as the total amount of variance accounted for. When all the year 1 measures were entered, the overall equation was not significant, $F(4, 31) < 1.80, p < .15$. On the other hand,

TABLE 3
Intercorrelations Among Variables

Variable	SES	Temperament (1 year)	Temperament (4 year)	Attachment (1 year)	Maternal Responsive (1 year)	Maternal Responsive (4 year)	Mother Psychosocial (1 year)	Mother Psychosocial (4 year)	BCL	PBQ
Medical risk	−.20†	−.01	.08	.32**	−.02	−.03	.12	.07	.13	.24†
SES		−.15	.08	.01	−.13	−.13	.06	−.13	−.06	−.09
Temperament (1 year)			.47**	−.10	.07	−.19	−.14	−.43**	.35*	.44**
Temperament (4 year)				−.14	−.11	.09	−.22†	−.33*	.57**	.10
Attachment (1 year)					.23*	−.10	.17	.14	−.05	−.04
Maternal Responsiveness (1 year)						.51**	.45**	.41**	.07	−.36*
Maternal Responsiveness (4 year)							.21	.36*	.26†	−.64**
Mother Psychosocial (1 year)								.51**	−.20	−.28*
Mother Psychosocial (4 year)									−.34**	−.61**
BCL										.02

†$p < .10$; *$p < .05$; **$p < .01$.

the equation including all year 4 measures was significant, accounting for a total of 37% of the variance, $F(3, 25) = 6.58$, $p < .002$.

Third, we were interested in how much additional information would be contributed by all the year 4 measures over and above all the year 1 measures, and how well a combination of years 1 and 4 measures predicted behavior problems. In this step, we reduced the measures for each age into a summary score by multiplying each score by its beta weight obtained in the previous regression analyses (step 1) and used the resultant sum. Thus, we had a summary score representing all year 1 measures and one representing all year 4 measures. In this way we reduced the number of measures to enter the final regression analyses as well as maximized the predictive power of each measure. These summary scores were then entered into the final regression analysis. Since year 1 chronologically preceded year 4, it was entered first. Once again, the significance of the overall equation and the amount of variance accounted for was calculated. The year 1 summary score accounted for a significant 21% of the variance, $\Delta F(1, 19) = 6.22$, $p < .02$, while the addition of year 4 summary score accounted for a significant 17%, $\Delta F(2, 18) = 6.26$, $p < .02$. Together the summary scores accounted for a significant total of 38% of the variance, $F(2, 18) = 7.11$, $p < .005$.

Thus, temperament at both ages was the best predictor of behavior problems reported by mother. Children who were reported as being more temperamentally difficult at ages 1 and 4 were also reported to have more behavior problems. While the other scores were not useful as individual predictors, summary scores did improve the prediction.

TABLE 4
Prediction of Mother Report of Behavior Problems (BCL Scores)

	R	R^2	Adjusted R^2	ΔR^2	ΔF	p	df
Status variables	.28	.08	.01	.08	1.18	.33	3,40
Year 1							
Temperament	.35	.12	.10	.12	4.81	.04	1,34
Remaining variables (forced)	.43	.19	.08	.06	0.83	.49	4,31
Year 4							
Temperament	.57	.33	.30	.33	13.10	.001	1,27
Remaining variables (forced)	.66	.44	.37	.11	2.56	.09	3,25
Summary scores							
Year 1	.50	.25	.21	.25	6.22	.02	1,19
Year 4	.66	.44	.38	.19	6.26	.02	2,18

Teacher report of behavior problems. (See Table 5). The numerals in parentheses refer to the steps outlined earlier. Of the year 1 variables, temperament and maternal responsiveness significantly entered the initial regression equation, both accounting for 31% of the variance, $F(2, 34) = 9.09$, $p<.001$. In year 4, maternal responsiveness and maternal well-being significantly entered the equation, accounting for 55% of the variance, $F(2, 26) = 17.9$, $p<.0001$. (2) When all four of the year 1 measures were entered, the total equation accounted for a significant 34% of the variance, $F(4, 32) = 5.61$, $p<.002$. When all three year 4 measures were entered, the total equation accounted for a significant 53% of the variance, $F(3, 25) = 11.48$, $p<.0001$, with a slight drop in the adjusted R^2 due to the addition of an extra variable. (3) The year 1 summary score accounted for a significant 38% of the variance, $\Delta F(1, 19) = 13.32$, $p<.002$, and the year 4 summary score added a significant 18% to the variance, $\Delta F(2, 18) = 8.67$, $p<.009$. Together the summary scores accounted for a significant total of 56% of the variance, $F(2, 18) = 13.69$, $p<.0002$.

In summary, for teacher reports of behavior problems on the PBQ, three of the predictor variables contributed to prediction of outcomes: maternal responsiveness at both age periods, temperament in year 1, and maternal well-being in year 4. For children whose mothers reported early difficult temperament, those with less responsive mothers and those with more problematic family situations were scored by teachers as having more problematic behaviors in school.

TABLE 5
Predictions of Teacher Report of Behavior Problems (PBQ Scores)

	R	R^2	Adjusted R^2	ΔR^2	ΔF	p	df
Status variables	.13	.02	−.06	.02	0.23	.88	3,41
Year 1							
Temperament	.44	.20	.17	.20	8.49	.006	1,35
Maternal responsiveness	.59	.35	.31	.15	8.00	.008	2,34
Remaining variables (forced)	.64	.41	.34	.06	1.73	.19	4,32
Year 4							
Maternal responsiveness	.64	.42	.39	.42	19.19	.0002	1,27
Family environment	.76	.58	.55	.16	10.13	.004	2,26
Remaining variables (forced)	.76	.58	.53	.00	.00	.99	3,25
Summary scores							
Year 1	.64	.41	.38	.41	13.32	.002	1,19
Year 4	.78	.60	.56	.19	8.67	.009	2,18

Testing the Model

The model depicted in Figure 1 entails several assumptions that were made for the following analyses. First, direct pathways from early measures were included only if they were not explained via the temporally intervening measures (Biddle & Marlin, 1987). Second, where there was continuity in measures from the same domain (e.g., temperament at year 1 correlating with temperament at year 4), the path of influence from year 1 was assumed to be via continuity with year 4. Third, continuity within a domain (auto-correlations) was given priority over correlations across time and domain (e.g., temperament year 1 predicting temperament year 4 took priority over temperament year 1 predicting maternal well-being in year 4). Paths across times and domain were considered only if they significantly added to the variance. Finally, where domains were interrelated and both predicted the outcome, they were entered in a stepwise regression to determine which ordering yielded the strongest prediction of outcome.

Figure 2 shows the final model and the beta weights for both teacher and mother reports of behavior problems. Maternal report of behavior problems was best predicted by temperament alone, while teacher report of behavior problems was predicted by maternal responsiveness and maternal well-being, as expected, but also indirectly by temperament. Thus, maternal report of behavior problems was predicted only by prior maternal report (of child behavior on temperament questionnaires). Teacher report of behavior problems was predicted by measures reflecting observation of mother and child (maternal responsiveness) and measures that combined maternal report plus clinician judgment (temperament, maternal well-being).

DISCUSSION

In these analyses, we examined four domains of risk and protective factors as predictors of mother and teacher reports of behavior problems at preschool age: medical, family environment, child temperament, and mother-child relationship. One major finding of the prediction analyses was that medical factors did not contribute to 4-year outcome measures. A second was that attachment status at 1 year was not a good predictor of subsequent behavior problems, although other measures of the quality of the mother-child relationship were good predictors. We will consider each of these in turn.

Our finding that medical factors were not good predictors must be qualified by the reminder that this population represents only a narrow range of variation in neonatal medical status. Infants were selected to be under 1,500 grams birthweight and to be free of obvious congenital problems. Second, we excluded from analyses children considered to be seriously handicapped. Third, as noted earlier, the current practice of routinely documenting intraventricular hemorrhages by use of ultrasound was not available at the time, and perhaps we missed the most important piece of medical information. At the same time, we should note that the present findings are consonant with both early (e.g., Drillen, 1964) and more recent (Sameroff & Chandler, 1975; Werner & Smith, 1982) evidence that indicates that medical status alone is not a good predictor of general developmental outcomes. Thus, while an identified medical condition (low birthweight premature birth) does increase vulnerability to behavior problems (as is the case in our sample with 46% identified as problematic on a screening instrument), it does not in and of itself account for poor outcomes. Thus, alternative pathways to later outcomes must amplify or minimize medical contributions to development of psychopathology.

The absence of a relationship between attachment status at year 1 and subsequent behavior problems may be considered unexpected for two reasons: (1) the tenet that disturbances in the mother-child relationship are a source of psychopathology is widely held; and (2) attachment quality has been shown to be a good predictor of a variety of social competencies to age 6 (e.g., Arend, Gove, & Sroufe, 1978; Lieberman, 1977; Main, Cassidy, & Kaplan, 1985; Sroufe, 1983). However, prior

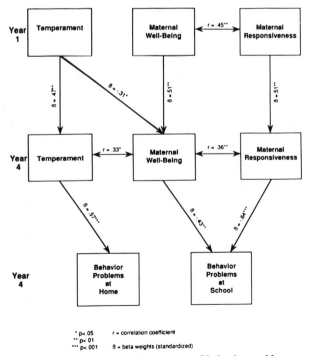

Figure 2. Prediction of mother and teacher reports of behavior problems

data on prediction of behavior problems from attachment status in the fullterm normally developing population have been equivocal. Erickson, Sroufe, and Egeland (1985) found that stable 12- to 18-month attachment status was a good predictor of observer-rated problem behavior at age 3½. Lewis, Feiring, McGuffog, and Jaskir (1984) reported a similar relation between early attachment status and mother-reported problems at age 6, but only for boys. In contrast, Bates and his colleagues (Bates & Bayles, 1988; Bates, Maslin, & Frankel, 1985) found, as we did, that attachment quality at 1 year did not predict scores on a behavior checklist at 3 or 4 years.

Since ours is the only study of the four that examined the relation between attachment and behavior problems in a medically compromised (high-risk) sample, it is important to consider the possibility that the standard classification scheme is not adequate for capturing attachment quality in these mother-child dyads. Indeed, we did encounter some difficulties in using the Strange Situation. First, although we saw infants at ages corrected for prematurity, it was our judgment that for many of the sample infants, motor skills were not yet robust enough to be taken for granted. Were we to repeat this study, we would not use the Strange Situation until 18 months. Second, our initial report of the attachment data included some anomalous findings (Goldberg, 1988; Goldberg et al., 1986). This led us to consider the need to review all of these assessments considering the Main and Solomon (1986) criteria for disorganization. While this review indicated that infants in the present sample were more disorganized than healthy controls (Goldberg et al., 1989), the new classifications did not significantly change the anomalous findings.

However, since Bates and his colleagues report similar data for a fullterm healthy sample, we must assume that the explanation cannot lie entirely with the assessment measures. Indeed, it seems reasonable to consider the likelihood that while attachment problems are probably implicated in some behavior disorders (e.g., oppositional disorder), there may well be others where there is no reason to suspect poor mother-child relationships as a causal factor.

We must also consider the limitations of our outcome measures, as neither mother nor teacher questionnaires yield psychiatric diagnoses. Furthermore, it is possible that the original classification scheme (A,B,C), which reflects more and less optimal attachment in the normal range, can be a good predictor of social competency, while potentially more pathological factors (e.g., disorganization) may be related to predicting pathology. Although attachment status per se did not predict behavior problems, other measures of the mother-child relationship were good predictors. Therefore, we cannot dismiss the role of the mother-child relationship because of lack of a relation between attachment and behavior problems. With these exceptions, our analyses showed that our predictors were generally related to outcomes in the manner we expected.

We then proceeded to test a specific model representing pathways of influence. Substantially different models emerged for mother and teacher reports of behavior problems. This was not entirely unexpected, since our prior report (Minde et al., 1989) indicated minimal agreement between mother and teacher reports—a finding that is consistent with a major recent survey of the prevalence of psychiatric disorders in children (Offord et al., 1987). However, our analyses suggest that maternal report of behavior problems is not predicted by any of the factors we examined other than temperament.

Our measure of temperament, like most current measures of temperament, is a parent report measure. Thus, the finding of a continuity from 1 to 4 years in temperament associated with maternal report of behavior problems may reflect a consistency in maternal perception of the child, a consistency in the child, or both. Nevertheless, it is of importance to know that mothers who consider their children to be difficult as infants are likely to report both difficult temperament and behavior problems at age 4. In contrast, mothers who report easy temperament in their infants report few problems at age 4. While it would be easy to dismiss these maternal reports as "subjective," it is well to bear in mind (a) that children presenting to mental health services at this age are most frequently brought by their parents, and (b) even where such a child is found on assessment to be "normal," the parent's perception that a problem exists may require some form of intervention. Thus, maternal report of problems continues to be an important indicator of service needs, whether corroborated by independent assessment or not.

Teacher report of behavior problems was predicted in a fashion generally consistent with our preliminary model. The exceptions were (a) medical factors did not contribute to prediction by either direct or indirect paths, and (b) the influence of temperament was indirect (via maternal well-being) rather than direct. It is of interest that teacher report (i.e., an outside observer's view of the child) was predicted well by other measures from outside observers: ratings of mother-child behavior in the home and clinical ratings from interview material concerning family environment.

Since this study was conducted with a specifically identified medical sample, it is not clear whether these models can be generalized to the population at large. While the study of high-risk populations is one of the valuable approaches in developmental psychopathology, we have yet to determine whether models developed in a high-risk population are readily transferable to low-risk populations or to other high-risk groups. In a prior review of outcomes of preterm birth, Goldberg and DiVitto (1983) found that factors affecting development of preterm infants generally appeared to be similar to those affecting healthy term infants. However whether the developmental pathways to specific outcomes are also similar remains to be discovered.

REFERENCES

Ainsworth, M.D.S., Bell, S.M.V., & Stayton, D.J. (1971). Individual differences in strange situation behaviors of one-year-olds. In H.R. Schaffer (Ed.), *The origins of human social relations*. London: Academic.

Ainsworth, M.D.S., Blehar, M.C., Waters, E., & Wall, S. (1978). *Patterns of attachment: A psychological study of the strange situation*. Hillsdale, NJ: Erlbaum.

Arend, R., Gove, F., & Sroufe, L.A. (1979). Continuity of individual adaptations from infancy to kindergarten: A predictive study of ego resiliency and curiosity in preschoolers. *Child Development, 50*, 950–959.

Bates, J.E., & Bayles, K. (1988). Attachment and development of behavior problems. In J. Belsky & Nezworski (Eds.), *Clinical implications of attachment*. Hillsdale, NJ: Erlbaum.

Bates, J.E., Maslin, C.A., & Frankel, K.A. (1985). Attachment security, mother-child interaction, and temperament as predictors of behavior problem ratings at age three years. In I. Bretherton & E. Waters (Eds.), *Growing points of attachment theory and research. Monographs of the Society for Research in Child Development, 50* (1–2, Serial No. 209).

Behar, L. (1977). The preschool behavior questionnaire. *Journal of Abnormal Child Psychology, 5*, 265–275.

Benton, A.L. (1940). Mental development of prematurely born children. *American Journal of Orthopsychiatry, 10*, 719–746.

Biddle, B.J., & Marlin, M. (1987). Causality, confirmation, credulity, and structural equation modeling. *Child Development, 58*, 4–17.

Breslau, N., Klein, N., & Allen, L. (1988). Very low birthweight: Sequelae at nine years of age. *Journal of the American Academy of Child and Adolescent Psychiatry, 27*, 605–612.

Bretherton, I., & Waters, E. (Eds.). (1985). Growing points of attachment theory and research. *Monographs of the Society for Research in Child Development, 50*, (1–2, Serial No. 209).

Broman, S.H., Nichols, P.L., & Kennedy, W.A. (1975). *Preschool IQ: Prenatal and early developmental correlates*. Hillsdale, NJ: Erlbaum.

Chess, S., & Thomas, A. (1982). Infant bonding: Mystique and reality. *American Journal of Orthopsychiatry, 52*, 213–222.

Crittenden, P.M. (1985). Social networks, quality of child-rearing, and child development. *Child Development, 56*, 1299–1313.

Dillon, W.R., & Goldstein, M. (1984). *Multivariate analysis: Methods and applications*. Toronto: Wiley.

Douglas, J.W.B. (1960). "Premature" children at primary school. *British Medical Journal, 1*, 1008–1013.

Drillien, C.M. (1964). *The growth and development of the prematurely born infant*. Edinburgh: Livingston.

Earls, F., & Jung, K.G. (1987). Temperament and home environment characteristics as causal factors in the early development of childhood psychopathology. *Journal of the American Academy of Child and Adolescent Psychiatry, 26*, 491–498.

Egeland, B., Taraldson, B., & Brunquell, D. (1977). *Observations of waiting room and feeding situations.* Unpublished manual. University of Minnesota, Minneapolis.

Erickson, M., Sroufe, L.A., & Egeland, B. (1985). The relationship between quality of attachment and behavior problems in a preschool high risk sample. In I. Bretherton & E. Waters (Eds.), *Growing points of attachment theory and research, Monographs of the Society for Research in Child Development*, 50(1–2, Serial No. 209).

Escalona, S. (1984). Social and other environmental influences on the cognitive and personality development of low birthweight infants. *American Journal of Mental Deficiency*, 88, 508–512.

Field, T.M., Dempsey, J., & Shuman, H.H. (1983). Five-year followup of preterm respiratory distress syndrome and post-term postmaturity in infants. In T.M. Field, & A. Sostek (Eds.), *Infants born at risk: Physiological, perceptual and cognitive processes.* New York: Grune & Stratton.

Fullard, W., McDevitt, S., & Carey, W. (1978). Assessing temperament in one-to-three-year-olds. *Journal of Pediatric Psychology*, 9, 205–217.

Goldberg, S. (1988). Risk factors in infant-mother attachment. *Canadian Journal of Psychology*, 42, 173–188.

Goldberg, S., & DiVitto, B. (1983). *Born too soon: Preterm birth and early development.* San Francisco: W.H. Freeman.

Goldberg, S., Fischer-Fay, A., Simmons, R., Fowler, R., & Levison, H. (1989). *Chronic illness and infant-attachment.* Paper presented in the Symposium on Use of the Strange Situation with Atypical Populations. Meetings of the Society for Research in Child Development. Kansas City, MO.

Goldberg, S., Lojkasek, M., Gartner, G., & Corter, C. (1989). Early maternal responsiveness and social development in low birthweight preterm infants. In M. Bornstein (Ed.), *Maternal responsiveness: Characteristics and consequences.* San Francisco: Jossey-Bass.

Goldberg, S., Perrotta, M., Minde, K., & Corter, C. (1986). Maternal behavior and attachment in low birthweight twins and singletons. *Child Development*, 57, 34–46.

Golden, M., & Birns, B. (1976). Social class and infant intelligence. In M. Lewis (Ed.), *Origins of intelligence: Infancy and early childhood.* New York: Plenum.

Hoy, E., Bill, J., & Sykes, D. (1988). Very low birthweight: A long term developmental impairment. *International Journal of Behavioural Development*, 11, 37–67.

Klein, N.K., Hack, M., & Breslau, N. (1989). Children who were very low birthweight: Development and academic achievement at nine years of age. *Journal of Developmental and Behavioral Pediatrics*, 10, 32–37.

Knobloch, H., Rider, R., Harper, P., & Pasamanick, B. (1956) Neuropsychiatric sequelae of prematurity. *Journal of the American Medical Association*, 161, 581–585.

Lewis, M., Feiring, C., McGuffog, C., & Jaskir, J. (1984).. Predicting psychopathology in six-year-olds from early social relations. *Child Development*, 55, 123–136.

Lieberman, A.F. (1977). Preschoolers' competence with a peer: Relations with attachment and peer experience. *Child Development*, 48, 1277–1287.

Lilienfeld, A., Pasamanick, B., & Rogers, M. (1955). Relationship between pregnancy experience and the development of certain neuropsychiatric disorders. *American Journal of Public Health*, 45, 637–645.

Main, M., Kaplan, N., & Cassidy, J. (1985). Security in infancy, childhood, and adulthood: A move to the level of representation. In I. Bretherton & E. Waters (Eds.), *Growing points of attachment theory and research. Monographs of the Society for Research in Child Development*, 50 (1–2, Serial No. 209).

McDevitt, S., & Carey, W. (1978). The measurement of temperament in 3- to 7-year-old children. *Journal of Child Psychology and Psychiatry*, 19, 245–253.

Minde, K. (1984). The impact of prematurity on the later behavior of children and on their families. *Clinics in Perinatology*, 11, 227–244.

Minde, K., Goldberg, S., Perrotta, M., Washington, J., Lojkasek, M., & Parker, K. (1989). Continuities and discontinuities in the development of 64 very low birthweight infants. *Journal of Child Psychology and Psychiatry*, 30, 391–404.

Minde, R., & Minde, K. (1977). Behavioural screening of preschool children: A new approach to mental health? In P.J. Graham (Ed.), *Epidemiological approaches in child psychiatry*. London: Academic.

Minde, K., Whitelaw, A., Brown, J., & Fitzhardinge, P. (1983). Effects of neonatal complications in premature infants on early parent-infant interactions. *Developmental Medicine and Child Neurology*, 25, 763–777.

Mohr, G.J., & Bartelme, P.F. (1934). Developmental studies of prematurely born children. In H.J. Hess, G.J. Mohr, & P.F. Bartelme (Eds.), *The physical and mental growth of prematurely grown children*. Chicago: University of Chicago Press.

Offord, D.R., Boyle, M.H., Szatmari, P., Rae-Grant, N., Links, P., Cadman, D.T., Byles, J.A., Crawford, J.W., Munroe-Blum, H., Bynne, C., Thomas, H., & Woodward, C.A. (1987). The Ontario Child Health Study: Prevalence of disorder and rates of service utilization. *Archives of General Psychiatry*, 44, 832–836.

Richman, N., & Graham, P.J. (1971). A behavioural screening questionnaire for use with three-year-old children: Preliminary findings. *Journal of Child Psychology and Psychiatry*, 16, 277–287.

Rutter, M., (1979). Protective favors in children's response to stress and disadvantage. In M.W. Kent & J.E. Role (Eds.), *Primary prevention of Psychopathology, Vol. 3: Social competence in children*. Hanover, NH: University Press of New England.

Rutter, M. (1987). Continuities and discontinuities from infancy. In J. Osofsky (Ed.), *Handbook of infant development* (2nd ed.) (pp. 1256–1296). New York: Wiley.

Sameroff, A.J., & Chandler, M.J. (1975). Reproductive risk and the continuum of caretaking casualty. In F.D. Horowitz, E.M. Hetherington, S. Scarr-Salapatele, & G.M. Siegel (Eds.), *Review of child development research* (Vol. 4, pp. 187–244). Chicago: University of Chicago Press.

Sameroff, A.J., Seifer, R., Barocas, B., Zax, M., & Greenspan, S. (1987). IQ scores of 4-year-old children: Social-environmental risk factors. *Pediatrics*, 79, 343–350.

Seidel, U.P., Chadwick, D.F.D., & Rutter, M. (1975). Psychological disorders in crippled children: A comparative study of children with and without brain damage. *Developmental Medicine and Child Neurology*, 17, 563–573.

Sroufe, L.A. (1983). Individual patterns of adaptation from infancy to preschool. In M. Perlmutter (Ed.), *Minnesota symposium on child psychology* (Vol. 16, pp. 41–81). Hillsdale, NJ: Erlbaum.

Thomas, A., Chess, S., & Birch, H. (1968). *Temperament and behavior disorders in children.* New York: New York University Press.

Werner, E., & Smith, R.S. (1982). *Vulnerable but invincible: Kanai's children come of age.* New York: McGraw-Hill.

Part II

STRESS AND VULNERABILITY

In recent years, increased attention has been directed toward the identification of factors influencing the vulnerability of children to stress. Subjects studied have included the children of mentally ill parents, children with cancer or other chronic illnesses (see Eiser's paper in Section V of this volume), children who have been exposed to traumatic events such as the Chowchilla kidnapping (*Annual Progress*, 1984), or a sniper attack in a school playground.

In the first paper in this section, Thompson's concern is not with a group of children exposed to one or another specific stressor, but more generally to all children who are subjects in non-therapeutic, developmental research studies. Current standards define minimal research risk as involving the potentiality of harm not greater than that ordinarily encountered in daily life or during the performance of routine physical or psychological examinations. Thompson finds this standard inadequate because it fails to define standards of decent treatment of minors who are research participants. By defining what is permissible in terms of what is normative in the child's life experience, the investigator is potentially able to act in ways that may be undermining to the child, because such experiences may be familiar to him or her. Rather, Thompson maintains that researchers should be hesitant to violate basic principles of respect for persons, autonomy, nonmaleficence, and justice in their treatment of the child, even though these principles may be regularly violated by others in everyday life. However, the search for alternative guidelines that better define standards of decent treatment of children in research settings is made difficult by the fact that children's vulnerability to research risk changes in complex ways over time. The importance of augmenting the conventional risk/benefit analysis with standards of decent treatment of children who participate in research is skillfully argued, and Thompson's suggestions for fostering this process within the research community deserve serious consideration.

Although previous research, most notably the Isle of Wight studies of Rutter, Tizard, and Whitmore, has shown that children with physical conditions involving the brain are at increased risk for psychopathology, it has been unclear whether brain dysfunction leads to disturbance directly or by increasing the children's vulnerability to environmental stress. Breslau addresses this question in the course of a methodologically sophisticated study.

Data was obtained from 157 brain-injured children and 339 controls similar in age, sex, and racial composition. Information about children's psychiatric symptoms came from direct interview with the children using the NIMH-Diagnostic Interview

Schedule of Children (DISC). Nosological and statistical considerations led to the decision to characterize psychiatric syndromes as dimensional rather than categorical variables. A dimensional approach takes advantage of the general consensus on the type of symptoms that characterize childhood disorders, but avoids disagreements surrounding precise definition of specific diagnoses. In addition, statistical analysis of continuous variables has greater power. The Family Environment Scale (FES) was used to elicit information from mothers about the social environment in the home and family. Hierarchical multiple-regression analysis was used to estimate and test the significance of main effects and their interaction. Physical disabilities were associated with significant increases in depressive symptoms and inattention. Family environment increased symptoms of depression to an equivalent degree in both brain-injured and control groups. With respect to symptoms of inattention, children with brain dysfunction were less vulnerable to environmental effects than other children. The pattern of findings has led Breslau to suggest that psychiatric sequelae of physical conditions that involve the brain might be of two types: symptoms that result directly from damage to the brain, and reactions to adversities associated with physical handicap. However, as Breslau emphasizes, in important respects children with brain dysfunctions have much in common with the general population of children. Specifically, their dysphoric reactions to being physically handicapped and living in adverse family environments are similar to those of children whose brain functions are unaffected by physical disease.

In the final paper in this section, Super, Herrera, and Mora report on the long-term effects of food supplementation and psychosocial intervention on the physical growth of Colombian infants at risk of malnutrition. The study is an elegantly designed and carefully executed large-scale intervention study wherein 280 children were assigned to one of four experimental groups formed by the presence/absence of two interventions: (1) food supplementation for the entire family, from mid-pregnancy until the target child was three years old, and (2) twice-weekly home-visiting program to promote cognitive development until age three. All families received free medical care and were studied prospectively at three and six years. Despite considerable sample attrition (25 percent at age three and 45 percent at age 6), extensive statistical analyses failed to reveal evidence of significant differential subject loss between experimental groups at either age period. At three years of age, children who had received food supplementation averaged 2.6 cm and 642 grams larger than controls. More important, home visiting and supplementation together reduced the number of children with severe growth retardation. Three years after intervention (age six) supplementation effects remained. Children in the home-visit condition had become larger than controls by 1.7 cm and 448 grams. The interactive effect to reduce stunting continued to be significant, but only marginally so. Three years after the interventions had ended, children in home-visited groups had higher levels of protein intake than their controls, although no differences were found for the average per capita level of adequacy in the family as a whole, suggesting channeling of protein to the target child. Channeling effects were absent in families that received supplementation.

The authors speculate that the "sleeper effect" of the home-visit intervention may have been mediated through changes in family function directed by parental understanding of, and attention to, developmental issues. The dietary data are strongly suggestive of changes in family functioning that would favor increased growth of the study child. Desirable as this might be, one can only wonder at whose expense? Nevertheless, the data provide unusually robust support for the conclusion that food supplementation in the early years of life, in connection with uniform medical care, can lead to a reduction in the occurrence of severe growth retardation and have significant and lasting effects on body size.

7

Vulnerability in Research: A Developmental Perspective on Research Risk

Ross A. Thompson

University of Nebraska, Lincoln

Child Development, *1990, 61, 1–16. Assessing potential risks to children who participate in developmental research is a challenging task because children are a heterogeneous population, varying in developmental competencies and in background characteristics. This essay offers a developmental perspective on research risk, emphasizing that children's vulnerability to research risk changes in complex ways: some risks decrease with increasing age, some increase as the child matures, others change in a curvilinear fashion, while some remain essentially stable with development. Because vulnerability in research does not simply decline linearly with age, assessments of research risk must entail multidimensional considerations that vary over developmental time. In a similar manner, individual characteristics of children at any age (e.g., maltreatment, at-risk status, etc.) may also heighten their vulnerability to certain risks which require special consideration by researchers. Finally, this discussion of developmental vulnerability and the principle underlying research ethics suggests that in addition to the*

Reprinted with permission from *Child Development*, 1990, Vol. 61, 1–16. Copyright © 1990 by the Society for Research in Child Development, Inc.

This paper was written as my contribution to a Work Group on Ethical Issues in Social and Behavioral Research with Minors convened and sponsored by the Office for Protection from Research Risk of the National Institutes of Health. I am grateful for the catalytic contributions and insights of other members of this group throughout our discussions of the past several years. Members of the work group were Judith Areen, Georgetown University; Thomas Grisso, University of Massachusetts; Ruth Macklin, Albert Einstein College of Medicine; Charles McKay, National Institutes of Health; Gary Melton, University of Nebraska; Mary Jane Rotheram, Columbia University; Joan Sieber, California State University at Hayward; Barbra Stanley, Columbia University (Chair); and Alexander Tymchuk, University of California at Los Angeles. This work was also advanced by my participation in a faculty seminar on Ethics and the Professions at the University of Nebraska. I am grateful for the comments and ideas provided by seminar participants, and also by the following colleagues: Robert Audi, Susan Crockenberg, Robert Levine, Ruth Macklin, Gary Melton, and Joan Sieber.

conventional risk/benefit analysis, researchers are in an optimal posi-
tion to establish and maintain standards of decent treatment of children
in research that safeguard their rights as research participants.
Suggestions for fostering this process in the research community are
outlined.

Consider the following research vignettes:

A 12-month-old infant and her mother are ushered into the research
playroom by a smiling lab assistant. After a few minutes of instructions, the two are left alone for the beginning of a 21-min procedure
designed to appraise the security of their attachment relationship.
During this period, a female stranger enters the room on two occasions
to play with the baby. The mother also leaves the room on two
occasions—once leaving the baby in the company of the stranger, and a
second time leaving the child alone—during which the baby becomes
markedly distressed. During the second reunion, the mother is disturbed to find that her child is not soothing, but instead alternates clinging with pushing away and angry crying. The child is still fussing when
the two leave the laboratory.

A 9-year old boy enters the empty school classroom with the
researcher who had been introduced to him just moments before. After
a few minutes of getting acquainted, the researcher tells the boy that she
is interested in his speed at completing jigsaw puzzles and gives him a
puzzle to complete. He does so quickly, and receives her admiration and
praise in return. She then gives him four more puzzles, and for each one
he is surprised to find that he is unable to finish it in the time provided.
The researcher then asks him some questions about how he evaluates
his abilities and efforts in completing puzzles, in finishing schoolwork,
and in other areas of achievement. Before he leaves, she notes that the
four puzzles were designed to be difficult to solve, so he should not feel
badly about his performance. He then returns to his classroom, where
he is in a special group for slow learners, wondering whether she told
him the truth.

A 13-year-old girl is observed from behind one-way windows while
she plays with the young baby who had been presented to her when she
arrived at the laboratory. After this 30-min observational session, she is
then escorted (without the infant) to an adjoining room where she com-
pletes several self-report measures concerning her personality, back-

ground, interests, and other characteristics. Among these measures is one in which she is asked to indicate the development of her secondary sexual characteristics by marking which of a series of photographs is most similar to her own breast size, pubic hair growth, and other physical features. She leaves the room wondering whether the researchers regarded her as underdeveloped for her age.

Procedures like these are representative of widely used methods in developmental and educational research that provide valuable information concerning early attachment relationships, achievement motivation, psychosexual development, and other topics. Procedures like these are regularly approved by university Institutional Review Boards (IRBs) because the relative balance of potential risks and benefits is judged to be favorable to conducting the research. Yet these procedures are also representative of some of the thorny ethical dilemmas many researchers encounter in their efforts to design sound practices in social and behavioral research involving children. By its nature, of course, the research process entails inherent risks to subjects, even though these risks are frequently minimal. The research process also yields, at times, important discoveries of broad social benefit, and thus one of the ethical considerations involved in the research process is assessing and balancing relative risks and benefits. This is not an easy task: most researchers are not trained to conduct the kind of ethical analysis required for a sensitive risk benefit assessment, and they commonly experience ethical review as a procedural obstacle to research progress that is distally related to ethical responsibility. Furthermore, members of IRBs are often discouraged from conducting a fine-grained appraisal of risks and benefits because of their limited expertise in the specific research field, members' reluctance to question their colleagues' ethical competence, and a bias in favor of approval incorporated into IRB guidelines (Williams, 1984). As a consequence, while procedures for ensuring privacy, confidentiality, and informed consent can be relatively well defined, assessing the potential risks and benefits of a research procedure is inherently more ambiguous and difficult, and this difficulty can undermine the ethical review process.

The purpose of this essay is not to ease the difficulty; rather, it is to introduce into the discussion of risk/benefit analysis two additional considerations. First, I will argue that a more thoroughgoing developmental perspective is required in judging research risks with children because children are a heterogeneous population, varying in developmental competencies as well as in background characteristics. Research risks vary in complex ways with the age of the child: some decrease with increasing age, some increase as the child matures, and others remain essentially stable over development. Because vulnerability in research does not simply decline linearly with age, the analysis of research risk must encompass these diverse changes in developmental vulnerability, as well as differences in background characteristics of the child. Second, I will also argue that judgments of research risk must be increasingly focused on establishing and maintaining standards of decent treatment of minors who are research participants. This involves a shift in emphasis from a primarily prohibitive (and minimalist) ethics of risk/benefit assessment to a more prescriptive ethics of treatment norms governing research, and derives both from existing shortcomings in prevailing methods of risk/benefit assessment as well as the special vulnerabilities of children as research participants.

Although much of this discussion is potentially applicable to biomedical clinical studies and other forms of research coupled with therapeutic intervention, there are also important ethical differences in the analysis of clinical compared to nonclinical research, and for present purposes, the concern is exclusively with research that does not have a therapeutic component. Moreover, this analysis also focuses on research in the social and behavioral sciences and will address prevailing methods and procedures in this field, which includes developmental psychology but also research in educational psychology, social psychology, sociology, anthropology, and other fields that entail procedures involving direct contact with children.

RISK/BENEFIT ASSESSMENT IN SOCIAL AND BEHAVIORAL RESEARCH WITH CHILDREN

A sensitive appraisal of research risks in relation to potential benefits is well instituted in the ethical guidelines of developmental researchers. The Ethical Standards for Research with Children of the Society for Research in Child Development specify, for example, that researchers should use no procedure that "may harm the child either physically or psychologically," although defining this is left to the investigator in consultation with colleagues. Although the Ethical Principles of Psychologists of the American Psychological Association include no special provisions concerning research with children, psychologists are mandated not to use research procedures "likely to cause serious or lasting harm to a participant" unless the research has "great potential benefit" and informed and voluntary consent is obtained.

Following the guidelines recommended in 1978 by the National Commission for the Protection of Human Subjects of Biomedical and Behavioral Research, the Department of Health and Human Services (DHHS) issued agency regulations in 1983 (45 CFR 46, Subparts A and D) specifically pertaining to research involving children. Various levels of research risk were established in these guidelines. "Minimal risk," for example, involves risk of harm not greater than that "ordinarily encountered in daily life or during the performance of routine physical or psychological examinations or tests" (45 CFR 46.102[g]), and research studies involving only minimal risk can be supported by DHHS contingent on the permission of the child's parents and the child's own assent. Research involving greater than minimal risk that does not directly benefit the child can be approved only with the additional finding by an IRB that the risk represents a "minor increase" over minimal risk, the procedure involves experiences that are commensurate with those involved in "actual or expected medical, dental, psychological, social, or educational situations," and the research is likely to yield "generalizable knowledge" that is of "vital importance" for the understanding of the subjects' condition (45 CFR 46.406). The kinds of procedures that constitute a "minor increase" over minimal risk are not defined in the regulations, although the National Commission recommended four guidelines: a common-sense estimation of risk, the researcher's prior experience with similar procedures, statistical data concerning these procedures, and the conditions of the research participants. Finally, research procedures that do not satisfy "minimal risk" or "minor increase" provisions may nevertheless be approved through additional review procedures by DHHS.

On the whole, these DHHS guidelines reflect most of the recommendations of the National Commission, but one recommendation was not adopted in the final DHHS regulations: that a child's objection to research participation constitutes a *binding* restriction, except in extraordinary circumstances, and thus that the assent of children age 7 and older be required, along with parental permission, for research participation (see Recommendation 7). Moreover, it is important to note that these regulations do not apply at all to certain classes of research involving children, such as those occurring in educational settings concerning instructional techniques or classroom management methods. This has been criticized by some commentators (e.g., Holder, 1988).

Ethical Basis for Risk/Benefit Analysis

On the surface, these professional and regulatory guidelines appear to mandate an act-utilitarian approach to risk/benefit analysis: judging research in terms of the relative balance of benefits and risks of the specific protocol. But the ethical bases for this analysis are considerably more complex because the regulations also require heightened thresholds of review for risky research and imply that there are certain general, unimpeachable requirements on the research process related to the limits of acceptable risk, informed consent, privacy, and confidentiality. Thus, a blend of utilitarian and deontological (i.e., Kantian) views seems to shape many of the existing guidelines concerning research ethics (Macklin, 1982).

Although utilitarian and Kantian perspectives each lead the ethical analysis in somewhat different directions, research ethicists often begin from a common principle of respect for persons (a chief aspect of which is autonomy): treating persons as ends in themselves, never solely as means to an end. This principle finds expression in Kant's (1785) categorical imperative, but it can also be defended within a rule-utilitarian analysis. The principle of respect for persons mandates that researchers guarantee the right of individual self-determination in the research process, and this includes respecting the wishes and decisions of research participants, as well as their values and beliefs. This principle thus underlies research regulations concerning informed consent, privacy, confidentiality, freedom to withdraw from participation, limits on deceptive research practices, and the importance of debriefing following research procedures.

A second principle underlying research ethics is the principle of nonmaleficence: that it is wrong to intentionally inflict harm on another. When considered together with the principle of beneficence—the positive obligation to remove existing harms and provide benefits to others—the ethical basis for the risk/benefit analysis becomes clear. Since researchers pursue their investigations with the general goal of improving human conditions through research knowledge (as well as advancing knowledge for its own sake), the principles of nonmaleficence and beneficence together incorporate into research ethics one overarching purpose of conducting research and apply them to the evaluation of specific research proposals. On a broad level, therefore, researchers must be able to justify their work in terms of the potential benefits it promises, especially when research entails risks to participants. Researchers are mandated to identify potential risks to research participation, describe potential benefits (direct, indirect, and societal) from the research, and struggle with their calculus.

Finally, a fourth ethical principle is commonly applied to research concerning justice: a fair distribution of goods, which entails the obligation to treat equally those who are equally situated and to treat differently those who differ in relevant ways. Distributive justice principles influence the research process concerning equitable subject selection and treatment, especially in studies evaluating potentially beneficial treatments, therapies, or social programs that may be denied control or placebo group members. Principles of justice mandate efforts to ensure that research participants suffer no undesirable consequences due to research involvement, and they also underlie efforts to treat research participants equitably in light of their backgrounds and characteristics. Finally, as we shall see below, distributive justice principles also figure into the risk/benefit assessment, especially concerning who benefits from the research process and who bears the risks. Many research ethicists would agree, for example, that a study whose benefits clearly outweighed its risks would nevertheless be morally impermissible if the risks were inequitably borne by individuals who enjoyed none of its benefits (e.g., MacIntyre, 1982).

An understanding of the ethical principles underlying the risk/benefit assessment in social and behavioral research does not contribute clarity to the specific considerations of researchers when planning a study. It does, however, provide a foundation for thinking consistently about researchers' ethical responsibilities toward subjects, the reasons for conducting ethical review, and the general considerations entailed in that review. In a sense, by becoming cognizant of the broader ethical principles underlying their responsibilities, researchers can think more comprehensively about their roles (vis-à-vis subjects, the profession, and society) and their research, and can thus more thoughtfully evaluate their proposed studies from this perspective.

Special Considerations for Children

Principles of justice do not mandate, of course, that all research participants be treated uniformly; on the contrary, justice requires that participants who differ in relevant ways (e.g., due to need or merit) be treated differently. It is because of justice concerns, therefore, that researchers take special precautions when children are participants in social and behavioral research. This is because the characteristics of children introduce several unique vulnerabilities to their roles as research participants.

First, young children are likely to have greater difficulty than older children and adults in understanding the research process because of their more limited cognitive competencies and experiential background. Consequently, their capacities to make reasoned decisions concerning research participation, to understand the consent procedure and their freedom to withdraw, and to resist intrusions on their rights as research participants are likely to be limited prior to the middle school-age years, and may not reach adult-like levels before mid-adolescence (see generally Weithorn, 1982, 1983). Moreover, limitations in cognitive competencies and experiential background may also constrain young children's understanding of the role of research participant, and this may influence the validity of research findings as well as ethical considerations.

These factors have given rise to a spirited debate concerning whether children should become involved as participants in research at all. On one extreme, Paul Ramsay (1970, 1976, 1977) has argued that because infants and children cannot consent in a voluntary, informed manner to research participation, their involvement in research that has no therapeutic benefit inevitably violates principles of respect for persons, and is thus morally wrong. Ramsay would prohibit children as research participants except when they might directly benefit from the research because, in his view, children are otherwise inevitably treated as means to an end (an object of research) rather than as ends in themselves (Kant's categorical imperative). To Ramsay, proxy consent does not alleviate these problems because this kind of consent procedure places children in the role of adults, freely volunteering (albeit through parental consent) to become research participants. At the other extreme, Richard McCormick (1974, 1976) has argued that when risk is minimal, children can become involved in research because, as humans, they possess a basic obligation to aid others by the knowledge gained through research, and thus their consent may be legitimately assumed. Arguing from a natural law perspective, McCormick notes that by their nature, humans desire the health and well-being of others as well as of themselves. Since research entailing minimal risk contributes to this goal and involves no personal harm, proxy consent simply affirms intrinsic values that are part of all human beings including children. In a sense, because of their nature, humans *should* participate in research involving minimal risk because doing so is *right,* and thus it can be presumed that infants and young children would consent to do so. Ramsay (1976), by contrast, replies that this requires treating children as adults by assigning moral obligations to them. Other philosophers have tried to devise alternative positions between the extremes taken by Ramsay and McCormick, including Bartholome (1976), who has argued that research participation may further children's moral education, and thus parents may legitimately give proxy consent because of these benefits for offspring. Bartholome would still restrict nonclinical research to children over the age of 5 (i.e., when, he argues, they can reasonably benefit morally from participation). Thus, the issue of whether research participation for young children can be justified, in view of their limited reasoning abilities and the demands of ethical principles in relation to informed consent, remains essentially unresolved by moral philosophers.

A second reason young children are uniquely vulnerable as research participants is their limited social power, which has been noted by classic (Piaget, 1932/1965) and contemporary developmental theorists. Parents and other adults exercise proxy consent for children, and children's institutionalization in extrafamilial care centers, schools, and other settings further reduces their power to exercise independent decision making concerning research participation. Although children's assent is encouraged by DHHS regulations, it may be difficult for children to dissent from participation because their invitation to participate typically occurs in a context of prior parental permission, institutional support, and researchers' interest in furthering the research enterprise. Indeed, consistent with the recommendation of the National Commission (although not adopted by DHHS), Pence (1980) has argued that because of the pressures to comply with the requests of social authorities like researchers, a child's dissent should be determinative in most research procedures. Even if this recommendation was adopted, however, it would remain true that in most situations children are more vulnerable to research risks because of their relative social powerlessness vis-à-vis adult authorities. These risks include not only coercion to participate but also pressures to act and respond in the research setting that may be inconsistent with the child's own wishes or desires, violative of the child's beliefs, or otherwise self-defeating.

Third, young children are uniquely vulnerable to research risks because of the special configuration of child, parental, and state interests relating to their research participation. Due to their legal status as minors, parents and other adults acting *in loco parentis* make fundamental decisions concerning children's health and welfare, including giving permission for their research participation and having access to research materials. It is unwise to assume that an identity between parental and child interests is always reflected in these decisions, but except in extreme circumstances the state is unlikely to intervene on behalf of children, and DHHS regulations include a number of provisions for waiving child assent requirements when parents consent to their participation. The reason for these circumstances is the ambiguous standing of children as "persons" before the law, a condition that fosters paternalistic interest in children's welfare but also undermines their independent decision making (see Baumrind, 1978; Melton, 1987). As a consequence, children have uniquely little control not only over their participation in research but also over the disposition of research materials, their withdrawal from research participation, and other decisions normally accompanying research participation.

Taken together, children are especially vulnerable as research participants because of both intrinsic and socially determined factors that make them unique social actors. As a consequence, the risk/benefit calculus must be determined differently for children than for adults, entailing a variety of considerations that normally are not applied to older populations.

DEVELOPMENTAL CHANGES IN RESEARCH VULNERABILITY

Of course, the term "children" encompasses a broad portion of the life span, and the risk-relevant capabilities and characteristics of children change markedly from infancy through adolescence. Research procedures that would be extremely stressful for an infant may have a negligible effect on an adolescent. As a consequence, it is necessary for researchers (and IRB members) to take a further step to consider how the children's *changing* characteristics alter their vulnerability to research risk (see Maccoby, 1983). The manner in which developmental changes in research vulnerability are portrayed can have a very significant influence on risk assessment in research involving minors.

The considerations outlined above reflect the prevailing portrayal of developmental changes in research vulnerability: infants and young children are the most vulnerable to research risks of various kinds, and with increasing age—and corollary increases in cognitive competencies, experiential background, and other changing capabilities—vulnerability to risk declines. From this developmental portrayal, there should be more stringent safeguards against research risk with younger subject populations, because young children are most susceptible to coerced consent, violations of confidentiality, research practices that are distressing, demeaning, or deceptive, and other risks that older individuals can better resist. Researchers are consequently mandated to think more carefully and conservatively in designing research procedures for younger participants. This portrayal of developmental changes in research vulnerability is essentially a linear one, with susceptibility to research risk declining in a uniform and straightforward fashion with increasing age.

However, alternative portrayals of developmental change in research vulnerability might also be proposed. Another linear model portrays research risk as *increasing*, rather than decreasing, with the child's growing maturity. Although this portrayal appears counterintuitive and contrary to the first, it is similarly based on some self-evident observations of the characteristics of children of various ages. For example, a very young child cannot easily be embarrassed or humiliated before she has acquired the cognitive capacities necessary for self-referent thinking. Threats to the self-concept are limited until the child has developed a coherent system of self-referent beliefs and can incorporate others' evaluations and social-comparison information into the system. Worries about what will happen next in a research procedure depend, to a great extent, on an ability to think within a past-present-future temporal context and on an experiential background that leads one to anticipate threatening future events in a research setting. Young children are unlikely to be stressed by a concern with the researcher's motives or intentions before the have acquired the ability to draw sophisticated psychological inferences about other people (although this also renders them more vulnerable to deceptive research practices). And, in general, the trust of infants and young children in their caregivers may reduce their vulnerability to certain stressors when those caregivers are present. Thus, an alternative portrayal of developmental vulnerability suggests that at younger ages, children are buffered against certain kinds of research risks because of limitations in their cognitive and experiential backgrounds, and that with increasing age (and corollary changes in self-understanding, inference processes, and other capabilities), vulnerability to these risks increases.

These alternative linear portrayals of developmental change in research vulnerability lead to very different guidelines concerning risk assessment in research with minors. The first model warrants greatest concern for research with young children, while the second model suggests that in some domains of risk, researchers should be most concerned with older children and adolescents. Taken together, they suggest that simple, straightforward linear models of uniform developmental changes in research vulnerability do not accurately portray the complex changes that occur with development and their implications for research risk. Nonlinear developmental models are necessary to more sensitively portray the kinds of risks to which children are likely to be vulnerable at different ages.

One kind of nonlinear developmental model is already instituted within DHHS guidelines. As noted above, regulations defining "minimal risk" and a "minor increase" over minimal risk comparably define these standards in relation to the child's everyday experiences. For example, minimal risk is evaluated in relation to the risk of harm ordinarily encountered in the child's daily life. From a developmental perspective, therefore, these regulations suggest that as a child's normative life experiences change with age—in accord with the child's growing competencies and experiential background—norms defining research risk must comparably be revised to encompass these changing experiences. By this guideline, research procedures that would ordinarily not be permitted at an early age (because they exceed the risk of harms which the child normally encounters at that age) might be permissible at a later age. For example, extended periods apart from parents with unfamiliar adults might be questionable in research with infants, but certainly not for older children and adolescents. Conversely, procedures that would be allowed with young children because they are part of that child's ordinary life experiences might not be permitted at later ages, when these experiences are not as typical.

The problem with this guideline is that it defends the use of research procedures that we might otherwise question on the basis of ethical principles (e.g., respect for persons, nonmaleficence, justice, etc.). For example, infants and toddlers commonly experience brief or prolonged separations from their caregivers (e.g., with a babysitter, in day-care, etc.), and they are often distressed by these experiences. By the "minimal risk" regulation, research involving infants' involuntary separations from their caregivers is permissible, even though some researchers are doubtful that this should be true (e.g., Rheingold, 1982). Young children regularly experience invasions of their bodily and personal privacy by parents, teachers, and other adults. It is unclear, however, whether this justifies privacy violations in the research context. Children and adolescents commonly encounter experiences at school that threaten their self-image, including unfavorable academic performance evaluations by teachers, teasing concerning personal or physical characteristics by peers, and spontaneous as well as elicited social comparison. But many would dispute whether these normative experiences provide a prima facie justification for considering comparable experiences to be "minimal risk" in a research context, because these experiences violate principles of nonmaleficence and respect for persons (e.g., autonomy). More generally, it is clearer that in studies with special populations of children and youth—such as those who are incarcerated, have been maltreated, or are substance abusers—researchers should not necessarily define standards of minimal risk in terms of the ordinary life experiences of children in these populations.

A portrayal of developmental change in research vulnerability that is based on the normative daily experiences of children at different ages fails because it does not adequately define standards of decent treatment of minors who are research participants. By defining what is permissible in terms of what is normative in the child's life experience, it potentially permits researchers to act in ways that undermine the child, even though these experiences may be familiar to the child. To put the issue somewhat differently, researchers should be hesitant to violate basic principles of respect for persons, autonomy, nonmaleficence, and justice in their treatment of the child, even though these principles may be regularly violated by others in the child's everyday life. In the search for alternative nonlinear portrayals of developmental change in research vulnerability, one must look elsewhere for guidelines that are sensitive to age-related changes in children's capabilities, experiences, and needs and that better define standards of decent treatment of children in research settings.

An Alternative Developmental Portrayal

A more adequate nonlinear portrayal must, unfortunately, be a more complex portrayal. In order to adequately describe the kinds of risks to which children are susceptible as research participants, different kinds of risks must be considered independently as well as developmentally. Because the changing competencies of children with increasing age provide new capacities for resiliency as well as vulnerability, it is no longer adequate to assume that vulnerability changes uniformly or linearly with developmental time. As noted earlier, some risks increase with the child's maturity, other risks decline, some remain stable, and others shift in a curvilinear fashion. Researchers (and IRB members) will benefit, therefore, from a more sensitive portrayal of developmental vulnerability to research risk in which different risks are considered independently along a developmental continuum.

This section offers the beginning to such a portrayal, albeit a limited one, by suggesting some general guidelines related to research vulnerability that appear to be supported by the research literature. It draws upon an incisive analysis by Maccoby (1983) to suggest examples of how susceptibility to different research risks varies with the child's development, although it is certainly not an exhaustive portrayal. These guidelines (in some cases, working hypotheses) are framed in terms of broad propositions.

1. *In general, the younger the child, the greater the possibility of general behavioral and socioemotional disorganization accompanying stressful experiences; with increasing age, the child's growing repertoire of coping skills permits greater adaptive functioning in the face of stress.* Although the research literature on coping and emotional self-regulation is very limited (see Kopp, in press, and Thompson, in press, for reviews), it portrays a general developmental transition from a reliance on extrinsic supports for emotional regulatory processes (e.g., the assistance of caregivers and other adults, use of security objects, etc.) to the growth of independent, self-regulatory coping capacities. While the young infant cries inconsolably until a nurturant adult intervenes, the toddler can use a rudimentary repertoire of self-soothing behaviors, the preschooler can reflect on and talk about her feelings, the gradeschool child can directly alter emotional arousal through strategic means (e.g., distracting mental imagery, altering goals, self-talk, etc.), and the adolescent has sufficient awareness of his own idiosyncratic emotional style to institute strategies that are well suited to regulating emotional experience. Because coping capacities change developmentally from a reliance on extrinsic supports to a growing repertoire of self-regulatory strategies, infants and young children are at greater risk for becoming overwhelmed with stressful research procedures at the moment they occur.

There are some corollary principles that follow from this general one. First, *at younger ages, the child's coping capacities depend more on the availability of trusted attachment figures than they do at later ages.* Thus, the presence and/or availability of the parent, relative, or surrogate caregiver in the research setting will provide greater support for a young child's coping with the demands of a research procedure than it will for an older child or adolescent. Second, *at younger ages, the child's coping capacities rely more on the familiarity of the setting and/or procedure, and on the availability of familiar objects, than they do at later ages.* Research procedures conducted at home or in the day-care center not only gain from ecological validity, but they also foster the child's coping with the demands of the research by permitting access to a structured environment with which the child is familiar (see Thompson & Limber [in press] for an example from studies of infant socioemotional development).

2. *Threats to a child's self-concept become more stressful with increasing age as children develop a more comprehensive, coherent, and integrated self-image, become more invested in an enduring identity, and acquire more sophisticated understandings of components of the self by which that self-concept becomes progressively modified and reshaped.* Although self-understanding exists in some form from shortly after birth, its content, organization, and structure change significantly from infancy through adolescence (see Damon & Hart [1982] and Harter [1983] for reviews of this research). Whereas the self-referent belief systems of preschoolers and young school-age children are predominantly physicalistic, concrete, and material—focusing on the child's physical or behavioral characteristics, activities, and possessions—the self-concepts of older school-age children and adolescents become more abstract, psychological, and integrated with increasing age. An important transition occurs between the ages of 7 and 9, according to researchers, when growing cognitive skills contribute to more characterological and personalistic self-referent belief systems, and when the evaluations of others become increasingly important to the child.

But these changes in the content of the self-concept are only part of the story. In addition, self-referent beliefs become increasingly more consolidated, differentiated, and hierarchically integrated with increasing age. Whereas the preschooler tends to provide self-evaluative judgments in an essentially all-or-none fashion and without integrating these judgments into a comprehensive self-concept, the older grade-school child attempts to find consistency among diverse self-attributes, and the adolescent begins to organize these self-referent beliefs into a broader, more abstract self-representational system (see Damon & Hart, 1982). The latter is, in some ways, a core component of the search for "identity," and it helps to explain both the importance of identity development for adolescents, as well as the self-consciousness of this period (Marcia, 1980). Moreover, with increasing age, the evaluations of others assume a greater role in shaping the child's self-perceptions. As a consequence, older children and adolescents are likely to be significantly more sensitive to the evaluative comments of others than are younger children.

Why do these developmental changes come about? According to Damon and Hart (1982) and Harter (1983), researchers have attributed them to growing cognitive competencies (e.g., the transition from preoperational to concrete-operational thought permitting greater systematization among self-referent beliefs, and the transition to formal-operational thought introducing greater abstraction and self-reflection to the self-concept), declining egocentrism and increased role-taking skills (allowing children to increasingly consider what others are thinking about the self), the growth of social comparison processes (see below), and other developmental capabilities. They also derive from changes in children's understanding of specific components of the self-system. For example, there is some evidence that preschoolers and young school-age children perceive ability as a changing attribute that is under personal control (like personal effort), and it is not until later in the school-age years that ability becomes more appropriately perceived as a relatively enduring personal quality (Nicholls, 1978). As a consequence, the meaning of statements from others concerning one's ability is likely to be much different to younger than older children, and younger children are more likely to remain optimistic in the face of negative ability attributions (see Dweck & Elliot, 1983, for a review).

These changes in the nature and structure of the self-concept have profound implications for developmental changes in vulnerability to research risk. They suggest, for example, that research experiences that have unfavorable implications for the self-concept are likely to be more stressful to older children and adolescents because they are more likely to be internalized, provoke worried self-reflection, and threaten broader aspects of self-esteem. While younger children may be sensitive to researchers' comments about their appearance and/or physical abilities, their confidence in the malleability of personal attributes (like ability) and the less-integrated quality of their self-referent beliefs may render these comments less portentous than they are at older ages. By contrast, older school-age children and adolescents are constructing broader and more coherent self-referent belief systems that incorporate psychological attributes, and thus their sensitivity to researchers' comments about a broader range of personal attributes renders them more vulnerable to threats to self-esteem. Moreover, in contrast to the unrealistic self-confidence of younger children, their more accurate understanding of the nature of these attributes (e.g., many personal qualities *cannot* be changed), combined with their own critical self-evaluations, may further increase their vulnerability to threats to self-esteem in research contexts.

3. *Social comparison information becomes a more significant mode of self-evaluation with increasing age.* As suggested above, one of the catalysts for developmental changes in the self-concept is the increasing role of social comparison information in self-evaluation (Dweck & Elliot, 1983). Although preschoolers are often aware of how their performances compare with those of others, this knowl-

edge plays comparatively little role in their general assessments of their skills and abilities. By contrast, older school-age children more regularly incorporate a comparative metric into their self-evaluations: performance is judged partly by the standards of others' performances (Ruble, 1983). As a consequence, older children may be more vulnerable to explicit or implied comparisons of their research performance with others, and may incorporate this information into their own evaluations of their abilities. Moreover, older children may also be more sensitive to the evaluations of others to whom their research performance is disseminated, such as parents and teachers.

4. *The capacity to make sophisticated psychological inferences of others' motives, attitudes, and feelings increases with age. This domain of psychological inferences includes inferences about others' reactions to oneself.* Of course, social comparison information may not be explicitly available to children but may be implicit in others' reactions. Although preschoolers exhibit a rudimentary awareness that others have psychological states that are different from their own, the capacity to draw accurate inferences of those psychological states increases significantly in breadth and scope throughout childhood and adolescence (Shantz, 1983). Most children in the late preschool years can offer simple psychological inferences concerning another's thoughts or feelings. But it is an especially difficult task conceptually for children to draw inferences about others' psychological judgments *about oneself* because doing so requires an ability to divorce one's own self-evaluation from the inferred evaluations of oneself by others, and current research suggests that this capacity begins to emerge in middle to late childhood (between 8 and 12 years of age) (Shantz, 1983). Thus, whereas a preschooler may not react to the researcher's raised eyebrow and questioning tone of voice following his answer, and the younger gradeschool child may notice it but not accurately infer what it means, the adolescent will correctly infer that he has provided an incorrect response and reevaluate her answer accordingly.

As this example suggests, the developing capacity to derive psychological inferences from others' behavior means that older children and adolescents are more vulnerable to implicit cues, demands, and judgments of their performance that may influence their behavior as research participants. While this is a concern for the validity of research findings, it also is an ethical concern insofar as they perceive researchers making unfavorable judgments of their performance or experience implicit pressures to act in a manner inconsistent with their wishes (e.g., to divulge confidential information). However, it is worth noting that this developing capacity is also a double-edged sword. In contrast to younger children, who are more likely to naively accept research tasks at face value, the older child's ability to speculate concerning another's motives and intentions may also contribute to greater skepticism concerning the true purpose of the research activity or the true intentions of the researcher. Thus, while older children may be somewhat more susceptible to implicit pressures and judgments, they may also approach the research task more skeptically than younger children do.

5. *Self-conscious emotional reactions—such as shame, guilt, embarrassment and pride—emerge later developmentally than do the primary emotions. But once they are acquired, young children may be more vulnerable to their arousal because of their limited understanding of these emotions.* In contrast to primary emotions such as happiness, sadness, fear and anger, self-conscious emotional reactions such as shame, guilt, embarrassment, and pride are not apparent in the first year of life but emerge early in the preschool years with the growth of self-understanding (Campos, Barrett, Lamb, Goldsmith, & Stenberg, 1983). But with their emergence in the early preschool years, there is evidence that young children overextend their meaning to apply to a broader range of circumstances than those for which they are appropriate. For example, preschoolers and young school-age children report feeling guilty in negative situations for which they are not responsible, perhaps because of exaggerated perceptions of personal agency, confusion concerning the nature of intentionality, or other social cognitive factors (Graham, Doubleday, & Guarino, 1984; Harter, 1983; Thompson, 1987). It is not until children are 7 or 8 years of age that they restrict feelings of guilt to more appropriate situations in which they are personally culpable for negative outcomes.

If this developmental transition applies also to other self-conscious emotions— such as shame and embarrassment—it suggests that once these emotions have emerged, young children may be especially vulnerable to their arousal in inappropriate or unexpected circumstances because of their immature understanding of the bases for these emotional experiences. However, there may also be another developmental resurgence in susceptibility to self-conscious emotional experiences—namely, in adolescence (Elkind, 1967)—which suggests that vulnerability to these emotions shows a curvilinear developmental trend. With respect to research participation, these findings suggest that when children experience negative outcomes for which they are not responsible, younger children may nevertheless be vulnerable to a variety of negative self-conscious emotions that reflect a negative self-assessment that may not be justified by the circumstances.

6. *Young children's understanding of authority renders them more vulnerable to coercive manipulations than older children, for whom authority relations are better balanced by an understanding of individual rights. Furthermore, young children's trust of authorities makes them more vulnerable to being deceived in research.* Students of social cognitive development have pointed out that children in the preschool and early gradeschool years regard authorities as legitimate and powerful individuals, mandating obedience because of their intrinsically superior qualities (Damon, 1977; Piaget, 1932/1965; Shantz, 1983). It is not until the late gradeschool years that children regard an authority's legitimacy as based in that person's training or experience, and obedience derives from respect for the authority rather than from

unilateral reverence. Authority relations increasingly become viewed as a cooperative, consensual compact adopted for the welfare of all.

Younger children are thus more likely to respond to authorities—including researchers—with immediate respect and obedience, even if the researcher makes unreasonable or illegitimate demands on the child. By contrast, older children's perceptions of the researcher's legitimacy may be undermined by inappropriate demands or requests, and the child's motivation to comply may be reduced as a result. Furthermore, young children are likely to be more susceptible to deceptive research practices because of their unquestioning compliance with the researcher's requests. Older children may be more skeptical because their understanding of authority relations involves consensual cooperation, and also because of a more sophisticated capacity to speculate about another's intentions and motives, as noted earlier.

7. *Privacy interests and concerns increase and become more differentiated as children mature, and broaden from an initial focus on physical and possessional privacy to include concerns with informational privacy.* As noted in a review of the research by Melton (1983), developmental changes in children's privacy interests are partly a by-product of how they are treated: preschoolers seldom have opportunities to exercise territorial or informational privacy rights, for example. However, the limited research evidence indicates that with increasing age, and especially with the transition to adolescence, privacy becomes increasingly important as a marker of independence and self-esteem. Children initially exercise greater concern with establishing a physical location of one's own (i.e., territorial privacy, such as one's bedroom) and the integrity of personal possessions (i.e., possessional privacy), but at later ages this concern extends to the control of others' knowledge of one's associations, activities, and interests (i.e., informational privacy) (e.g., Wolfe, 1978). In this sense, the transition from physical, material markers of personal privacy concerns to more psychologically oriented privacy interests reflects the child's developing self-representational system, as noted above. Importantly, however, these findings suggest that children may become increasingly vulnerable to privacy intrusions in research settings with increasing age. Whereas younger children may feel comfortable divulging personal information to a researcher upon request, older children and especially adolescents are likely to experience certain inquiries as unduly intrusive and threatening. Moreover, to the extent that researchers gain access to personal information about research participants without their consent (e.g., data from school records via parental permission), adolescents are especially likely to experience this as a breach of informational privacy.

8. *Owing to their more limited conceptual skills, younger children may benefit less from feedback during the research experience, including dehoaxing and debriefing procedures, than do older children and adolescents.* In some studies, children are provided with false feedback concerning their performance on a task,

and are subsequently told during a dehoaxing procedure that the task had been designed to be difficult, and thus they should not feel badly about their performance. There are several reasons to doubt the efficacy of this procedure with young children. First, understanding deception tactics requires recursive reasoning (e.g., "I knew that you would think this way when I did . . ."), which is conceptually demanding for preschoolers and early grade-school children. Second, deception tactics may themselves be difficult for young children to understand because of their complexity, especially when they involve dehoaxing a set of convincing instructions or procedures instituted by the researcher that children trusted to be true. Finally, because young children often have difficulty reevaluating past performance in light of a subsequent standard, they may not spontaneously reevaluate their critical evaluations of earlier performance in light of what they are subsequently told about the nature of the study. For example, having been earlier convinced that they performed poorly on a task, a subsequent dehoaxing procedure may not fully change their earlier critical self-evaluation based on false performance feedback.

Taken together, these considerations suggest that young children may not benefit fully from the dehoaxing procedures that follow deceptive research practices. Insofar as these procedures are used to reduce the risks inherent in research deception, alternative approaches may be necessary. However, contrary to older children and adolescents, younger children may nevertheless be *less* vulnerable to heightened future sensitivity to deceit in research because of their continuing trust in authorities (see above). By contrast, older children may experience undermined trust in research authorities—and a questioning of their legitimacy—as a consequence of having been earlier deceived as a research participant. More generally, these considerations suggest that younger children are less likely to understand postresearch debriefing as a whole following research participation, whether debriefing involves dehoaxing, a broader explanation of the research purposes and goals, or assurance that the child had performed satisfactorily. This is true, in part, because of their limited understanding of the research process and the purposes of research activity. As a consequence, young children are less likely to experience debriefing as a benefit from research participation.

9. *With increasing age, children are likely to become more sensitive to cultural and socioeconomic biases in research that reflect negatively on the child's background, family, or previous experiences.* With developmental changes in the breadth and coherence of the self-concept, children are likely to increasingly identify themselves as members of broader social groups, including racial, ethnic, and socioeconomic groups. As a consequence, their vulnerability (and sensitivity) to overt and subtle biases in the research process is likely to increase with age.

Taken together, these guidelines illustrate how the child's vulnerability to different domains of research risk vary in different ways in developmental analysis. For some kinds of risk, children become increasingly vulnerable as they mature, while for other risk factors, vulnerability decreases with increasing age, and for some kinds of risk (e.g., susceptibility to embarrassment) curvilinear developmental changes may be normative. These considerations thus mandate a more complex, but more sensitive, analysis of developmental vulnerability to research risk to guide ethical decision making in research with minors. In this approach, a somewhat different set of considerations may be preeminent in ethical analysis of research with children of one age compared to another. Moreover, in longitudinal studies, new research risks may emerge for consideration by researchers as the cohort under study increases in age. In general, while this developmental portrayal significantly increases the complexity of the analysis of research risk for studies involving children, it also promises a more acute analysis that is likely to ultimately benefit the children who participate.

Individual Differences

Just as the term "children" embraces a very heterogeneous developmental population, so also the term encompasses a diverse range of backgrounds, characteristics, and prior experiences for children of any age. Characteristics of the subject population must thus also shape ethical decision making, especially in social and behavioral research concerning children.

Consider, for example, the special ethical considerations involved in research with maltreated infants, children, and adolescents. Because maltreating parents may not be reliable advocates for their offspring's interests and may also seek to avoid detection of their abusive behavior, issues of proxy consent by parents must be reconsidered in studies focused on children who have been maltreated or who are at risk for abuse. Additional or substitute consent procedures may be necessary, involving other adults acting in the child's interests. In the research setting, the young child's coping with the demands of the research may be undermined rather than supported by the parent's presence because maltreated children are typically insecurely rather than securely attached to their parents and experience other difficulties in the parent-child relationship (Cicchetti, in press). Maltreated children also share other characteristics that are likely to make them more vulnerable to certain research procedures: they exhibit an acute sensitivity to aggressive stimuli and may be more prone to perceive ambiguous situations as threatening, they have diminished self-esteem and impaired perceptions of personal competence, and they respond atypically to novel adults, sometimes showing aloof disinterest, at other times exhibiting clingy dependency (see Cicchetti, in press, for a comprehensive review of this research). These characteristics suggest that maltreated children are likely to experience various aspects of the research process as more stressful then do nonmaltreated children. Moreover, just as the consequences of maltreatment change with increasing age, so also the research vulnerabilities of maltreated children vary with their developmental status (Aber & Cicchetti, 1984; Cicchetti, in press). As a consequence, researchers studying this special population must take care to safeguard against the more unique vulnerabilities these children experience.

Other kinds of research risks also merit special attention. When at-risk populations of children are identified for study (e.g., adolescent substance abusers, offspring of adults with emotional disturbances, etc.), researchers must ensure that the perceptions of these children by custodians from whom permission is sought (e.g., school personnel, daycare workers, etc.) are not biased by the description of the selection criteria. Children can be victimized by the research process if they become labeled in disadvantageous ways. In some cases, children are enmeshed in a special web of power relations that can undermine obtaining truly voluntary consent to research participation. In Grisso's (1981) study of incarcerated juveniles, for example, most youths believed (despite disclaimers) that researchers were part of the juvenile justice system, and their assent to participate reflected, for some, a concern with potentially unfavorable reactions from the court should they decline. This research reveals how important it is for researchers to carefully examine subjects' implicit assumptions about the role of the researcher in the power network. Not only children but also families under stress must be considered in ethical decision making. Parents of special children (e.g., AIDS or cancer victims, children who have suffered traumatic experiences, etc.) may regard *any* contact with professionals as a means of helping the child, and this has important implications for the nature of informed consent as well as participants' implicit expectations concerning research benefits (see Fisher & Rosendahl, in press, for a discussion of these and related issues). Finally, special care must be taken with children experiencing intellectual deficits (e.g., Down syndrome children) to ensure that the child's assent is meaningfully obtained (if possible), the child's freedom to withdraw is fully understood, and that dehoaxing (when deception is used) and debriefing procedures are appropriate to the child's level of comprehension.

Thus, a developmental perspective to research vulnerability is additionally complicated by the necessity of considering seriously the special vulnerabilities (or, at times, unusual resiliency) of the populations of children under study. This is because what constitutes "minimal risk" or "decent treatment" of children from special populations is likely to vary from what is true of normative developmental populations, and this is especially true of social and behavioral research on sensitive issues. And as the study of maltreatment has indicated, these vulnerabilities may vary with developmental time. Clearly, doing a careful ethical analysis of research risk in studies with children is a difficult, demanding task.

RISKS IN RELATION TO BENEFITS

Professional and federal guidelines for social and behavioral research indicate, of course, that risk assessment must be considered in relation to the potential benefits of research findings. In contrast to the risks of physical harm, disability, or infection that may occur in biomedical research, potential threats of embarrassment, diminished self-esteem, or pressures to cooperate encountered in social and behavioral research seem benign by comparison,and this is especially so when these potential risks are weighed against possible research benefits (e.g., potential social utility, advancing knowledge, etc.). As a consequence, researchers are encouraged to approach the ethical review process as a threshold concern: can the level of risk to children be justified by the anticipated benefits of research results? Once a researcher (and an Institutional Review Board) can answer affirmatively, institutional requirements of ethical review are satisfied.

But this analysis of children's vulnerability in research suggests that developmental researchers are also uniquely sensitive to and responsible for establishing and maintaining standards of *decent treatment* of children alongside a risk/benefit calculus. That is, researchers should be concerned with minimizing stresses to children who participate, however minimal they may be, as part of their ethical obligations to subjects (i.e., respect for persons). One reason is that an emphasis on a prescriptive ethics of decent treatment underscores the researcher's obligation to consider diverse aspects of research risk to subjects, even if the study as a whole passes the threshold test. Even when research is considered minimal risk, for example, researchers should still exercise care to design procedures that reduce potential harm that could occur to children. A prescriptive ethics of decent treatment underscores this obligation by making ethical analysis a graded rather than a threshold concern.

Another reason for emphasizing standards of decent treatment of children in research is that the risk/benefit calculus is a problematic basis for the ethical analysis of research. The reason is that this calculus requires the comparison of things that are *not* comparable, and thus cannot be balanced against each other. Risks, for example, are borne largely by research participants, but in nonclinical research participants seldom benefit directly from their involvement, especially if they are children. Principles of justice mandate that a risk/benefit calculus is calibrated according to who are the bearers of risk and who enjoy its benefits (MacIntyre, 1982), and many research studies provide very few direct benefits to those who bear the risks. In most instances, in other words, risks are proximal to research participants, while benefits are distal.

Other factors also distinguish risks from benefits and complicate their comparison. One concerns their estimation: it is much easier to accurately predict the risks posed to research participants than to predict the benefits research will provide. To some extent, this is inherent in the research process. Risks to research participants can be estimated as soon as research procedures have been designed, but benefits are contingent on the outcome of the study, and thus involve a prediction of unknowns at the time the research is proposed. There are other reasons that potential benefits are difficult to predict. The social utility of behavioral research findings is often applied years after research insights have been generated, and is sometimes contingent on corollary research findings, trends in scholarly activity, and timing of social needs and concerns. Often research studies are conducted that yield essentially no identifiable social benefits because of unexpected methodological difficulties, resource constraints to continuing the research, and/or publication obstacles to the dissemination of findings. Finally, it must be acknowledged that many social and behavioral studies have no direct, foreseeable social applications, but are designed to advance knowledge on a topic of special interest and concern within the scholarly community. Although the latter is a valuable goal, it alters the assessment of benefits in significant ways.

For these reasons, comparing risks with benefits in ethical analysis is like comparing apples and oranges. To be sure, risk/benefit analysis is a useful heuristic when research of great social import must be conducted at some risk to participants. But in these instances, and increasingly when benefits are less clear and predictable, risk/benefit analysis must be combined with ethical principles of respect for persons and justice that underlie standards of decent treatment of children as research participants. And researchers are themselves in an optimal position for identifying and maintaining these treatment standards.

CONCLUSION

Two considerations in ethical decision making in nonclinical research involving children have been discussed in this essay. The first concerns the need for a more thoroughgoing developmental analysis of research risk that takes into account children's changing vulnerabilities with increasing age, as well as the special risks involved in their background characteristics. The second concerns the need for ethical guidelines to be increasingly framed around norms of decent treatment of children as research participants to supplement the prevailing risk/benefit analysis. Taken together, these considerations significantly complicate the ethical review of social and behavioral research involving children.

For various reasons, members of Institutional Review Boards are ill-equipped to conduct such a sensitive analysis: they are seldom trained in human development, and because many IRB members are from biomedical fields they are unacquainted with the domains of psychological risk commonly encountered by children in developmental, educational, social,and other fields of behavioral research. The professionals who *can* claim such expertise are researchers themselves, who are for that reason uniquely equipped to foster more creative and thoughtful collegial interaction on ethical research concerns. Instruction on the philosophical and professional ethical obligations of researchers in graduate curricula, discussions of methodological alternatives to prevailing research practices that might unduly stress the children who participate, and constructive critique of existing research protocols can easily be accommodated within this collegial dialogue. Moreover, the constructive contributions of behavioral researchers to the institutional review processes—as consultants and IRB members—might substantially inform this review procedure.

Research is, in many respects, a limited knowledge-gathering tool. It is limited by prevailing methodological alternatives, available data-gathering technology, data-analysis techniques, existing scientific theories, and, of course, the ethics of using humans as research subjects. Yet this final limitation is perhaps the most telling in light of the overarching goal of science to advance human welfare. The limitations that scientists accept on the research enterprise in the interests of safeguarding human rights are descriptive of the values underlying their efforts. When children are research participants, researchers' obligations are especially great.

REFERENCES

Aber, J.L., & Cicchetti, D. (1984). The socioemotional development of maltreated children: An empirical and theoretical analysis. In H.E. Fitzgerald, B.M. Lester, & M.W. Yogman (Eds.), *Theory and research in behavioral pediatrics* (Vol. **2**, pp. 147–205). New York: Plenum.

Bartholome, W.G. (1976). Parents, children, and the moral benefits of research. *Hastings Center Report*, December, 44–45.

Baumrind, D. (1978). Reciprocal rights and responsibilities in parent-child relations. *Journal of Social Issues*, **34**, 179–196.

Campos, J.J., Barrett, K.C., Lamb, M.E., Goldsmith, H.H., & Stenberg, C. (1983). Socioemotional development. In M.M. Haith & J.J. Campos (Eds.), P.H. Mussen (Series Ed.), *Handbook of child psychology: Vol. **2**. Infancy and developmental psychobiology* (pp. 783–915). New York: Wiley.

Cicchetti, D. (in press). The organization and coherence of socioemotional, cognitive, and representational development: Illustrations through a developmental psychopathology perspective on Down syndrome and child maltreatment. In R.A. Thompson (Ed.), *Nebraska symposium on motivation: Vol. **36**. Socioemotional development*. Lincoln: University of Nebraska Press.

Damon, W. (1977). *The social world of the child*. San Francisco. Jossey-Bass.

Damon, W., & Hart, D. (1982). The development of self-understanding from infancy through adolescence. *Child Development*, **53**, 841–864.

Dweck, E.S., & Elliot, E.S. (1983). Achievement motivation. In E.M. Hetherington (Ed.), P.H. Mussen (Series Ed.), *Handbook of child psychology: Vol. **4**. Socialization, personality, and social development* (pp. 643–691). New York: Wiley.

Elkind, D. (1967). Egocentrism in adolescence. *Child Development*, **38**, 1025–1033.

Fisher, C.B., & Rosendahl, S. (in press). Psychological risks and remedies of research partic- ipation. In C.B. Fisher & W.W. Tryon (Eds.), *Ethics in applied developmental psychol- ogy*. Norwood, NJ: Ablex.

Graham, S., Doubleday, C., & Guarino, P.A. (1984). The development of relations between perceived controllability and the emotions of pity, anger, and guilt. *Child Development,* **55,** 561–565.

Grisso, T. (1981). *Juveniles' waiver of rights: Legal and psychological competence.* New York: Plenum.

Harter, S. (1983). Developmental perspectives on the self-system. In E.M. Hetherington (Ed.), P.H. Mussen (Series Ed.), *Handbook of child psychology: Vol.* **4.** *Socialization, personality, and social development* (pp. 275–385). New York: Wiley.

Holder, A.R. (1988). Constraints on experimentation: Protecting children to death. *Yale Law and Policy Review,* **6,** 137–156.

Kant, I. (1785). *Foundations of the metaphysics of morals.* New York: Macmillan, 1959.

Kopp, C.B. (in press). Regulation of distress and negative emotions: A developmental view. *Developmental Psychology.*

Maccoby, E.E. (1983). Social-emotional development and response to stressors. In N. Garmezy & M. Rutter (Eds.), *Stress, coping, and development in children* (pp. 217–234). New York: McGraw-Hill.

MacIntyre, A. (1982). Risk, harm, and benefit assessments as instruments of moral evalua- tion. In T.L. Beauchamp, R.R. Faden, R.J. Wallace, Jr., & L. Walters (Eds.), *Ethical issues in social science research* (pp. 175–189). Baltimore: Johns Hopkins University Press.

Macklin, R. (1982). The problem of adequate disclosure in social science research. In T.L. Beauchamp, R.R. Faden, R.J. Wallace, Jr., & L. Walters (Eds.), *Ethical issues in social science research* (pp. 193–214). Baltimore: Johns Hopkins University Press.

Marcia, J.E. (1980). Identity in adolescence. In J. Adelson (Ed.), *Handbook of adolescent psy- chology* (pp. 159–187). New York: Wiley.

McCormick, R.A. (1974). Proxy consent in the experimental situation. *Perspectives in Biology and Medicine,* **18,** 2–20.

McCormick, R.A. (1976). Experimentation in children: Sharing in sociality. *Hastings Center Report,* December, 41–46.

Melton, G.B. (1983). Minors and privacy: Are legal and psychological concepts compatible? *Nebraska Law Review,* **62,** 455–493.

Melton, G.B. (1987). The clashing of symbols: Prelude to child and family policy. *American Psychologist,* **42,** 345–354.

Nicholls, J.G. (1978). The development of the concepts of effort and ability, perception of aca- demic attainment, and the understanding that difficult tasks require more ability. *Child Development,* **49,** 800–814.

Pence, G.E. (1980). Children's dissent to research—a minor matter? *IRB: A Review of Human Subjects Research,* **2,** 1–4.

Piaget, J. (1965). *The moral judgment of the child* (M. Gabain, Trans.). New York: Free Press. (Original work published 1932)

Ramsay, P. (1970). *The patient as person.* New Haven, CT: Yale University Press.

Ramsay, P. (1976). The enforcement of morals: Nontherapeutic research on children. *Hastings Center Report,* August, 21–30.

Ramsay, P. (1977). Children as research subjects: A reply. *Hastings Center Report,* April, 40–42.

Rheingold, H.L. (1982). Ethics as an integral part of research in child development. In R. Vasta (Ed.), *Strategies and techniques of child study* (pp. 305–324). New York: Academic Press.

Ruble, D.N. (1983). The development of social-comparison processes and their role in achievement-related self-socialization. In E.T. Higgins, D.N. Ruble, & W.W. Hartup (Eds.), *Social cognition and social development* (pp. 143–157). Cambridge University Press.

Shantz, C.U. (1983). Social cognition. In J.H. Flavell & E.M. Markman (Eds.), P.H. Mussen (Series Ed.), *Handbook of child psychology: Vol.* **3.** *Cognitive development* (pp. 495–555). New York: Wiley.

Thompson, R.A. (1987). Development of children's inferences of the emotions of others. *Developmental Psychology,* **23,** 124–131.

Thompson, R.A. (in press). Emotion and self-regulation. In R.A. Thompson (Ed.), *Nebraska symposium on motivation: Vol.* **36.** *Socioemotional development.* Lincoln: University of Nebraska Press.

Thompson, R.A., & Limber, S.P. (in press). "Social anxiety" in infancy: Stranger and separation anxiety. In H. Leitenberg (Ed.), *Handbook of social anxiety.* New York: Plenum.

Warwick, D.P. (1982). Types of harm in social research. In T.L. Beauchamp, R.R. Faden, R.J. Wallace, Jr., & L. Walters (Eds.), *Ethical issues in social science research* (pp. 101–124). Baltimore: Johns Hopkins University Press.

Weithorn, L.A. (1982). Developmental factors and competence to make informed treatment decisions. In G.B. Melton (Ed.), *Legal reforms affecting child and youth services* (pp. 85–100). New York: Haworth.

Weithorn, L.A. (1983). Children's capacities to decide about participation in research. *IRB: A Review of Human Subjects Research,* **5,** 1–5.

Williams, P.C. (1984). Why IRBs falter in reviewing risks and benefits. *IRB: A Review of Human Subjects Research,* **6,** 1–4.

Wolfe, M. (1978). Childhood and privacy. In I. Altman & J.F. Wohlwill (Eds.), *Children and the environment* (pp. 175–222). New York: Plenum.

8

Does Brain Dysfunction Increase Children's Vulnerability to Environmental Stress?

Naomi Breslau

University of Michigan, Ann Arbor

Previous research has shown that children with physical conditions involving the brain are at increased risk for psychopathology. It is unclear whether brain dysfunction leads to disturbance directly or whether it does so by increasing the children's vulnerability to environmental stress. I examined the vulnerability hypothesis in a sample of 157 children with cerebral palsy, myelodysplasia, or multiple handicaps and in 339 randomly selected controls. Data on psychopathology came from direct interviews with the children; data on the family environment came from mothers' reports. Physical disabilities were associated with significant increases in depressive symptoms and inattention. Family environment had a significant main effect on depressive symptoms; effect on disabled children was not significantly different from effect on controls. Family environment had no significant effects on symptoms of inattention in disabled children. The findings provided no support for the hypothesis that brain dysfunction renders children vulnerable to environmental stress.

The effect of environment on psychopathology in children and adults has been consistently observed to vary markedly across individuals. To explain this phenom-

Reprinted with permission from *Archives of General Psychiatry*, 1990, Vol. 47, 15–20. Copyright © 1990 by the American Medical Association.

This investigation was supported in part by grant HD16821 from National Institutes of Health, Bethesda, MD, and Research Scientist Development Award K02MH-00380 from the National Institute of Mental Health, Bethesda, Md.

The helpful comments of Helen Orvaschel, PhD, and Glenn C. Davis, PhD, are gratefully acknowledged.

144

enon, researchers have postulated the people's responses to environmental stressors are contingent on their level of vulnerability.[1-3] According to this explanation, psychopathology results from an interaction of individual predispositions and factors in the social environment. Despite the plausibility of the interaction hypothesis, little empirical evidence has been produced in its support. Although some vulnerability hypotheses, especially those formulated to explain depression, have been the focus of extensive inquiry, conflicting findings have been reported.[4-7] In this study, I examined a variant of the vulnerability model. Specifically, I tested whether brain dysfunction renders children vulnerable to environmental stress.

In 1970, Rutter et al[8] reported that the prevalence of psychiatric disorder in children with physical conditions involving the brain exceeded that in the general population of children by 3.6 times. Because the survey was of a geographically defined population (the Isle of Wight, England), there could be confidence that selection biases that had characterized previous studies of clinical populations did not affect the estimates of psychiatric risk generated in that study. While the coexistence of psychiatric problems in children with neurologic abnormalities had long been observed clinically, the Isle of Wight study clarified the specificity of brain dysfunction as the cause, by demonstrating that rival explanations of the association were unlikely. Most importantly, psychiatric disturbance could not be attributed to adaptational stress arising from the children's physical crippling, as the effect of being physically handicapped appeared to be relatively small. Subsequent studies confirmed these findings.[9-12]

Two general hypotheses about the mechanisms that might explain how brain dysfunction leads to psychiatric disorder have been proposed. The first hypothesis postulated a direct disorganizing effect of brain damage on behavior. The likelihood of psychiatric disorder, according to this hypothesis, is thought to be influenced by characteristics of the lesion, chiefly its locus, severity, or clinical features.[8,13-15] According to the second hypothesis, an increased risk for psychiatric disorder in children with brain dysfunction is thought to result from the children's vulnerability to environmental stress.[8,12,15]

The notion that home and family environmental factors have a significant causal influence on children's psychopathology is a dominant theme in the psychiatric and psychologic literature. Chronic adversities, chiefly marital discord and psychiatric disturbance in a parent, have been found to increase the risk for all types of childhood disorder, ranging from conduct disorder to depression.[16,17] Studies of stressful events, that is, acute rather than ongoing stressors, have also reported increased risks for a variety of psychiatric disorders in children.[18] Recent reviews have underscored the implication of genetic confounding for the reported correlations between family environment and children's behavior. Despite reductions in the correlations when genetic confounding is controlled, the remaining association between environmental factors and behavior suggests that the environment does exert a causal influence on children's behavior, although the size of the influence is considerably smaller.[19] Thus, to the extent that undesirable environments contribute to children's psychopathology, vulnerability to such environmental effects could potentially explain the increased psychiatric risk observed in children with brain abnormality.

To date, the vulnerability hypothesis has not been put to proper empirical test, although findings relevant to it have been presented.[11-13,15] Such a test requires evidence on whether the power of environmental factors to cause psychopathology is greater in children with brain abnormalities than in the general population of children. In statistical terms, support for the vulnerability hypothesis hinges on evidence of a significant interaction effect. The mere observation that brain-damaged children are more likely to develop psychiatric disorders when there is discord in the family or when a parent is mentally ill does not support the vulnerability hypothesis, unless these associations are demonstrated to be significantly stronger than corresponding associations in the general population of children.

In previous reports, I have demonstrated that children with physical conditions involving the brain are at increased psychiatric risk relative to children with physical conditions that do not involve the brain, as well as children who are physically healthy.[9,10] The primary objective of the present study was to investigate whether the effect of the family environment on psychiatric symptoms in children with conditions involving the brain is significantly different from its effect in the general population of children. To address this question, data from two sources were used: those on children's psychopathology were obtained directly from the children, and those on the family environment were obtained from the mothers. Because the two sets of data are operationally uncontaminated, estimates of the associations between factors in the family and child's behavior are unconfounded.

The notion that brain-damaged children are vulnerable to environmental disadvantage was tested in my study as one of several alternative hypotheses about the potential role of the environment in psychiatric sequelae of brain damage. Environmental effects can be conceptualized as taking the following forms: First, an adverse family environment can be hypothesized to be the intervening variable between brain dysfunction and psychopathologic problems: the presence of a disabled child in the home may have determined effects on the family social environment, and the deteriorated family environment, in turn, may contribute to psychopathologic problems in the child. A rationale for this hypothesis is provided by the available evidence that, compared with the general population, mothers of disabled children are more psychologically distressed and are at increased risk for marital dissolution.[20,21] Second, the effects of undesirable family environments can be hypothesized to be modified by (or interact with) the children's brain abnormality. The vulnerability hypothesis, which postulates an exacerbation of environmental effects in brain-damaged children, is one form of this general hypothesis. Third, the effects of adverse environments can be hypothesized to be unrelated to brain dysfunction, exerting the same influence on psychopathology in brain-damaged children as they do in the general population of children, that is, exerting only main effects.

SAMPLE AND METHODS

Samples

Data were obtained from a follow-up study of children with cerebral palsy, myelodysplasia, and multiple physical handicaps, all conditions involving the brain, and from randomly selected controls. (Data on a subset of children with cystic fibrosis, a condition that does not involve brain dysfunction, were not included in this analysis.) The disabled children were patients of pediatric specialty clinics in two teaching hospitals in Cleveland, Ohio, whose caseloads were representative of area children with these conditions. (See previous reports from this study for a fuller description of this sample.)[9,10] Of 351 children 3 to 18 years of age, 292 (83%) complete interviews were obtained at initial assessment, in 1978. For a control group, a three-stage probability sample was used to represent all Cleveland-area children of comparable ages. From 530 children 3 to 18 years of age, 454 (86%) complete interviews were obtained at their initial assessment, in 1979. Five years later, the two samples were reassessed, the disabled children in 1983 and the controls in 1984. At time of follow-up, the sample of 292 children with conditions involving the brain was reduced by death (n = 20) to 240, of whom 229 (95%) were reevaluated. The sample of 454 controls was reduced by relocation to 424, of whom 360 (85%) were reevaluated.

This report is on 157 disabled children and 339 controls, for whom data were available from face-to-face diagnostic interviews. Of the total sample of 229 disabled children for whom follow-up data from mothers were available, information from direct interviews was missing on 72 children, most of whom (n = 62) were unable to be interviewed because of moderate or severe mental retardation secondary to cerebral palsy or multiple physical handicaps.

The sociodemographic characteristics of the samples are depicted in Table 1. The two samples of children were similar in age, sex, and racial compositions. Verbal IQ, measured by the Peabody Picture Vocabulary Test, described below, was markedly lower in the disabled children than in the controls, replicating earlier findings about IQ deficits associated with brain abnormality, even within affected children who are not mentally retarded.[12] Mother's education, an indicator of the families' social class, was somewhat lower in the sample of disabled children than in the controls. The sample of disabled children consisted of 53 children with cerebral palsy, 61 with myelodysplasia, and 43 with multiple handicaps.

Measurement

Interviews were conducted with mothers and children separately in their homes by trained lay interviewers. Data on children's psychiatric symptoms came from direct interviews with the children in which the National Institute of Mental Health-Diagnostic Interview Schedule for Children (DISC) was used.[22] A parallel parent version of the interview—the DISC-Parent—was administered to mothers about their children. The DISC was designed to elicit information necessary to yield DSM-III diagnoses in children. An interview schedule for adults would have been more appropriate for those 18 to 23 years of age, given the conventional boundary between childhood and adulthood in psychiatry. However, the DISC was used on the entire age range to provide uniform data on psychiatric symptoms in the sample. The DISC is a fully structured interview schedule, which specifies the exact wording and sequence of questions and provides a complete set of categories for classifying respondents' answers. The highly structured format is intended to minimize the need for clinical judgment in ascertaining the presence of criterial symptoms and can be used reliably by trained lay interviewers. Test-retest and interrated reliabilities and comparisons with other diagnostic approaches were reported by Orvaschel.[23]

Analysis was performed on psychiatric syndromes as dimensional rather than categorical variables. The selection of a dimensional approach was based on nosologic and statistical considerations. A dimensional approach takes advantage of the general consensus on the type of symptoms that characterize childhood disorders but avoids the disagreements surrounding the precise definition of specific diagnoses.[24] Additionally, statistical analysis of continuous variables has greater power for finding true effects than analysis of dichotomized variables.

Symptom scales were constructed by adding DISC items that inquire about

TABLE 1
Sociodemographic Characteristics of Samples*

Variable	Disabled Children (n = 157)	Controls (n = 339)
Age, y	15.16 ± 4.42	15.51 ± 4.74
Sex, %		
M	49	43
F	51	57
IQ (standardized)	83.22 ± 21.90	99.68 ± 18.09
Race, %		
B	25	29
W	75	71
Mother's education, y	12.0 ± 2.1	12.7 ± 2.1

*Values for age, IQ, and mother's education are expressed as mean ± SD.

criterial symptoms for specific *DSM-III* diagnoses, or clinically defined clusters of symptoms within diagnoses (eg, suicidal cluster in depression).[25] Each item is coded 0 if negative, 1 if probable, and 2 if positive. Thus, a scale's score ranges between 0 and twice the number of items that constitute it. A depression scale, with 38 items, comprised four subscales, each measuring a clinically defined domain: affective (13 items, eg, sadness, anhedonia, worthlessness, self-blame, and irritability), cognitive (6 items, eg, boredom, confusion, and indecision), vegetative (10 items, eg, loss of appetite, sleep disturbance, loss of energy, and weight fluctuations), and suicidal (9 items, eg, hopelessness, thoughts of death, and suicidal thoughts, plans, and attempts). Additionally, analysis covered data on scales measuring overanxious disorder (14 items), separation anxiety (22 items), oppositional disorder (14 items), inattention (7 items), impulsivity (8 items), and hyperactivity (8 items).

The Peabody Picture Vocabulary Test-Revised[26] was administered to all the children. The Peabody Test is a receptive vocabulary test, used widely as a quick estimate of general mental ability or intelligence.[27] In the analysis, standardized Peabody Test scores were employed.

The Family Environment Scale (FES)[28] was used to elicit information from mothers about the social environment in the home and family. The FES consists of 90 true-false questions covering dimensions of family relationship, personal growth, and family organization. The psychometric characteristics of the FES are adequate,[28,29] and the scale is used with increasing frequency in research on the relationship of family environment and psychiatric disorders in children and adults.

The Center for Epidemiologic Studies-Depression Scale[30] was used to measure depressive symptoms in mothers. The Center for Epidemiologic Studies-Depression Scale consists of 20 items selected from existing depression scales, such as the Zung Depression Scale, Beck's Depression Inventory, and the Minnesota Multiphasic Personality Inventory. The scale includes items on depressed mood, feelings of worthlessness, hopelessness, loneliness, loss of appetite, sleep disturbance, concentration problems, and psychomotor retardation. Respondents are asked to rate each symptom on a scale of 0 to 3, according to the frequency with which they experienced the symptom during the past week.

Analysis

To test the research hypotheses, I used hierarchical multiple-regression analysis, designed to estimate and test the significance of main effects and their interaction.[31] The term *interaction* in analysis of variance means a conditional relationship. In this study, the effect of family environment on child psychiatric symptoms are hypothesized to depend on whether the child was disabled. Hierarchical multiple regression provides linear regression results equivalent to the results produced by analysis of variance, except that it permits the analysis of continuous independent variables and can assess exact tests of significance for main and interaction effects, even with unequal cells. The results of three successive regressions are presented in this study. The first estimates the effect of disability on child psychiatric symptoms, controlling for child's age, sex, and IQ. The second adds family cohesion to the equation. The third regression adds the two-way interaction, represented by the product of the two variables (disability multiplied by family cohesion), from which the main effects have been partialled out. The second and third regression together provide the test for the interaction and main effects hypotheses described above.

A comparison of the coefficients of the variable "sample," in the first and second regressions, that is, before and after family cohesion was added, can show whether family cohesion acts as an intervening variable between disability and psychiatric symptoms, as postulated in the first hypothesis. Specifically, evidence that the introduction of family cohesion in the second step obliterates the relationship between disability and psychiatric symptoms, as estimated in the first step, would support the hypothesis that the family environment is an intervening mechanism.

RESULTS

Psychiatric Symptoms in Disabled Children vs. Controls

In Table 2 appear the comparisons of disabled children and controls on symptom scales constructed from children's responses, elicited in interviews using the National Institute of Mental Health-DISC. Disabled children scored higher than controls on all seven symptom scales covered in the study, that is, depression,

TABLE 2
Psychiatric Symptoms Reported by Disabled Children vs. Controls

Symptom Scales	Disabled Children* (n = 157)	Controls* (n = 339)	t
Depression	17.99 ± 9.88	15.54 ± 9.25	2.68†
Overanxious	10.93 ± 6.61	10.94 ± 6.15	0.04
Separation anxiety	8.89 ± 8.61	7.26 ± 6.70	2.16‡
Oppositional	5.04 ± 4.68	4.85 ± 4.54	0.50
Inattention	4.57 ± 3.34	3.32 ± 2.76	4.08§
Impulsivity	2.94 ± 3.00	2.29 ± 2.45	2.35‡
Hyperactivity	2.91 ± 3.06	2.81 ± 3.64	0.34

*Values are expressed as mean ± SD.
†*P*<.007.
‡*P*<.05.
§*P*<.0001.

overanxiousness, separation anxiety, oppositionalism, inattention, impulsivity, and hyperactivity. On two scales, depression and inattention, differences were statistically significant at .007, an α level set to correct for the increased probability that any one of the multiple interrelated comparisons would be significant by chance alone. On two other scales, those measuring symptoms of separation anxiety and impulsivity, differences between the samples revealed a trend toward significance (.007<*P*<.05). The association between type of physical condition and psychiatric symptoms was examined by a series of analyses of variance. Differences across cerebral palsy, myelodysplasia, and multiple handicaps were not statistically significant in any symptom domain. Similar findings were reported earlier from comparisons of mothers' reports of children's symptoms.[9,10]

Further analysis, depicted in Table 3, showed that the excess in depressive symptoms in disabled children was accounted for chiefly by the more common reports of cognitive and suicidal symptoms in disabled children compared with controls. Differences in the affective and vegetative symptom clusters were small and not significant.

I tested whether the effects of disability on psychopathologic problems varied significantly between two age categories, 8 to 17 years vs 18 to 23 years. No significant interaction between age and disability was detected. The power to find a significant interaction at *P*<.05 was .81 for an effect size of 1.6% or greater. Subsequent analyses were performed on the entire sample.

Family Environment and Psychiatric Symptoms

I turned next to examine the effects of factors in the family environment on psychiatric symptoms and to test the hypotheses outlined above. The analysis focuses on depression and inattention, the two domains in which children with physical conditions involving the brain manifested significant excess symptoms. Children's ages, sex, and IQ were included in the analysis to control for their effects, so that more

TABLE 3
Depression Subscores in Disabled Children vs. Controls*

Subscales	Disabled Children (n = 157)	Controls (n = 339)	*t*
Affective	8.56 ± 4.60	8.02 ± 3.96	1.25
Cognitive	3.19 ± 2.41	2.53 ± 2.13	3.07†
Vegetative	3.95 ± 3.43	3.42 ± 3.28	1.78
Suicidal	2.11 ± 2.99	1.36 ± 2.44	2.76†

*Values are expressed as mean ± SD.
†*P*<.005.

accurate estimates could be made of the effects of the independent variables of interest, namely, brain dysfunction and family environment.

To select empirically the most efficient combination of family measures, stepwise multiple-regression analysis was used. The strategy was used to maximize the statistical power of the multivariate analysis by limiting the total number of independent variables.[32] The data used in this analysis were mothers' reports on the FES subscales that measure family cohesion, family conflict, family repertoire of social-recreational and cultural activities, and maternal depressive symptoms (Center for Epidemiologic Studies-Depression Scale). Family cohesion, a subscale of the FES, was the best environmental predictor of children's self-reported symptoms and, after cohesion was selected in the stepwise multiple regression, none of the other family measures added a significant increment to explained variance in children's symptoms. I also tested whether family factors other than cohesion (although insignificant in explaining symptoms across the combined sample) had differential effects on disabled children and controls. The results showed that, controlling for family cohesion and its interaction with child disability, interactions of other family factors were not significant. Family cohesion was used, therefore, in the analysis below as an indicator of the family social environment. Mean scores ($\pm$SD) on the family cohesion subscale in the sample of disabled children was similar to that of the controls (7.38 ± 1.66 vs 7.54 ± 1.69, respectively; not significant).

Depression. In Table 4 appear successive results from the hierarchical multiple-regression analysis of depressive symptoms, using the combined sample of disabled children and controls. In the first column it can be seen that when age, sex, and IQ were controlled, brain dysfunction, represented by the variable "sample" (coded as 1 if the child were disabled and 0 if the child were in the control group), was associated with a significant excess in depression score. Age had a significant association with depression, whereas child's sex and IQ were unrelated to symptoms in this

TABLE 4
Hierarchical Multiple Regression for Depression*

	1	2	3
Sample (disabled children vs controls)	2.262†(0.955)	2.176†(0.932)	2.086 (3.977)
Age, y	0.438†(0.090)	0.426†(0.088)	0.426†(0.087)
Sex (0 M, 1 F)	1.231 (0.835)	1.418 (0.816)	1.417 (0.818)
IQ (standardized)	−0.023 (0.020)	−0.017 (0.020)	−0.017 (0.020)
Family cohesion	. . .	−1.217†(0.241)	−1.220†(0.291)
Sample × cohesion	. . .	. . .	0.012 (0.521)
R^2	.07	.12	.12

*Values are unstandardized regression coefficients, with SEs in parentheses.
†The coefficient exceeds twice its SE.

domain. An examination of the second column shows that family cohesion had a significant inverse association with depressive symptoms and increased by 5% the total explained variance. The introduction of family cohesion did not obliterate, or even reduce materially, the association between brain dysfunction and depression: the coefficient of the variable "sample" remained significant and nearly unchanged, 2.26 vs. 2.18, before and after family cohesion was introduced, respectively. Thus, the hypothesis that the family social environment is an intervening variable between brain dysfunction and psychiatric symptoms received no support in these data.

The interaction hypothesis was tested by adding in the third step a product termed sample × cohesion. The results, which appear in the third column, provide no support for this hypothesis because the interaction term was not significant. The amount of variance explained by the interaction was less than 1%. In other words, the effect of cohesion on depression in disabled children was not significantly stronger (or weaker) than its effect in physically healthy controls. Because the interaction term was not significant, it can be concluded that the model presented in the second regression fits the data best. Estimates of the additive effects of disability and family cohesion are provided in that regression. Depressive symptoms were influenced by brain dysfunction as well as by family environment, each contributing its own share of risk independently of the other. Thus, disabled children in adverse family environments (ie, low cohesion) were subject to the additive risk of both factors, whereas those in beneficial family environments (ie, high cohesion) were at risk only by virtue of their brain dysfunction. (Note that the results of the third regression should not be interpreted as evidence that the effect of child disability, as represented by the variable "sample," was in any way no longer significant. The figure associated with the variable sample in these results is an estimate of the regression slope of depression on the variable sample at a point where family cohesion is equal to 0, because

TABLE 5
Hierarchical Multiple Regression for Inattention*

	1	2	3
Sample (disabled children vs controls)	0.733†(0.300)	0.718†(0.298)	−1.887 (1.266)
Age, y	−0.034 (0.028)	−0.036 (0.028)	−0.036 (0.028)
Sex (0 M, 1 F)	−0.896†(0.262)	−0.865†(0.261)	−0.895†(0.261)
IQ (standardized)	−0.027†(0.006)	−0.026†(0.006)	−0.025†(0.006)
Family cohesion	. . .	−0.202†(0.077)	−0.312†(0.092)
Sample × cohesion	. . .	. . .	0.351†(0.165)
R^2	.09	.10	.11

*Values are unstandardized regression coefficients, with SEs in parentheses.
†The coefficient exceeds twice its SE.

the effect of changes in the slope associated with varying levels of cohesion was partialled out by the inclusion of the interaction term.)

Inattention. The analysis of symptoms of inattention is presented in Table. 5. As can be seen in the first column, brain dysfunction significantly increased symptoms of inattention when age, sex, and IQ were controlled. IQ had a significant inverse association with inattention, and female subjects had significantly fewer symptoms than male subjects. Findings pertinent to the hypothesis that family environment is an intervening variable between disability and symptoms of inattention appear in the second column. As in the depression results, there is no support for this hypothesis. The introduction of family cohesion into the analysis did not cause the association between child disability and inattention to vanish or even diminish.

The third column shows the results on the interaction hypothesis. In contrast to the depression results, these results show a significant interaction between disability and family cohesion. However, they show that disability did not amplify the power of family environment to cause symptoms but rather that it attenuated it. Specifically, the regression of inattention on cohesion in the controls, as estimated by the coefficient of the variable cohesion after the interaction term was partialled out, is equal to − .312 (that is, a point of increase in cohesion is associated with a drop of .312 in inattention score). The regression of inattention on cohesion in the disabled sample can be estimated by the sum of the coefficients of cohesion (− .312) and the interaction term (.351), which measures the difference in the effect of cohesion between the two samples. The sum of the two coefficients is near 0(.039). Thus, although the results show a significant interaction, they provide no support for the vulnerability hypothesis. The findings provide evidence for the opposite case, that is, that with respect to symptoms of inattention, children with brain dysfunction were less vulnerable to environmental effects than other children.

COMMENT

Analysis of data from direct interviews with disabled children and randomly selected controls revealed the following: (1) Physical disabilities involving brain dysfunction were associated with significant increases in symptoms in two domains: depression and inattention. (2) Although inattention was related to IQ, the association with brain dysfunction remained significant even when the effect of IQ was partialled out. (3) Depressive symptoms were associated also with an adverse family environment (low cohesion). Brain dysfunction and family environment did not interact in their effect on depressive symptoms. Their effects were additive. (4) Brain dysfunction and family environment interacted in their effect on inattention. However, compared with other children, children with brain dysfunction were not more, but rather were less, vulnerable to family environmental stress. (5) Family environment was not an intervening mechanism between brain dysfunction and either depression or inattention.

The interpretation of the results should take into account the exclusive reliance on mothers' and children's reports for the measurement of key variables, namely, family environment and children's psychiatric symptoms. Observational data on family environment and clinical evaluations of children's psychiatric symptoms would have strengthened my confidence in the findings. It should be noted that inferences are limited to psychopathology defined dimensionally rather than as discrete diagnoses. Although both sets of symptoms are criterial features of specific psychiatric disorders, neither depressive symptoms nor symptoms of inattention can be directly translated into psychiatric diagnoses. Because children with mental retardation were not interviewed, the generalizability of the data is limited to those children who were not retarded. Additional analysis of data gathered from mothers on the National Institute of Mental Health-DISC-Parent version suggests that brain-injured children who were mentally retarded manifested more externalizing symptoms of oppositionalism, hyperactivity, and impulsivity than brain-injured children whose intellectual abilities were within the normal range. No differences emerged, however, in mothers' reports of symptoms of inattention.

Several important strengths of this study deserve mention. This study used a large sample of children with conditions involving brain dysfunction, who were unselected for psychiatric sequelae, and geographically based probability sample of the general population of children. The validity of the results is enhanced by the high follow-up rate, which is a condition necessary for maintaining the initial representativeness of the sample. Data on children's psychopathology were obtained directly from the children, whereas those on the family environment were elicited from mothers. Consequently, any correlation between children's psychopathology and the social environment is free of the confounding introduced when a common source of information is used. Most importantly, the statistical technique used in this analysis is appropriate for testing interactions.[32] Previous studies that reported findings about associations between psychopathology and environmental stressors in brain-injured children did not test whether the effect of the environment on psychopathology in these children was significantly different from its effect in the general population.

The results of this analysis provide no support for the hypothesis that the high risk for psychopathology associated with brain dysfunction is due to the children's vulnerability to stress. When family environment was found to be related to psychiatric symptoms in these children, the effect was additive. In this respect, the findings are in accord with recent reports on another type of interaction between ostensibly stable personal characteristics and the environment, that is, between temperament and the family social environment as they affect behavior problems in children.[33] One example of this hypothesis is the proposition that "difficult" children are more sensitive to the adverse effect of unstable family environments than other children. Until recently, the temperament-environment interaction hypothesis had not been rigorously tested.[32] Plomin and DeFries[29] have recently published detailed results on tests of temperament-environment interactions, using hierarchical multiple-regression analysis, a statistical technique used in the present study. They found no evidence to support the hypothesis that children with difficult temperaments are more vulnerable to adverse environments.

Children with brain dysfunction in this study reported excess symptoms in two domains: depression and inattention. Low family cohesion had no effect on their symptoms of inattention but increased their symptoms of depression. Being disabled as well as having low family cohesion, each independent of the other, contributed a significant increment to the overall level of a child's depressive symptoms. These observations suggested that depressive symptoms in these children might be an instance of psychologic distress, seen in persons who are exposed to a variety of stressors, including social devaluation and other negative experiences associated with being chronically ill or handicapped,[34-36] as well as general environmental adversities, such as family discord. In contrast, symptoms of inattention might be linked in these children more distinctly to their brain abnormalities. Additional support for this interpretation comes from previously reported data from this study, which indicated that children with cystic fibrosis, a condition that does not involve the brain, manifested more depressive symptoms than controls, but not more symptoms of inattention.[37] In sum, psychiatric sequelae of physical conditions that involve the brain might be of two types: reactions to adversities associated with physical handicap and symptoms that result directly from damage to the brain.

The results of this analysis suggest a reformulation of the interaction hypothesis. With respect to psychiatric sequelae of a distinctly organic origin, the effect of the social environment might be attenuated rather than exacerbated. Severe brain dysfunction might insulate children from the effects of the social environment, whereas moderate or mild brain dysfunction might leave children more permeable to environmental effects. It should, however, be emphasized that, in important respects, children with brain dysfunctions are not unlike the general population of children. Specifically, their dysphoric reactions to being physically handicapped; and living in adverse family environments are similar to those of children whose brain functions are unaffected by physical disease.

The lack of support for the hypothesis that brain-damaged children are vulnerable to environmental stress calls for a reassessment of research findings that had served as the scientific background for the hypothesis. Researchers had observed the following: (1) Despite their markedly increased risk for disorder, only a minority of brain-damaged children are psychiatrically disturbed. (2) With few exceptions, there is no specific pattern of psychopathology associated with brain damage. (3) The "dose-response" relationship between brain damage and psychopathology is relatively weak and inconsistent. (4) Factors other than the characteristics of the brain lesion, primarily factors in the family environment, appear to influence the likelihood of psychiatric sequelae. Taken together, these observations were interpreted as evidence that the causal association between brain damage and psychiatric disorder in children is indirect, rather than direct,[11] and led investigators to ask whether brain damage lowers children's threshold of vulnerability to adverse environments.[13] A reassessment of these findings must take into account our limited knowledge of general brain-behavior relationships, especially knowledge concerning structural organizations that govern affect and drives. Additionally, direct connections between characteristics of brain lesions and behavioral aberrations might have been obscured by the inadequacy of methods used for detecting and diagnosing damage to the brain. Recent advances in brain mapping technologies might shed new light on these questions. Other mechanisms that might explain psychiatric sequelae of brain damage include cognitive impairments other than a lowered general intelligence, as well as the brain-damaged child's lowered threshold for genetically heritable psychiatric symptoms and disorders.

REFERENCES

1. Brown GW, Harris TO. *Social Origins of Depression: A Study of Psychiatric Disorder in Women*. New York, NY: Free Press; 1978.
2. Seligman MEP, Peterson C. A learned helplessness perspective on childhood depression: theory and research. In: Rutter M, Izard CE, Read PB, eds. *Depression in Young People: Developmental and Clinical Perspectives*. New York, NY: Guilford Press; 1986:223–249.
3. Rutter M. Stress, coping, and development: some issues and some questions. In: Garmezy N, Rutter M, eds. *Stress, Coping and Development in Children*. New York, NY: McGraw-Hill International Book Co; 1983: chap 1.
4. Brown GW, Harris T. Stressor, vulnerability and depression: a question of replication. *Psychol Med*. 1986;16:739–744.
5. Costello CG, Social factors associated with depression: a retrospective community study. *Psychol Med*. 1982:12:329–339.
6. Solomon Z, Bromet E. The role of social factors in affective disorder: an assessment of the vulnerability model of Brown and his colleagues. *Psychol Med*. 1982;12:123–130.
7. Tennant C, Bebbington P. The social causation of depression: a critique of the work of Brown and his colleagues. *Psychol Med*. 1978;8:565–575.
8. Rutter M, Tizard J, Whitmore K. *Education, Health and Behavior*. London, England: Longman Group Ltd; 1970.
9. Breslau N. Psychiatric disorder in children with physical disabilities. *J Am Acad Child Psychiatry*. 1985;24:87–94.
10. Breslau N, Marshall IA. Psychological disturbance in children with physical disabilities: continuity and change in a 5-year follow-up. *J. Abnorm Child Psychol*. 1985:13:199–216.

11. Brown G, Chadwick O, Shaffer D, Rutter M, Traub M.A prospective study of children with head injuries, III: psychiatric sequelae. *Psychol Med.* 1981;11:63–78.

12. Seidel U, Chadwick O, Rutter M. Psychological disorders in crippled children: a comparative study of children with and without brain damage. *Dev Med Child Neurol.* 1975:17:563–573.

13. Shaffer D, Chadwick O, Rutter M. Psychiatric outcome of localized head injury in children. In: Porter R. FitzSimons DW, eds. *Outcome of Severe Damage to the Central Nervous System.* Amsterdam, the Netherlands: Elsevier Science Publishers; 1975;191–214.

14. Sollee NN, Kindlon DJ. Lateralized brain injury and behavior problems in children. *J. Abnorm Child Psychol.* 1987;15:479–491.

15. Rutter M. Brain damage syndrome in childhood: concepts and findings *J Child Psychol Psychiatry.* 1977;18:1–21.

16. Robins LN. Sturdy childhood predictors of adult antisocial behavior: replications from longitudinal studies. *Psychol Med.* 1978;8:611–622.

17. Rutter M. *Children of Sick Parents: An Environmental and Psychiatric Study.* New York, NY: Oxford University Press; 1966.

18. Goodyer IM, Kolvin I, Gatzains S. The impact of recent undesirable life events on psychiatric disorders in childhood and adolescence. *Br J Psychiatry.* 1987;151:179–184.

19. Sines JO. Influence of the home and family environment on childhood dysfunction. In: Lahey BB, Kazdin AE, eds. *Advances in Clinical Child Psychology.* New York, NY: Plenum Publishing Corp; 1978;10:1–54.

20. Breslau N, Davis GC. Chronic stress and major depression. *Arch Gen Psychiatry.* 1986;43:309–314.

21. Jessop DJ, Riessman CK, Stein REK. Chronic childhood illness and maternal mental health. *J Dev Behav Pediatr.* 1988;9:147–156.

22. Costello AJ, Edelbrock C, Dulcan MK, Kalas R, Klaric SH. *Development and Testing of the NIMH Diagnostic Interview Schedule for Children in a Clinic Population.* Rockville, MD: Center for Epidemiologic Studies, National Institute of Mental Health; 1984.

23. Orvaschel H. Psychiatric interviews suitable for use in research with children and adolescents. *Psychopharmacol Bull.* 1986;21:737–745.

24. Rutter M, Shafer D. DSM-III: a step forward or back in terms of the classification of child psychiatric disorders? *J Am Acad Child Psychiatry.* 1980;19:371–394.

25. Edelbrock C, Costello AJ, Dulcan MK, Kalas R. Conover NC. Age differences in the reliability of the psychiatric interview of the child. *Child Dev.* 1985;56:265–275.

26. Dunn LM, Dunn LM. PPVT, *Peabody Picture Vocabulary Test-Revised.* Minneapolis, Minn: American Guidance Service; 1981.

27. Robertson GJ, Eisenberg JL. Technical supplement. In: Dunn LM, Dunn LM. PPVT, *Peabody Picture Vocabulary Test-Revised.* Minneapolis, Minn: American Guidance Service; 1981.

28. Moss RH, Moss BS. *Family Environment Manual.* Palo Alto, Calif: Consulting Psychologists Press; 1981.

29. Plomin R, DeFries JC. *Origins of Individual Differences in Infancy: The Colorado Adoption Project.* Orlando, Fla: Academic Press Inc; 1985.

30. Radloff LS. The CES-D scale: a self-report depression scale for research in the general population. *Appl Psychol Measurement.* 1977;1:385–401.

31. Cohen J, Cohen P. *Applied Multiple Regression/Correlation Analysis For the Behavioral Sciences.* 2nd ed. Hillsdale, NJ: Lawrence Erlbaum Associates Inc Publishers; 1983.

32. Plomin R, Daniels D. The interaction between temperament and environment: methodological considerations. *Merrill Palmer Q.* 1984;30:149–162.

33. Thomas A, Chess S. *Temperament and Development.* New York, NY: Brunner/Mazel Inc; 1977.

34. Akiskal HS. Dysthymic disorder. psychopathology of proposed chronic depressive subtypes. *Am J Psychiatry.* 1983;140:11–20.

35. Cassileth BR, Lusk EJ, Strouse TB, Miller D, Brown L, Cross P, Tengalia AN. Psychosocial status in chronic illness: a comparative analysis of six diagnostic groups. *N. Engl J Med.* 1984;311:506–511.

36. Wells KB, Golding JM, Burnam MA. Psychiatric disorder in a sample of the general population with and without chronic medical conditions. *Am J Psychiatry.* 1988;145:976–981.

37. Breslau N. Chronic physical illness. In: Burrows GS, ed. *Handbook of Studies in Child Psychiatry.* New York, NY: Elsevier Science Publishing Co. Inc; 1989.

9

Long-Term Effects of Food Supplementation and Psychosocial Intervention on the Physical Growth of Colombian Infants at Risk of Malnutrition

Charles M. Super, M. Guillermo Herrera, and José O. Mora
Harvard School of Public Health

Colombian infants at risk of malnutrition were randomly assigned to 1 of 4 experimental groups formed by the presence/absence of 2 interventions: (1) food supplementation for the entire family, from mid-pregnancy until the target child was 3 years old, and (2) a twice-weekly home-visiting program to promote cognitive development, from birth until age 3. All families received free medical care and were studied prospectively. At 3 years of age, children who had received food supplementation averaged 2.6 cm and 642 grams larger than controls. Home visiting and supplementation together reduced the number of children with severe growth retardation. 3 years after intervention (age 6), supplementation effects remained. Children in the home visit condition had become larger than controls, by 1.7 cm and 448 grams. The interactive effect to reduce stunting was marginally significant at this age, and the overall distribution of scores was improved. Other results suggest that changes in family functioning as well as biological mechanisms account for the observed pattern of results.

Reprinted with permission from *Child Development*, 1990, Vol. 61, 29–49. Copyright © 1990 by the Society for Social Research in Child Development, Inc.

The work reported here was funded in part by the National Institute of Child Health and Human Development (grant no. HD06774); the Ford Foundation; the Colombian Institute of Family Welfare; and the Fund for Research and Teaching, Department of Nutrition, Harvard School of Public Health. All statements made and opinions expressed are the sole responsibility of the authors.

Research over the past few decades on malnutrition in children has been dominated by three issues: (1) How much of the complex syndrome of "malnutrition"—operationally defined as reduced growth—is a direct effect of the biological deficits in energy and protein intake, and how much is caused by coincident morbidity and deficits in the psychosocial environment of the family and community? (2) To what degree are the effects of undernutrition early in life irreversible, that is, is there a "critical" or "sensitive period" during which the child is especially vulnerable to loss of potential for growth? (3) Is the simple provision of foodstuffs an effective, and cost-effective, intervention to reduce the incidence of malnutrition and its sequelae? These three questions are intricately related, and they have posed complex problems in the design and execution of field-based research and policy evaluation (see Beaton & Ghassemi, 1982; Brozek & Schurch, 1984; Joos & Pollitt, 1984; Martorell, Lechtig, Yarbrough, Delgado, & Klein, 1976).

Until the late 1960s, the major strategy for field research on these questions was to compare retrospectively the development of malnourished and control infants, but this approach entailed considerable difficulties in matching the two groups on economic and social background (e.g., Cravioto, Birch, De Licardie, Rosales, & Vega, 1969). Large-scale projects were undertaken in the late 1960s and early 1970s to address these problems, but they too experienced self-selection by subjects, differences in baseline measures, and complications in defining the exact nature of the interventions (Chavez, Martinez, & Yachine, 1975; Gopalan, Swaminathan, Kumari, Rao, & Vijayaraghavan, 1973; Graves, 1976; Taylor, Kielmann, De Sweemer, & Uberoi, 1978).

Among those concerned with social policy and direct intervention, the exact allocation of cause has often seemed less important than finding ways to interrupt the process of malnutrition, for the human problem is immense. It has been estimated that 100 million, or 18%, of the world's children are malnourished (De Maeyer, 1976). In poor countries, where large portions of the population are malnourished, the formation of human capital and ultimately the course of national development are thought to be impeded by the consequences in health and learning (Horton, 1984; Townsend, 1984). The most straightforward intervention—providing food—has entailed enormous costs and administrative difficulties, and the actual gains in growth, when evaluated, have proven modest at best (Beaton & Ghassemi, 1982; Joos & Pollitt, 1984; Martorell et al., 1976).

The Bogotá Study of Malnutrition, Diarrheal Disease, and Child Development is a quasi-experimental field project started in 1973 in Bogotá, Colombia, as a collaborative effort by the Harvard School of Public Health Department of Nutrition and the Colombian Institute of Family Welfare. The two interventions reported on here, which were carried out from the last trimester of pregnancy to age 36 months, were designed to evaluate simultaneously the independent effects of food supplementation and of psychosocial stimulation on subsequent growth and development, as well as to address policy questions of cost-effective intervention. The present report focuses on physical growth as an outcome, updating earlier analyses of growth through the end of the interventions at 3 years of age (Mora, Herrera, Suescun, de Navarro, & Wagner, 1981; Mora, Sellers, Suescun, & Herrera, 1981), and adding new data on the long-term growth effects in the subsequent 3 years. Additional dietary and family functioning data are also reported here in order to explore one explanation of unanticipated growth results. Reports of other outcomes and analyses of individual variation in responsiveness have been presented elsewhere or are in process (Christiansen, 1984; Christiansen, Mora, de Navarro, & Herrera, 1980; Christiansen et al., 1977; Herrera et al., 1980; Herrera, Mora, de Paredes, & Wagner, 1979; Herrera, Super, & Mora, 1989; Lutter et al., 1989; Mora, Clement, Christiansen, Suescun, Wagner, & Herrera, 1978; Mora, de Navarro, Clement, Wagner, de Paredes & Herrera, 1978; Mora et al., 1979; Mora, Herrera, Sellers, & Ortíz, 1981; Overholt, Sellers, Mora, de Paredes, & Herrera, 1982; Sellers, Mora, Super, & Herrera, 1982; Super et al., 1981; Super, Herrera, & Mora, 1987a, 1987b; Super, Sellers, Mora, de Paredes, & Herrera, 1989; Vuori et al., 1979, 1980; Waber et al., 1981).

METHOD

Sample

Subjects of the study came from poor neighborhoods in southern Bogotá. Families were located by door-to-door surveys of the target neighborhoods. To be selected for the study the mother had to be in the first or second trimester of pregnancy, with at least one living child, and at least half of her living children under age 5 years had to be below 85% in weight for age of the corresponding age- and sex-specific Colombian standards (Reuda-Williamson, Luna-Jaspe, Ariza, Pardo, & Mora, 1969), thus selecting for high risk of malnutrition for the study child. In addition, it was required that the subject's father be coresident. Four successive waves of surveys, at 6-month intervals starting in 1974, were used to locate 552 families meeting these criteria.

Treatment

All families were provided free obstetric and pediatric health care. This was done in order to assure access to medical services and thus minimize variance in this regard, to obtain health information on the pregnant mother and infant under study, and to provide an incentive for families to remain in the study.

Two interventions were undertaken to alter food availability at the household level and to increase environmental stimulation for the target child's cognitive growth, independently of other factors. They were (1) food supplementation for the entire family, and (2) a program of home visits by "facilitators" trained in a curriculum for promoting early cognitive development.

The nutrition intervention. Food supplements were provided in amounts sufficient to close the gap between baseline dietary intake (as established by survey) and the Colombian recommended dietary allowance for each member of the family over 1 year of age (Ariza, 1967). Supplements were in the form of familiar foods: enriched bread, powdered skim milk, and vegetable cooking oil for all family members over 1 year of age, and whole powdered milk and a commercial high-protein vegetable mixture ("Duryea") for children from 3 months (or at weaning if earlier) to 12 months (see Table 1). In addition, vitamin and mineral tablets were given to the mothers supplemented during pregnancy, and ferrous sulfate and vitamin A were given daily to supplemented children until 12 months of age, semi-annually from 1 to 3 years. Further detail on the supplements can be found in Herrera et al. (1980).

The supplements were distributed weekly to the families at special centers resembling neighborhood shops for consumption at home. A nutritionist taught mothers how to prepare the dry milk, and emphasis was given to the hygienic handling and storage of foodstuffs. Practical demonstrations were given frequently and were followed up with visits to the home. Families were instructed to continue eating their usual diet in addition to the supplement. This family-based intervention constituted an experimental manipulation of risk factors for the target children, with the ultimate goal of increasing their protein, calorie, and other nutrient intake. Most simply, therefore, the outcome constitutes an evaluation of a food supplementation program. We have presented elsewhere evidence from 24-hour recall assessments that nutrient intake was higher in the supplemented group than among controls (Mora, de Navarro et al., 1978). It is logical to attribute group differences in consumption to

TABLE 1
Nutrient Composition of the Supplementation

Source	Grams Supplied	Calories (no.)	Protein (g)	Fat (g)
Each family member:				
Dry skim milk	60	214	21.6	.6
Enriched bread	75	233	8.4	2.6
Vegetable oil	20	176	0	20.0
Total		623	30.0	23.2
Additional for mother:				
Enriched bread	75	233	8.4	2.6
Total for mother	. . .	856	38.4	25.8

NOTE.—Values for micronutrients are given in Herrera et al. (1980).

the experimental intervention, and increments in growth at least in part to improved nutrition.

The home visiting intervention. One goal of the early education program carried out during home visits was to stimulate learning and development of the target child through direct intervention by a trained home visitor. This was a means of pursuing a second, more important goal: to modify caretaker-child interaction such that stimulation would become self-sustaining in the absence of intervention personnel. During the first 3 years of life, the child's family was visited twice weekly by a specially trained paraprofessional home visitor (a secondary school graduate with experience in teaching) who interacted with the child and the principal caretaker. Individual treatments were deliberately varied in response to the mother's style and initial understanding.

The intervention was guided by a substantial body of research and theory on parent education and was based on close collaboration with the High/Scope project in Ypsilanti, Michigan. Their curriculum (Lambie, Bond, & Weikart, 1974) was followed, with suitable modifications for the Colombian sample. A written plan was prepared by the home visitor in advance of each household visit, and for every hour of subject contact there was an hour of supervision by a program coordinator to ensure uniformity of progress toward a common and clearly conceptualized goal. Although the curriculum included suggested activities appropriate to different developmental stages that were intended to extend and reinforce certain behaviors, the program did not restrict its focus to training in specific skills. General problem-solving abilities were emphasized. The home visitor served not only as educational specialist but also as a flexible and sensitive observer who assumed specific interactive and supportive roles in order to help further the child's development. Nevertheless, every effort was made to limit the content of interactions to the domain of cognitive functioning in the target child (and any siblings present). The curriculum contained no instruction on nutrition, hygiene, or other health-related topics, and any questions in this regard were referred to the project health team, who were available to all participants. We have analyzed the nature of the interactions between the home visitors and the mothers, and have demonstrated at the group level changes in family interaction patterns that are in accord with the goals of the intervention: for example, tutored mothers were more playful with and responsive to their babies (Super et al., 1981).

Design

Families were assigned to one of six experimental groups, as listed below.

Group A, nonintervened control. These families received only obstetric and pediatric care, but they participated in all scheduled evaluations.

Group B, late supplementation. These families received food supplementation from the time the target child was 6 months old until he or she reached 36 months.

Group C, early supplementation. These families received the standard supplements from the time of enrollment during pregnancy until the child was 6 months old. Groups B and C were included to evaluate the effect variation in the timing of supplementation, and their results are reported elsewhere (Herrera et al., 1989).

Group D, full supplementation. These families were given supplementation for the full period of intervention, from week 26 of pregnancy until 36 months of age.

Group A1, home visit. Mothers in this group received intensive tutoring by a home visitor in order to increase the level of cognitive and social stimulation directed toward the target child. There was no food supplementation.

Group D1, full supplementation and home visit. These families received both types of intervention from enrollment until age 36 months.

The experimental groups can be combined in several ways for analytical purposes. The analysis here contrasts, in a 2 × 2 analysis of variance design, groups A and A1 (without food supplementation) to D and D1 (supplemented), and also A and D (without home visits) to A1 and D1 (with visits). Thus the present report forms a simple two-factor randomized trial, each factor contrasting a treatment and a no-treatment control group. (In most analyses, sex was also included as a third factor in the ANOVA, yielding a 2 × 2 × 2 design.)

Assignment to groups was random, with two types of exceptions. First, in order to avoid contamination of treatments across experimental group, households in the same city block were assigned as a unit. This procedure might in theory decrease the variance within groups, but the analysis of background measures described below suggests that the bias, if any, was of marginal importance.

Second, assignment to experimental group was not equally probable within the four waves of recruitment. Because the home visit intervention was conceived and introduced only after the first two waves had been recruited, only children from the last two waves were assigned to groups A1 and D1. In addition, logistical issues delayed the implementation of food distribution procedures, briefly postponing assignment to groups D and D1 (and C, not reported here). Hence, children in group A were born, on average, 5 months earlier than those in group D, and nearly 10 months earlier than those in A1 and D1. To the degree, therefore, that secular trends existed in any of the phenomena studied, the home visit comparison could be influenced by factors other than the experimental manipulation. It is known, for example, that economic inflation was rapid during this time, requiring adjustments to monetary-based measures (e.g., income). In addition, the four waves of recruitment covered contiguous but distinct neighborhoods, and subtle neighborhood differences could in theory contaminate the experimental paradigm. Analyses described below were undertaken to evaluate the results of the secular and geographic biases in group assignment.

Longitudinal Evaluations

The children and families were monitored at regular intervals. Standard anthropometric techniques (Jelliffe, 1966) were used to assess height (or length, for infants under 2 years), weight, head circumference, and triceps skinfold of the study child at birth and at 18 subsequent ages, ending at 73 months (6 years). All measures were taken by the same team of experienced anthropometrists. Because there was some variation in actual age at the time of measurement, recorded values for height/length and weight were converted to age-appropriate z scores by use of computer software distributed by the Centers for Disease Control (Jordan & Staehling, 1986), using standards compiled by the National Center for Health Statistics (U.S. Public Health Service, 1976). Our earlier reports (Mora, Herrera, Suescun et al., 1981; Mora, Sellers et al., 1981) did not include this refinement, and adjusted values at 3 years are presented here.

Maternal anthropometry was monitored at several points, but only baseline measures (at 26 weeks gestation) are used here in order to avoid contamination by intervention effects (see Table 2).

Standardized maternal interviews conducted by a Colombian field worker provided broad information about family life and household facilities at the beginning of the study (26 weeks of pregnancy), near the time of birth of the study child, and at several points thereafter. The interview items were designed to sample domains known to be related to variation in child growth and development, specifically, family demographic characteristics, household sanitation, economic status and functioning, child-rearing attitudes and practices, parental education and literacy, and social supports and stressors. From the dozens of derived measures available, the 34 listed in Table 2 were selected for use as background variables in the present analysis on the basis of satisfactory statistical properties, representation of these conceptual domains, and minimal redundancy. Unless otherwise noted, they were taken from baseline visits before the birth of the target child.

Dietary intake for all members of the household was estimated at several points in time through an interview with the mother that covered the previous 24-hour period (see Lechtig, Yarbrough, Martorell, Delgado, & Klein, 1976). Estimates were converted to energy and protein values by use of appropriate food-composition tables, and the results were compared to the recommended Colombian standards. Only data when the target child was 6 years old are presented here, but previous reports document differences in nutrient intake for mothers and target children in the supplemented groups compared to those in the nonsupplemented groups (Mora, de Navarro, et al., 1978; Mora, de Paredes et al., 1979; Sellers et al., 1982).

TABLE 2
Background Measures

1. *Mother's age* in years
2. *Mother's education* in years of schooling
3. *Mother's literacy* as demonstrated by a short reading test
4. *Mother's years of residence in Bogotá* (categorized to obtain adequate distribution)
5. *Father's age* in years
6. *Father's education* in years of schooling
7. *Father's literacy* as demonstrated by a short reading test
8. *Father's years of residence in Bogotá* (categorized to obtain adequate distribution)
9. *Second caretaker*: the availability, or not, of a secondary caretaker in the household, for example, an older sister or aunt
10. *Number of siblings*: total number of mother's living offspring prior to the study child's birth
11. *Number of household members*: total number of family members living in the household
12. *Marital status*: maternal coresidence with husband, when the target child was born
13. *Income*: total household income in constant Colombian pesos ($1 US = $25 Colombian, adjusted to January 1973 to control for inflation)
14. *Possessions*: an index of wealth constructed by counting the presence of seven items: radio, television, clock, door with lock, closet, dining table, more than one bed
15. *Floor area* of the living quarters, in square meters
16. *Number of rooms* in the living quarters
17. *Sanitary facilities*: a count of six household sanitary facilities present, such as running water and indoor plumbing for waste
18. *Neighbor's help*: mother's report of feeling that she had neighbors or kin nearby that she could rely on when necessary
19. *Friends nearby*: mother's rating of how many friends lived close by
20. *Social contacts*: the number of recent visits between the mother and friends, neighbors, and kin (raw counts were categorized to obtain adequate distribution)
21. *Mother's life dissatisfaction*: mothers' responses to two questions that tap dissatisfied or depressed feelings: "In recent weeks have you felt dissatisfied or bored (*aburrida*) at times?" and "Would you like your life to continue as it is, or change considerably?"
22. *Mother's marital dissatisfaction* as expressed to the interviewer
23. *Orderliness* of the household, as rated by home visitor
24. *Mother smokes* cigarettes (4-point scale)
25. *This pregnancy interval*: the time in months between the birth of the target child and the adjacent elder sibling
26. *Average pregnancy interval*: the average interbirth interval, in months
27. *Number of previous pregnancies*
28. *Number of mother's children who died* after live birth
29. *Number of miscarriages*
30. *Mother's height*
31. *Mother's weight*
32. *Mother's weight/height*
33. *Mother's triceps skinfold*
34. *Mother's head circumference*

Subject Loss

Twenty-five and 45% of the cases were not available for anthropometric assessment at ages 3 and 6 years; respectively. Although the remaining numbers are adequate in their own right, the possibility of differential loss in the experimental groups prompted the following analyses. First, subject loss itself was analyzed with the $2 \times 2 \times 2$ design, using logistic regression instead of ANOVA, in light of the dichotomous dependent variable (0/1, for subject loss). No group effects on loss were found. Second, subject loss was correlated with the 34 baseline measures listed in Table 2. Loss was found to be nonrandom with regard to several background factors. Third, these correlations were repeated within the two contrasting groups across each factor (supplementation and home visits) and the results were examined for differences. Variables that appeared to correlate differently with subject loss in the two groups were selected for use in a stepwise logistic regression. In this procedure, a new score was constructed to represent each variable's interaction with the intervention term; that is, the individual's score on the predictor variable was multiplied by 0 or 1 depending on whether or not the family received the intervention. The predictor variables and their interaction scores were all included in the pool of independent variables in a stepwise logistic procedure to predict subject loss. Stepping was continued until the residual chi-square became insignificant ($p > .05$). Variables whose intervention-interaction terms were significant ($p \leq .05$) in predicting subject loss would then be available as covariate controls in the analyses of physical growth. In the end, however, no evidence of significant differential subject loss was found.

RESULTS

Baseline Conditions

The social environment in the neighborhoods (*barrios*) of southern Bogotá included features of poverty, overcrowding, and poor sanitation found in many urban populations that have grown rapidly with the influx of rural migrants. Two-thirds of the study families lived in simple shacks, usually with limited access to running water and hygienic waste disposal. The remaining third of the families lived in rented rooms in small buildings where they shared the water and cooking facilities with others. Mean family size in the subset of families reported here was 5.4 at the outset of the study (SD = 2.0), of whom 2.9 were children. Mothers averaged 26.5 years in age (SD = 6.4) and had an average of 3.6 years of schooling (SD = 2.8). Male heads of household, typically 28.1 years old (SD = 6.1), had an average of 4.5 years in school (SD = 3.3). Their most frequent occupations were as day laborer in construction and painting, shoe repair, factory work, and taxi driver, but job stability was low and unemployment was high. The average monthly income per capita was approximately US $9.07 (in 1973 dollars), with an average of 70% of it spent on food. Around these typical values there was considerable variation. There were a few families living in two-or three-bedroom homes, and where the father had stable employment; there were also families in which neither parent had ever been to school and the per capita income was less than US $3 per month.

The dietary survey at the beginning of the study (26 weeks of pregnancy) confirmed the low energy intake and substandard nutritional quality of the diets (see Mora, de Navarro et al., 1978, for more detail): maternal energy intake averaged 82 percent of recommended levels (1,568 kcal daily) and protein intake averaged 80% (367 grams daily).

Bias in Group Assignment

Analysis of the groups at enrollment in the study indicates overall comparability, with a few noteworthy exceptions. Of the 34 baseline variables listed in Table 2, 23 showed no significant ($p < .05$) "effects" (i.e., assignment bias) of supplementation, home visiting, or sex in analysis of variance, either alone or in interaction with each other. Three variables yielded a significant interaction term of sex with home visiting (father's years in Bogotá and number of household members) or supplementation (sanitary facilities). These were presumably chance occurrences since sex of the study child was not known at the time of group assignment. The remaining eight background measures differed significantly between intervention groups. Home-visited families lived in slightly larger dwellings, as indexed by floor area, $F(1,270) = 13.45, p = .003$, and had more material possessions, $F(1,270) = 5.38, p = .02$, than those that were not visited. There was also a significant interaction of supplementation with home visiting in income, such that the nonintervened group (A) had unexpectedly high income, $F(1,218) = 3.90, p = .05$. We believe these differences are true reflections of the neighborhoods represented in the home visit intervention. Other findings have less obvious interpretations. Supplemented children had fewer siblings (2.7 vs. 3.2, $F[1,270] = 6.46, p = .01$) and shorter maternal residence in Bogotá, $F(1,270) = 7.47, p = .01$, than unsupplemented ones. Home-visited mothers were more depressed (maternal life dissatisfaction) at the onset of the study, $F(1,270) = 4.40, p = .04$, than their controls. In addition to these contrasts in sociodemographic conditions, there were two significant differences in maternal anthropometry. Mothers in the home-visited condition had less body fat (smaller triceps skinfold) than their comparison group (13.5 vs. 14.7 mm, $F[1,266] = 6.33, p = .01$), and those who were to receive supplementation had marginally larger head circumference (before supplementation) than those who were not (53.2 cm vs. 52.8 cm, $F[1,213] = 3.71, p = .06$).

With the exception of housing and material possessions, we believe all the observed differences to be chance occurrences and without general import for the interpretation of results. As specific differences, however, they could distort the interpretation of outcome if they differentially mediated the effects of the interventions. With this in mind, all the parametric analyses below have been computed with seven covariate adjustments: mother's years in Bogotá, number of siblings, mother's life dissatisfaction, family possessions, floor area of house, mother's head circumference, and mother's triceps skinfold. This procedure is conservative in the sense of potentially underestimating true effects of the interventions: any variance shared with the interventions is automatically assigned to the covariates. On the other hand, reducing variance that is uniquely associated with the background measures only makes more obvious any variation independently effected by the interventions. Thus the covariate adjustments could in principle either damage or enhance the identification of true experimental effects. In the end, as indicated below, the covariate adjustments for assignment bias did not alter the major conclusions.

Subject Loss

Ninety-six (17%) of the 552 qualifying families never entered the study: 39 migrated from the area, 34 pregnancies were aborted, and 23 families declined to participate. Of the 456 enrolled subjects, 280 were assigned to the four groups presented here; 209 of these, or 75%, were available for anthropometric measurement at age 3 years, the conclusion of the intervention phase. Fifty-five had moved and were lost to the project, 12 refused further cooperation, one had died, and three remained in the study but were not available for these particular procedures. In addition, 19 cases were omitted from covariate analysis (Table 4) because they lacked one or more of the background measures.

Baseline correlates of subject loss indicate an association with smaller, poorer, and more isolated families. These correlations are reliable (generally $p = .05$) but are of low power ($r = .15$). While noting these relations is important for specifying the subsample reported on, they do not by themselves affect the experimental rigor of the study if subject loss is equally distributed across groups.

In order to evaluate the possibility of unequal subject loss between intervention groups, dummy (0/1) variables were constructed to represent absence/presence of anthropometry measurement at ages 36 and 73 months. A logistic regression was carried out on the results, using dummy variables to imitate the supplementation $\times$ home visiting $\times$ sex model in the analyses of variance. The overall model approached statistical significance, $\chi^2(7) = 13.54$, $p = .06$, but no individual effect or interaction was even marginally significant.

A second analysis was undertaken to explore the possibility that the correlates of dropout might differ slightly across groups: The dummy variable for subject loss was correlated with the 34 background measures listed in Table 2, separately for each level of supplementation and for each level of home visiting. There are, in fact, a few noticeable differences in the correlations between intervention groups. They are generally not statistically reliable but are large enough (e.g., $r = .36$ vs. .15) to warrant care in the final analyses, for what amounts to an interaction of group assignment and characteristics of dropout would destroy the experimental logic. It could lead, for example, to the available data sets for supplemented and unsupplemented children to differ also in parental education.

For subject loss at 3 years with regard to supplementation, only two variables were judged potentially relevant (i.e., differences in the intervention-group correlations greater than .20): mother's life dissatisfaction and the previous pregnancy interval. However, in a stepwise logistic regression containing these two measures and their interaction terms with the intervention, none of the interaction terms (nor the background measures) proved significantly related to subject loss. For the home visit intervention, father's age, mother's age, income, number of previous pregnancies, and number of miscarriages (and their interactions with the home visiting) were used for the stepwise logistic regression. Again, no interaction term (nor background measure) was able to be entered into the model (alpha was set to .05).

At 6 years of age, 153 (55%) of the subjects were available for anthropometric measurement. Thirteen of these lacked background measures for covariate analysis. Again logistic regression indicated no effect of supplementation, home visit, sex, or their interactions on subject loss. Baseline correlates of dropout at 73 months suggest that we disproportionally lost smaller, younger, and more isolated families, as well as those with higher education—essentially the same picture as 3 years earlier. The correlations are about the same size and significance as at 3 years.

Once again, visual inspection suggested that the correlates of dropout might differ across groups, at about the same level as at 3 years of age. The same procedure was followed to identify potential confounding variables (in interaction with the interventions) and to test their significance with stepwise logistic regression. For subject loss with regard to supplementation, eight variables had correlations that differed between intervention groups by more than .20 and thus were used in the stepwise regression along with their interaction terms: father's years in Bogotá, mother's social contacts, number of family members, number of siblings, mother's age, father's age, household possessions, and friends nearby. Although household possessions, mother's age, and mother's social contacts proved significantly related to subject loss ($p = .007, .004,$ and .022, respectively), none of them had significant interactions with supplementation in predicting subject loss. For the home visit intervention, family possessions, father's age, mother's age, and number of rooms were used in the stepwise logistic regression. Mother's age and household possessions were significantly related to subject loss ($p = .003$ and .004), but no background measure interacted with home visiting in predicting subject loss.

In summary, extensive analyses failed to produce evidence of significant differential subject loss between experimental groups at either age period. The final samples, however, are not fully representative of the poorer, smaller, younger, and more isolated families in the original baseline sample. Because the interventions might be most powerful for such relatively needy families, one can speculate that the obtained results slightly underestimate what would have been found without the subject losses.

Anthropometry at Three Years

Average scores of the four groups (and combined into the two interventions) at age 3 years are presented in Table 3; these results include the covariate adjustments described above. Differences from the results of unadjusted analyses are trivial and in almost all cases are restricted to the last reported decimal place of the z score. The results of analysis of variance, with the covariate adjustments, are presented in Table 4; reanalysis without adjustments yields essentially the same conclusions, but in most cases with lower levels of significance.

Comparison with our earlier published results for height and weight, which did not adjust for variation in age or for assignment bias, reveals a few minor differences, but the conclusions are essentially the same: Supplementation significantly increased height and weight, by 2.6 cm and 642 grams, respectively. In addition, the effect of supplementation on head circumference was marginally significant, and there was no effect on skinfold thickness or weight for height. Home visits had no effect by themselves, but one can see in the group means a small interaction with supplementation to produce especially large results in the group that received both interventions; in contrast to our earlier analysis, however, the ANOVA interaction term does not reach the .05 level of statistical significance. Home visiting is associated with lesser skinfold thickness at a marginal level of significance, which might simply reflect the already cited difference in maternal anthropometry. Aside from the sex difference in head circumference and skinfold (the values for which were not adjusted through comparison with sex-specific standards), the only other noteworthy result is a three-way interaction effect on head circumference, reflecting unexpectedly large values for girls who received home visits but not supplementation. We can find no meaningful interpretation for this result.

Of more importance than shifts in the group average is what happens at the lower tail of the distribution, that is, among those children who were not only small, but so small as to indicate severe curtailing of growth. Each of the three measures used here, adjusted for age and sex, has a different meaning in this regard. Extremely short stature (stunting) reflects a long-term growth deficiency, as might be caused by chronic malnutrition; extremely low weight might only reflect the same linear growth retardation revealed in short stature, or it could indicate acute malnutrition;

Continued p. 175

TABLE 3
Group Statistics at 3 Years

Group	n	Weight		Height		Wt/Ht	Head Circumference	Skinfold
		kg	z	cm	z	z	(mm)	(mm)
A (control)	59	11.890	−1.62	85.4	−2.40	−.20	46.7	9.3
D (supplemented)	58	12.260	−1.38	87.5	−1.85	−.31	47.1	9.1
A1 (home visited)	32	11.702	−1.75	85.3	−2.43	−.37	46.8	8.9
D1 (both)	41	12.615	−1.16	88.5	−1.57	−.19	47.1	8.5
D + D1 (supplemented)	99	12.438	−1.27	88.0	−1.71	−.25	47.1	8.8
A + A1 (not supplemented)	91	11.796	−1.68	85.4	−2.41	−.30	46.8	9.1
A1 + D1 (home visited)	100	12.156	−1.45	86.9	−2.00	−.28	46.9	8.7
A + D (not home visited)	90	12.075	−1.50	86.5	−2.13	−.27	46.9	9.2

TABLE 4
ANOVA Results at 3 Years (Covariance Adjusted for Assignment Bias)

Variable	Weight for Age (z)		Height for Age (z)		Weight for Height (z)		Head Circumference		Skinfold Thickness	
	F	p	F	p	F	p	F	p	F	p
Supplementation	11.87	.001	21.89	.000	.23	.631	2.76	.099	1.57	.213
Home visiting	.19	.667	.67	.415	.01	.927	.10	.753	3.10	.080
Sex	2.16	.144	.10	.753	.47	.496	28.39	.000	.11	.742
Supplementation × home visit	2.26	.135	1.22	.271	1.61	.207	.02	.895	.18	.671
Supplementation × sex	.04	.841	.00	.956	.14	.712	.05	.830	.13	.723
Home visit × sex	.91	.343	.60	.439	.47	.496	1.43	.233	.07	.796
Supplementation × home visit × sex	.03	.865	.00	.965	.02	.888	6.80	.010	3.98	.048
Mother's years in Bogotá	.57	.452	1.99	.160	.20	.658	.36	.548	2.07	.152
Number of siblings	5.22	.024	7.32	.008	.57	.450	.48	.490	.89	.347
Mother's life dissatisfaction	2.39	.124	.94	.334	1.42	.234	.23	.634	1.88	.172
Floor area of house	.77	.380	1.67	.198	.01	.926	1.03	.312	.25	.619
Family possessions	4.39	.038	12.32	.001	.10	.749	2.09	.150	.81	.370
Mother's head circumference	11.10	.001	2.12	.147	12.47	.001	23.34	.000	2.39	.125
Mother's skinfold thickness	.30	.582	.12	.727	1.71	.192	.68	.410	.00	.961

Note.—$df = 1/175$, except for skinfold thickness, $df = 1/173$.

weight for height helps differentiate these two possibilities and indicates how well proportioned the child is, regardless of absolute size (for a more detailed discussion see Waterlow, 1977, or World Health Organization, 1983). The criterion of severe growth retardation used here, for each of the three anthropometric measures, was a z score less than -2 (i.e., the child's score would fall in the lowest 2.3% of the reference population).

Unlike the situation for the parametric analyses of z scores above, where shifts in the mean resulting from covariate adjustment were of no importance, analysis of the lower tail would be distorted by adjustments that alter the percent of children with $z < -2$. Therefore, the present analysis does not include the covariate adjustments for assignment bias; in light of the small differences found in the two versions of the analyses of variance, this omission is judged to be of minor importance.

A logistic regression with a dummy variable for $z < -2$ or $z \geq -2$ was used to mimic the $2 \times 2 \times 2$ ANOVA. For weight for age at 3 years, 54 of the 209 cases had z scores below -2. Because of several cells with very low expected frequencies, however, the initial analysis did not arrive at satisfactory mathematical convergence (even with tolerance set to .01). A second analysis was then conducted without sex or any interaction terms involving sex. Because the scores are adjusted for sex in the use of reference standards, and because sex had no overall effect in the analysis of variance, this procedure carries little risk of yielding distorted conclusions. Table 5 presents the derivatives for the independent variables and their associated probability statistics. The overall model for weight for age is highly significant, $\chi^2(3) = 21.69$, $p < .01$, and the interaction term of supplementation $\times$ home visiting is significant in its own right. As indicated by the derivative values, receiving both interventions, compared to receiving neither, shifts the probability of having a z score for weight < -2 by .45. The actual percents are 34 for 1, for neither and both interventions, respectively.

One hundred two of the 3-year-olds had a height-for-age score less than -2, compared to 107 with scores above this. Although the full $2 \times 2 \times 2$ model for dichot-

TABLE 5
Analysis of Severe Growth Retardation at 3 Years

Variables	t	p	Derivative
Weight for age:			
Supplementation	$-.879$	.38	$-.054$
Home visiting	.096	.92	.007
Supplementation $\times$ home visit	-2.439	.02	$-.450$
Height for age:			
Supplementation	-1.982	.04	$-.175$
Home visiting	.344	.73	.038
Supplementation $\times$ home visit	-1.726	.09	$-.267$

omized height for age did converge successfully, only a two-factor analysis parallel to that for weight is presented (in this case, sex and its interactions were seen to have no effect before reducing the number of independent variables). Again, the overall model is highly significant, $\chi^2(3) = 19.34, p < .01$. Supplementation significantly reduces the probability of stunting (a shift of .18), but more power lies in the supplementation $\times$ home visit interaction (a shift of .27, but only marginally significant): the percent of children who are stunted is 61 without any intervention, and 23 with both interventions.

There were no children who were severely underweight for their height.

A reduction in extremely poor growth scores could result from two separate mechanisms. If the interventions simply moved the entire distribution upward to the higher mean, this shift upward would naturally carry with it the lower tail, thereby reducing the number of children, with z scores under -2. The preceding analysis, in this case, would be only a second way of seeing the same effect revealed in the parametric analyses. Alternatively (or in addition), the actual shape of the distribution of scores could be changed by the interventions, with the lower tail extending less far or being less densely populated. Evidence in support of this possibility is provided by both statistical and graphical analysis.

For the statistical evaluation, the two distributions (with and without intervention) were first standardized to equal means and variances. The control distribution (A) was then categorized into tenths, the frequencies of which served as expected values for the experimental distribution, tabulated into the same categories. Goodness-of-fit of the two distributions was calculated following the procedure outlined by Edwards (1964, pp. 384–387).

For all three outcomes (weight, height, and weight for height), the shape of the distribution of supplemented children (group D) is significantly different from that of the controls: for weight, $\chi^2(7) = 30.96, p < .01$; for height, $\chi^2(7) = 28.68, p < .01$; for weight for height, $\chi^2(7) = 25.87, p < .01$. Figure 1, a quantile-quantile plot (Gnanadesikan, 1977) for height for age, illustrates that the source of difference lies in the tails: without supplementation, the lower tail is elongated and more dense, while with supplementation the upper end of the distribution is more full. Were the two distributions similarly shaped, points in the quantile-quantile plot would fall approximately along a straight line (the regression line is drawn in Fig. 1 for visual comparison). At 36 months of age, therefore, supplementation not only shifts the entire population upward in height (see the ANOVA means), but it also minimizes the stunting effect (analysis of $z < -2$), even relative to its own mean (this analysis). Similarly, supplementation encourages positive deviations even when the overall variance is equated. The quantile-quantile plots for weight for age and weight for height reveal similar effects, although in the latter case the pattern is less regular. In both the ANOVA and the analysis of extreme growth retardation, the influence of home visiting is significant only in interaction with supplementation. In the present analysis of the overall distribution, home visiting is seen to be effective in its own right. Figure 2 presents the quantile-quantile plot of height for age in group A versus group A1, and it is evident that the same phenomenon occurs as with supplementation alone. The effect is statistically significant for height: for weight, $\chi^2(7) = 13.04$, $p = .07$; for height, $\chi^2(7) = 40.40$, $p < .01$; for weight and height, $\chi^2(7) = 6.6$, $p = .39$.

The powerful interaction effect found in the earlier analysis is also present here, and Figure 3, comparing the distributions of group A versus group D1, provides the clearest picture of all the intervention effects, with the lower tail extended in the control group and the upper tail extended and fuller for those who received both supplementation and home visiting. Goodness-of-fit testing indicates that the differences are reliable for all three measures, although the pattern of effect is less easily summarized for body proportion: for weight, $\chi^2(7) = 28.51$, $p < .01$; for height, $\chi^2(7) = 19.14$, $p < .01$; for weight and height, $\chi^2(7) = 29.40$, $p < .01$.

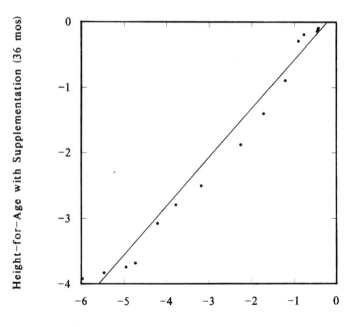

Height-for-Age without Supplementation (36 mos)

Figure 1. Quantile-quantile plot of height for age at 36 months, with and without supplementation

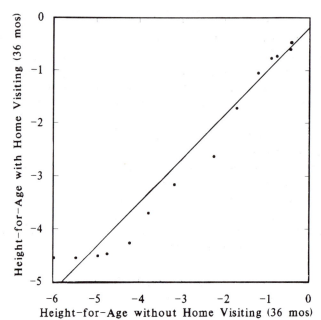

Figure 2. Quantile-quantile plot of height for age at 36 months, with and without home visiting.

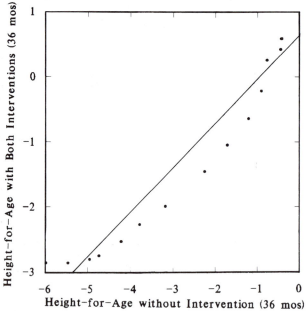

Figure 3. Quantile-quantile plot of height for age at 36 months, without intervention and with both interventions.

Anthropometry at Six Years

At 6 years, the supplemented children had essentially retained their absolute advantage in height and weight, now 2.3 cm and 536 grams (see Table 6), and the effect remained statistically significant (marginally so for weight, see Table 7). At this point, however, 3 years after termination of the interventions, children who had been visited at home were also larger than controls, by 1.7 cm and 448 grams (Table 6). The effect for height is significant (Table 7). Reanalysis of the same subgroup of children at age 3 years does not reveal any significant effects of home visit at that age. Hence the effect at 6 years cannot be attributed to differences in the subsamples used. There were no intervention effects on head circumference and skinfold, except for the same three-way interaction for head circumference cited at 3 years.

Table 8 reveals that the earlier effects of intervention in reducing extreme growth retardation persist only weakly at age 6 years. Neither of the factors nor their interaction reliably effects a reduction in extremely low weight, but supplementation and its interaction with home visiting reduce the incidence of stunting at a marginal level of significance. With neither intervention, 55% of the children were stunted in their growth, compared to 17% of those who received both supplementation and home visiting.

As at 36 months, quantile-quantile plots and goodness-of-fit tests were used to examine the shape of distribution of scores with and without intervention. The effects of either supplementation or home visiting alone at 73 months were found to be similar to those 3 years earlier, but weaker; only the effect on height is significant for supplementation, $\chi^2(7) = 15.94, p = .03$; for weight, $\chi^2(7) = 10.79; p = .15$; for weight for height, $\chi^2(7) = 12.75, p = .08$. For home visiting, differences in the distribution of both linear measures are marginally significant: for weight, $\chi^2(7) = 12.90, p = .08$; for height, $\chi^2(7) = 12.37, p = .09$; for weight for height, $\chi^2(7) = 9.41, p = 9.41, p = .22$. When both interventions were applied, however, the differences in distribution (again, most evident at the tails) are significant for the two linear measures: for weight, $\chi^2(7) = 28.02, p < .01$; for height, $\chi^2(7) = 24.38, p < .01$; for weight for height, $\chi^2(7) = 4.95, p = .64$.

Summary of Growth Effects

Although there are minor differences in the conclusions from the three major approaches to analysis of growth effects, the pattern of results is cohesive. Table 9 presents a summary of the statistical significance of the three procedures (ANOVA, logistic regression for z score < -2, and chi-square comparison of the shape of distributions) for the two major outcomes, height for age and weight for age. Both interventions, especially in interaction, reduced the frequency of low growth scores at both the end of the interventions and 3 years later. The average score was signifi-

TABLE 6
Group Statistics at 6 Years

Group	n	Weight		Height		Wt/Ht	Head Circumference	Skinfold
		kg	z	cm	z	z	(mm)	(mm)
A (control) 40		17.124	−1.46	105.1	−2.34	−.04	49.0	9.1
D (supplemented) 42		17.649	−1.20	107.7	−1.74	−.14	49.2	9.1
A1 (home visited) 23		17.561	−1.25	107.1	−1.90	−.06	49.0	9.7
D1 (both) 35		18.108	−1.04	109.2	−1.48	−.12	49.4	9.1
D + D1 (supplemented) 77		17.878	−1.12	108.4	−1.61	−.13	49.3	9.1
A + A1 (not supplemented) 63		17.342	−1.35	106.1	−2.12	−.01	49.1	9.4
A1 + D1 (home visited) 58		17.834	−1.15	108.1	−1.69	−.09	49.2	9.4
A + D (not home visited) 82		17.386	−1.33	106.4	−2.04	−.05	49.1	9.1

TABLE 7
ANOVA Results at 6 Years
(Covariance Adjusted for Assignment Bias)

Variable	Weight for Age (z)		Height for Age (z)		Weight for Height (z)		Head Circumference		Skinfold Thickness	
	F	p	F	p	F	p	F	p	F	p
Supplementation	3.34	.070	11.22	.001	.95	.332	1.70	.194	.67	.413
Home visiting	2.09	.151	5.39	.022	.13	.720	.02	.902	.60	.440
Sex	2.36	.127	2.51	.116	.44	.506	20.33	.000	10.71	.001
Supplementation × home visit	.04	.842	.38	.541	.24	.626	.24	.628	1.18	.280
Supplementation × sex	.00	.957	.01	.934	.09	.770	.00	.951	.48	.488
Home visit × sex	.05	.829	.06	.800	.27	.607	.02	.903	.24	.625
Supplementation × home visit × sex	.23	.635	.09	.770	.13	.720	3.68	.057	.40	.530
Mother's years in Bogotá	1.56	.214	2.33	.129	.01	.911	.03	.862	.61	.435
Number of siblings	1.14	.287	3.37	.069	.09	.760	1.76	.188	.01	.905
Mother's life dissatisfaction	.04	.847	.19	.667	.43	.511	.74	.392	.03	.855
Floor area of house	.07	.790	.09	.768	.56	.456	1.33	.251	.74	.391
Family possessions	.70	.406	4.38	.038	1.03	.312	2.70	.103	1.03	.311
Mother's head circumference	10.47	.002	4.22	.042	5.93	.016	15.56	.000	.16	.686
Mother's skinfold thickness	.03	.872	.27	.606	.09	.766	.75	.388	.51	.476

NOTE.—$df = 1/125$.

cantly greater with supplementation at both ages; with home visiting, the group mean was greater only at the older age.

Diet at Six Years

To what degree are the long-term growth effects a reflection of lasting differences in dietary intake? A three-way ANOVA (supplementation × home visiting × sex) at age 6, 3 years after interventions had ended, indicates that children in the home-visited groups had higher levels of protein intake than did their controls: they averaged 103% of the Colombian recommended daily allowance for protein (RDA), compared to 88%, $F(1,160) = 5.82$, $p = .02$. For calories, the effect (67% vs. 62%) was not significant. No differences were found for the average per capita level of adequacy in the family as a whole, suggesting channeling of protein to the target child. Further analysis of the difference between the family and target child's adequacy measures confirms this suggestion: Home visiting (compared to no home visiting) produced a difference of +9% versus –1% RDA advantage to the target child in protein intake, $F(1,159) = 8.57$, $p = .004$. This effect remained essentially unchanged when the assignment bias covariate adjustments were made. The difference in protein intake was not simply the result of larger children demanding more to eat, since supplemented children showed the same degree of growth advantage at age 6 years as did the children in the home-visited families, but the channeling effect was absent, $F(1,159) = 0.29$, $p = .59$. Channeling of calories was in the same direction but not significant (–11% vs. –8% RDA, home visited vs. control, $F[1,159] = 2.37, p = .13$). Home visit effects on dietary intake at age 3 in the same subsample were in the same direction as these results, but not statistically significant.

TABLE 8
Analysis of Severe Growth Retardation at 6 Years

Variables	t	p	Derivative
Weight for age:			
Supplementation	−1.222	.21	−.072
Home visiting	−.919	.35	−.065
Supplementation × home visit	−.963	.34	−.136
Height for age:			
Supplementation	−1.765	.08	−.180
Home visiting	.382	.71	.046
Supplementation × home visit	−1.667	.11	−.297

Paternal Involvement

The preceding results, especially the unexpected effect of home visiting on dietary intake, prompted a review of available measures of family functioning. Beyond those reported by Christiansen (1984) concerning changes in contraceptive use and alcohol consumption, it was found here that home visiting increased paternal involvement with the target child. In the vast majority of cases, the mother or sister accompanied the target children to the laboratory during testing and measurement sessions. In up to a dozen cases at any age, however, it was the father who brought in the child. These cases were predominantly in the home visiting group. Fisher's Exact Test was used to test each of the interventions at each age (logistic regression was precluded by so many expected values of 0), and only home visiting was found to affect the probability of paternal escort. This effect is first evident at 18 months ($p = .08$) and was significant at 24 ($p = .01$) and 36 months ($p = .03$). The effect had dissipated by 54 and 67 months, the only later ages at which this measure is available.

DISCUSSION

The persistent effect of supplementation 3 years after termination of the interventions is impressive. It is consistent in size with the results seen at age 3, and somewhat larger than results from other studies, as might be expected from the quantity, duration, and local familiarity of the supplementation (Edozien, Switzer, & Bijan, 1979; Gopalan et al., 1973; Joos & Pollitt, 1984; Martorell, Klein, & Delgado,

TABLE 9
Summary of Significance of Major Intervention Effects on Weight for Age
and Height for Age

	ANOVA		$z < -2$		SHAPE	
	wt	ht	wt	ht	wt	ht
At 36 months:						
Supplementation	.00	.00	.38	.04	<.01	<.01
Home visiting	.67	.42	.92	.73	.07	<.01
Supplementation × home visit	.13	.27	.02	.09	<.01	<.01
At 73 months:						
Supplementation	.07	.00	.21	.08	.15	.03
Home visiting	.15	.02	.35	.71	.08	.09
Supplementation × home visit	.84	.54	.34	.11	<.01	<.01

1980; Rao & Nadamuni, 1977; Taylor et al., 1978). The human significance of the average gains produced by the food supplements—2.3 cm and 536 grams—is small. In contrast, the effect of supplementation in interaction with home visiting is more considerable: at 6 years of age, a full 3 years after cessation of the intervention, more than half of the nonintervened children were stunted in their growth, compared to less than 20% of the previously supplemented and visited children. A similar effect of approximately the same magnitude, not previously identified due to differences in data treatment, is now found at 3 years. The stability of this effect over 3 years without further interventions suggests the possibility that the gains may be preserved into adolescence. By this measure, therefore, the supplementation intervention, in conjunction with home visiting, achieved results that could be of major public health significance.

The effects of home visits on physical growth are more surprising and somewhat different. Although we have now identified at 3 years a reduction in the incidence of growth retardation similar to though somewhat smaller than that for supplementation, it remains true that home visits did not affect the typical pattern of growth by the time of termination of direct intervention. There was an effect on the overall distribution of scores, however, with the lower tail of the distribution proving more sparse. Three years later, more direct effects are visible: The children whose mothers had been given tutoring in cognitive and social stimulation showed an average growth advantage over controls about three-quarters as great as those whose families had been given food. The synergistic effect of home visiting and food supplementation together in reducing the incidence of severe growth retardation is of theoretical and programmatic importance. The fact that the home visit effects increased over time, most evidently after interventions terminated, suggests that the mechanism of causation became established either in the child or the ecology, that is, the causal mechanisms had been created and instituted rather than merely supplied contemporaneously by the intervention.

Other studies have found similar patterns of delayed treatment effects (see Clarke & Clarke, 1981, and Seitz, 1981, for a related discussion). Follow-up evaluations of 11 early interventions in the United States, based on curricula related to the one used here, found that program children were more successful in school and showed greater orientation toward education and achievement than controls; similarly, the mothers of program children had higher educational and vocational goals (Lazar & Darlington, 1982). The best documented evidence in those studies concerns what are presumed to be internal characteristics of the individual, namely, IQ and attitudes. One can speculate that the present home visit intervention resulted in more active and more confident children who were more aggressive in locating and exploiting resources for growth.

The U.S. studies have relatively little information on family processes but offer interesting hints concerning, for example, maternal aspirations. The dietary data presented here are strongly suggestive of changes in family functioning that would favor increased growth of the study child. The increase in paternal involvement, at least in the one available measure of public escort, supports this interpretation, as do previously published findings that home visiting increased the use of contraceptive practices by the mothers and decreased reported alcohol abuse by the fathers (Christiansen, 1984). During the period of active intervention, the home visitors reported a variety of anecdotes indicating increased maternal enthusiasm for the child's early development and greater paternal involvement (e.g., returning home early from work to be present for the home visits). Although the home visit intervention did not include any programmatic material on health of nutrition, it seems likely that the study child's overall development would gain increased salience in the family and that increased resources, social and economic, might follow. Synergistic effects of a changing child and reoriented environment would be consistent with current theories of environmental regulation of developmental processes and the conviction that the appropriate unit of analysis is the child in context (e.g., Harkness & Super, in press; Kessen, 1979; Sameroff & Chandler, 1975; Super & Harkness, 1986).

The pattern of growth seen in both experimental and control groups—short and light but not, on average, emaciated children—is the pattern commonly found in populations suffering chronic undernutrition (Anderson, 1979; Keller, Donoso, & De Maeyer, 1976; Martorell et al., 1980). We have reported earlier that children in the present study passed through a period of moderate relative emaciation during the second year of life, but that following that phase their overall growth had become adapted to the level of resources available in the environment: they became short in stature and low in weight, but appropriately proportioned in weight for height (Mora, Herrera, Suescun et al., 1981). Clearly this adaptation has generally persisted through age 6. It is noteworthy, however, that even children in the most favored groups average one or more standard deviations below the reference population in size. The more general power of poverty, intergenerational effects on body size, and genetic factors may all contribute to this.

The near randomization of assignment and specificity of interventions in the Bogotá study are unusual among large-scale field studies. Possible shortcomings caused by temporal and geographic bias, and other compromises in design (e.g., it was not "double blind"), appear to be minimal and within reasonable control. As a consequence, the results reported here provide unusually robust answers to the guiding questions. Food supplementation in the opening years of life, in connection with uniform medical care, can have significant and lasting effects on body size, presumably through biological influence at a sensitive period of growth. Of particular importance is the large reduction in the number of cases of severe growth retardation. In addition, the "sleeper effect" of the home visit intervention on growth suggests other mechanisms of influence, namely, through family function as directed by parental understanding of or attention to development. The enmeshment of malnutrition-related growth retardation in a web of biosocial factors exacerbates the problems of isolating its causes and consequences, but it also provides a variety of opportunities for lasting intervention.

REFERENCES

Anderson, M. A. (1979). Comparison of anthropometric measures of nutritional status in preschool children in five developing countries. *American Journal of Clinical Nutrition, 32,* 2339–2345.

Ariza, J. (1967). Recommendacion diaria de calorias y nutrientes para la poblacion colombiana. *Archivos Latinoamericanos de Nutricion, 17,* 255–263.

Beaton, G. H., & Ghassemi, H. (1982). Supplementary feeding programs for young children in developing countries. *American Journal of Clinical Nutrition, 35,* suppl.

Brozek, J., & Schurch, B. (Eds.). (1984). *Malnutrition and behavior: Critical assessment of key issues.* Lausanne: Nestle Foundation.

Chavez, A., Martinez, C., & Yachine, T. (1975). Nutrition, behavioral development, and mother-child interaction in young rural children. *Federation Proceedings, 34,* 1574.

Christiansen, N. (1984). Social and economic effects of supplementation and stimulation. In J. Brozek & B. Schurch (Eds.), *Malnutrition and behavior: Critical assessment of key issues* (pp. 520–530). Lausanne: Nestle Foundation.

Christiansen, N., Mora, J. O., de Navarro, L., & Herrera, M. G. (1980). Effects of nutritional supplementation upon birth weight: The influence of pre-supplementation diet. *Nutritional Reports International, 21,* 615–624.

Christiansen, N., Vuori, L., Clement, J., Herrera, M. G., Mora, J. O., & Ortíz, N. (1977). Malnutrition, social environment, and cognitive development of Colombian infants and preschoolers. *Nutrition Reports International, 16,* 93–102.

Clarke, A. B. D., & Clarke, A. M. (1981). "Sleeper effects" in development: Fact or artifact? *Developmental Review, 1,* 344–360.

Cravioto, J., Birch, H. G., De Licardie, E., Rosales, L., & Vega, L. (1969). The ecology of growth and development in a Mexican preindustrial community, Report I: Method and findings from birth to one month of age. *Monographs of the Society for Research in Child Development, 34*(5, Serial No. 129).

De Maeyer, E. M. (1976). Protein-energy malnutrition. In G. Beaton & J. Bengoa (Eds.), *Nutrition in preventative medicine* (WHO Monograph Ser. No. 62) (pp. 23–54. Geneva: World Health Organization.

Edozien, J. C., Switzer, B. R., & Bijan, R. B. (1979). Medical evaluation of the special supplemental food program for women, infants, and children. *American Journal of Clinical Nutrition, 32,* 677–692.

Edwards, A. L. (1964). *Statistical methods for the behavioral sciences.* New York: Holt, Rinehart & Winston.

Gnanadesikan, R. (1977). *Methods for statistical data analysis of multivariate observations.* New York: Wiley.

Gopalan, C., Swaminathan, M. C., Kumari, V. K. K., Rao, D. H., & Vijayaraghavan, K. (1973). Effect of calorie supplementation on growth of undernourished children. *American Journal of Clinical Nutrition, 26*, 563–566.

Graves, P. (1976). Nutrition, infant behavior, and maternal characteristics: A pilot study in West Bengal, India. *American Journal of Clinical Nutrition, 29*, 305.

Harkness, S., & Super, C. M. (in press). The developmental niche as a framework for analyzing the household production of health. *Social Science and Medicine.*

Herrera, M. G., Mora, J. O., Christiansen, N., Ortíz, N., Clement, J., Vuori, L., Waber, D., de Paredes, B., & Wagner, M. (1980). Effects of nutritional supplementation and early education on physical development. In R. R. Turner & H. W. Reese (Eds.). *Life-span developmental psychology: Intervention* (pp. 149–184). New York: Academic Press.

Herrera, M. G., Mora, J. O., de Paredes, B., & Wagner, M. (1979). Maternal weight/height and the effect of food supplementation during pregnancy and lactation. In *Maternal nutrition during pregnancy and lactation* (pp. 252–263). Lausanne: Nestle Foundation.

Herrera, M. G., Super, C. M., & Mora, J. O. (1989). *The long-term effects of food supplementation in early and late infancy.* Manuscript in preparation.

Horton, S. (1984). Malnutrition and human capital. In J. Brozek & B. Schurch (Eds.), *Malnutrition and behavior: Critical assessment of key issues* (pp. 621–629). Lausanne: Nestle Foundation.

Jelliffe, D. B. (1966). *The assessment of the nutritional status of the community.* Geneva: World Health Organization.

Joos, S., & Pollitt, E. (1984). Comparison of four supplementation studies. In J. Brozek & B. Schurch (Eds.), *Malnutrition and behavior: Critical assessment and key issues* (pp. 507–519). Lausanne: Nestle Foundation.

Jordan, M., & Staehling, N. (1986). *Anthropometric statistical package, version 3* [computer program]. Atlanta: Centers for Disease Control.

Keller, W., Donoso, G., & DeMaeyer, E. M. (1976). Anthropometry in nutritional surveillance: A review based on results of the WHO collaborative study on nutritional anthropometry. *Nutrition Abstracts Review, 46*, 591–609.

Kessen, W. (1979). The American child and other cultural interventions. *American Psychologist, 34*, 815–820.

Lambie, D. Z., Bond, J. T., & Weikart, D. P. (1974). *Home teaching with mothers and infants.* Ypsilanti, MI: High/Scope Research Foundation.

Lazar, I., & Darlington, R. (1982). Lasting effects of early education: A report from the consortium for longitudinal studies. *Monographs of the Society for Research in Child Development, 47* (2-3, Serial No. 195).

Lechtig, A., Yarbrough, C., Martorell, R., Delgado, H., & Klein, R. (1976). The one-day recall dietary survey: A review of its usefulness to estimate protein and calorie intake. *Archivos Latinoamericanos de Nutricion, 26*, 243–271.

Lutter, C. K., Mora, J. O., Habicht, J. P., Rasmussen, K. M., Robson, D. S., Sellers, S., Super, C. M., & Herrera, M. G. (1989). Nutritional supplementation: Effects on child stunting because of diarrhea. *American Journal of Clinical Nutrition, 50*, 1–8.

Martorell, R., Klein, R., & Delgado, H. (1980). Improved nutrition and its effects on anthropometric indicators of nutritional status. *Nutrition Reports International, 21,* 219–230.

Martorell, R., Lechtig, A., Yarbrough, C., Delgado, H., & Klein, R. E. (1976). Protein-calorie supplementation and postnatal physical growth: A review of findings from developing countries. *Archivos Latinoamericanos de Nutricion, 26,* 115–128.

Mora, J. O., Clement, J., Christiansen, N., Suescun, J., Wagner, M., & Herrera, M. G. (1978). Nutritional supplementation and the outcome of pregnancy: III. Perinatal and neonatal mortality. *Nutritional Reports International, 18,* 167–175.

Mora, J. O., de Navarro, L., Clement, J., Wagner, M., de Paredes, B., & Herrera, M. G. (1978). The effect of nutritional supplementation on calorie and protein intake of pregnant women. *Nutritional Reports International, 17,* 217–228.

Mora, J. O., de Paredes, B., Wagner, M., de Navarro, L., Suescun, J., Christiansen, N., & Herrera, M. G. (1979). Nutritional supplementation and the outcome of pregnancy: I. Birth weight. *American Journal of Clinical Nutrition, 32,* 455–462.

Mora, J. O., Herrera, M. G., Sellers, S. G., & Ortíz, N. (1981). Nutrition, social environment, and cognitive performance of disadvantaged Colombian children at three years. In *Nutrition in health and disease and international development: Symposia from the XII International Congress of Nutrition* (pp. 403–420). New York: Liss.

Mora, J. O., Herrera, M. G., Suescun, L., de Navarro, L., & Wagner, M. (1981). The effects of nutritional supplementation on physical growth of children at risk of malnutrition. *American Journal of Clinical Nutrition, 34,* 1885–1892.

Mora, J. O., Sellers, S. G., Suescun, J., & Herrera, M. G. (1981). The impact of supplementary feeding and home education on physical growth of disadvantaged children. *Nutritional Research, 1,* 213–225.

Overholt, C., Sellers, S., Mora, J. O., de Paredes, B., & Herrera, M. G. (1982). The effects of nutritional supplementation on the diets of low-income families at risk of malnutrition. *American Journal of Clinical Nutrition, 36,* 1153–1161.

Rao, D. H., & Nadamuni, N. A. (1977). Nutritional supplementation—whom does it benefit most? *American Journal of Clinical Nutrition, 30,* 1612–1616.

Reuda-Williamson, R., Luna-Jaspe, H., Ariza, J., Pardo, F., & Mora, J. O. (1969). Estudio seccional de crecimiento, desarrollo y nutricion en 12, 138 ninos de Bogotá, Colombia: I. Tablas de peso y talla en ninos colombianos. *Pediatria, 10,* 335–345.

Sameroff, A. J., & Chandler, M. J. (1975). Reproductive risk and the continuum of caretaking casualty. In F. D. Horowitz (Ed.). *Review of child development research* (Vol. 4, pp. 187–244). Chicago: University of Chicago Press.

Seitz, V. (1981). Intervention and sleeper effects: A reply to Clarke and Clarke. *Developmental Review, 1,* 361–373.

Sellers, S. G., Mora, J. O., Super, C. M., & Herrera, M. G. (1982). The effects of nutritional supplementation and home education on children's diets. *Nutrition Reports International, 26,* 727–741.

Super, C. M., Clement, J., Vuori, L., Christiansen, N., Mora, J. O., & Herrera, M. G. (1981). Infant and caretaker behavior as mediators of nutritional and social intervention in the barrios of Bogotá. In T. Field, P. H. Leiderman, & P. Vietze (Eds.), *Culture and early interaction* (pp. 171–188). Hillsdale, NJ: Erlbaum.

Super, C. M., & Harkness, S. (1986). The developmental niche: A conceptualization at the interface of child and culture. *International Journal of Behavior Development, 9*, 545–569.

Super, C. M., Herrera, M. G., & Mora, J. O. (1987a). *The long-term effects of nutritional supplementation and psychosocial intervention on preschool achievement test scores.* Manuscript in preparation.

Super, C. M., Herrera, M. G., & Mora, J. O. (1987b). *Culture, psychosocial intervention, and developmental quotients in Colombian infants.* Manuscript in preparation.

Super, C. M., Sellers, S. G., Mora, J. O., de Paredes, B., & Herrera, M. G. (1989). *Weaning, diarrhea, and the transition to a family diet among Colombian infants at risk of malnutrition.* Manuscript submitted for publication.

Taylor, C. E., Kielmann, A. A., De Sweemer, C., & Uberoi, I. S. (1978). The Narangwal experiment on interactions of nutrition and infections: I. Project design and effects upon growth. *Indian Journal of Medical Research, 68*, 1–20.

Townsend, J. W. (1984). Social significance of nutrition-related programs. In J. Brozek & B. Schurch (Eds.), *Malnutrition and behavior: Critical assessment of key issues* (pp. 615–620). Lausanne: Nestle Foundation.

U.S. Public Health Service, Health Resources Administration. (1976). *NCHS growth charts* (HRA 76-1120, 25, 3). Rockville, MD: U.S. Government Printing Office.

Vuori, L. N., Christiansen, N., Clement, J., Mora, J. O., Wagner, M., & Herrera, M. G. (1979). Nutritional supplementation and the outcome of pregnancy: II. Visual habituation at 15 days. *American Journal of Clinical Nutrition, 32*, 463–469.

Vuori, L. N., de Navarro, L., Christiansen, N., Mora, J. O., & Herrera, M. G. (1980). Food supplementation of pregnant women at risk of malnutrition and their newborns' responsiveness to stimulation. *Developmental Medicine and Child Neurology, 22*, 61–71.

Waber, D. P., Vuori, L., Ortíz, N., Clement, J., Christiansen, N., Mora, J. O., Reed, R. B., & Herrera, M. G. (1981). Nutritional supplementation, maternal education, and cognitive development of infants at risk of malnutrition. *American Journal of Clinical Nutrition, 34*, 807–813.

Waterlow, J. C. (1977). The presentation and use of height and weight data for comparing the nutritional status of groups of children under the age of 10 years. *Bulletin of the World Health Organization, 55*, 489–498.

World Health Organization. (1983). *Measuring change in nutritional status.* Geneva: World Health Organization.

Part III

LANGUAGE STUDIES

In the first paper in this section, Pennington summarizes converging lines of evidence indicating that dyslexia, broadly defined as unexpected difficulty in the acquisition of reading and spelling skills, is a developmental language disorder that mainly affects the phonological domain of language. Heritable differences in spoken language skills, especially awareness of phonemic segments in words, lead to problems in the phonological coding of written language, which is a key prerequisite for skill in single word recognition and spelling. Dyslexia runs in families, and recent twin studies have specifically examined the heritability of different aspects of reading and spelling skill. Of particular interest is that although single word reading and spelling in dyslexia were found to be genetically influenced independent of IQ, reading comprehension was not. Verbal short-term memory as assessed by Digit Span was found to be genetically influenced, but measures of perceptual and motor speed were not. Genetic analyses directed to the elucidation of the mode of transmission or gene location have, to date, been less informative, although available evidence points to both linkage and genetic heterogeneity. As behavioral genetic studies require accurate diagnosis of adult family members, further advances in this area are dependent on the identification of a subclinical marker for dyslexia in compensated adults in order to validate a diagnosis based on history.

The longitudinal study by Scarborough adds a developmental perspective to the increasing consensus that dyslexia is a developmental language disorder. The meticulous research design allowed for the study of three groups of children who were first studied at 30 months of age: 20 children from families in which other members were dyslexic and who subsequently became dyslexic themselves; 12 children from dyslexic families who became normal readers; and 20 other normal children selected to resemble the dyslexic group closely in IQ, socioeconomic status, and sex. At 30 months of age, children who later developed reading disabilities were deficient in the length, syntactic complexity, and pronunciation accuracy of their spoken language, although not in lexical or speech discrimination skills. As three-year-olds, these children began to show deficits in receptive vocabulary and object-naming abilities, and as five-year-olds they displayed weaknesses in object naming, phonemic awareness, and letter-sound knowledge that have characterized kindergarteners who became poor readers in other studies. The language deficits of dyslexic children were unrelated to maternal reading ability and were not observed in children from dyslexic families who became normal readers. Although the number of children studied is small, the findings are striking. A thoughtful discussion considers implications for etiologic theories of dyslexia.

Lederberg and Mobley examine yet another facet of early language development—its relation to attachment during the toddler years. Forty-one hearing-impaired and 41 hearing toddlers, who were between 18 and 25 months of age, were observed together with their hearing mothers in the Ainsworth Strange Situation during free play. Analysis of the behavior of mothers and children during free play revealed that hearing-impaired toddlers and their mothers were judged to miscommunicate significantly more frequently than hearing toddlers and their mothers. In addition, hearing-impaired toddlers and their mothers spent less time interacting than hearing toddlers and their mothers. Despite these effects on communication and quantity of interaction, hearing impairment did not affect the quality of the relationship between mother and toddler. Ratings of the quality of maternal and toddler behavior during free play were similar for hearing-impaired and hearing dyads. Moreover, no differences in ratings of attachment existed between the groups. Fifty-six percent of the hearing-impaired children were securely attached as compared with 61 percent of the hearing children. In addition, mother-toddler interaction and security of attachment were related in similar ways for both hearing-impaired and hearing toddlers. The discussion amplified the authors' conclusion that the development of a secure attachment and maintenance of good mother-toddler relationship does not depend on normal language development during the toddler years.

10

Annotation: The Genetics of Dyslexia

Bruce F. Pennington
University of Denver

Dyslexia is a common, specific developmental disorder in which considerable progress has been made in the last 10 years in defining both the genetics and the behavioral phenotype. The pathophysiology of dyslexia below the level of behavior is less well understood, though there is evidence for left hemisphere brain dysfunction. Dyslexia may be simply defined as unexpected difficulty in the acquisition of reading and spelling skills. Generally accepted prevalence rates for dyslexia are 5–10%, with a male : female sex ratio of 3.5–4.0 : 1. The sex ratio in familial samples is considerably lower, about 1.8–2.0 : 1 (DeFries, 1989). The sex difference in prevalence rates of dyslexia could be explained by a polygenic model with a lower threshold for males or by a major locus model with a sex difference in expressibility. X-linked inheritance does not fit the available family data.

These prevalence estimates, of course, depend on how the disorder is defined. As is true for other behaviorally-defined disorders, there is disagreement about the diagnostic definition of this disorder. One of the key themes of this review is how behavior, genetic and experimental analyses can help in defining both the phenotypic core and the phenotypic boundaries of a complex developmental disorder like dyslexia (Pennington & Smith, 1988).

Converging evidence indicates that dyslexia is a developmental language disorder which mainly affects the phonological domain of language. Heritable differences, in particular spoken language skills—especially awareness of phonemic segments in words—lead to

Reprinted with permission from *Journal of Child Psychology and Psychiatry*, 1990, Vol. 31, No. 2, 193–201. Copyright © 1990 by the Association for Child Psychology and Psychiatry.

This research was supported by the following grants to the author: a NIMH RSDA (MH00419) and project grants from NIMH (MH38820), NICHD (HD19423), the March of Dimes (12-135) and the Orton Dyslexia Society.

problems in the phonological coding of written language, which is a key prerequisite for skill in single word recognition and spelling. In this review, we will consider some of the evidence that points to this broad conclusion.

Conceptually, genetic analyses proceed in a series of linked steps considering in turn the questions of familiality, heritability, mode of transmission, *and* gene locations. *The first part of the review will be organized accordingly. Then I will consider the issues of* heterogeneity *and* behavioral phenotype.

FAMILIALITY

Familial aggregation in dyslexia was soon noticed after the disorder was first described by Kerr (1897) and Morgan (1896). It was reported in a number of case studies (Fisher, 1905; Hinshelwood, 1907, 1911; Stephenson, 1907; Thomas, 1905) that children with dyslexia often had an affected relative. Of these, Thomas's (1905) report of two affected brothers and another child with an affected sister and mother was the first to note the familial tendency in dyslexia. Stephenson (1907) reported a three-generation family history affecting five females and one male. These early reports documented a number of aspects of the clinical presentation of dyslexia which have been substantiated by subsequent research: early manifestations often include difficulty in learning letter names; affected children are frequently good at mathematics and spatial tasks; severity varies across those affected; and the deficit persists into adulthood, either as a problem with both reading or spelling, or just spelling.

The magnitude of familial risk for dyslexia has not been measured in a representative population sample until recently. In a selected sample of families, Hallgren (1950) had found the risk to first-degree relatives to be 41%, which is considerably higher than the population risk (5–10%). However, Hallgren's (1950) diagnoses of affected family members were not based on testing, and ascertainment biases may have led to the selection of families with higher than normal proportions of affected relatives. Vogler, DeFries and Decker (1985) measured familial risk for dyslexia in the Colorado Family Reading Study (CFRS) sample, which was a representative population sample, and found the risk to a son of having an affected father is 40% and of having an affected mother is 35%, a five- to seven-fold increase in risk over that found in sons without affected parents. For daughters, the risk of dyslexia of having an affected parent of either sex was 17–18%, a 10- to 12-fold increase over that found in daughters without affected parents. These risk figures are somewhat lower than Hallgren's (1950), but still substantially elevated, and clearly demonstrate familiality.

Similar estimates of familial risk (range 36–45%) have also been reported by Klasen (1968), Naidoo (1972), Zahalkova, Vrzal and Kloboukova (1972), and Finucci, Guthrie, Childs, Abbey and Childs (1976). The magnitude of familial risk for dyslexia is clinically significant in that family history could be used to help screen for children at high risk for this disorder.

HERITABILITY

The next question to consider is whether this familiality indicates genetic transmission. Twin studies have been mainly used to address this question in dyslexia. Earlier twin studies, which indicated substantial heritability of dyslexia, had methodological problems, such as biases of ascertainment, failure to limit the dyzogotic (DZ) twin comparison group to same sex twins, and lack of objective diagnostic criteria. Two well-designed twin studies have recently been conducted which avoided these methodological problems.

One study (Stevenson, Graham, Fredman & McLaughlin, 1986) examined a large population cohort of adolescent twins in London, only some of whom (naturally) were dyslexic. The authors tested for the heritability of both reading and spelling skill in the whole population, as well as specific reading and spelling retardation in a subset of the population. They found only modest heritability for reading ability and disability, but significant heritability for spelling ability and disability. Their results for reading are discrepant from all other twin studies and may be due to the older age of their sample.

The second study was conducted by John DeFries and colleagues at the Institute for Behavior Genetics in Boulder. They have developed a new, multiple regression technique for testing heritable and common environmental contributions to extreme low scores on a continuous trait in a twin study. This method assumes that at least one twin in each monozygotic (MZ) or DZ pair is disabled, as do traditional twin studies. But instead of examining differential (categorical) concordance rates, this technique examines differential regression to the population mean in the co-twin, thus making full use of the information available in a continuous variable, like reading scores. To the degree that the condition is heritable, there should be greater regression to the mean in the DZ co-twin scores (because their degree of relationship is 0.50, whereas that in MZ twins is 1.00). An expanded version of this model (LaBuda, DeFries & Fulker, 1986) can estimate both heritability and shared environmental influences. With a large enough data set, this model can also test for major gene effects.

These investigators used this technique to test for the heritability of reading, spelling and related cognitive skills in a sample of 64 MZ and 55 DZ twins, in which at least one member of each pair was reading disabled (DeFries, Fulker & LaBuda, 1987). Significant heritability was found for PIAT Reading Recognition, PIAT

Spelling and WISC-R Digit Span; whereas it was not found for PIAT Reading Comprehension, WISC-R Coding or the Colorado Perceptual Speed test. The estimate of heritability for a composite discriminant score was 0.29, suggesting about 30% of the cognitive phenotype in reading disability is attributable to heritable factors. It is important to note that this result was not simply due to the heritability of IQ, since IQ was controlled in these analyses.

The pattern of scores across different measures in this study begins to provide information about which components of reading are genetically influenced in dyslexia. Single word reading and spelling in dyslexia were found to be genetically influenced independent of IQ, but reading comprehension was not. In the area of reading-related skills, a measure of verbal short term memory (Digit Span) was found to be genetically influenced, but measures of perceptual and motor speed were not. These results fit with a growing consensus that dyslexics are more deficient in single word recognition skills than in comprehension skills and that the precursor to this deficit in single word reading is in the domain of phonological processing skills.

Olson, Wise, Conners and Rack (1989) analyzed the heritability of phonological versus orthographic coding in single word reading in the dyslexic twin sample studied by DeFries *et al.* (1987). Quite strikingly, Olson *et al.* (1989) found significant heritability (about 0.46) for a phonological coding measure (i.e. oral non-word reading accuracy). In contrast, a measure of orthographic coding skill in single word reading was not found to be heritable. Moreover, the contribution of phonological coding to the heritability of reading in these twins was 0.93 ± 0.39, whereas the contribution of orthographic coding was essentially zero. Other evidence argues against problems in orthographic coding being a causal deficit in dyslexia (Olson, 1985; Pennington *et al.* 1986), whereas the evidence supporting a deficit role for phonological coding is strong. Thus it is quite interesting that the deficient component is likewise the heritable component.

The next key question of interest is which phonological processing skills at the level of spoken language are a heritable precursor to this heritable deficit in the phonological coding of written language. Olson *et al.* (1989) found significant ($p < 0.05$) heritability estimates for the correlation between two different phoneme awareness measures, rhyming fluency (h2 $= 0.99 \pm 0.86$) and pig Latin (h2 $= 0.81 \pm 0.75$) and the heritable non-word reading measure. These investigators pointed out that the large confidence intervals on these estimates meant these results need to be confirmed by future studies. Nonetheless, the pattern of results is consistent with the overall argument we have been developing at Denver. We expect that the heterogeneous etiologies that lead to dyslexia do not affect reading directly, but instead alter the development of spoken language skills important for later reading development. These behavior genetic analyses are consistent with the view that the heritable component in dyslexia at the written language level is in phonological coding and the heritable precursor to this deficit in phonological coding is a deficit in phoneme awareness.

MODES OF TRANSMISSION

While twin or adoption studies are informative about the presence of genetic influences, they do not ordinarily address the issue of the mode(s) of genetic transmission. A number of different modes of transmission have been proposed in dyslexia, including autosomal dominant transmission (Hallgren, 1950; Zahalkova *et al.*, 1972), but there has been really only one model complex segregation analysis performed on this disorder (Lewitter, DeFries & Elston, 1980).

This study included 133 nuclear families, all members of which were tested. Rather than a discrete phenotype definition, a continuous phenotype measure based on a discriminant analysis was employed. A shortcoming of this study is that adults with a positive history of dyslexia but normal test scores (compensated adults) were not counted as affected.

In the population as a whole, no support was found for a single major locus (autosomal dominant, autosomal recessive, or co-dominant transmission), but the null hypothesis of no vertical transmission was likewise rejected. These investigators also tested different models of transmission in subpopulations, including families with probands of a given sex, families with severely affected probands, and children considered alone, because of possible unreliability of the measure in adults. Autosomal recessive inheritance could not be rejected in families with female probands and codominant inheritance was supported when children were considered alone. The authors concluded that their results most likely indicated genetic heterogeneity. This conclusion is similar to that reached by Finucci *et al.* (1976) in a well-documented study of 20 extended families, all members of which were tested. Unfortunately, this sample was too small to permit a formal, complex segregation analysis.

In short, the existing data support genetic heterogeneity in the transmission of dyslexia but do not converge on which different modes of transmission are operating. There is clearly a need for more data on this issue, especially a segregation analysis of a large sample of dyslexic families which employs several different phenotype definitions (including compensated adults) and which uses a more sophisticated segregation analysis program, such as POINTER (Lalouel, Rao, Morton & Elston, 1983).

GENE LOCATIONS

We have been conducting linkage studies of dyslexia at Denver for about 10 years now, and the main results are: firstly, significant evidence for linkage between dyslexia and chromosome 15 heteromorphisms in a minority of families with apparent autosomal dominant transmission (Smith, Kimberling, Pennington & Lubs, 1983); and secondly, significant evidence of genetic heterogeneity (Smith, Pennington, Kimberling & Ing, 1990). We are currently testing the linkage to chromosome 15 with DNA polymorphisms in the same region as the original marker and we are looking for a possible second dyslexia locus on another chromosome in the majority of families who are not linked to chromosome 15. A clue about where to look for a second locus has been provided by the association we and others have found between dyslexia and immune disorders (Geschwind & Behan, 1982; Pennington, Smith, Kimberling, Green & Haith, 1987). We are currently testing for a possible second locus on chromosome 6 near the HLA region.

In the original study (Smith *et al.*, 1983), which found significant linkage between dyslexia and chromosome 15 heteromorphisms, there was one family which had substantial negative LOD scores for markers on chromosome 15, arguing against linkage in that family. However, a test for heterogeneity was not significant. Since then we have doubled the number of families in the sample and more than doubled the N. We now have linkage data on 245 individuals in 21 extended families. When we tested this larger sample for genetic heterogeneity using Ott's (1985) HOMOG program, the hypothesis of heterogeneity was supported over two competing hypotheses: that of homogeneity and that of no linkage (Smith *et al.*, 1990). HOMOG estimated that dyslexia is linked to chromosome 15 in about 20% of the families. The range of LOD scores in the entire sample of families spans six orders of magnitude, from negative LOD scores less than -3.0 (i.e. 1000 : 1 odds against linkage to 15) to a positive LOD score of 3.2 (i.e. 1000 : 1 odds in favor of linkage to 15), which by itself indicates linkage to chromosome 15 in one family.

A Danish study (Bisgaard, Eiberg, Moller, Niebuhr & Mohr, 1987) failed to find linkage between dyslexia and chromosome 15 heteromorphisms. Since only five families were studied, this apparent non-replication may only be due to heterogeneity (since dyslexic families linked to 15 appear to be rarer than those not so linked). In addition, there were other problems with this study. Only nuclear families were studied and the diagnosis of dyslexia was based on questionnaire rather than test data. However, confirmation of our original linkage result by both different investigators and by different markers on chromosome 15 is obviously important.

The results of the linkage work on dyslexia are similar to the results emerging from linkage studies of other complex behavioral disorders, including schizophrenia, bipolar illness and Alzheimer's disease. That is, there is evidence for both linkage and genetic heterogeneity. What is currently unclear is how common are the single major locus forms of these disorders. Nonetheless, it is certainly true that single gene effects are turning out to be more important in understanding psychiatric disorders than was previously thought.

HETEROGENEITY

Both the results of segregation and linkage analyses support the not too surprising conclusion that dyslexia is genetically heterogeneous. Additional support for this conclusion is provided by the finding of a high rate of dyslexia among boys with a 47, XXY karyotype (Pennington, Bender, Puck, Salbenblatt & Robinson, 1982); this sex chromosome anomaly is too rare (about 1/1000 male births) to account for much of the genetic influence on dyslexia.

But heterogeneity in etiology does not necessarily indicate heterogeneity in pathophysiology; there may not be a 1 : 1 mapping between etiologic and phenotypic subtypes. In fact, the evidence for discrete phenotypic subtypes in developmental dyslexia is much less compelling than it once appeared. Current evidence supports the view that the vast majority of developmental dyslexics have an underlying problem in the phonological coding of written language. While there are individual differences in this and other component reading processes within the dyslexic population, there is little evidence for discrete subgroups (Olson, 1985).

Thus, at the level of behavior, the final common pathway in most of developmental dyslexia is a deficit in phonological coding. We know virtually nothing about the role of biochemistry in the pathophysiology of dyslexia. More is known about neuroanatomy and neurophysiology, although much remains to be discovered. The general consensus is that dyslexia involves dysfunction in the left cerebral hemisphere (Galaburda, Sherman, Rosen, Aboitiz & Geschwind, 1985). The more interesting question of how a developmental disorder affecting the left hemisphere largely spares conversational speech and language has hardly been addressed.

BEHAVIORAL PHENOTYPE

There has been considerable progress within the last 10 years or so in defining the behavioral phenotype in developmental dyslexia. The work of Vellutino (1979) and others established clearly that the main deficit in most developmental dyslexics is linguistic rather than visual. As discussed above, more recent work has shown that within the linguistic domain, it is the phonological level of language that is critically affected. For conceptual clarity, we divide these phonological problems into those that involve spoken language skills (such as phonemic segmentation) and those that involve written language (such as non-word reading). We have presented some of the evidence for the view that the spoken language precursor to the phonological coding deficit in written language is a deficit in phonemic segmentation and awareness skills; other relevant articles include Bradley & Bryant (1978, 1983), Pratt and Brady (1988), and Wagner and Torgesen (1987). Reading experience also facilitates phoneme awareness (Morais, Cary, Alegria & Bertelson, 1979). Thus, the relationship between reading skill and phoneme awareness appears to be one of reciprocal causation.

The phenotypic core of dyslexia is becoming well defined, but we are less certain about phenotypic boundaries. Dyslexics have other problems with phonological processing in spoken language, such as problems with speech production (Catts, 1986, 1988), name retrieval (Katz, 1986), and verbal short term memory (Jorm, 1983; Stanovich, 1982a,b). What is unclear at this point is what is the causal relation of these other phonological processing problems to dyslexia. Are they other manifestations of the underlying cause, correlates of the underlying cause, a result of poor reading or just incidental to the syndrome?

Recent results from our laboratory (Pennington, Van Orden, Kirson & Haith, 1990) and from others (Conners & Olson, 1990; Mann & Ditunno, 1990) support the view that these various phonological processing skills are not a unitary domain, nor do they all have a similar causal relation to reading skill. In these studies, measures of phoneme awareness loaded on a separate factor from measures of verbal STM and accounted for much more unique variance in reading skill. Thus it appears that the deficits in verbal STM often found in dyslexic populations are more likely to be a correlate or a result of reading problems than a cause, whereas the evidence for a causal relation for problems in phoneme awareness is fairly strong.

Similar questions about the causal relation to dyslexia exist for characteristics more distant from the phenotypic core, such as left-handedness, attention problems, and problems with self-esteem and depression. There is also an association between dyslexia and immune disorders (Geschwind & Behan, 1982; Pennington *et al.*, 1987), the basis for which is not well understood. In other words, how do we interpret evidence for co-morbidity in dyslexia? It seems likely that problems with self-esteem and depression are a result of dyslexia. Since left-handedness and attention problems are not found in every dyslexic sample, these symptoms may have an incidental or artifactual relation to dyslexia. But we really lack good data on these questions.

The techniques of behavior genetics can help to answer these questions about phenotype boundaries, just as they have helped to define the phenotypic core. For instance, co-heritability analyses can address the issue of whether an associated symptom is causally or artifactually related to the phenotype of dyslexia. Pauls *et al.* (1986) have used these analyses to clarify which associated symptoms are part of the phenotype in Tourette's syndrome (chronic tics and obsessive compulsive disorder) and which are not (attention problems).

A final issue of considerable interest for genetic studies is whether there exists a subclinical marker for dyslexia. Since some adults compensate for their earlier dyslexia, do they nonetheless have persisting behavioral characteristics which could be used to validate a diagnosis based on history? This is an important question for behavior genetic studies in which there is a need to diagnose adult family members.

What little research there is suggests that problems in phonological coding and phoneme awareness are among the most persistent features of the disorder (Campbell & Butterworth, 1985), but more work is needed to see whether such problems will be useful as subclinical markers.

REFERENCES

Bisgaard, M. L., Eiberg, H., Moller, N., Niebuhr, E. & Mohr, J. (1987). Dyslexia and chromosome 15 heteromorphism: negative lod score in a Danish material. *Clinical Genetics,* **32,** 118–119.

Bradley, L. & Bryant, P. E. (1978). Difficulties in auditory organisation as a possible cause of reading backwardness. *Nature,* **271,** 746–747.

Bradley, L. & Bryant, P. E. (1983). Categorizing sounds and learning to read—a causal connection. *Nature,* **301,** 419–421.

Campbell, R. & Butterworth, B. (1985). Phonological dyslexia and dysgraphia in a highly literate subject: a developmental case with associated deficits of phonemic awareness and processing. *Quarterly Journal of Experimental Psychology,* **37,** 435–475.

Catts, H. W. (1986). Speech production/phonological deficits in reading disordered children. *Journal of Learning Disabilities,* **19,** 504–508.

Catts, H. W. (1988). Phonological processing deficits and reading disabilities. In S. Kamni & H. Catts (Eds), *Reading disabilities: A developmental language perspective* (pp. 101–132). San Diego: College Hill Press.

Conners, G. & Olson, R. K. (1990). Reading comprehension in dyslexic and normal readers: a component-skills analysis. In D. A. Balota, G. B. Flores d'Arcais & K. Rayner (Eds), *Comprehension processes in reading.* Hillsdale, NJ: Erlbaum (in press).

DeFries, J. C. (1989). Gender ratios in reading-disabled children and their affected relatives: a commentary. *Journal of Learning Disabilities,* **22,** 544–545.

DeFries, J. C., Fulker, D. W. & LaBuda, M. C. (1987). Reading disability in twins: evidence for a genetic etiology. *Nature,* **329,** 537–539.

Finucci, J. M., Guthrie, J. T., Childs, A. L., Abbey, H. & Childs, B. (1976). The genetics of specific reading disability. *Annual Review of Human Genetics,* **40,** 1–23.

Fisher, J. H. (1905). Case of congenital word-blindness (inability to learn to read). *Ophthalmological Review,* **24,** 315.

Galaburda, A. M., Sherman, G. F., Rosen, G. D., Aboitiz, F. & Geschwind, N. (1985). Developmental dyslexia: four consecutive patients with cortical anomalies. *Annals of Neurology,* **18,** 222–232.

Geschwind, N. & Behan, P. O. (1982). Left-handedness: association with immune disease, migraine, and developmental learning disorder. *Proceedings from the National Academy of Science, U.S.A.,* **79,** 5097–5100.

Hallgren, B. (1950). Specific dyslexia (congenital word-blindness): a clinical and genetic study. *Acta Psychiatrica et Neurologica,* Supplement 65, 1–287.

Hinshelwood, J. (1907). Four cases of congenital word-blindness occurring in the same family. *British Medical Journal,* **2,** 1229–1232.

Hinshelwood, J. (1911). Two cases of hereditary word-blindness. *British Medical Journal*, **1**, 608–609.

Jorm, A. F. (1983). Specific reading retardation and working memory: a review. *British Journal of Psychology*, **74**, 311–342.

Katz, R. B. (1986). Phonological deficiencies in children with reading disability: evidence from an object-naming task. *Cognition*, **22**, 225–257.

Kerr, J. (1987). School hygiene, in its mental, moral, and physical aspects. Howards Medical Prize Essay. *Journal of the Royal Statistical Society*, **60**, 613–680.

Klasen, E. L. (1968). *Legasthenia*. Bern: Huber.

LaBuda, M. C., DeFries, J. C. & Fulker, D. W. (1986). Multiple regression analysis of twin data obtained from selected samples. *Genetic Epidemiology*, **3**, 425–433.

Lalouel, J. M., Rao, D. C., Morton, N. E. & Elston, R. C. (1983). A unified model for complex segregation analysis. *American Journal of Human Genetics*, **35**, 816–826.

Lewitter, F. I., DeFries, J. C. & Elston, R. C. (1980). Genetic models of reading disability. *Behavior Genetics*, **10**, 9–30.

Mann, V. A. & Ditunno, P. (1990). Phonological deficiencies: effective predictors of future reading problems. In G. Pavlides (Ed.), *Dyslexia: A neuropsychological and learning perspective*. New York: Wiley (in press).

Morais, J., Cary, L., Alegria, J. & Bertelson, P. (1979). Does awareness of speech as a sequence of phonemes arise spontaneously? *Cognition*, **7**, 323–331.

Morgan, W. P. (1986). A case of congenital word-blindness. *British Medical Journal*, **2**, 1543–1544.

Naidoo, S. (1972). *Specific dyslexia*. London: Pitman.

Olson, R. K. (1985). Disabled reading processes and cognitive profiles. In D. B. Gray & J. K. Kavanaugh (Eds), *Biobehavioral measures of dyslexia* (pp. 215–244). Parkton, MD: York Press.

Olson, R., Wise, B., Conners, F. & Rack, J. (1989). Specific deficits in component reading and language skills: genetic and environmental influences. *Journal of Learning Disabilities*, **22**, 339–348.

Ott, J. (1985). Estimation of the recombination fraction in human pedigrees: efficient computation of the likelihood for human studies. *American Journal of Human Genetics*, **26**, 588–597.

Pauls, D. L., Hurst, C. R., Kruger, S. D., Leckman, J. F., Kidd, K. K. & Cohen, D. J. (1986). Gilles de la Tourette's syndrome and attention deficit disorder with hyperactivity: evidence against a genetic relationship. *Archives of General Psychiatry*, **43**, 1177–1179.

Pennington, B. F., Bender, B., Puck, M., Salbenblatt, J. & Robinson, A. (1982). Learning disabilities in children with sex chromosome anomalies. *Child Development*, **53**, 1182–1192.

Pennington, B. F., McCabe, L. L., Smith, S. D., Lefly, D. L., Bookman, M. O., Kimberling, W. J. & Lubs, H. A. (1986). Spelling errors in adults with a form of familial dyslexia. *Child Development*, **57**, 1001–1013.

Pennington, B. F. & Smith, S. D. (1988). Genetic influences on learning disabilities: an update. *Journal of Consulting and Clinical Psychology*, **56**, 817–823.

Pennington, B. F., Smith, S. R., Kimberling, W., Green, P. A. & Haith, M. M. (1987). Left-handedness and immune disorders in familial dyslexics. *Archives of Neurology,* **44,** 634–639.

Pennington, B. F., Van Orden, G., Kirson, D. & Haith, M. M. (1990). What is the causal relation between verbal STM problems and dyslexia? In S. Brady & D. Shankweiler (Eds), *Phonological processes in literacy.* Hillsdale, NJ: Lawrence Erlbaum Associates (in press).

Pratt, A. & Brady, S. (1988). The relationship of phonological awareness to reading disability in children and adults. *Journal of Educational Psychology,* **80,** 319–323.

Smith, S. D., Kimberling, W.J., Pennington, B. F. & Lubs, H. A. (1983). Specific reading disability: identification of an inherited form through linkage and analysis. *Science,* **219,** 1345–1347.

Smith, S. D., Pennington, B. F., Kimberling, W. J. & Ing, P. S. (1990). Familial dyslexia: use of genetic linkage data to define subtypes. *Journal of the American Academy of Child Psychiatry* (in press).

Stanovich, K. (1982a). Individual differences in the cognitive processes of reading. II. Text-level processes. *Journal of Learning Disabilities,* **15,** 485–493.

Stanovich, K. (1982b). Individual differences in the cognitive processes of reading. II. Text-level processes. *Journal of Learning Disabilities,* **15,** 549–554.

Stephenson, S. (1907). Six cases of congenital word-blindness affecting three generations of one family. *Ophthalmoscope,* **5,** 482–484.

Stevenson, J., Graham, P., Fredman, G. & McLoughlin, V. (1986). A twin study of genetic influences on reading and spelling ability and disability. *Journal of Child Psychology and Psychiatry,* **28,** 231–247.

Thomas, C. J. (1905). Congenital 'word-blindness' and its treatment. *Ophthalmoscope,* **3,** 380–385.

Vellutino, F. R. (1979). *Dyslexia: Theory and research.* Cambridge, MA: MIT Press.

Vogler, G. P., DeFries, J. C. & Decker, S. N. (1985). Family history as an indicator of risk for reading disability. *Journal of Learning Disabilities,* **18,** 419–421.

Wagner, R. K. & Torgesen, J. K. (1987). The nature of phonological processing and its causal role in the acquisition of reading skills. *Psychological Bulletin,* **101,** 192–212.

Zahalkova, M., Vrzal, V. & Kloboukova, E. (1972). Genetical investigations in dyslexia. *Journal of Medical Genetics,* **9,** 48–52.

11

Very Early Language Deficits in Dyslexic Children

Hollis S. Scarborough

Brooklyn College, City University of New York

At 2½ years of age, children who later developed reading disabilities were deficient in the length, syntactic complexity, and pronunciation accuracy of their spoken language, but not in lexical or speech discrimination skills. As 3-year-olds, these children began to show deficits in receptive vocabulary and object-naming abilities, and as 5-year-olds they exhibited weaknesses in object-naming, phonemic awareness, and letter-sound knowledge that have characterized kindergartners who became poor readers in other studies. These late preschool differences were related to subsequent reading status as well as to prior language skills, but early syntactic proficiency nevertheless accounted for some unique variance in grade 2 achievement when differences at age 5 were statistically controlled. The language deficits of dyslexic children were unrelated to maternal reading ability and were not observed in children from dyslexic families who became normal readers. The implications of the results for etiological issues are discussed.

"Dyslexia," or "reading disability," refers to severe reading problems that cannot be attributed to sensory, intellectual, emotional, or socioeconomic handicaps or to other known impediments to learning to read. By definition, therefore, dyslexics are not identified until they have tried and failed to learn to read in school. By that time,

Reprinted with permission from *Child Development*, 1990, Vol. 61, 1728–1743. Copyright © 1990 by the Society for Research in Child Development, Inc.

This research was supported in part by grants from the National Institute of Child Health and Human Development and the March of Dimes Birth Defects Foundation. Maria Hager, Janet Wyckoff, and Wanda Dobrich assisted with data collection and analysis, and Martin Braine, Virginia Mann, Adele Abrahamsen, Bruce Pennington, Guy Van Orden, and two anonymous reviewers provided helpful comments on the paper. Thanks are also extended to the families who participated in this study for their patience and goodwill.

it is difficult to determine whether observed differences between reading-disabled children and their classmates reflect direct causes, or merely consequences, of reading failure. To circumvent this problem, one can take a prospective approach, whereby children are examined before they try to learn to read. In the study to be reported, the role of language-processing deficits in the etiology of dyslexia was investigated in a long-term prospective study of 2-year-olds who later were identified as disabled readers.

By studying such young children it was possible to look for early precursors to dyslexia that would be relatively unconfounded by the effects of preschool reading instruction and consequent differences in "preliteracy" achievement. Most prior prospective studies of reading disability have been conducted with children who are initially between the ages of 4½ and 6 years, when they are about to begin formal schooling or are in the first year of school. One consistent finding of those studies has been that many of the best predictors of later reading achievement are measures of skills very similar to those involved in reading itself: recognizing and naming letters, matching sounds to letters, writing one's name, and so forth (e.g., Jansky & deHirsch, 1972; Mann, 1984; Share, Jorm, Maclean, & Matthews, 1984). Because differences in the preliteracy skills of normal and disabled readers are already established by the late preschool years, to discover more fundamental antecedents of dyslexia required the examination of even younger children.

Early language development was chosen as the focus of the present investigation because prospective and retrospective studies have consistently found that language-processing abilities are deficient in kindergartners and older children with poor literacy skills, while most nonverbal cognitive abilities of disabled readers are unimpaired. Accordingly, virtually every recent review has judged that a language-based origin for reading disabilities is most consistent with available findings (e.g., Kamhi & Catts, 1989; Kavanagh & Yeni-Komshian, 1985; Perfetti, 1985; Stanovich, 1988; Vellutino, 1979).

A broad range of linguistic impairments has been observed in prior prospective studies of reading disability. Kindergartners and prekindergartners who later exhibit low reading achievement exhibit weaknesses in receptive vocabulary (e.g., Share et al., 1984; Stanovich, Cunningham, & Feeman, 1984), object naming (e.g., Share et al., 1984; Wolf & Goodglass, 1986), syntax comprehension (e.g., Share et al., 1984), syntax production (e.g., Butler, Marsh, Sheppard & Sheppard, 1985), phonological production (e.g., Butler et al., 1985; Silva, McGee, & Williams, 1985), syntactic awareness (e.g., Tunmer, Herriman, & Nesdale, 1988), and phonemic awareness (e.g., Lundberg, Olofsson, & Wall, 1980; Mann, 1984; Mann & Ditunno, 1990; Stanovich, Cunningham, & Cramer, 1984; Stuart & Coltheart, 1988).

Some or all of these linguistic deficits may also be evident in dyslexic children at even younger ages. Very recently, for instance, Bryant, Bradley, Maclean, and Crossland (1989) showed that the ability of 40-month-olds to recite nursery rhymes was predictive of their emerging phonological awareness skills and letter knowledge (and thereby, indirectly, of grade 1 reading). The early emergence of differences between dyslexic and nondyslexic children is also suggested by retrospective parental reports of early language deficits in children who became disabled readers (e.g., Ingram, Mason, & Blackburn, 1970; Rutter & Yule, 1975) and by follow-up studies showing a high incidence of later reading problems in samples of preschoolers who were treated for language impairment (Weiner, 1985).

Although many linguistic weaknesses have been shown to antedate reading disabilities, it is not clear whether a specific aspect of language ability (e.g., impaired phonological processing) or a more general linguistic deficiency is most directly responsible for reading failure (Bowey & Patel, 1988; Kamhi & Catts, 1989; Stanovich, 1988; Vellutino, 1979). Among the language measures associated with dyslexia, the strongest predictors of subsequent reading achievement are usually those that require the representation, retrieval, or metalinguistic analysis of phonological information (e.g., Share et al., 1984; Stanovich, Cunningham, & Cramer, 1984; Stuart & Coltheart, 1988; Wagner & Torgesen, 1987). Furthermore, some have argued that purported measures of lexical and syntactic proficiency may actually reflect a child's difficulties with phonological or memory processing aspects of the task (e.g., Fowler, 1988; Shankweiler & Crain, 1986). On the other hand, a specific deficit in phonological processing does not account well for the findings of some recent studies, in which reading was more successfully predicted by more general language assessments (e.g., Bowey & Patel, 1988; Butler et al., 1985). The issue of specificity is further clouded by the possibility that the scope of impairment is likely to vary according to the criteria used to classify reading disabilities and is likely to broaden over time as a consequence of the cognitive, instructional, and motivational changes brought about by the child's reading difficulties (Stanovich, 1988). In the present study, assessments of syntactic and lexical as well as phonological skills were made at a very early age so that the nature and breadth of the dyslexic children's presumed early language deficits could be evaluated with respect to this etiological issue.

METHOD

Subjects

Three groups of 30-month-old children were studied: 20 children from "dyslexic families" (see below) who subsequently became disabled readers, 12 children from dyslexic families who became normal readers, and 20 other normal children selected so as to resemble the dyslexic group closely in IQ, socioeconomic status, and sex (see Table 1). All 52 subjects were from lower- to upper-middle-class (Hollingshead & Redlich, 1958) monolingual families residing in central New

Jersey, and none had any gross visual, audiological, or neurological deficits. The subjects were all participants in a larger investigation of the relations between preschool development and later reading achievement; pursuant to the goals of that study, the reading abilities of members of the children's immediate families were evaluated, and the children's reading status at grade 2 (age 8.0 years) was assessed.

Family incidence of dyslexia. Dyslexia tends to run strongly in families (e.g., DeFries, Vogler, & LaBuda, 1985). Therefore, preschoolers with dyslexic relatives are more likely than other youngsters to develop reading problems, and the sample for the study was selected so as to overrepresent such children. Subjects were recruited in 1979–1981 through advertisements and referrals that encouraged families with 2-year-old children, "especially those families in which someone has experienced a severe childhood reading problem," to make confidential inquiries. All willing respondents who reported cases of dyslexia in the family, plus a subset of the many other respondents, were included in an original sample of 88 children; 10 families subsequently withdrew due to geographic relocation or loss of interest.

Of the 78 subjects remaining in the study, 34 were from dyslexic families. These children each had at least one parent or older sibling who exhibited low reading achievement despite normal IQ. The immediate families of the other 44 participants

TABLE 1
Comparability of Contrasted Groups

	Disabled Readers from Dyslexic Families	Normal Readers from Control Families	Normal Readers from Dyslexic Families
Number of children	20	20	12
Boys : girls	11:9	9:11	5:7
Cases with dyslexic mothers (%)	55	0	50
Cases with dyslexic fathers (%)	45	0	50
Family members dyslexic (%)	55.3 (21.9)	0	53.3 (26.1)
Socioeconomic status[a]	2.95 (.89)	2.95 (.89)	2.50 (.85)
IQ at 36 months[b]	107.0 (13.5)	110.5 (11.5)	113.9 (12.0)
IQ at 60 months[c]	112.1 (11.9)	115.7 (11.2)	116.0 (10.4)
IQ at grade 2[d]	110.0 (10.2)	114.4 (10.4)	117.4 (10.5)
Grade 2 reading[e]	479.2 (7.9)	502.0 (7.3)	501.8 (6.4)
Grade 2 math[f]	75.5 (19.5)	82.4 (24.9)	74.0 (22.2)

NOTE.—Standard deviations are shown in parentheses.

[a] On a 5-point scale based on parental education and occupational prestige (Hollingshead & Redlich, 1958); lower values represent higher status.

[b] Short form of the McCarthy Scales (Kaufman, 1977).

[c] McCarthy Scales of Preschool Abilities (McCarthy, 1972).

[d] Wechsler Intelligence Scale for Children—revised (Wechsler, 1974).

[e] Reading Cluster of the Woodcock-Johnson Psychoeducational Battery (Woodcock & Johnson, 1977).

[f] Percentile on a school-administered nationally standardized test.

had no reading-disabled members. The criteria used to classify family members have been described in detail previously (Scarborough, 1984, 1989a).

Outcome reading status. The Reading Cluster of the Woodcock-Johnson Psychoeducational Battery (Woodcock & Johnson, 1977) and the Wechsler Intelligence Scale for Children—Revised (Wechsler, 1974) were administered to 66 of the 78 subjects (31 from dyslexic families and 35 from nondyslexic families) at the end of grade 2. The reading status of the other 12 children was estimated from scores earned on school-administered nationally standardized tests of reading achievement and scholastic aptitude.

As previously described (Scarborough, 1989a), expected reading levels for this suburban New Jersey sample were based on analyses of the achievement scores of subjects from *non*dyslexic families. A cutoff of 1.5 SD below the mean of this group was used, and any child in the entire sample whose achievement score was more than 1.5 SD below the control mean was designated as reading disabled. There were 24 such cases in the entire sample; their z scores ranged from -1.5 to -5.8 ($M = -2.68$).[1]

Outcomes were strongly determined by family type. Of the 34 children from dyslexic families, 22 (65%) developed reading problems. This incidence level is considerably higher than that of Finucci, Gottfredson, and Childs (1985), who found that 36% of alumni of a school for dyslexic adolescents reported (in a follow-up questionnaire) having at least one reading-disabled offspring. This disagreement between studies may result from differences in recruitment or diagnostic methods, or simply from sampling variation. For the present analyses of linguistic differences at age 30 months, two of the 22 reading-disabled subjects had to be excluded for lack of preschool data at that age, resulting in a sample size of 20 for the dyslexic group.

In contrast, all but two (95%) of the other 44 children became normal readers. From these 42, 20 normal readers from normal families were selected to form a comparison group that would be as similar as possible to the reading-disabled group with regard to sex, SES, and IQ. This was done by first making all possible one-to-one matches between dyslexic children and those in the pool of possible controls (which could be done for 11 of the 20 cases) and then selecting nine others who were dissimilar to a dyslexic child only in sex (two cases), SES (four cases, in two of which the SES was higher for the reading-disabled child), or IQ (three cases, in all of which IQ was more than 7 points higher for the control child). Choices among potential control subjects who were equally well matched to a dyslexic case were made by random drawing.[2] As shown in Table 1, the resulting groups were

---

[1]On average, the reading scores of these 24 cases were 2.64 SE below levels defined by a regression of reading on IQ within the subsample from nondyslexic families (Scarborough, 1989a).

[2]The 22 other normal readers from nondyslexic families were 15 girls and seven boys whose mean SES was 1.91 (SD 0.31). Their mean reading score was 502.5 (SD 5.4), and mean IQs were 114.6 (SD 11.4) at age 36 months, 118.8 (SD 10.1) at 60 months, and 125.7 (SD 9.9) at grade 2.

very similar in the distribution of sex,[3] SES, and IQ but could not be analyzed as matched pairs of individuals.

One-way analyses of variance with planned pairwise contrasts between groups revealed no differences in grade 2 math achievement, SES, or IQ, although the IQ difference between the two groups from dyslexic families approached statistical significance at age 36 months, $F(1,49) = 2.976$, $p = .091$. IQ was thus controlled for in all analyses.

Procedures

In the larger project of which this study is a part, six evaluations of preschool development were conducted between the ages of 2 and 5 years. Language proficiency at age 30 months was the major focus of the present analyses, but some test scores obtained at other ages were also analyzed for this report so as to clarify the interpretation of the findings at 30 months.

At age 30 months ($\pm$ 2 weeks), each child was seen at home, in the presence of one or both parents, for a single session lasting about 2 hours. Seven measures of early language skill were analyzed for this study, including three test scores and four measures of natural language production during a 30-min mother-child play session.

Language tests. Vocabulary recognition, naming vocabulary, and speech discrimination were assessed using the Peabody Picture Vocabulary Test (PPVT; Dunn, 1965), Boston Naming Test (BNT; Kaplan, Goodglass, & Weintraub, 1978), and Phoneme Discrimination Series (PDS), respectively. On each PPVT trial, the child must indicate which of four line drawings corresponds to a spoken word. On successive trials of the BNT, the child must name pictured objects of increasing difficulty. On each of 24 PDS trials, the child must indicate which of two similarly named objects (e.g., bear/pear) is the one whose name has been spoken. Two children from the dyslexic group would not cooperate on the BNT, and one of them also refused to take the PDS, as did one child from each of the other two groups. Analyses involving these measures were carried out using available scores only.

The PDS was readministered at age 36 months, and the PPVT and BNT at age 42 months. A third administration of the BNT was also included in a readiness assessment (see below) at age 60 months.

Natural language production. Language samples were drawn from videorecorded mother-child play sessions with age-appropriate materials supplied by the examin-

---

[3]Although the ratio of dyslexic boys to girls is often less than 2:1, when classifications are based on test scores rather than school placement (Finucci & Childs, 1981; Naiden, 1976), the ratio obtained in the present project was nevertheless lower than expected. Perhaps this is due to other differences in ascertainment bias from study to study or is a consequence of the mode of familial transmission (DeFries, in press). Sex differences in adult reading ability have been discussed previously (Scarborough, 1984).

ers. All maternal and child utterances during play were transcribed along with contextual notes, and every transcript was reviewed for accuracy by a second transcriber prior to analysis. Four language production measures were derived from each child's transcript.

Two measures of productive syntax were coded for each child from a corpus of 100 successive intelligible child utterances within each transcript, excluding imitations, self-repetitions, and routines (such as counting or singing). Mean length of utterance (MLU) was computed according to conventional guidelines for counting morphemes (Brown, 1973). MLU is widely used to estimate a young child's general syntactic performance level, but the validity and interpretation of this measure have sometimes been questioned (Crystal, 1974; Klee & Fitzgerald, 1985). Thus, the Index of Productive Syntax (IPSyn; Scarborough, 1990) was also used as a measure of grammatical complexity. IPSyn scores are derived by crediting the occurrence of up to two unique tokens of 56 types of constructions, including noun phrase elaborations, verb phrase constructions, inflectional morphemes, interrogative and negative forms, and simple and complex sentence structures. IPSyn scores thus reflect the diversity of syntactic and morphological forms produced by the child.

As an index of phonological production ability, the child's consonant pronunciation error rate was based on the accuracy of the child's pronunciation of the first 100 identifiable words in the corpus, excluding determiners, pronouns, auxiliary verbs, proper nouns, and yes/no responses.[4] The number of omissions, additions, substitutions, and transpositions of consonant phonemes in those words was tallied for each child.

Last, lexical diversity was scored as the number of distinct lexical types (i.e., the number of different words) produced among the first 250 identifiable words (tokens) in the transcript. Richards (1987) has argued that this approach to scoring productive vocabulary is more stable and less confounded by syntactic proficiency than more traditional type-token scores based on a fixed number of utterances or a smaller number of lexical tokens.[5]

For each language-production measure, 10% to 25% of the corpora were coded independently by two scorers, and at least 92% of coding judgments were found to be in agreement in each case.

Assessment of readiness skills at age 60 months. The subjects were evaluated at age 60 months (when most had not yet begun kindergarten) with respect to some known precursors to reading achievement. As reported previously (Scarborough,

---

[4]This was done so that highly frequent words (like *Mommy, no, this, there,* and *what*) would not be the predominant productions scored for pronunciation, and so that words used primarily by more syntactically advanced 2-year-olds (like *the* and auxiliary verbs) would not confound the assessment of phonological production. Vowel pronunciation was not scored because of possible dialect differences and anticipated difficulties in achieving reliable transcription and coding.

[5]A more traditional lexical diversity measure was used in previous analyses of this sample (Scarborough, 1989b, 1989c).

1989a), only the BNT and the Sounds and Letters Test (which includes eight letter-identification terms, 16 letter-sound correspondence items, and 20 phonological awareness items requiring rhyme matching or first-sound matching of spoken words) of the Stanford Early School Achievement Test, Level 1 (Madden, Gardner, & Collins, 1981) were predictive of grade 2 reading achievement (with IQ controlled). Hence just these scores were included in the present analyses.

Feedback to parents. Parents who requested it were given information about their child's performance on standardized instruments only and were advised to interpret these scores cautiously in light of the questionable predictive validity of preschool instruments. In only one case was a child's productive language deficit at age 30 months noticed by the examiners who made the in-home recording; when this was brought to the parent's attention, their response was to disregard it.

RESULTS

Group Differences in Early Language Proficiency

The mean scores of the three groups on language measures at age 30 months are provided in Table 2, and intercorrelations among the seven measures in Table 3. Substantial correlations among the three test scores were obtained even when shared variance with IQ was partialed out. However, with IQ controlled, the test scores were not significantly related to the natural production measures other than MLU. Lexical diversity was weakly correlated with IPSyn, and not with other aspects of productive language. Pronunciation error rate was moderately correlated with both syntax measures, which were very closely related. A principal components factor

TABLE 2
Language Proficiency of Groups at Age 30 Months

Measure	Disabled Readers from Dyslexic Families		Normal Readers from Control Families		Normal Readers from Dyslexic Families	
	M	SD	M	SD	M	SD
Language tests:						
PPVT	25.2	11.1	31.2	12.9	33.1	6.1
BNT	8.6	2.8	9.1	3.2	10.2	3.4
PDS	19.9	2.3	20.3	3.6	21.7	2.1
Natural production:						
MLU	2.35	.58	2.89	.48	2.97	.66
IPSyn	46.6	13.4	61.7	11.7	58.8	11.9
Consonant errors ...	43.0	17.9	27.5	16.0	26.3	14.2
Lexical diversity	83.5	10.8	84.1	11.0	86.3	9.7

TABLE 3
Correlations Among Language Measures at Age 30 Months

Measures	1	2	3	4	5	6	7
1. PPVT		.48***	.66***	.47***	.39**	−.24	.31*
2. BNT	.44**		.54***	.37**	.32*	−.31*	.34*
3. PDS	.60***	.50***		.39**	.27	−.22	.20
4. MLU	.36**	.39**	.32*		.85***	−.44**	.23
5. IPSyn	.22	.25	.16	.83***		−.56***	.39*
6. Consonant errors	−.09	−.28	−.15	−.38**	−.50***		−.13
7. Lexical diversity	.23	.27	.15	.15	.31*	−.05	

NOTE.—Simple correlations among measures are shown above the diagonal, and partial correlations with IQ at age 36 months controlled are below the diagonal.

* $p < .05$.
** $p < .01$.
*** $p < .001$.

analysis of MLU and IPSyn was thus used to derive a single factor score for syntactic production.

To test the main hypothesis that early language deficits would be exhibited by children who become disabled readers, multivariate analyses of covariance (MANCOVA), with IQ at 36 months as the covariate, were carried out. Because they appeared to tap relatively independent facets of early language proficiency, test scores and natural language production measures were analyzed separately with respect to group differences. A MANCOVA with PPVT, BNT, and PDS test scores as the predictors revealed no significant group effect: Wilks's lambda = .907, $F(6,84) = 0.704, p = 0.65$; this analysis included only the 48 children for whom all three test scores were available.

A second MANCOVA, with consonant error rate, lexical diversity, and the syntax factor as predictors, yielded a significant group effect, Wilks's lambda = .730, $F(6,92) = 2.618, p = .022$. Planned pairwise contrasts between groups indicated that there was no difference at age 30 months between the two groups who became normal readers, Wilks's lambda = .990, $F(3,46) = 0.160, p = .922$. The dyslexic group, however, differed from the normal readers from nondyslexic families, Wilks's lambda = .753, $F(3,46) = 4.229, p = .004$, and from the normal readers from dyslexic families, Wilks's lambda = .836, $F(3,46) = 2.795, p = .050$. Univariate results indicated that the syntax factor, $F(2,48) = 6.421, p = .003$, and consonant error rate, $F(2,48) = 4.620, p = .015$, differed among groups, but that lexical diversity did not, $F(2,48) = 0.065, p = .937$.

These results established, as hypothesized, that early language skills of the dyslexic group were poorer than those of the other two groups, which did not differ from each other. The inclusion of two equivalent groups would necessarily make subsequent variance analyses of the relation of preschool differences to reading outcomes less meaningful and less powerful. Thus, the two groups of children who became normal readers were collapsed into a single group in the remaining analyses.

Three analyses of covariance were carried out to determine which aspect(s) of language production—syntax, phonology, or vocabulary—contributed uniquely to the difference between children who became disabled readers and children who became normal readers. In successive analyses, each language-production measure in turn served as the predictor, and the other two measures served as covariates in addition to IQ. Not surprisingly, in view of the univariate results of the MANOVA described above, there was no difference between dyslexic and normal groups in lexical diversity after variance due to IQ, the syntax factor, and consonant error rate was removed, $F(1,47) = 0.528, p = .471$. Likewise, when IQ, the syntax factor, and lexical diversity were controlled, consonant error rate accounted for no significant additional variance in outcomes, $F(1,47) = 2.818, p = .100$. The syntax score, however, did significantly differentiate the groups even with IQ, consonant errors, and lexical diversity controlled, $F(1,47) = 6.450, p = .014$. Thus the phonological differences between groups, revealed in the univariate MANOVA results, accounted for no unique variability in outcomes beyond that accounted for by syntactic differences.

Family Incidence of Reading Disability

The finding that children from dyslexic families who did not develop reading disabilities resembled the other normal readers, rather than the other children from dyslexic families, suggests that the early language deficits of reading-disabled children did not stem only from being reared in a family with dyslexic members. This suggestion was supported by other analyses of the data.

The 32 children from dyslexic families had an average of 1.63 older family members (55% of household) with reading disability. If verbal communication patterns within such families are unusual, preschoolers from dyslexic families might be exposed to qualitatively or quantitatively different language input. Of particular importance to language development might be the input provided by the child's mother, who was the child's primary caretaker—and hence probably the major language model—in nearly all of the families in the present sample.

One might thus expect that children who became disabled readers would be more likely to have reading-disabled mothers or to have a higher incidence of reading disability in their immediate families than the children from dyslexic families who became normal readers. As shown in Table 1, this was not the case in the present sample. It might also be hypothesized that the severity—rather than the incidence—of a child's weaknesses might be influenced by the mother's status. That is, even if genetic transmission (or some other nonenvironmental factor) was responsible for the language and reading problems observed in the children who became disabled readers, environmental differences might ameliorate or exacerbate a child's predisposition to have difficulty acquiring language and reading. If so, one would expect that, within the dyslexic group, the 11 children with dyslexic mothers might have more severe deficits than the nine children whose mothers are normal readers. However, no large or significant differences between these two subgroups in IQ, in language scores at age 30 months, or in reading ability at grade 2 were observed (all p's > .10). Ongoing analyses of maternal language will potentially yield direct evidence of whether the linguistic input to dyslexic children is atypical, but until those results are available, no firm conclusions can be drawn. Thus the present results are consistent with, but do not provide a clear test of, the hypothesis that dyslexia is a genetically transmitted disorder. Considerable evidence for the heritability of dyslexia has been found in recent studies in behavioral genetics (e.g., DeFries, Fulker, & LaBuda, 1987; Olson, Wise, Conners, Rack, & Fulker, 1989; Smith, Kimberling, Pennington, & Lubs, 1983).

Language and Readiness Skills in the Later Preschool Years

Analyses of covariance, with IQ as the covariate, were carried out to examine differences between the dyslexic and normal groups on subsequent scores on the three language tests that had been given at 30 months. Table 4 shows group means (separately for the two normal groups) on these follow-up tests and provides partial correlations with the prior administration of each test, with IQ controlled. Scores for one normal reader on the PDS at age 36 months and for two normal readers on the BNT and PPVT at 42 months were not available.

The PDS, when readministered at age 36 months, again failed to differentiate the children who became disabled readers from the children who became normal readers, $F(1,48) = 0.571$, $p = .454$. However, language test scores obtained 6 months earlier were strongly correlated with PDS scores at 36 months, and consonant pronunciation was the only language-production measure related to subsequent phoneme discrimination ability. Thus, although PDS scores were unrelated to outcomes at either age, this test was apparently sensitive to individual differences that were also tapped by other measures.

TABLE 4

Performance on Readministrations of the Phoneme Discriminations Series (PDS), Peabody Picture Vocabulary Test (PPVT), and Boston Naming Test (BNT)

	PDS, 36 Months	PPVT, 42 Months	BNT, 42 Months
Comparison of groups (means):			
Disabled readers from dyslexic families	20.6	39.1	13.9
	(2.5)	(10.4)	(5.3)
Normal readers from control families	21.3	46.6	17.4
	(2.3)	(8.8)	(4.4)
Normal readers from dyslexic families	22.0	45.0	18.5
	(2.0)	(12.7)	(4.8)
Partial correlations[a] with earlier language measures:			
30-month language tests:			
PPVT	.42**	.48***	.44**
BNT	.50***	.72***	.58***
PDS	.63***	.38**	.21
30-month natural production:			
MLU	.22	.40**	.30*
IPSyn	.17	.33*	.38**
Consonant errors	−.36*	−.35*	−.36**
Lexical diversity	.11	.31*	.14

NOTE.—Standard deviations are in parentheses.
[a] Controlling for IQ at 36 months.
* $p < .05$.
** $p < .01$.
*** $p < .001$.

In contrast, both of the vocabulary test scores at age 42 months were significantly lower for the reading-disabled group: PPVT, $F(1,47) = 4.038$, $p = .050$; BNT, $F(1,47) = 5.770$, $p = .020$. These two measures were again strongly intercorrelated ($r = .62$, $p < .001$). Moreover, BNT and PPVT scores were related not only to vocabulary test scores obtained 1 year earlier but also to earlier syntactic and phonological production abilities.

As Table 5 shows, the children who became disabled readers also did more poorly as 5-year-olds. Analyses of covariance, with IQ at 60 months serving as the covariate, were carried out for language and preliteracy tests administered at age 60 months. Group differences on the BNT were again found, $F(1,47) = 5.139$, $p = .028$, and scores on this test were correlated with language tests, IPSyn scores, and

TABLE 5
Language and Preliteracy Skills at Age 60 Months

| | BOSTON NAMING TEST | SOUNDS AND LETTERS TEST | | | |
		Letter-Recognition Items	Phoneme Awareness Items	Letter-Sound Items	Total Score
Comparison of groups (means):					
Disabled readers from dyslexic families ...	24.8	6.3	10.8	6.5	23.5
	(6.8)	(1.7)	(4.0)	(3.8)	(8.6)
Normal readers from control families	29.7	7.4	13.7	8.5	29.6
	(7.0)	(1.0)	(3.7)	(4.9)	(7.8)
Normal readers from dyslexic families	30.9	7.2	14.3	11.5	32.9
	(8.4)	(.8)	(3.0)	(4.5)	(5.2)
Partial correlations[a] with early language measures:					
30-month language tests:					
PPVT	.37**	.19	.32*	.05	.13
BNT	.70***	.18	.36*	.08	.20
PDS	.29*	−.07	.19	.06	.10
30-month natural production:					
MLU	.27	.43**	.40**	.22	.38**
IPSyn	.32*	.51***	.36**	.23	.40**
Consonant errors	−.50***	−.49***	−.34*	−.37**	−.44**
Lexical diversity	.26	.08	.15	.19	.19

NOTE.—Standard deviations are in parentheses.
[a] Controlling for IQ at 36 months.
* $p < .05$.
** $p < .01$.
*** $p < .001$.

consonant error rates of the children 3 years earlier. As expected, the Sounds and Letters Test also revealed substantial differences in favor of the children who became normal readers, $F(1,47) = 9.383, p = .004$. Moreover, each of the readiness skills assessed in subsections of this test was weaker for the dyslexic group: letter identification, despite an apparent ceiling effect in the normal group, $F(1,47) = 6.936, p = .011$; phonemic awareness, $F(1,47) = 4.072, p = .049$. MLU, IPSyn, and consonant errors at age 30 months all predicted letter recognition, phonemic awareness, and total Sounds and Letters scores at age 5, but only early consonant production skill was also related to subsequent abilities on items requiring knowledge of letter-sound correspondences. In contrast, early vocabulary test scores were correlated solely with the phonemic awareness subtest.

As described above, early syntactic and phonological production abilities were strongly predictive of outcome reading status in the sample. To see whether these differences at age 30 months were directly related to grade 2 classifications, or only indirectly through intervening differences in readiness skills at age 60 months (which were also strongly related to outcomes), analyses of covariance were carried out with IQ, BNT, and Sounds and Letters scores at age 60 months as the covariates. A significant effect of group was still obtained for the syntax factor score, $F(1,45) = 5.103, p = .029$, but not for consonant error rate, $F(1,45) = 2.336, p = .133$. These results suggest that the relation of early syntactic deficits to reading disabilities was not simply mediated by problems with language and preliteracy in the late preschool years.

DISCUSSION

Precursors of Reading Disabilities

Because dyslexia is usually defined in terms of reading achievement, the condition cannot be diagnosed until a child's difficulties in reading become apparent during the school years. As reviewed earlier, prospective research studies have often shown that such children often have poor *pre*literacy skills even before they begin kindergarten. Preliteracy weaknesses were also a precursor of subsequent reading disability in the present sample at age 60 months, suggesting that these children resembled those in other prospective studies despite differences in recruitment methods. Having learned less about letters and letter-sound correspondences as preschoolers, the children were already exhibiting problems with learning to read.

Previous prospective studies have further demonstrated that these children's preliteracy deficits are accompanied by oral language difficulties that are also related to subsequent progress in reading. This, too, was seen in the present sample; as 5-year-olds, the children with poor letter-sound knowledge and who later became poor readers were also deficient in object-naming and phonemic awareness skills. Very

recent work (Bryant et al., 1989) has revealed that some oral vocabulary and phonological processing differences among children as young as 40 months are related to
future reading achievement, although those effects appear to be mediated by late
preschool metaphonological skills. The present study identifies even earlier characteristics that distinguish children who become disabled readers from those who
become normal readers and confirms prior findings that weakness in language skill
is a precursor to reading disability.

The main focus of the study was oral language proficiency at 30 months of age.
At that time, normal language development typically undergoes rapid improvements
in syntactic complexity, pronunciation accuracy, and vocabulary size (e.g., Dale,
1976). In the present sample, syntactic differences among 2-year-olds corresponded
most closely with the children's eventual outcomes, but phonological production was
also substantially impaired in the children who were later identified as poor readers.
Not surprisingly, these productive language skills are often deficient in kindergartners who later develop reading problems (Butler et al., 1985; Silva et al., 1985) and
in dyslexic schoolchildren (Catts, 1986; Donahue, Pearl, & Bryan, 1982; Feagans &
Short, 1984; Siegel & Ryan, 1984; Taylor, Lean, & Schwartz, 1989). Syntactic
complexity and speech accuracy are correlated in young normal children (e.g.,
Dobrich & Scarborough, 1984) and in children with expressive language impairments (e.g., Wolfus, Moscovitch, & Kinsbourne, 1980). The interdependence of
these two facets of language development is further suggested by Panagos, Quine,
and Klich's (1979) demonstration that more speech errors tend to be made during a
child's production of complex than simple syntactic forms.

On the other hand, some early linguistic abilities were apparently intact in the children who became disabled readers. For example, there was no evidence of early
receptive phonological impairment, a result that is consistent with Mann and
Ditunno's (1990) recent finding that kindergartners' speech discrimination abilities
were not predictive of reading achievement. It is thus unlikely that the early syntactic
and phonological production problems of the children who became dyslexic can be
explained simply on the basis of incomplete or distorted perception of language input.

There was also little evidence for very early problems in vocabulary development
among the children who later developed reading disabilities. At age 30 months,
diversity of words in natural conversation, elicited object-naming abilities (on the
BNT), and recognition of spoken words (on the PPVT) were not closely related
either to concurrent productive syntactic and phonological deficits or to future reading abilities in the sample. Vocabulary deficits, of course, *have* often been associated
with reading problems in prior prospective studies (e.g., Bryant et al., 1989; Share
et al., 1984; Stanovich, Cunningham, & Feeman, 1984; Wolf & Goodglass, 1986),
and this result was also observed in the present sample—but not until the children
were 42 months old.

This observed change in the relation of vocabulary skill to later reading achievement was probably not due merely to the methods of assessment used. Floor effects were not apparent for either the BNT or PPVT at 30 months, and moderate across-age and concurrent correlations were observed among these scores, so it is unlikely that the vocabulary tests were just insensitive to early lexical differences among the groups. On the other hand, lexical diversity during natural conversation was not strongly related to any concurrent or subsequent measures in the study, and it is not yet known whether this measure will, like tested vocabulary skills, also emerge as a predictor of reading disability at older ages. Although the type-token ratio has long been used as a clinical tool and has been associated with reading achievement differences among schoolchildren (Fry, Johnson, & Muehl, 1970; Idol-Maestas, 1980), little is actually known about what such scores tell us about individual differences in productive vocabulary development (Richards, 1987). When more longitudinal data on natural language development become available for the sample, the validity of this measure will be examined closely.

Nevertheless, the BNT and PPVT test results indicate that vocabulary deficits may not emerge as precursors to reading disabilities at as early an age as do syntactic and phonological production deficits. Conceivably, vocabulary problems could be consequences of earlier structural language deficiencies. Even if syntactic and phonological production problems are initially quite specific and compartmentalized, this disruption of the normal interdependence among developing components of the language faculty might impede the further progress of other components, including vocabulary growth. Such a diffusion in the scope of language impairment over time might also occur if conversational partners adjusted their speech to the perceived ability level of the child, thus providing less enriching input. For whatever reasons, by age 42 months some vocabulary deficits of children who become disabled readers appear to predict their later reading problems.

In sum, the picture that emerges from research on the precursors of dyslexia is one of a child who not only has difficulty with reading and language during the school years but who also typically experiences problems with preliteracy skills during the late preschool period; exhibits vocabulary deficiencies, poor rhyme recitation skills, and phonemic awareness deficits from the age of 3 or 4 years; and produces shorter, syntactically simpler sentences and less accurate pronunciations of words than other 2-year-olds.

The Etiology of Reading Disability

Although early deficits in syntactic and phonological processing appear to be precursors to reading disabilities many years later, and although even broader language deficits are associated with inadequate literary skills from the time children usually start learning letter names and letter-sound correspondences, these findings do not mean that a dyslexic child's difficulty in learning to read is necessarily brought about by these linguistic weaknesses. Several approaches to explaining dyslexia will be considered in light of the present findings.

Explaining reading failure. What causes dyslexia? When dyslexia is defined as primarily a reading failure, then the central etiological goal is to explain what goes awry during the process of learning to read, and to determine to what extent the deficient language skills a child brings to the learning situation may impede that process. It is generally agreed that the major task facing the beginning reader is to decode grapheme strings into recognizable phonemic sequences. To do this, an appreciation of the fact that *spoken* words are composed of sequences of phonemes (which often correspond in regular ways to letter sequences) is of great help to the learner, much more so perhaps than sophisticated syntactic and vocabulary skills. Phonological processing abilities at the time that formal instruction in decoding begins may thus play an important role in the acquisition of reading (Liberman, Shankweiler, Fischer, & Carter, 1974).

In contrast, the syntactic and lexical skills of kindergartners who become disabled readers are probably not so impaired as to impede their understanding of the relatively simple words and sentences found in primers. The children's poor performance in tasks that purportedly assess lexical and syntactic skills may often instead primarily reflect their phonological limitations, including difficulties with verbal coding for short-term memory and with retrieval of stored phonological information (Fowler, 1988; Shankweiler & Crain, 1986). Although poor oral language skills could adversely affect teacher-student communication, and thereby reduce the effectiveness of instruction, the fact that the reading-disabled children's achievement problems do not extend to math suggests that the source of their reading problems is probably not merely a failure to understand and be understood by their teachers.

Consequently, most contemporary views reject the notion that general language deficits are directly responsible for reading difficulties in favor of the hypothesis that a more specific deficit in phonological—or, more narrowly, in *meta*phonological—skill is the more likely proximal cause of poor reading achievement, at least in the early school years (e.g., Kamhi & Catts, 1989; Stanovich, 1988; Wagner & Torgesen, 1987). In support of this hypothesis, correlations between phonological skills and future reading achievement have been demonstrated in many prior prospective studies of preschoolers, as noted earlier. Moreover, training in phonemic awareness skills has been shown to be effective, although not dramatically so, in improving reading acquisition (e.g., Blachman, 1989; Bradley & Bryant, 1983; Williams, 1980). The present findings of impaired phonemic awareness and name-retrieval skills in 5-year-olds who became disabled readers are consistent with the conclusion that phonological processing is the aspect of language skill most closely related to outcomes, with only secondary contributions, if any, from more general language deficiencies.

Plausible though this hypothesis might be, it may not provide a complete explanation of reading failure. There is abundant evidence that the reading difficulties of dyslexic children begin to emerge from the time that they start learning to recognize letters and to appreciate letter-sound correspondences. Moreover, the relation between metaphonological and literacy skills is apparently one of reciprocal causation, such that phonological proficiency facilitates the learning of letter-sound correspondences, which in turn enhances phonological skill and awareness (e.g., Ehri, 1985; Morais, Carey, Alegria, & Bertelson, 1979; Stuart & Coltheart, 1988). To explain reading failure in terms of these phonological skills, therefore, may say little more than that a child's success in early literacy achievement is predictive of subsequent progress in reading, and raises the question of what underlies the early deficits in literacy and phonological processing to begin with (Kamhi, 1989; Tunmer et al., 1988).

The relevance of syntactic and lexical deficits to reading acquisition also cannot be ruled out entirely, despite the greater weight of evidence for strong correlations between phonological performance and subsequent reading scores. Bowey and Patel (1988), for instance, have shown that when general language abilities are carefully assessed, metaphonological abilities do *not* account for any unique variance in reading achievement. Also, several follow-up studies of samples of clinically identified language-impaired preschoolers, reviewed by Weiner (1985), have shown that children with broad deficit profiles are at much greater risk for reading disabilities than children with only phonological impairments. Finally, the present finding that some additional variance in outcomes was predicted by very early syntactic abilities, above and beyond the contributions of phonemic awareness and early literacy skills at age 60 months, suggests that the prevailing explanation of reading disability may be overly narrow, and that it might be fruitful to consider a different etiological approach.

Explaining developmental dyslexia. The answer to the question, "What causes dyslexia?" may depend on whether one takes the traditional view of dyslexia as fundamentally a reading problem, or instead defines it as a broader condition of which reading problems are merely the most evident—and most debilitating—symptom. Dyslexia, that is, may be a disorder (or an extreme of natural variation) that emerges even before any literacy demands are made on the child (Catts, 1989; Kamhi & Catts, 1989). If so, the sentence-production and pronunciation deficits at age 30 months in the present study would be early symptoms of dyslexia, as would many of the preschool characteristics that have so far been called "precursors" to dyslexia. Reading failure itself would also be a symptom of the disorder. The observed relations among early and late symptoms would thus arise, at least in part, because each reflected persisting individual differences along the more fundamental underlying dimension. Of course, the earlier symptoms could also contribute to the development or expression of the later ones.

What might this hypothesized underlying condition be? The possibilities are many, given that so little is yet known about early symptoms. Possible exogenous conditions would include child-rearing patterns that could adversely affect early language development and that might occur more often in dyslexic families than in others, such as infrequent verbal interchanges in the household, low parental expectations regarding progress in language development, or decreased emphasis on language-related activities, including reading. This possibility cannot be entirely ruled out, especially since the early deficits identified in this study all involved measures of performance during mother-child interaction, but is counterindicated by the present findings that the children from dyslexic families who did not develop reading problems exhibited normal early language proficiency, and that equally severe language deficits occurred in children whose mothers were dyslexic as in children with normal mothers. Furthermore, any differences in child-rearing patterns cannot be so broad as to affect *all* aspects of the child's future development, since most of the affected subjects in this study and others have exhibited normal nonverbal processing and adequate math achievement.

Possible endogenous conditions would include a variety of cognitive or personal characteristics (and associated neurological substrates). A genetically transmitted trait, of course, would most readily account for the extent to which dyslexia runs in families. Differences in temperament, health, sociability, attention, and the like might conceivably lead to the symptoms observed in dyslexic children, but the normal nonverbal development of these children might not as easily be explained. A more plausible hypothesis is that the underlying dimension of difference involved an intrinsic limitation in some verbal-cognitive capacity that constrains language processing to a greater extent than other aspects of development.

Along these lines, Kamhi and Catts (1989) have argued that the process of representing or retrieving phonological information may be the fundamental source of difficulty. This notion would account particularly well for name-retrieval, verbal memory, and phonological deficits associated with reading disabilities but would not as readily explain the present findings of syntactic deficits and unimpaired lexical skills (including name retrieval) at age 30 months.

Instead, the nature of syntactic and phonological rule systems may make them particularly difficult for dyslexic children to acquire and use efficiently. For both of these "structural" components of a language (and arguably for few, if any, other human faculties), the child must discover rules that govern the order-dependent combination of abstract formal elements (phonemic and syntactic categories) into higher-order structures of which only the surface features are uttered and perceived. Moreover, the generation and comprehension of these multiple levels of abstract structural relations go on simultaneously during speaking and listening, making the acquisition problem even more difficult. A limitation in dealing with any of various aspects (abstractness, low redundancy, order sensitivity, duality of structure, etc.) of acquiring and using such a system might conceivably later impede the acquisition of letter-sound correspondence rules as well. There is indeed some evidence that the decoding problems of dyslexic schoolchildren are attributable, in part, to such rule-learning difficulties (Manis et al., 1987; Morrison, 1987).

In addition, early structural language deficits themselves might affect the quality of linguistic models provided by conversational partners, or alter the child's tendency to engage in language-dependent preschool activities. These or other imaginable consequences of early structural language problems could in turn produce short- and long-term developmental effects (on vocabulary acquisition, memory processing strategies, and metalinguistic awareness) above and beyond the initial underlying problem. Some such consequences might be preventable, even if the intrinsic underlying limitation and early symptoms are not.

In conclusion, the present results reveal that potentially important differences between children who do and do not become disabled readers are evident by the third year of life. The causal relations between these early symptoms and eventual reading problems are probably complex and often indirect. A clearer etiological picture may emerge when more is learned about the preschool development of the present sample from ongoing analyses of their productive language skills at other ages, of the maternal language input they receive, of their emerging attitudes toward literacy, and of their attentional and motivational characteristics.

REFERENCES

Blachman, B. A. (1989). Phonological awareness and word recognition: Assessment and intervention. In A. G. Kamhi & H. W. Catts (Eds.), *Reading disabilities: A developmental language perspective* (pp. 133–158). Boston: Little, Brown.

Bowey, J. A., & Patel, R. K. (1988). Metalinguistic ability and early reading achievement. *Applied Psycholinguistics, 9,* 367–383.

Bradley, L., & Bryant, P. E. (1983). Categorizing sounds and learning to read—a causal connection. *Nature, 301,* 415–421.

Brown, R. (1973). *A first language: The early stages.* Cambridge, MA: Cambridge University Press.

Bryant, P. E., Bradley, L., Maclean, M., & Crossland, J. (1989). Nursery rhymes, phonological skills and reading. *Journal of Child Language, 16,* 407–428.

Butler, S. R., Marsh, H. W., Sheppard, M. J., & Sheppard, J. L. (1985). Seven-year longitudinal study of the early prediction of reading achievement. *Journal of Educational Psychology, 77,* 349–361.

Catts, H. W. (1986). Speech, production/phonological deficits in reading-disordered children. *Journal of Learning Disabilities, 19,* 504–508.

Catts, H. W. (1989). Defining dyslexia as a developmental language disorder. *Annals of Dyslexia, 39,* 50–64.

Crystal, D. (1974). A review of Brown's *A first language. Journal of Child Language,* **1,** 289–307.

Dale, P. (1976). *Language development.* New York: Holt, Rinehart & Winston.

DeFries, J. C. (in press). Gender ratios in reading-disabled children and their affected relatives: A commentary. *Journal of Learning Disabilities.*

DeFries, J. C., Fulker, D. W., & LaBuda, M. C. (1987). Evidence for a genetic etiology in reading disability in twins. *Nature,* **329,** 537–539.

DeFries, J. C., Vogler, G. P., & LaBuda, M. C. (1985). Colorado family reading study: An overview. In J. L. Fuller & E. C. Simmel (Eds.), *Behavior genetics: Principles and applications* (Vol. **2,** pp. 357–368). Hillsdale, NJ: Erlbaum.

Dobrich, W., & Scarborough, H. S. (1984). Form and function in early communication: Language and pointing gestures. *Journal of Experimental Child Psychology,* **38,** 475–490.

Donahue, M., Pearl, R., & Bryan, T. (1982). Learning disabled children's syntactic proficiency on a communicative task. *Journal of Speech and Hearing Disorders,* **47,** 397–403.

Dunn, L. M. (1965). *Peabody Picture Vocabulary Test.* Circle Pines, MN: American Guidance Service.

Ehri, L. C. (1985). Effects of printed language acquisition on speech. In D. R. Olson, N. Torrance, & A. Hildyard (Eds.), *Literacy, language, and learning* (pp. 333–367). Cambridge: Cambridge University Press.

Feagans, L., & Short, E. J. (1984). Developmental differences in the comprehension and production of narratives by reading-disabled and normally achieving children. *Child Development,* **55,** 1727–1736.

Finucci, J. M., & Childs, B.(1981). Are there really more dyslexic boys than girls? In A. Ansara, N. Geschwind, A. Galaburda, M. Albert, & N. Gartrell (Eds.), *Sex differences in dyslexia* (pp. 1–9). Towson, MD: Orton Dyslexia Society.

Finucci, J. M., Gottfredson, L. S., & Childs, B. (1985). A follow-up study of dyslexic boys. *Annals of Dyslexia,* **35,** 117–136.

Fowler, A. E. (1988). Grammaticality judgments and reading skill in grade 2. *Annals of Dyslexia,* **38,** 73–94.

Fry, M. A., Johnson, C. S., & Muehl, S. (1970). Oral language production in relation to reading achievement among selected second graders. In D. J. Bakker & P. Satz (Eds.), *Specific reading disability: Advances in theory and method* (pp. 123–146). Rotterdam: Rotterdam University Press.

Hollingshead, A.B., & Redlich, F. C. (1958). *Social class and mental illness.* New York: Wiley.

Idol-Maestas, L. (1980). Oral language responses of children with reading difficulties. *Journal of Special Education,* **14,** 385–404.

Ingram, T. T. S., Mason, A. W., & Blackburn, I. (1970). A retrospective study of 82 children with reading disability. *Developmental Medicine and Child Neurology,* **12,** 271–281.

Jansky, J., & deHirsch, K. (1972). *Preventing reading failure.* New York: Harper.

Kamhi, A. G. (1989). Causes and consequences of reading disabilities. In A. G. Kamhi & H.

W. Catts (Eds.), *Reading disabilities: A developmental language perspective* (pp. 67–99). Boston: Little, Brown.

Kamhi, A. G., & Catts, H. W. (1989). *Reading disabilities: A developmental language perspective.* Boston: Little, Brown.

Kaplan, E., Goodglass, H., & Weintraub, S. (1978). *Boston Naming Test.* Boston: published by the authors.

Kaufman, A. S. (1977). A McCarthy short form for rapid screening of preschool, kindergarten, and first-grade children. *Contemporary Educational Psychology, 2,* 149–157.

Kavanagh, J. F., & Yeni-Komshian, G. (1985). *Developmental dyslexia and related reading disorders.* Bethesda, MD: National Institute of Child Health and Human Development.

Klee, T., & Fitzgerald, M. D. (1985). The relation between grammatical development and mean length of utterance in morphemes. *Journal of Child Language, 12,* 251–269.

Liberman, I., Shankweiler, D., Fischer, F., & Carter, B. (1974). Explicit syllable and phoneme segmentation in young children. *Journal of Experimental Child Psychology, 18,* 201–212.

Lundberg, I., Olofsson, A., & Wall, S. (1980). Reading and spelling skills in the first school years predicted from phonemic awareness skills in kindergarten. *Scandinavian Journal of Psychology, 21,* 159–173.

Madden, R., Gardner, E. F., & Collins, C. S. (1981). *Stanford Early School Achievement Test.* New York: Psychological Corp.

Manis, F. R., Savage, P. L., Morrison, F. J., Horn, C. C., Howell, J. J., Szeszulski, P. A., & Holt, L. K. (1987). Paired associate learning in reading-disabled children: Evidence for a rule-learning deficiency. *Journal of Experimental Child Psychology, 43,* 25–43.

Mann, V. A. (1984). Longitudinal prediction and prevention of early reading difficulty. *Annals of Dyslexia, 34,* 117–136.

Mann, V. A., & Ditunno, P. (1990). Phonological deficiencies: Effective predictors of future reading problems. In G. Pavlides (Ed.), *Perspectives on dyslexia* (Vol. 2, pp. 105–131). New York: Wiley.

McCarthy, D. (1972). *McCarthy Scales of Children's Abilities.* New York: Psychological Corp.

Morais, J., Carey, L., Alegria, J., & Bertelson, P. (1979). Does awareness of speech as a sequence of phonemes arise spontaneously? *Cognition, 7,* 323–331.

Morrison, F. J. (1987). The nature of reading disability: Toward an integrative framework. In S. J. Ceci (Ed.), *Handbook of cognitive, social, and neuropsychological aspects of learning disabilities* (pp. 33–62). Hillsdale, NJ: Erlbaum.

Naiden, N. (1976, February). Ratio of boys to girls among disabled readers. *Reading Teacher,* 439–442.

Olson, R., Wise, B., Conners, F., Rack, J., & Fulker, D. (1989). Specific deficits in component reading and language skills: Genetic and environmental influences. *Journal of Learning Disabilities, 22,* 339–348.

Panagos, J. M., Quine, M. E., & Klich, R. J. (1979). Syntactic and phonological influences on children's articulation. *Journal of Speech and Hearing Research, 22,* 841–848.

Perfetti, C. A. (1985). *Reading ability.* New York: Oxford University Press.

Richards, B. (1987). Type/token ratios: What do they really tell us? *Journal of Child Language,* **14,** 201–209.

Rutter, M., & Yule, W. (1975). The concept of specific reading retardation. *Journal of Child Psychology and Psychiatry,* **16,** 181–197.

Scarborough, H. S. (1984). Continuity between childhood dyslexia and adult reading. *British Journal of Psychology,* **75,** 329–348.

Scarborough, H. S. (1989a). Prediction of reading disability from familial and individual differences. *Journal of Educational Psychology,* **81,** 101–108.

Scarborough, H. S. (1989b, June). *Reading disabilities and early language deficits: A longitudinal study.* Paper presented at the meeting of the American Psychological Society, Alexandria, VA.

Scarborough, H. S. (1989c, June). *Early language deficits of two-year-olds who became disabled readers.* Paper presented to the Joint Conference on Learning Disabilities, Ann Arbor, MI.

Scarborough, H. S. (1990). Index of productive syntax. *Applied Psycholinguistics,* **11,** 1–22.

Shankweiler, D., & Crain, S. (1986). Language mechanisms and reading disorder: A modular approach. *Cognition,* **24,** 139–168.

Share, D. L., Jorm, A. F., Maclean, R., & Matthews, R. (1984). Sources of individual differences in reading acquisition. *Journal of Educational Psychology,* **76,** 1309–1324.

Siegel, L. S., & Ryan, E. B. (1984) Reading disability as a language disorder. *Remedial and Special Education,* **5,** 28–33.

Silva, P. A., McGee, R., & Williams, S. (1985). Some characteristics of 9-year-old boys with general reading backwardness or specific reading retardation. *Journal of Child Psychology and Psychiatry,* **26,** 407–421.

Smith, S. D., Kimberling, W. J., Pennington, B. F., & Lubs, H. A. (1983). Specific reading disability: Identification of an inherited form through linkage analyses. *Science,* **219,** 1345–1347.

Stanovich, K. E. (1988). The right and wrong places to look for the cognitive locus of reading disability. *Annals of Dyslexia,* **38,** 154–177.

Stanovich, K. E., Cunningham, A. E., & Cramer, B. B. (1984). Assessing phonological awareness in kindergarten children: Issues of task comparability. *Journal of Experimental Child Psychology,* **38,** 175–190.

Stanovich, K. E., Cunningham, A. E., & Feeman, D. J. (1984). Intelligence, cognitive skills, and early reading progress. *Reading Research Quarterly,* **19,** 278–303.

Stuart, M., & Coltheart, M. (1988). Does reading develop in a sequence of stages? *Cognition,* **30,** 139–181.

Taylor, H. G., Lean, D., & Schwartz, S. (1989). Pseudoword repetition ability in learning-disabled children. *Applied Psycholinguistics,* **10,** 203–219.

Tunmer, W. E., Herriman, M. L., & Nesdale, A. R. (1988). Metalinguistic abilities and beginning reading. *Reading Research Quarterly,* **23,** 134–158.

Vellutino, F. R. (1979). *Dyslexia: Theory and research.* Cambridge, MA: MIT Press.

Wagner, R. K., & Torgesen, J. K. (1987). The nature of phonological processing and its causal role in the acquisition of reading skills. *Psychological Bulletin,* **101,** 192–212.

Wechsler, D. (1974). *Wechsler Intelligence Scale for Children—revised.* New York: Psychological Corp.

Weiner, P. (1985). The value of follow-up studies. *Topics in Language Disorders,* **5,** 78–92.

Williams, J. P. (1980). Teaching decoding with an emphasis on phoneme analysis and phoneme blending. *Journal of Educational Psychology,* **72,** 1–15.

Wolf, M., & Goodglass, H. (1986). Dyslexia, dysnomia, and lexical retrieval: A longitudinal study. *Brain and Language,* **28,** 154–168.

Wolfus, B., Moscovitch, M., & Kinsbourne, M. (1980). Subgroups of developmental language impairment. *Brain and Language,* **10,** 152–171.

Woodcock, R. W., & Johnson, M. B. (1977). *Woodcock-Johnson Psychoeducational Battery.* Boston: Teaching Resources Corp.

12

The Effect of Hearing Impairment on the Quality of Attachment and Mother-Toddler Interaction

Amy R. Lederberg

Georgia State University, Atlanta
Caryl E. Mobley
College of Nursing, Texas Woman's University

In the present study, 41 hearing impaired and 41 hearing toddlers together with their hearing mothers were observed in Ainsworth's Strange Situation and during free play. Both security of attachment and ratings of maternal and toddler behavior during free play were remarkably similar for the hearing impaired and hearing dyads. In addition, security of attachment was related to the ratings of maternal and toddler behavior in a similar way for the hearing impaired and hearing toddlers. The results suggest that development of a secure attachment and maintaining a good mother-toddler relationship does not depend on normal language development during the toddler years.

Over 90% of hearing impaired children are born to hearing parents who have had little or no previous contact with hearing impairment. In these families, both educators and researchers have hypothesized that the development of a normal mother-child relationship is disrupted by the inability of the child to understand his or her

Reprinted with permission from *Child Development*, 1990, Vol. 61, 1596–1604. Copyright © 1990 by the Society for Research in Child Development, Inc.

This research was partially supported by grants from the Office of Special Education ($265,035, or 76% of total cost) and the March of Dimes Foundation to the first author. We thank Vicki Everhart, Catherine Manning, Cynthia McIntyre, Lisa Meek, Margaret Owen, Karen Smith, James Stahlecker, and Kathleen Wincorn for their aid in data collection and coding; Margaret Owen and Deborah Vandell for their helpful comments on earlier drafts; and the mothers, toddlers, and parent advisors that made this study possible. Portions of this paper were presented at the meeting of the Society for Research in Child Development, held in Baltimore, MD, 1987.

mother's normal means of communication (Harris, 1978; Moores, 1982; Schlesinger & Meadow, 1972; Wedell-Monnig & Lumley, 1980). In support of this hypothesis, hearing mothers of deaf 3–5-year-olds have been rated as more controlling, intrusive, didactic, rigid, disapproving, and negative with their children than mothers of hearing children. Deaf preschoolers have been rated as less responsive, creative, happy, and positive with their mothers than were hearing preschoolers (Schlesinger & Meadow, 1972). Other researchers have also found mothers of hearing impaired preschoolers less positive (Goss, 1970), more controlling or directive (Brinich, 1980; Henggeler & Cooper, 1983; Henggeler, Watson, & Cooper, 1984), and dominant (Nienhuys, Horsborough, & Cross, 1985) than mothers of hearing preschoolers. Meadow, Greenberg, Erting, and Carmichael (1981) found that deaf preschoolers had shorter interactions with their mothers than did hearing preschoolers. Deaf preschoolers initiated interactions less frequently than did hearing preschoolers.

Although the effect of child hearing impairment on preschoolers' mother-child relationship has been studied, little is known about younger deaf children's relationship with their mothers. There are a few small-scale studies (n = 3–6 hearing impaired subjects) that suggest that this relationship may be less problematic than that of preschoolers. Mothers of hearing impaired infants still seem to dominate interaction. They initiated more and controlled the topic of interaction more than mothers of hearing infants (Spencer & Gutfreund, in press; Wedell-Monnig & Lumley, 1980). On the other hand, mothers and their hearing impaired infants were as responsive to each other as hearing infants and their mothers (Spencer & Gutfreund, in press; Wedell-Monnig & Lumley, 1980). In addition, the synchrony of face-to-face interaction is within the norms for hearing infants and their mothers (Nienhuys & Tikotin, 1985).

While this research is suggestive, any conclusions based on it must be tentative. Generalizing from small sample sizes is especially problematic among the hearing impaired population, where large individual differences in social and communicative competence occur (Greenberg, 1980). In addition, these studies are limited to examining differences in the frequency of behaviors. The major difference between deaf and hearing preschool dyads seems to be in the quality of the interaction (Schlesinger & Meadow, 1972). The primary goal of the present study was to contrast the relationships between hearing impaired toddlers and their hearing mothers with those of a matched group of hearing toddlers and their mothers. Toddlers were studied rather than infants because hearing impairment is rarely identified during infancy.

The mother-toddler relationship was measured in two ways. First, the quantity and quality of mother-toddler interaction during free play was examined using coding procedures similar to the ones used with deaf preschoolers (Greenberg, 1980; Schlesinger & Meadow, 1972).

Second, the quality of the attachment relationship between mother and toddler was examined using the Strange Situation paradigm (Ainsworth, Blehar, Waters, & Wall, 1978). During the past decade, assessment of the security of the attachment bond, as described by Bowlby (1969) and Ainsworth (1973), has become a widely accepted way to describe the quality of the early mother-child relationship. Research suggests that security of attachment is related to the mother's sensitivity to the infant/toddler's needs and signals (Ainsworth et al., 1978). In addition to being an indicator of the mother-child relationship, the attachment relationship predicts social competence during the preschool years (Sroufe, 1988).

The only published study on the attachment relationship between hearing impaired children and their hearing parents used a modification of Ainsworth's procedure to examine the development of attachment among deaf preschoolers (Greenberg & Marvin, 1979). Deaf preschoolers who communicated poorly with their mothers were more delayed in the development of a mature (goal-directed partnership) attachment relationship and more likely to show behaviors indicative of an insecure attachment than deaf preschoolers who communicated well with their mothers (Greenberg & Marvin, 1979). Similarly, deaf children of *deaf* parents (and thus with high communication skills) developed attachment similar to hearing children (Meadow, Greenberg, & Erting, 1985). This research suggests that only deaf children with poor communication skills are at risk for developing insecure attachments. However, this conclusion is tentative because these studies did not include hearing children, nor did they use the traditional classification system for assessing attachment security.

Hearing impaired toddlers with hearing parents might be at risk for developing insecure attachments for several reasons. First, poor communication between hearing impaired toddlers and their mothers may lead to insecure attachments. Hearing impaired toddlers may perceive their mothers as being insensitive because their mothers respond to them with speech or vocalizations that the toddlers do not hear (Blacher & Meyer, 1983). Second, mothers of hearing impaired toddlers seem to dominate or control interaction (Spencer & Gutfreund, in press; Wedell-Monnig & Lumley, 1980). Deaf children may perceive this control as insensitivity. Finally, parents of hearing impaired children experience more stress than parents of hearing children (Friedrich, Greenberg, & Crnic, 1983), and maternal stress has been associated with attachment security (Vaughn, Egeland, Sroufe, & Waters, 1979).

On the other hand, there are some reasons to expect that hearing impaired toddlers are not at risk for developing insecure attachments. Hearing impaired infants/toddlers and their mothers seem to be as responsive to each other as hearing infants/toddlers and their mothers (Spencer & Gutfreund, in press; Wedell-Monnig & Lumley, 1980). In addition, hearing impaired toddlers may not need to hear their mothers' voice because spoken responses are frequently redundant with non-verbal visual communication. This is probably why interaction between hearing impaired infants and their mothers appears synchronous (Nienhuys & Tikotin, 1985). Finally, research with other "at risk" infants suggests that the early attachment relationship may only be affected by extreme risk factors (Easterbrooks, 1989; Goldberg, 1988; Shapiro, Sherman, Calamari, & Koch, 1987; Sierra, 1989; Stahlecker & Cohen, 1985; Wasserman, Lennon, Allen, & Shilansky, 1987).

In summary, the impact of child hearing impairment on the mother-toddler relationship was examined by assessing security of attachment and the quality and quantity of mother-toddler interaction during free play. The subjects included almost all hearing impaired toddlers enrolled in parent education programs in a major metropolitan area over a 5-year period. The results, therefore, are able to be generalized to hearing impaired toddlers enrolled in parent education programs. To ensure that results also apply to subgroups of this population, two additional analyses were conducted. One compared the mother-toddler relationship of 30 profoundly deaf toddlers with that of a matched group of hearing toddlers. The second examined the impact of age identification and intervention on the mother-toddler relationship.

METHOD

Subjects

Hearing impaired toddlers and their hearing mothers (hearing impaired dyads). The study included 41 hearing impaired toddlers who were between 18 and 25 months of age (*M* age = 22 months) and their hearing mothers.[1] All hearing impaired children and their mothers were enrolled in one of six public school parent education programs for hearing impaired children in a major metropolitan area. This represented all the urban and suburban schools in the area. Once an infant or toddler was identified as hearing impaired, he or she was referred to the public schools and enrolled in one of these six programs. Because these programs were free and consisted entirely of home visits, the participation rate was high. Parent advisors referred to us all hearing impaired children under the age of 24 months who were not multiply handicapped and whose parents were hearing. Only three mothers referred to us refused to participate. Nine toddlers, on the average, were referred during a year, with data collected over a 5-year period.

The subjects included 20 boys and 21 girls; 33 were white, 7 black, and 1

---

[1]Eighteen months is the usual age used for assessing toddler attachment. However, we would have had a much smaller sample if we had used 18 months as our cutoff for assessments. Ten of our 41 subjects were not enrolled in an intervention program until 18 months or older. Twenty-five months was used in order to obtain the largest sample of deaf children possible and still be able to use the Strange Situation.

Hispanic. Thirty-seven came from intact families; there were 3 single mothers and 1 divorced mother. Nineteen mothers were employed full-time, 20 were not employed, and 2 worked part-time. One mother had a grade school education, 1 had some high school education, 10 had graduated high school, 26 had attended college, and 3 had attended graduate school. The sample clearly included a broad range of families.

On the average, the children were identified as hearing impaired at 10 months (range = 1–21 months) and had been enrolled in an intervention program for 8 months (range = 0–22 months) at the time of the study. Thirty had a severe to profound hearing loss, 7 had a moderate to severe loss, and 4 had a mild to moderate loss. Causes of hearing impairment included genes ($n = 3$), meningitis ($n = 12$), pneumonia ($n = 2$), atresia and birth complications ($n = 1$ each), and unknown ($n = 22$). At the time of data collection, 8 mothers were using some sign language; 11 had some training in using an oral approach; 22 mothers used only speech with their children, but had not yet decided on the type of linguistic approach they wanted to use. During the 15-min free play, the model number of verbal utterances (either speech or sign) the children used was 0 (range = 0–69).

Hearing toddlers and their hearing mothers (hearing dyads). The study included 41 hearing toddlers who were the same age as the hearing impaired toddlers (age range = 18–25 months; M age = 22 months). The hearing dyads were matched with the hearing impaired dyads on sex of child, ethnicity, family status, maternal employment, and education. The Hodge-Siegel-Rossi Index (1972) was used to assign prestige scores for maternal and paternal occupations. There were no significant differences between the two groups on maternal occupation and on paternal education and occupation. Maternal and paternal occupation ranged from blue collar to professional. The hearing toddlers were recruited through referrals from mothers of the hearing impaired toddlers ($n = 6$), church groups, and personal contacts. The number of utterances of the hearing children was higher than that of the hearing impaired children; on the average, they used 37 utterances during the 15 min of free play (range = 10–164).

Procedure

Each dyad was seen for two visits approximately 1 week apart. During the first visit, mothers were asked to play with their toddlers for 15 min in a playroom equipped with age-appropriate toys "as they would at home." During the second visit, the toddlers were observed in the standard Strange Situation procedure (Ainsworth et al., 1978). During both visits, interactions were videotaped using two cameras hidden behind one-way mirrors. A special effects generator was used to combine the pictures from the two cameras into a single split-screen image.

During the second visit, the Denver Developmental Screening Test (excluding the language test) was administered. None of the children were delayed in the three areas administered.

Coding Procedures

The mother-toddler relationship was assessed in three ways: quality of attachment, quantity of interaction, and quality of interaction.

Attachment. From the videotapes of the Strange Situation, security of attachment was classified into three forced-choice groups—Avoidant (A), Secure (B), and Resistant (C)—using Ainsworth's standard classification scheme (Ainsworth et al., 1978). Researchers have recently questioned the appropriateness of this traditional scheme for assessing the attachment of handicapped children (Goldberg, Fisher-Fay, Simmons, Fowler, & Levison, 1989; Sierra, 1989; Stahlecker & Cohen, 1985). Classifying attachment of handicapped children as A, B, or C was more difficult in these studies than classifying nonhandicapped children. To see if this was also true with hearing impaired toddlers, coders were asked to categorize the tapes as difficult or not. In addition, attachment was further classified as disorganized/disordered (D) or organized (Main & Solomon, 1966). Tapes were coded by two developmental psychologists who were highly trained in scoring attachment from the Strange Situation (Margaret Owen and James Stahlecker). The latter also has extensive experience with deaf children. The two coders had established high reliability with each other on a different sample of handicapped children prior to this study. The tapes were randomly distributed between the two coders. Thirteen hearing impaired toddlers and 11 hearing toddlers were judged difficult to classify and were therefore classified independently by the other coder. This distribution of "difficult tapes" suggests that the coding of the hearing impaired and hearing toddlers' attachment was of equal difficulty. Interrater reliability on these difficult tapes was 83%. Differences were resolved by conferencing.

Quantity of interaction. Mother-toddler interaction during free play was coded using an event sample coding procedure (Lederberg, 1984). Frequency and success rate of initiations, frequency and reason for terminations were coded. An initiation was defined as the first socially directed behavior that occurred after a 3-sec period of noninteractive activity. An initiation was successful if it received a social response within 3 sec. An interaction started with a successful initiation and continued until there was a 3-sec period without any socially directed behaviors. The person who did not respond to the last socially directed act of an interaction was coded as the terminator of that interaction. The frequency with which terminations occurred because the communication was not received by the partner (e.g., a gesture out of visual range) was also noted.

A third pair of researchers, blind to attachment classifications, coded the quantity of interaction. After all play sessions were coded, 20 randomly selected play sessions, evenly distributed between hearing impaired and hearing dyads, were recorded by the same coders. Interrater reliability, calculated using the formula agreements/disagreements + agreements, for the above described variables ranged from 79% to 95%, with a mean of 86%.[2]

Quality of interaction. The quality of mother-toddler interaction was coded using 5-point Likert-like rating scales adapted from ones by Schlesinger and Meadow (1972) and Crawley and Spiker (1983). Two researchers independently coded all tapes for maternal behavior and the dyadic scale for communicative competence. Another two researchers independently coded all tapes for toddler behavior and two dyadic scales. All research assistants were blind to the toddlers' attachment classifications. Interrater reliability for exact agreement between members of the pairs of coders, calculated using Cohen's kappa, is noted below.

Maternal behavior was coded along the following nine dimensions: didactiveness (use of a formal teaching style, $\kappa = .95$), directiveness (degree of direct guidance the mother offers the child, $\kappa = .99$), stimulation value (cognitive stimulation value of maternal behavior, $\kappa = .98$), developmental appropriateness of play (appropriateness of activities for the child's abilities, $\kappa = 1.00$), positive affect (amount of positive feelings expressed, $\kappa = .91$), negative affect (amount of negative feelings expressed, $\kappa = .99$), positive reinforcement (frequency and intensity of appropriate reinforcement of the child's behavior, $\kappa = .93$).

Toddler behavior was rated along the following nine dimensions: social initiative (frequency and intensity of initiations, $\kappa = .86$), social responsiveness (child compliance to maternal initiations and requests, $\kappa = .75$), affective sharing (the amount of enthusiasm and interest the child shows in interactions with mother, $\kappa = .75$), positive affect (amount of positive feelings expressed, $\kappa = .79$), negative affect (amount of negative feelings expressed, $\kappa = .93$), attention span/distractibility (degree the child is persistent in attempting tasks, whether successful or not, $\kappa = .61$), object initiative (amount of object-directed behavior the child engages in, independent of maternal prompting, $\kappa = .76$), pride in mastery (the expression of positive affect and pride following task accomplishment, $\kappa = .92$), and creativity (imagination and creativity of child's play, $\kappa = .84$).

In addition, the dyad was rated along three dimensions: mutuality (degree to which interactions are harmonious and in sync, $\kappa = .80$), dominance (degree to which mother or child dominates interaction, $\kappa = .77$), and communication competence (the degree that both mother and child display mutual and reciprocal understanding of each other's communicative acts, $\kappa = .97$).

---

[2]Percentage agreement, rather than Cohen's kappa, was used because of the difficult in unitizing to determine agreement for noncoded events in an event sample code.

TABLE 1
Attachment Classification for Hearing Impaired
and Hearing Toddlers

| | | ATTACHMENT CLASSIFICATION | |
| | | Insecure | |
TODDLERS	Secure	Avoidant	Ambivalent/ Resistant
Hearing impaired	23	9	9
Hearing	25	13	3

RESULTS

Quality of Attachment

A 3 (attachment security) $\times$ 2 (hearing status) chi-square analysis indicated no significant differences in the distribution of A, B, and C type attachments for the hearing impaired and hearing toddlers, $\chi^2(2, N = 82) = 3.81, p < .15$ (see Table 1). In fact, the number of securely and insecurely attached hearing impaired and hearing toddlers was almost identical. There were also no significant differences in the number of D classifications for the hearing impaired and hearing toddlers, $\chi^2(1, N = 82) = 3.10, p < .10$ ($n = 10, 4$, respectively). For further analyses, D classifications were force classified as A, B, or C type attachments (hearing impaired = 3 As, 1 B, 6 Cs; hearing = 2 A, 1 B, 1 C).

Mother-Toddler Interaction

The next series of analyses tested the effect of hearing impairment on mother-toddler interaction and explored the possibility that mother-toddler interaction is affected by an interaction between hearing status and attachment security.

Quantity of interaction. To test for effects on the quantity of interaction, 2 (hearing impaired vs. hearing) $\times$ 2 (secure-B vs. insecure-A & C attachment) ANOVAs were conducted on the following variables: frequency, average duration, and success rate of both maternal and child initiations; proportion of interactions terminated by child; and proportion of interactions terminated because the child did not receive the communication.[3]

Hearing status affected the quality of interaction in three ways. First, hearing

---

[3]All variables were not calculated for all 82 dyads. For a few subjects ($n = 8$), interaction started before the camera was started and/or continued until the end of the session, resulting in no coded initiations and/or terminations. In order not to reduce all variables to an N of 74, ANOVAs rather than MANOVAs were conducted.

impaired toddlers and their mothers spent less time interacting than did hearing toddlers and their mothers, $F(1,78) = 6.55, p < .01$ ($M = 682$ sec and 764 sec, respectively). Perhaps to try to compensate for this decrease in interaction, mothers of hearing impaired toddlers initiated more to their children than did mothers of hearing toddlers, $F(1,73) = 12.24, p < .001$ ($M = 11.46$ and 6.82, respectively). Finally, hearing impaired toddlers were much more likely to terminate an interaction because they did not see or hear the last communication by their mothers than were hearing toddlers, $F(1,70) = 20.75, p < .0001$ ($M = 18\%$ and 0% of terminations by hearing impaired and hearing toddlers, respectively). There were no significant differences in any of the other measures.

None of the measures showed a significant interaction between hearing status and attachment, nor a significant effect of attachment.

Quality of interaction. Ratings of mother-toddler interaction were analyzed using three 2 (hearing status) × 2 (attachment security) multivariate analyses of variance (MANOVAs). One MANOVA included the nine ratings of maternal behavior, one included the nine ratings of toddler behavior, and one included the three ratings of dyadic behavior. The ANOVAs were computed for individual ratings when the overall MANOVA was significant.

Hearing impairment exerted only a minimal impact on the global ratings of mother-toddler interaction, either as a main effect or in interaction with attachment security. Only the dyadic MANOVA showed a significant effect for hearing status, $F(3,76) = 3.51, p < .02$. Hearing impaired dyads were less communicatively competent ($M = 2.7$) than hearing dyads ($M = 3.5$), $F(1,78) = 10.55, p < .01$. There were no other significant multivariate or univariate differences between hearing impaired and hearing toddlers or between their mothers. Security of attachment and hearing status showed a significant interaction only for maternal behavior, $F(10,69) = 1.98, p < .05$, with only a significant univariate effect for negative affect, $F(1,78) = 6.20, p < .05$. Mothers of insecurely attached hearing toddlers expressed more negative affect than mothers of insecurely attached hearing impaired toddlers, securely attached hearing impaired toddlers, and securely attached hearing toddlers.

Security of attachment showed significant but minimal effects on maternal behavior, $F(9,70) = 2.02, p < .05$, and more extensive effects on toddler behavior, $F(9,70) = 2.03\ p < .05$. Mothers of securely attached toddlers reinforced their children more than did mothers of insecurely attached toddlers, $F(1,78) = 16.56, p < .01$. Securely attached toddlers initiated more, $F(1,78) = 4.57, p < .05$, and responded more to their mothers, $F(1,78) = 4.62, p < .05$, showed more affective sharing, $F(1,78) = 5.32, p < .05$, had a longer attention span, $F(1,78) = 10.27, p < .001$, than insecurely attached toddlers.[4]

---

[4]An additional series of analyses was conducted. To test for sex differences, all analyses were repeated

Analyses with Deaf Toddlers

In order to ensure that the results could be generalized to profoundly deaf toddlers, all the analyses were repeated using only data from 30 deaf toddlers and 30 matched hearing toddlers. There were no differences between these results and those reported previously. Security of attachment did not differ between the profoundly deaf and hearing dyads, $\chi^2(1, N = 60) = .28 \, p < .59$ ($n = 17, 19$, respectively), nor did the number of disorganized attachments differ significantly ($n = 4, 2$, respectively). As with the whole sample, the only effect of deafness dyadic communicative competence. Finally, deaf dyads interacted for less time, had more maternal initiations, and had more terminations due to miscommunication than hearing dyads.

Ages of Identification and Intervention

To determine whether differences in attachment were related to either the age that children were identified as hearing impaired or the number of months enrolled in intervention, t tests (secure vs. insecure attachment) were conducted using these two variables as dependent variables. In addition, age of identification and months in intervention were correlated with all interaction measures. Ages of identification and intervention were not significantly related to attachment or any measure of mother-toddler interaction.

DISCUSSION

As expected, hearing impairment affected the ability of mother and toddler to communicate effectively. Hearing impaired toddlers and their mothers were judged to miscommunicate much more frequently than hearing toddlers and their mothers. Consistent with this global rating, hearing impaired toddlers frequently did not respond to their mothers' communication because they did not seem to hear or see it. These problems probably result from the need to communicate visually. Unlike hearing children who can listen to speech while visually attending to objects, deaf children have to divide their visual attention between the environment and the communicator in order to receive the communication. Learning to coordinate their visual attention appropriately is one of the major learning tasks that hearing impaired children have to accomplish, and it may not be completed until well into the preschool years (Wood, Wood, Griffiths, & Howarth, 1986). In addition hearing parents have to learn to coordinate their communication with their child's attention

---

with sex as an additional factor. No main or interaction effects were found.

(Spencer & Gutfreund, in press). The hearing impaired toddlers and their mothers spent less time interacting than hearing toddlers and their mothers. This may also have been caused by the hearing impaired toddlers' difficulty attending to their mother while playing with the toys in the room. Finally, similar to past research (Wedell-Monnig & Lumley, 1980), mothers of hearing impaired toddlers initiated interactions more than mothers of hearing toddlers. Others have interpreted this increase in maternal initiation as an increase in maternal directiveness or dominance (e.g., Jones, 1980; Wedell-Monnig & Lumley, 1980). However, in the present study, mothers of hearing impaired and hearing toddlers did not differ on qualitative ratings of dominance or directiveness. Thus, although mothers of hearing impaired toddlers may have been more responsible for starting an interaction, these mothers were as likely as mothers of hearing children to allow their child to set the topic and to control the interaction. Given that an initiation is defined as the first social behavior following noninteraction, mothers of hearing impaired toddlers may just have had more opportunity to initiate interactions because the dyads spent less time interacting.

Despite these effects on communication and quantity of interaction, hearing impairment did not affect the quality of the relationship between mother and toddler. Ratings of the quality of maternal and toddler behavior during free play were similar for the hearing impaired and hearing dyads. Thus, the two groups of mothers did not differ on affect, sensitivity, control, or teaching behavior. The hearing impaired and hearing toddlers did not differ on initiative, compliance, affect, attention span, pride in mastery, or creativity. Consistent with the lack of differences in quality of interaction, there were no differences in the hearing impaired and hearing toddlers' security of attachment to mother.

Unlike other handicapped populations, hearing impaired children were not more difficult to classify and did not show significantly more disorganized attachments than hearing toddlers. In addition, mother-toddler interaction and security of attachment were related in similar ways for both hearing impaired and hearing toddlers. Securely attached toddlers were happier and more socially interactive and compliant, and had longer attention spans and showed more pride in mastery than insecurely attached toddlers. Mothers of secure toddlers reinforced them more than mothers of insecure toddlers. The fact that relations between attachment and maternal-toddler behavior were the same for both hearing impaired and hearing toddlers and are consistent with attachment theory suggests that both the Strange Situation and the standard coding procedure were a valid assessment of the hearing impaired toddlers' quality of attachment.

Thus, despite their communicative difficulties and their delayed language development, hearing impaired toddlers were as likely to establish a positive, reciprocal, secure relationship with their mothers as were hearing toddlers. This was true for the sub-sample of profoundly deaf toddlers as well as for the whole sample. The results, together with past research, suggest that "sensitive caregivers can adapt to a variety of special needs of their infants/toddlers in such a way as to make their children feel secure in their care. Caregivers seem to be able to adapt to the needs of children who are hearing impaired, premature, neurologically impaired, physically impaired, or have difficult temperaments (Goldberg, 1988; Stahlecker & Cohen, 1985; Vaughn, Lefever, Seifer, & Barglow, 1989; Wasserman et al, 1987). As Goldberg (1988) points out, this supports Ainsworth's hypothesis that the quality of the early attachment relationship is more dependent on maternal than infant characteristics (Ainsworth et al., 1978).

With hearing impaired children, maternal adaptation probably entails using enough visual and physical communication that hearing impaired toddlers feel that their needs are being met. Thus, for example, the hearing impaired toddler would not need to hear their mother's comforting voice because their mother is also communicating that comfort visually and physically through body language. It is likely, even before the mother knows her child is hearing impaired, that the infant shapes appropriate responses from her by not being comforted by responses that are solely auditory. These adaptations did not seem to be due to educational intervention since the number of months the dyads were enrolled in intervention programs did not relate to any measure of interaction.

The findings in the present study, together with past research with preschool children (Meadow et al., 1981; Schlesinger & Meadow, 1972), suggest that the impact of hearing impairment on mother-child interaction increases from toddlerhood to preschool. This change may be due to a developmental change in the importance of language for normal mother-child interaction. The poor quality of interaction between deaf preschoolers and their mothers seems to be due to communication problems (Greenberg, 1980; Schlesinger & Meadow, 1972). In contrast, in the present study, although hearing impairment affected communication, this effect did not, in turn, affect the mother-toddler social relationship in a major way. The inability to communicate effectively and to use language may become more disruptive to the mother-child relationship as the children get older because age-appropriate activities become more dependent on language and good communication.

On the other hand, differences between our results and those with preschoolers may be caused by differences in the characteristics of the hearing impaired children studied. In the present study, by necessity, only hearing impaired toddlers already identified as such and enrolled in an intervention program were studied. There may be more insecure attachments and worse social interaction patterns between hearing impaired toddlers and parents who are not sensitive enough to notice or to seek help for a hearing problem until that child is older. Unlike the present study, the studies with preschool children included children who were identified after 2 years of age. Thus, the apparent deterioration of the mother-child relationship may just be caused by inclusion of these late identified children in the preschool studies. In support of this explanation, in the research by Greenberg and colleagues (Greenberg, 1980; Greenberg & Marvin, 1979; Meadow et al., 1981), the average age of identification of the high communicatively competent children was 13 months (similar to the present study), while the average age of identification for the low communicatively competent children was 21 months. It was the latter children that seemed to account for most of the effects of hearing impairment. This possibility highlights the importance of longitudinal research for understanding developmental changes in the impact of hearing impairment on the mother-child relationship. We are at present collecting such data.

REFERENCES

Ainsworth, M. D. (1973). The development of infant-mother attachment. In B. M. Caldwell & H. N. Ricciuti (Eds.), *Review of child development research* (Vol. 3, pp. 1–95). Chicago: University of Chicago Press.

Ainsworth, M. D., Blehar, M., Waters E., & Wall, S. (1978). *Patterns of attachment.* Hillsdale, NJ: Erlbaum.

Blacher, J., & Meyer, C. E. (1983). A review of attachment formation and disorder of handicapped children. *American Journal of Mental Deficiency, 87,* 359–371.

Bowlby, J. (1969). *Attachment and loss: Vol. 1 Attachment.* New York: Basic.

Brinich, P. M. (1980). Childhood deafness and maternal control. *Journal of Communication Disorders, 13,* 75–81.

Crawley, S. B., & Spiker, D. (1983). Mother-child interactions involving two-year-old Down syndrome: A look at individual differences. *Child Development, 54,* 1312–1323.

Easterbrooks, M. A. (1989). Quality of attachment to mother and to father: Effects of perinatal risk status. *Child Development, 60,* 825–830.

Friedrich, W. N., Greenberg, M. T., & Crnic, K. (1983). The Revised Questionnaire on Resources and Stress: QRS-R. *American Journal of Mental Deficiency, 88,* 41–48.

Goldberg, S. (1988). Risk factors in infant-mother attachment. *Canadian Journal of Psychology, 42,* 173–188.

Goldberg, S., Fischer-Fay, A., Simmons, R., Fowler, R., & Levison, H. (1989, April). Effects of chronic illness on infant-mother attachment. In R. Marvin (Chair), *Assessing attachment in special populations using Ainsworth Strange Situation.* Symposium conducted at the meeting of the Society for Research in Child Development, Kansas City, MO.

Goss, R. N. (1970). Language used by mothers of deaf children and mothers of hearing children. *American Annals of the Deaf, 115,* 93–96.

Greenberg, M. (1980). Social interaction between deaf preschoolers and their mothers: The effects of communication method and communicative competence. *Developmental Psychology, 16,* 465–474.

Greenberg, M., & Marvin, R. (1979). Attachment patterns in profoundly deaf preschool children. *Merrill-Palmer Quarterly, 25,* 265–279.

Harris, A. (1978). The development of the deaf individual and the deaf community. In L. Liben (Ed.), *Deaf children: Developmental perspectives* (pp. 217–234). New York: Academic Press.

Henggeler, S. W., & Cooper, P. F. (1983). Deaf and child-hearing mother interaction: Extensiveness and reciprocity. *Journal of Pediatric Psychology, 8,* 83–95.

Henggeler, S. W., Watson, S. M., & Cooper, P. F. (1984). Verbal and nonverbal controls in hearing mother-deaf child interaction. *Journal of Applied Developmental Psychology, 5,* 319–329.

Hodge, R. W., Siegel, P. M., & Rossi, P. (1972). Occupational prestige in the United States. In P. Blaumberg (Ed.), *The impact of social class* (pp. 231-246). New York: Harper & Row.

Jones, O. H. M. (1980). Prelinguistic communication skills in Down's syndrome and normal infants. In T. Field, S. Goldberg, D. Stern, & A. Sostek (Eds.), *High-risk infants and children* (pp. 205–247). New York: Academic Press.

Lederberg, A. (1984). Interaction between deaf preschoolers and unfamiliar hearing adults. *Child Development, 55,* 598–606.

Main, M., & Solomon, J. (1986). Discovery of an insecure disorganized/disoriented attachment pattern: Procedures, findings, and implications for the classification of behavior. In T. B. Brazelton & M. Yogman (Eds). *Affective development in infancy* (pp. 95–124). Norwood, NJ: Ablex.

Meadow, K. P., Greenberg, M. T., & Erting, C. (1985). Attachment behavior of deaf children of deaf parents. In S. Chess & A. Thomas (Eds.), *Annual progress in child psychiatry and child development,* 1984 (pp. 176–187). New York: Brunner/Mazel.

Meadow, K. P., Greenberg, M. T., Erting, C., & Carmichael, H. (1981). Interactions of deaf mothers and deaf preschool children: Comparisons with three other groups of deaf and hearing dyads. *American Annals of the Deaf, 126,* 454–568.

Moores, D. F. (1982). *Educating the deaf: Psychology, principles and practices,* 2d ed. Boston: Houghton-Mifflin.

Nienhuys, T. G., Horsborough, K. M., & Cross, T. G. (1985). A dialogic analysis of interaction between mothers and their deaf or hearing preschoolers. *Applied Psycholinguistics, 6,* 121–140.

Nienhuys, T. G., & Tikotin, J. A. (1985, August). *Mother-infant interaction: Prespeech communication in hearing and deaf babies.* Paper presented at the XVII International Congress on Education of the Deaf, Manchester, UK.

Schlesinger, H. S., & Meadow, K. P. (1972). *Sound and sign: Childhood deafness and mental health.* Berkeley: University of California Press.

Shapiro, T., Sherman, M., Calamari, G., & Koch, D. (1987). Attachment in autism and other developmental disorders. *Journal of American Academy of Child and Adolescent Psychiatry, 26,* 480–484.

Sierra, A. (1989, April). The assessment of attachment in infants with mild to moderate cerebral palsy. In R. Marvin (Chair), *Assessing attachment in special populations using Ainsworth Strange Situation.* Symposium conducted at the meeting of the Society for Research in Child Development, Kansas city, MO.

Spencer, P. S., & Gutfreund, M. K. (in press). In D. Moores & K. Meadow-Orlans (Eds.)

Research on Educational and Developmental Aspects of Deafness. Washington, DC: Gallaudet University Press.

Sroufe, L. A. (1988). The role of infant-caregiver attachment in development. In J. Belsky & T. Nezworski (Eds.), *Clinical implications of attachment* (pp. 18–38). Hillsdale, NJ: Erlbaum.

Stahlecker, J., & Cohen, M. C. (1985). Application of the strange situation attachment paradigm to a neurologically impaired population. *Child Development, 85,* 502–507.

Vaughn, B. E., Egeland, B., Sroufe, L. A., & Waters, E. (1979). Individual differences in infant-mother attachment at twelve and eighteen months: Stability and change in families under stress. *Child Development, 50,* 971–975.

Vaughan, B. E., & Lefever, G. B., Seifer, R., & Barglow, P. (1989). Attachment behavior, attachment security, and temperament during infancy. *Child Development, 60,* 728–737.

Wasserman, G., Lennon, M., Allen, R., & Shilansky, M. (1987). Contributors to attachment in normal and physically handicapped infants, *Journal of American Academy of Child and Adolescent Psychiatry, 26,* 9–15.

Wedell-Monnig, J., & Lumley, J. (1980) Child deafness and mother-child interaction. *Child Development, 51,* 766–774.

Wood, D., Wood, H., Griffiths, A., & Howarth, I. (1986). *Teaching and talking with deaf children.* New York: Wiley.

Part IV

TEMPERAMENT STUDIES

Over the past ten years there has been an explosion of research on aspects of temperament. As the contributions in this section reflect, interest in temperament as an important consideration in the understanding of both psychopathology during childhood and normal developmental processes continues unabated. In introducing their study, Maziade, Caron, Côté, Boutin, and Thivierge note that the association between an extremely difficult temperament and the appearance of clinical disorders in children is well established. If difficult temperaments predispose children to serious developmental and psychiatric disorders, then children with extremely difficult temperaments should be overrepresented among children referred to child psychiatric clinics.

The authors tested this hypothesis by comparing measures of temperament in a consecutive sample of children (N = 814) referred to a child psychiatric center with normative values for temperament obtained in previously studied random samples of the general population of children in Quebec City. Diagnoses of externalizing disorders, developmental delays, and mixed disorders were derived from a review of hospital records by raters blind to temperament scores.

The hypothesis was confirmed in that children with difficult temperaments were indeed overrepresented in the child psychiatric population. Moreover, the findings suggested a specificity in the relationship between particular temperamental factors and the type of clinical problem. The temperamental cluster of withdrawal from new stimuli, low adaptability, high intensity, and negative mood was found more likely to be associated with disruptive behavior disorders; whereas the triad of low persistence, high-sensory threshold, and high mobility was found to be associated more with specific developmental delays. Most important, a large proportion of children referred for a psychiatric disorder did not present with an extreme temperament. Although some have suggested that common psychiatric disorders of children, with the exception of syndromes such as autism, psychosis, or serious eating disorders, are an expression of an extreme form of temperament, these results provide empirical evidence to the contrary by clearly establishing the non-equivalence of extreme temperament and clinical disorder.

The report by Biederman, Rosenbaum, Hirshfeld, Faraone, Bolduc, Gersten, Meminger, Kagan, Snidman, and Reznick examines the psychiatric correlates of behavioral inhibition in two groups of young children: offspring of parents with panic disorder and agoraphobia (N = 30) and the offspring of parents who were free of manifest psychiatric disorder (N = 41). Each group contained roughly equivalent numbers of inhibited and uninhibited children. The assessment of child psychopathology was based on interviews with mothers using the Diagnostic Interview for Children and Adolescents-Parent Version.

The findings indicate that inhibited children irrespective of parentage had higher rates of multiple anxiety disorders (two or more anxiety disorders per child) suggesting an association between behavioral inhibition and childhood anxiety disorders. High rates of multiple anxiety disorders were found only among inhibited children (22.2 percent of those whose parents had anxiety disorders and 18.2 percent of those whose parents were without disorder). Interestingly, inhibited children whose parents were anxious had higher rates of major depression and oppositional disorder than the uninhibited children of anxious parents. No such pattern was found among inhibited children whose parents were not psychiatrically ill. The findings, although preliminary, suggest that behavioral inhibition may be one of multiple risk factors contributing to the development of childhood anxiety disorders. Moreover, it appears as if the risk of psychiatric disorder is increased more generally among inhibited children exposed to familial psychopathology. Clearly, more investigation is required to further elucidate these relationships.

In a longitudinal study, Kyrios and Prior develop a "stress resilience" model of temperamental influence on behavioral functioning during the preschool period. The relation of childhood stress, child health, parental adjustment, language abilities, child-rearing practices, and other developmental influences as well as temperament to behavioral adjustment at three to four years of age and again 12 months later are examined by Path analysis.

The results suggest that temperamental characteristics exhibit the most predictive independent relationships with measures of early childhood behavioral adjustment, both concurrently and prospectively. Maladjustment within the parental subsystem also played an important role both directly and indirectly. Child-rearing practices and rate of development were limited in their prediction of children's adjustment, and children's stress and health problems, sex, and verbal intelligence did not directly relate to children's adjustment. The authors explore several alternative explanations for the findings. Of particular interest is the suggestion that whereas "difficult" temperament can predispose children to negative outcomes, positive temperamental characteristics can act to protect a child from the effects of an adverse environment.

The clearly conceived and implemented study by Mangelsdorf, Gunnar, Kestenbaum, Lang, and Andreas addresses the debate over the relative contributions of maternal sensitivity and infant temperament to the development of secure and insecure attachment. Sixty-six mother-infant pairs were studied when the infants were nine and 13 months of age. The report examines relations between infant proneness-to-distress, a temperamental dimension; maternal personality characteristics; and mother-infant attachment.

The complex array of findings can be summarized as follows: infant proneness-to-distress appears to be related to both maternal personality and behavior to attachment classifications derived from the Strange Situation. Instead, security of attachment could be predicted from an interaction between infant and mother characteristics. Maternal personality factors had a greater effect on the attachment behavior of infants who rated high on temperamental proneness-to-distress. This pattern of findings is interpreted as pointing to a need to consider goodness-of-fit models in relating maternal and infant characteristics to attachment security.

13

Extreme Temperament and Diagnosis: A Study in a Psychiatric Sample of Consecutive Children

Michel Maziade

Université Laval Robert-Giffard, Quebec

Chantal Caron

Hôtel-Dieu du Sacré-Coeur de Jésus, Quebec

Robert Côté, Pierrette Boutin, and Jacques Thivierge

Université Laval Robert-Giffard, Quebec

We report on an epidemiological-clinical study of the New York (NY) Longitudinal Study temperament model in a consecutive sample of children (N = 814) referred to a child psychiatric center. Temperament comparisons in this clinical population were made by using temperament normative values obtained in previous random samples of the general population in the greater Quebec City (Canada) area. Different clinical diagnostic groups (externalized disorders, developmental delays, and mixed disorders) were derived from a review of the entire hospital charts in which the interrater reliability was tested and performed "blind" to temperament scores. The diagnostic groups were confirmed through discriminant function analyses. The results (1) replicated, in this child psychiatric population, two factors of temperament similar to those previously found in random samples of our general population; (2) showed, in the psychiatric population of children, an overproportion of difficult temperaments on both factors; (3) confirmed

Reprinted with permission from *Archives of General Psychology*, 1990, Vol. 47, 477–484. Copyright © 1990 by the American Medical Association.

This study has reported on the epidemiological data from the general and child psychiatric populations, and these studies were supported by grants from the Fonds de Recherche en Santé du Québec, Montreal, the Canadian Psychiatric Research Foundation, Toronto, and Health and Welfare Canada (National Health Research Development Program), Ottawa.

conversely that a large proportion of children referred for a disorder did not present with an extreme temperament, and, therefore, an extreme temperament and a clinical disorder were not equivalent; and (4) suggested a specificity in the relationship between particular temperament factors and the type of clinical problem. Temperament factor 1 (withdrawal from new stimuli, low adaptability, high intensity, and negative mood) was found to be more associated with externalized disorders (opposition, conduct, or attention-deficit disorders), whereas temperament factor 2 (low persistence, high sensory threshold, and high mobility) was found to be more associated with specific developmental delays. The findings provided leads for future clinical research on temperament, family functioning, and child psychiatric diagnoses.

The association between an extremely difficult temperament and the appearance of clinical disorders in children now has been well documented in random samples of the general population in Quebec, Canada,[1,2] and in other samples. [3-5] If difficult temperaments predispose children to serious developmental and psychiatric disorders, then one should observe an overproportion of extremely difficult temperaments among children referred to child psychiatric clinics. Moreover, looking at the distribution of different temperament components in clinical populations of children also should throw light on possible specificities in the relationship between some types of clinical diagnoses and particular temperamental patterns. With regard to the often raised question as to whether an extremely difficult temperament would not just be the same as a clinical behavior disorder in children,[6,7] the study of the types of temperaments, along with the types of clinical disorders, in a population of children referred to a child psychiatric center might provide answers.

To our knowledge, no research, to date, has investigated temperaments through a consecutive sample of all children referred to a regional child psychiatric center within a specific period. Some studies[8-14] have turned to schools or other environments to look into temperamental differences in small samples of children who present with developmental disorders. One study used a group of aggressive children who were referred to a hospital clinic compared with children with behavior disorders in school and with controls.[15] It is difficult to draw a conclusion from these studies because of the differences on the definitions of temperament and of developmental or behavior disorders and also because of the differences in the samplings or in the rates of nonrespondents. We were in a position to benefit from temperament normative values that were standardized at different age levels in our general population, and we used them to sustain comparisons of temperaments in a child psychiatric population.

Four or five models of temperament are now under study in different countries.[16] With regard to the New York (NY) Longitudinal Study (NYLS) model, many transcultural replications of a temperament phenomenology that resembles the NYLS "easy-difficult" cluster now have been obtained through parental questionnaires from infancy to the age of 7 years.[17,18] The traits of adaptability, approach/ withdrawal, mood, and intensity were found to be aggregated in a first factor that was drawn from a principal-component analysis (PCA) in random samples of the general population at 4 to 8 months of age[17] and at 7 years of age,[18] and in other normal solicited samples.[19] Recent results have shown that despite a "subjective" component related to maternal and environmental characteristics, this temperamental factor, measured through parental questionnaires, displays a good concordance with "objective" measurements in the laboratory.[20] A second orthogonal factor, mainly characterized by a low persistence and a high sensory threshold, also has been observed in infancy[17] and at the age of 7 years in the general population.[18] To our knowledge, these temperament factors have never been replicated in a population of children referred to a child psychiatric clinic.

The present study was aimed at answering the following questions: Can we reproduce in a child psychiatric population the same temperamental typologies that are found at different age levels in the general population of Quebec, and will we find the same type of relationship with socioeconomic status (SES) and sex? Will we find, in a child psychiatric population, an overproportion of children presenting with an extremely difficult temperament on these typologies, and if so, what will distinguish the clinical sample of children who present with an extremely difficult temperament from the clinical sample of children who do not have a difficult temperament? Are certain types of extreme temperaments associated with particular types of clinical problems?

PROCEDURE

Sample

The target population consisted of all the children, at intake, at the Hôtel-Dieu du Sacré-Coeur de Jésus de Québec, which is a multidisciplinary center of child and adolescent psychiatry. The hospital provides outpatient and inpatient services to the urban and suburban areas of Quebec (population, 600,000). Children were referred by medical physicians, schools, social services, and parents themselves (Table 1).

We selected all the 3- to 12-year old children who presented within a specific period. According to their chronology of entry, all the subjects were assigned a hospital staff psychiatrist and his or her multidisciplinary team. Sixty-five percent of the psychiatrists agreed to have their patients assessed for the study (N = 881); the sample was not biased by this percentage because the allocation of subjects to psychiatrists was done according to the order in which the subjects presented themselves without reference to the type of problem. Of the 881 subjects targeted, 814

TABLE 1
Description of the Child Psychiatric Sample*

Variable	No. (%)	No. (%)
Age levels, y		
<3	7 (1)	...
3-4	202 (25)	...
5-6	190 (23)	...
7-8	178 (22)	...
9-10	143 (18)	...
11-12	94 (11)	...
Socioeconomic status (Hollingshead)	Child Psychiatric Sample	General Population Sample†
Class I	29 (4)	118 (10)
Class II	85 (11)	134 (11)
Class III	120 (15)	259 (21)
Class IV	287 (37)	413 (33)
Class V	252 (33)	306 (25)
Missing information	41	...
Family status		
Single parents	235 (30)	...
Intact families	547 (70)	...
Missing information	32	...
Referral sources		
Physicians	319 (39)	...
School	162 (20)	...
Parents	93 (12)	...
Other specialists	90 (11)	...
Social services	44 (5)	...
Missing information	106 (13)	...
Diagnoses	3-7 y (N = 502)	8-12 y (N = 312)
Externalized disorders	81 (26)	80 (44)
Developmental delay	89 (29)	19 (10)
Externalized and developmental delay	56 (18)	14 (8)
Internalized disorders	13 (4)	26 (14)
Mixed disorders	14 (5)	14 (8)
Mental retardation‡	30 (10)	10 (5)
Autism and pervasive developmental disorders	4 (1)	...
No disorders	22 (7)	21 (11)
Subjects without chart§	69	38
Insufficient information‖	124	90

*Total sample: N = 814 (573 boys and 241 girls).
†Numbers taken from combination of two random samples of our general population: one aged 7 years and one aged from 8 to 12 years.
‡Mental retardation associated or not with another disorder.
§Subjects whose temperament and demographic data were obtained at intake but who withdrew while on waiting list for clinical assessment.
‖Information insufficient in the hospital chart to make a definite diagnosis.

parents filled in the temperament measurements that totaled 92% of the respondents. Table 1 describes the sample. Unsurprisingly, we observe a high ratio of boys to girls. Consistent with what also has been found for other consecutive child psychiatric samples,[21] the SES structure (the Hollingshead two-factor index taken from the higher scores of the two parents)[22] of our clinical sample was found to be only slightly different from that of the general population (Table 1), even though the difference was statistically significant ($\chi^2 = 41.63$, $df = 4$, and $p = .001$); the observable difference in the psychiatric sample resided only in the extremes of the SES distribution that showed a slight overproportion of poor and uneducated parents (class V) and fewer highly educated and wealthy parents (class I). The SES, the family status, the age at consultation, the referral sources, and the types of disorders were homogeneously distributed in boys and girls. According to Table 1, the numbers in the different analyses will vary with each research question.

Instruments

In this child psychiatric population, we assessed temperaments through instruments that previously were standardized in random samples (N = 980 and N = 640) of our general population: the Thomas, Chess, and Korn Parent Temperament Questionnaire[4] for the 3- 7-year-old children and the Middle Childhood Temperament Questionnaire[23] for the 8- 12-year-old children. The reliability, the normative values, and the demographic correlates of the French version of these instruments have been detailed elsewhere.[18,24] For a questionnaire to be acceptable, we defined criteria as follows: (1) at least 64 of the total 72 items in the Thomas, Chess, and Korn Parent Temperament Questionnaire had to be answered, and there had to be no more than 2 unanswered items in a category; and (2) 89 of the total 99 items in the Middle Childhood Temperament Questionnaire had to be answered, and there had to be no more than 3 unanswered items in any category. Of the 814 questionnaires (458 Thomas, Chess, and Korn Parent Temperament Questionnaires and 268 Middle Childhood Temperament Questionnaires), 726 met these criteria. The subjects with an unacceptable questionnaire were not found to be different from the rest of the sample on the different variables (sex, SES, family status, age at consultation, and diagnosis). The parents completed the temperament questionnaires while the child was on the waiting list.

We obtained the child's diagnosis by means of a semistructured review of the hospital charts that contained (1) clinical information taken by the psychiatric nurse from the school, the parents, and social services; and (2) observations by the staff psychiatrist and by professionals of other disciplines (speech therapists, social workers, psychometricians, etc) who had contact with the child and the parents. According to the criteria defined in Table 2, a judgment was made on the presence of a clinical disorder by using Rutter's definition of a disorder[25]; once a child was classified as having a disorder, his or her condition was diagnosed as an external-ized, internalized, or mixed disorder, a developmental delay, or mental retardation. Some children had a combination of disorders. The externalized/internalized catego-rization was less sophisticated than the *DSM-III* nosology, but it has been validated in children by many investigators.[26] The data from the medical charts were not suf-ficiently refined to use the *DSM-III* categories reliably, whereas the charts fulfilled the research requirements to categorize the externalized and internalized disorders in addition to the other diagnoses mentioned in Table 2. Externalized disorders cor-responded somewhat to *DSM-III* diagnoses, such as attention-deficit, oppositional-defiant, and conduct disorders; internalized disorders corresponded to *DSM-III* diagnoses, such as anxiety, anxious, dysthymic, inhibited, and neurotic disorders.

A severity scale also was used when a disorder was present, ie, the National Institute of Mental Health Global Impression Scale.[27] All the hospital charts were reviewed by an experienced psychologist (P.B.) from our research team, and the concordance was verified through an independent chart review by a child psychia-

TABLE 2

Definitions of Disorder and of Diagnoses in the Review of Hospital Charts

Definitions and Diagnoses
A child was considered as presenting with a disorder when behavior or symptoms were judged deviant enough to disturb the personal, social, or school environment or functioning and warrant consultation. The ECDEU* clinical global impression of severity[27] was also rated when a disorder was present.
Once judged as present, the disorder was categorized as follows:
Internalized: Clinical manifestations characterized ($\geq$80%) by neu-rotic or emotional symptoms, eg, fears, phobia, social inhibition, tic, sleep disturbances, anxiety, and somatization. If externalized symptoms were present, they did not have to account for more than 20% of the clinical picture for a child to be assigned to this category.
Externalized: Clinical manifestations characterized ($\geq$80%) by act-ing-out type of behaviors, conduct problems, oppositional behav-iors, aggressivity, and overactivity. If internalized symptoms were present, they did not have to account for more than 20% of the symptoms.
Mixed: Clinical manifestations in which externalized and internalized behaviors were mixed in about the same proportions, and that were or were not associated with a developmental delay.
Developmental delay: The Diagnostic Criteria for Specific Develop-mental Disorder on *DSM-III* Axis II were used, ie, disorders in specific areas of development not due to another disorder, such as infantile autism or mental retardation. Specific disorders are developmental reading disorder, developmental arithmetic disorder, developmental language disorder, developmental articulation dis-order, and mixed specific developmental disorder.
Mental retardation: Subaverage general intellectual functioning is defined as an IQ of 70 or below on an individually administered IQ test.

*Adapted from Guy.[27]

trist (M.M.). The interrater reliability on the review of the full hospital charts was done on 73 subjects: a concordance level of 93% was obtained for the presence or absence of disorders, and a concordance level of 79% was found for the types of diagnoses (Table 2). The interrater concordance of the chart review was verified at regular intervals across the study. This review was done blind to the temperament scores. The proportions of each diagnosis in our child psychiatric samples are reported in Table 1. Thirteen percent (n = 107) of the referred children had their temperament assessed at presentation, but the parents later canceled so that we had no clinical information on those children. Another 9% (n = 43) of referred children were found to have no disorder that was important enough to warrant a consultation. The children with insufficient information to make a definite diagnosis (n = 214) were not found to be different from the rest of the sample in terms of temperament, SES, sex, family status, and age at consultation.

Statistical Analysis

As a first analysis, a PCA (SAS program) without an iteration and without a rotation was performed to verify the temperament factorial structure in this child psychiatric sample. To analyze the relationship between the temperament components and the type of clinical problems we used, as in our previous work, two complementary strategies: (1) a categorical analysis based on the extremes of temperament, and (2) a continuous analysis in which all the subjects were characterized by their temperament factor scores distributed on a continuum. Concerning the first strategy, an analysis of the distribution of the temperament extremes (on each component) in the different clinical diagnosis groups was achieved by means of χ^2 statistics to test the null hypothesis of the homogeneity of the distributions. In this analysis, the subjects were defined according to the extreme centile cutoffs on the temperament categories that loaded strongly on the factors found at the Principal Component Analysis (PCA). The temperament centile ranks were based on the normative data obtained from the previous assessments of the age-appropriate random samples of the general population. Our second strategy used discriminant analyses (SPSS-X program) on the different clinical diagnosis groups as independent variables; all the subjects were characterized by their factor scores derived from the PCA, and temperament was used as a dependent variable along with other variables, such as SES, sex, age, and family status. This second strategy was complementary in that it verified whether or not the results obtained from the analysis of the extremes were dependent on the arbitrary cutoff points used. The first strategy on the extremes gave clinicians and epidemiologists a better estimate of the magnitude of the associations found.

RESULTS

Temperament Factorial Structure in the Clinical Population

To answer the first research question as to whether the temperament clusters found in the general population were reproducible in the child psychiatric population, a PCA (SAS program) without an iteration and without a rotation was run on the means of the nine categories in the clinical sample of children aged 3 to 7 years (n = 458). Table 3 shows the comparison between the factor structure in the clinical population and that in the general population: in the clinical population, we found a first factor that explained 30% of the total variance and in which the five temperament categories that had the higher loadings were the same as those previously found in the first factor (PCA) in our general population (ie, the traits of adaptability, approach/withdrawal, intensity, mood, and distractibility). Interestingly, the second factor found in children aged 3 to 7 years in the present clinical population also displayed a strong similarity with the second factor (PCA) that previously was found in our general population at this age level (Table 3): a low persistence, a high sensory threshold, and a high activity level all loaded strongly on the adverse pole of factor 2; there was only a slight difference with the general population on the loading for rhythmicity. Thus, the first factor found in the 3- to 7-year-old children who were referred to the clinic showed the same degree of similarity with the easy-difficult cluster of Thomas and Chess[4] and with the first factor that we previously had found in the general population at that age. The PCA that was run on the clinical sample of 8- to 12-year-old children (n = 268) also showed that the temperament categories that loaded strongly on factor 1 at this age level and that explained 37% of the total variance were the same as those found in factor 1 in the general population at that age (Table 3). Thus, the age (3 to 7 years) factor structure was distinct from the age (8 to 12 years) structure; the age (3 to 7 years) factor 1 structure, which was similar to the NYLS cluster, disappeared at the age of 8 to 12 years in the child psychiatric population, as this was observed in our previous studies of the general population.[24] Both factors 1 and 2 were found to be only slightly associated with SES at ages of 3 to 7 years ($r = .17$ and $P = .005$); $r = .17$ and $P = .0003$, respectively) and independent of SES at the ages of 8 to 12 years ($r = .02$ and $r = .05$). Factors 1 and 2 were dependent on sex in the subsample of children aged 3 to 7 years (for factor 1, Wilcoxon $z = 2.65$ and $P = .008$; for factor 2, Wilcoxon $z = 2.16$ and $P = .03$). Boys were more represented on the negative pole of the factors, as we also found in the general population.[18]

TABLE 3

Temperament Factorial Structure in the Clinical Population and Comparison with the General Population*

| | Principal Component Analysis | | | |
| | Ages, 3-7 y (n = 458) | | Ages, 8-12 y (n = 268) | |
Categories	Factor 1†	Factor 2‡	Factor 1	Factor 2
Distractibility	0.79 (0.72)	0.0 (0.08)	0.46 (0.37)	−0.63 (0.65)
Adaptability	0.73 (0.75)	−0.12 (0.01)	0.74 (0.79)	0.33 (−0.22)
Intensity	−0.66 (−0.66)	−0.22 (−0.11)	0.65 (0.61)	−0.32 (0.44)
Mood	0.62 (0.58)	0.13 (−0.11)	0.68 (0.77)	0.42 (−0.19)
Approach/withdrawal	0.49 (0.61)	0.16 (0.02)	0.05 (0.21)	0.82 (−0.58)
Threshold	−0.03 (−0.04)	0.75 (0.72)	0.32 (0.23)	0.01 (0.54)
Rhythmicity	0.39 (0.33)	−0.52 (−0.23)	0.65 (0.71)	0.12 (−0.26)
Persistence	−0.41 (−0.33)	−0.49 (−0.62)	0.77 (0.79)	0.0 (−0.25)
Activity	−0.43 (−0.29)	0.42 (0.55)	0.72 (0.77)	−0.23 (0.24)
Eigenvalue	2.72 (2.53)	1.35 (1.28)	3.29 (3.55)	1.53 (1.52)
% of total variance	30.2 (28.1)	15.0 (14.2)	36.5 (39.4)	17.0 (16.9)

*In parentheses are the loadings from the principal component analysis on two different random samples of the general population, at 7 (18) and at 8 to 12 years of age (24) assessed with the same instruments as those used in the clinical sample.

†On the difficult pole of factor 1 at age 3 to 7 years, low adaptability, high intensity, negative mood, withdrawal from new stimuli, and low distractibility cluster in the clinical and general populations.

‡On the adverse pole of factor 2 at age 3 to 7 years, high activity, low persistence, and high sensory threshold cluster in the clinical and general populations.

Proportions of Subjects With Extreme
Temperament in the Clinical Population

Given the replication of the factorial structure in the child psychiatric population, we considered whether we would find an overproportion of children with an extremely difficult temperament on factor 1, and also on factor 2, in the clinical population of 3- to 7-year-old children. To this end, we first used a categorization of extreme levels that had already been used in our previous work on temperament.[1,18] For each of the temperament categories, each subject was characterized by his or her temperament centile rank by using the normative values taken from our general population at appropriate age levels.[18,24] A subject was defined as presenting with an extremely difficult temperament on factor 1 if he or she presented with a centile less than 30 (>70 for intensity) for at least four of the five categories that loaded strongly on factor 1: they were subjects with a low adaptability, proneness to withdrawal from new stimuli, intense emotional reactions, a general level of negative mood, and a low distractibility. As shown in Table 4, 24% of the children aged 3 to 7 years in the clinical population met these extreme temperament criteria in comparison with 9% in the general population ($z = 6.75$ and $P < .001$). The same centile criteria (on the categories of approach/withdrawal, adaptability, intensity, mood, and distractibility) were applied for the 8- to 12-year-old children, and Table 4 shows a similar, though less important, overproportion (16% vs 7%, $z = 3.35$ and $P < .001$). We must note that our temperament norms from the younger sample in the general population were based on children aged approximately 7 years, whereas our subjects in the clinical sample were aged from 3 to 7 years. This does not preclude the comparison because other studies have shown that norms do not vary from 3 to 7 years of age,[28,29] and our own comparison of a sample of 80 four-year-old children in the general population with the normative sample of 7-year-old children showed negligible differences.

Since we observed, in this clinical population, a similar aggregation of traits on factor 2 (sensory threshold, persistence, and activity) as that found in the general population at the age of 7 years, we also examined the proportion of children with an extreme temperament on factor 2 (low persistence, high sensory threshold, and high activity) in the present clinical population. To do so, we identified the subjects with a temperament centile greater than 70 for activity and threshold and less than 30 for persistence by using the normative values from the general population. We again found an overproportion of an extremely difficult temperament on factor 2 in the population of children (Table 4) who were referred to a child psychiatric center (11% vs 4%, $z = 4.60$ and $P < .001$; 16% vs 4%, $z = 4.84$ and $P < .001$). The same trends, but inverted, were observed for the proportions of an extremely easy temperament on factors 1 and 2 in the clinical population in comparison with the general population. Other cutoffs on the temperament distribution were used to compare the pro-

TABLE 4

Comparison of Proportions of Extremely Difficult Temperaments in the Child Psychiatric Population with Those in the General Population According to Age Levels

Type of Extremely Difficult Temperament	Proportions in Population, No. (%)					
	Child Psychiatric			General*		
	Total†	Boys	Girls	Total	Boys	Girls
On factor 1‡						
3-7 y	112/477 (24)	80/324 (25)	32/153 (21)	78/879 (9)	53/453 (12)	25/426 (6)
8-12 y	42/271 (16)	34/207 (16)	8/64 (13)	37/514 (7)	20/245 (8)	17/269 (6)
On factor 2§						
3-7 y	54/477 (11)	42/324 (13)	12/153 (8)	35/879 (4)	26/453 (6)	9/426 (2)
8-12	43/271 (16)	37/207 (18)	6/64 (9)	22/514 (4)	16/245 (7)	6/269 (2)

*For the comparison, we used the normative values from two different random samples of our general population whose temperament was assessed with the same instruments at age 7 years (18) and at age 8 to 12 years (24).

†Total sample size is increased by 22 (726 to 748) because of the inclusion of the subjects with temperament questionnaires meeting the criteria of acceptability on the categories of the factor under study but with unacceptable ratings in the categories of the factor not under study.

‡Extreme subjects on the adverse pole of factor 1 were situated under centile 30 (>70 for intensity) for at least four of the five categories loading strongly on factor 1 (low adaptability, very withdrawing, negative mood, very intense, and low distractibility). This was also applied to the 8- to 12-year-old subjects.

§Extreme subjects on the adverse pole of factor 2 were situated under centile 30 for persistence and greater than 70 for activity and threshold, ie, the three categories loading strongly on factor 2 (low persistence, high sensory threshold, and high activity level). This was also applied to the 8- to 12-year-old subjects.

portion of extremes in the clinical population with that in the general population, and this yielded congruent results.

Extreme Temperament and Type of Clinical Diagnosis

Given the observed overproportion of extreme temperaments on both factors 1 and 2 in the children who were referred to a child psychiatric center, we were in a position to test whether it was merely the extreme characteristics of temperament in general that were associated with any kind of disorders or whether there existed a specificity in the relationship between the extreme levels on special features of temperament and certain kinds of disorders. To this end, a contingency table was built in which the two columns were the extreme temperaments on factor 1 and the extreme temperaments on factor 2 by using the same centile cutoff points as were used previously. The three rows represented the subjects with only an externalized disorder, the subjects with only a developmental delay, and the subjects who presented with a combination of these two diagnoses. The distribution of disorders in the different temperament groups was not homogeneous ($\chi^2 = 7.91$, $df = 2$, and $P = .02$): an overproportion of externalized disorders was found in the extreme temperaments on factor 1, and an overproportion of developmental delays was found in the extreme temperaments on factor 2. The combined disorders were distributed in about the same proportions in both groups with extreme temperaments (Table 5. For this analysis, we used the subsample of children aged 3 to 7 years to be able to use the temperament factor scores on factors 1 and 2 and because of the small numbers of developmental delays in the older part of the sample of children aged 8 to 12 years. We excluded other combinations of disorders and also the internalized disorders because of the small numbers in those categories at the ages of 3 to 7 years. Table 5 also shows that the subjects with insufficient information to make a diagnosis were evenly distributed in the temperamental groups. However the sizes of the proportion differences make clear that temperament is far from being the only variable that contributes to the variance that differentiates the diagnostic groups. Other cutoffs points to define the extremes of temperament were used and yielded similar results.

As a complement to this analysis at the extremes and to confirm the distinction between the three diagnostic groups, we ran discriminant function analyses (SPSS-X program) and then stepwise discriminant analyses (SAS program) in which the dependent variables were the age (3 to 7 years) temperament factor 1 (with the subjects being characterized by their factor score on factor 1 from the PCA), the age (3 to 7 years) temperament factor 2 (with the subjects being characterized by their factor score on factor 2), sex, SES, child's age at consultation, and family status (single or intact family); the independent variables were the diagnostic groups. We took into account, in the statistical analysis, the unequal sizes of the groups. A discriminant function was derived to distinguish between the diagnostic

TABLE 5

Distribution of the Different Disorders in the Extreme Temperamental Groups on Factors 1 and 2 in the 3- to 7-Year-Old Subsample

Temperament	Type of Disorders, No. (%)				
	Externalized Disorders	Developmental Delays	Externalized and Developmental Delays	Insufficient Information	Total
Extreme subjects on factor 1*	23 (33)	9 (13)	17 (25)	20 (29)	69 (100)
Extreme subjects on factor 2†	3 (10)	9 (29)	9 (29)	10 (32)	31 (100)
Others‡	53 (22)	65 (28)	25 (11)	90 (39)	233 (100)
Total§	79 (24)	83 (25)	51 (15)	120 (36)	333 (100)

*Extreme subjects on factor 1 were situated under centile 30 (>70 for intensity) for at least four of the five categories loading strongly on factor 1 (low adaptability, very withdrawing, negative mood, very intense, and low distractibility).

†Extreme subjects on factor 2 were situated under centile 30 for persistence and greater than 70 for activity and threshold, ie, the three categories loading strongly on factor 2 (low persistence, high sensory threshold, and high activity).

‡All other subjects who were not extreme of temperament either on factor 1 or factor 2.

§Unacceptable questionnaires on temperament explain the different total numbers of disorders (are missing n = 2 externalized, n = 6 developmental delays, n = 5 combined disorders, and n = 4 insufficient information on disorders).

groups that were compared one to one. Concerning the externalized disorders (n = 76) and the developmental delays (n = 78), the function significantly discriminated the two groups (eigenvalue = .71), Wilks' λ = .58, df = 6, and P < .0001) and had 80% (true externalized disorders) and 83% (true developmental delays) of classification accuracy. The coefficients of the six variables that contributed to this function were –.66 for age, .61 for temperament factor 1, .42 for family status, –.10 for SES, .08 for temperament factor 2, and –.07 for sex. The function was largely defined by the first two variables; older children in the group aged 3 to 7 years and children who were highly difficult on factor 1 were more likely to present with externalized disorders. In the discriminant function analysis on the group with externalized disorders alone (n = 76) vs the group with externalized disorders plus developmental delays (n = 44), the function also significantly discriminated both groups (eigenvalue = .21, Wilks' λ = .82, df = 6, and P = .001) and had 83% and 48% of classification accuracy; the age at consultation and temperament factor 2 contributed most to the function(–.62 and .59, respectively). In the analysis on the group with developmental delays alone (n = 78) vs the group with externalized disorders plus developmental delays (n = 44), the function discriminated significantly (eigenvalue = .37, Wilks' λ = .73, df = 6, and P < .00001) and had 85% and 60% of classification accuracy; temperament factor 1 contributed most to the function (.65). As expected, the analysis better distinguished from each other the two groups with pure disorders than it distinguished each pure disorder from the group that presented with a combination of these disorders.

These results confirmed, to some degree, that our three clinical diagnostic groups were different groups. Additionally, we performed three stepwise discriminant analyses (SPSS-X program) that compared the diagnostic groups to look at the possible variables (especially temperament factors 1 and 2) that would distinguish the groups in the sense that the selected variables would explain more intergroup variance than all the others; our hypothesis was that externalized disorders would again be more difficult on factor 1, and the developmental delays would be more adverse on factor 2. In the stepwise discriminant analysis on the externalized disorders (n = 76) vs the developmental delays (n = 78), the age at consultation in step 1 (R = .49, F = 46.88, and P = .0001), the temperament factor 1 in step 2 (R = .42, F = 32.35, and P = .0001), and the family status in step 3 (R = .26, F = 10.88, and P = .001) composed the model that distinguished best the two groups; children with externalized disorders were more likely to be older, to be difficult on factor 1, and to live in intact families. In the stepwise analysis on the group with externalized disorders (n = 76) vs the group with externalized disorder plus developmental delays (n = 44), the age at consultation in step 1 (R = .26, F = 9.47, and P = .003) and the temperament factor 2 in step 2 (R = .24, F = 7.95, and P = .006) distinguished the groups. In the analysis on the group with developmental delays (n = 78) vs the group with externalized disorders plus developmental delays (n = 44), the temperament factor 1 in step

1 ($R = .37$, $F = 19.20$ and $P = .0001$ and the age at consultation in step 2 ($R = .24$, $F = 7.39$, and $P = .008$) distinguished the two groups.

Thus, consistent with our previous analyses on the extremes, this analysis showed that (1) temperament factors 1 or 2 distinguished between the diagnostic groups; (2) the externalized disorders were more difficult on temperament factor 1 than the developmental delays; (3) among the children in the clinical sample with externalized disorders, those who additionally presented with developmental delays were more adverse on temperament factor 2; and (4) among the children in the clinical sample with a developmental delay, those who additionally presented with an externalized disorder were more difficult on temperament factor 1.

All this is congruent with the suggestion borne by Table 5: temperament (age range, 3 to 7 years) factor 1 was more associated with an externalized disorder, whereas temperament (age range, 3 to 7 years) factor 2 was more associated with a developmental delay. Our results also showed that, on the continuum on temperament factor 2, the group characterized by an externalized disorder alone was the least adverse (average factor score, -0.17), the group characterized by a developmental delay alone was intermediate (average factor score, -0.01), and the group characterized by a developmental delay combined with an externalized disorder was in the most adverse position (average factor score, 0.45). There also was a trend toward the children with a developmental delay being referred at a younger age (mean age at referral, 4.82 years for the group with a developmental delay alone; 5.44 years for the group with developmental delay plus an externalized disorder; and 6.29 years for the group with an externalized alone.

As Table 5 also indicates, despite the significant association found between extremely difficult temperament on factor 1 (age range, 3 to 7 years) and externalized disorders, a large proportion of externalized disorders (53/79; 67%) presented with no extremely difficult temperament. It was thus warranted to investigate, through another stepwise discriminant analysis, the possible differences between these two groups: those externalized disorders associated with an extremely difficult temperament on age (3 to 7 years) factor 1 below the 20th centile on temperament factor scores distribution; $n = 27$) vs those externalized disorders without such a difficult temperament (above the 50th centile on temperament distribution; $n = 22$); among variables, such as sex, age at consultation, family size, and child's rank, SES, family status, and severity of disorder, only the degree of severity distinguished the two groups ($R^2 = .10$, $F = 5.27$, and $P = .03$). When a difficult temperament was present, the externalized disorders were more severe.

COMMENT

The present findings raise many important issues for clinicians and for future clinical research: (1) in their current practice, clinicians in child psychiatry are likely to find themselves in the presence of a considerable number of children with an extremely difficult temperament as defined by our age (3 to 7 years) factor 1; (2) even though a significant overproportion of children with an extreme temperament are referred to child psychiatric centers, not all children referred to clinicians display an extreme temperament; (3) specific temperament components are associated with particular clinical problems; and (4) future clinical research must address the distinction between an extreme temperament and a clinical disorder and the intricate relationship between the two.

Replication of Temperament Clusters in the
Child Psychiatric Population

First, we replicated, in a child psychiatric population, through a PCA, a first temperament cluster that was similar to the one found in infancy[17] and at the age 7 years[18] in our general population and that resembled the NYLS "easy-difficult" factor. The difference, recurrently found with the NYLS cluster, resides in rhythmicity being substituted by distractibility. Thus, this first factor even remains consistent when questionnaires are answered by parents who have problems either with their child or in their family and who are referred to or request a consultation. Epidemiological studies already have demonstrated that this temperament factor, composed mainly of adaptability, approach/withdrawal, intensity, mood, and distractibility, is independent of SES[24] in random samples of the general population, and that it is consistent transculturally and identifiable in the general population from infancy to the age of 7 years.[17,18] This temperament factor is no more identifiable in the general population at ages of 8 to 12 years.[24]

Does this additional replication of the factorial structure up to the age of 7 years, which is independent of the fact that parents are selected from a clinical population or from a general population, argue against a strong objective component in this questionnaire factor (ie, temperament questionnaire would mainly tap subjective characteristics in the parent instead of qualities within the child)? We are inclined to believe so, but only studies of the possible correlations of this temperament factor with biological parameters will ultimately resolve the issue. As it was recently demonstrated, this factor, obtained by questionnaire, presents a stronger association with objective laboratory measurement than with maternal or environmental characteristics.[20] This result supports our previous and present epidemiological findings that this temperamental factor is not strongly linked to demographic or environmental parameters. The present findings also reproduce, in the child psychiatric population, a second temperament factor that is similar to the one observed in the general population.

Overproportion of Extreme Temperament in the Referred Children

Second, we found an overproportion of extremely difficult temperaments in the referred children, especially in the younger ones. Some evidence previously had shown that an extremely difficult temperament, as assessed by factor 1 in the general population, longitudinally predisposes the development of clinical disorders in a child, especially the oppositional or externalized type.[1] We formerly demonstrated that this extremely difficult temperament (factor 1), based on the NYLS model, is not totally equivalent to a clinical disorder in children. For instance, in our longitudinal cohorts in the general population, even if children presenting with an extremely difficult temperament on factor 1 at the age of 4.5 years[2] or from the ages of 7 to 12 years[1] were more prone to present with a disorder, disorders (as measured by interviews conducted independently by two psychiatrists[30]) did not develop in a large proportion of these temperamentally extreme children, even those keeping their extreme temperamental qualities throughout many years.

The present data, being congruent with the former, confirm that more children with an extremely difficult temperament are found in the population of children referred to a child psychiatric clinic. They also show, however, that a large proportion of children who present with disorders, even externalized, and referred to a child psychiatric clinic, do not present with an extremely difficult temperament. This provides further evidence that an extreme temperamental phenomenology is not automatically equivalent to a clinical behavior disorder in childhood and vice versa; this, to a certain extent, goes against the argument of some researchers[6] that common childhood psychiatric disorders (with the exception of syndromes, such as autism, psychosis, or serious eating disorders) are mostly the expression of an extreme form of temperament qualities. Of course, our present data cannot eliminate the possibility, if measurements of temperament had been taken at recurrent occasions in the years surrounding the period of referral, that we could have observed a more important association between an extreme temperament and disorders. However, this latter possibility clearly is not supported, as previously mentioned, by the results of our longitudinal studies of extreme temperamental groups in the general population in preschool years[31] or in middle childhood[30]: disorders developed in only approximately one half of the extremely difficult children during the 4 to 9 years of follow-up. Moreover, the stable occurrence of temperament factor 1 early at the ages of 4 and 8 months in random samples of our general population[17] and the complex relationship between extreme temperament in infancy and disorders at 4 years of age[31] also argue against an equivalence or a strong direct relationship between extreme levels on the temperament continuum and childhood behavior disorders. So far, our epidemiological findings rather support the view that an extremely difficult temperament on factor 1 is a precursor of disorders and not the same entity or a parallel phenomenology in which the extreme levels are disorders on one end and a normal human personality on the other.

Relationship Between Each Temperament Component and Types of Clinical Problems

Third, our present findings indicate a degree of specificity in the relationship between different temperament components and particular types of disorders. As it is consistent with our previous longitudinal findings in cohorts of the general population whereby a more externalized behavior disorder developed in temperamentally extreme subjects on factor 1 comparatively with other developmental deviancies,[1,2] the present data show that children with extreme temperaments on factor 1 in a child psychiatric population aged 3 to 8 years (low adaptability, withdrawal in the face of new stimuli, intensity of emotional reactions, negative mood, and low distractibility) also are more likely to have been referred for externalized disorders. Also, the temperamentally extreme subjects on factor 2 (low persistence, high threshold, and high activity) are more likely to have been referred to a child psychiatric center for developmental delays. However, the association is not exclusive, ie, the type of temperament is not the only factor that distinguishes the diagnostic groups, as it might have been expected from clinical experience. In other words, the present data provide evidence that there is more than just a general extremeness of temperament that is linked to any type of developmental or behavioral deviancies: a temperament-diagnosis specificity might exist. The present finding also suggests that, if we had also selected extremes on factor 2 in addition to extremes on factor 1 in our previous longitudinal cohorts in the general population, the two types of temperament would have led to a different clinical outcome. This specificity should be tested in future longitudinal studies.

How would an adverse temperament on (age 3 to 7 years) factor 1 lead to decompensation into externalized disorders in children of the general population and in those children referred to the clinic? We previously observed that it was in the presence of dysfunctional parental attitudes of discipline or behavior control that externalized oppositional disorders were more likely to develop in 12-year-old children who had presented with an extremely adverse temperament on factor 1 at the age of 7 years.[1] Conversely, in terms of behavior control, disorders developed up to adolescence in almost none of the temperamentally adverse children on factor 1 who lived in a superiorly functioning family. As we have previously hypothesized,[32] these children who are temperamentally withdrawing from new stimuli, poorly adaptable, intense, and presenting a negative mood, could present with intrinsic tendencies toward opposition to rules and demands. Therefore, when the family rules lack clarity and are not characterized by parental consensus and consistency,[1,2] the excessive solicitation of these children on some parents' insufficient abilities to control their behaviors would progressively lead to clinical decompensation.

Leads for Future Clinical Research

Fourth, such findings provide leads for further clinical studies to investigate the mechanisms that involve different temperamental components in the development of different clinical deviancies. For instance, what differentiates the externalized disorders associated with a difficult temperament on factor 1 from the externalized disorders without such a difficult temperament? Are there differences in terms of the symptoms, the family functioning, or the mechanisms that are involved in the appearance of disorders? Among the variables that we assessed, the only difference that we now find between these two groups is the degree of severity of the externalized symptoms. The referred children with an externalized disorder, associated with an extremely difficult temperament, present with more severe disorders; this could imply a serious impact on the outcome or on the course of treatment. Further studies must address the possible differences between these two groups in terms of more precise diagnostic categories (oppositional, conduct, and attention-deficit disorders), the environmental specificity of the symptoms, the type of family dysfunction, and the prognosis.

Fifth, the two temperamentally different subgroups of children in the clinical sample presenting with a combination of externalized disorders and developmental delays (the sub-group that was extreme on temperament factor 1 and the one that was extreme on temperament factor 2) pose challenging questions; researchers must investigate a possible heterogeneity with respect to the mechanisms of the appearance of this combination of disorders.

Finally, we should point out possible biases generated by our methods that might bring caution in interpreting our results: for instance, the possibility of a strong confounding or circularity effect that involved the assessment of temperament and that of diagnosis. This could arguably originate, on the one hand, from the fact that the mother filled in the temperament measurement, and on the other hand, that the hospital chart reviews contained information from the parents. We cannot eliminate this possibility, but we think it is unlikely for several reasons. First, for most hospital charts, the information used was obtained from many respondents, including the school, and from the child's clinical observations by a number of mental health professionals. Second, the charts review was done blind to the temperament scores, and the charts contained no clinical description of temperamental traits per se. Third, our results themselves rather argue against such a confounding effect: the temperament traits (for instance, factor 2: high activity level, low persistence, and high threshold), which would have been expected to be associated mostly to externalized disorders, were those found to be especially related to developmental delays in our clinical sample. It was the factor 1 component that was more associated to the externalized problems.

Another question could be raised: is it the occurrence of a developmental delay that renders the child's temperament less persistent and more active with a higher sensory threshold, or is it the temperament traits that predispose to developmental delays? With regard to temperament factor 1, we already have some evidence that the difficult traits antedate the appearance of disorders[1]; however, for temperament factor 2, the issue is less clear. The occurrence of two similar temperamental factors at such a young age as 4 and 8 months,[17] in the general population, rather supports the idea that they are precursors of disorders rather than secondary effects of them. We believe that only longitudinal multivariate studies of extreme temperament levels, clinical status, and environmental parameters, along with biophysiological markers, will enlighten the issue. Of course, the question as to what physiological markers to target is a complex one because one has, as yet, few empirical leads to rely on. In that respect, the developmental studies of extreme temperamental features and physiological reactivity conducted by Kagan and his group[33,34] and the ones conducted on monkeys by Suomi[35,36] on social reactivity and cortisol levels are promising; such methods could be incorporated in the design of longitudinal and epidemiological-clinical studies in children.

The present results suggest future clinical studies of these different subgroups in child psychiatric samples, with an emphasis on the combined use of standardized interviews to make *DSM-III* diagnoses and measurements of temperament and family and cognitive functioning. The inclusion of biophysiological measures also will be necessary since they will constitute the ultimate reliable mean to differentiate temperament, as we usually assess it, from the different clinical disorders according to present nosologies.

REFERENCES

1. Maziade M, Capéraà P, Laplante B, Boudreault M, Thivierge J, Côté R, Boutin P. Value of difficult temperament among 7-year-olds in the general population for predicting psychiatric diagnosis at age 12. *Am J Psychiatry.* 1985; 142:943–946.

2. Maziade M, Côté R, Thivierge J, Boutin P, Bernier H. Significance of extreme temperament at 4–8 months for predicting diagnosis at 4.7 years. *Br J Psychiatry.* 1989; 154:535–543.

3. Earls F, Jung KG. Temperament and home environment characteristics as causal factors in the early development of childhood psychopathology. *J Am Acad Child Adolesc Psychiatry.* 1987;26:491–498.

4. Thomas A, Chess S. *Temperament and Development.* New York, NY: Brunner/Mazel Inc; 1977.

5. Graham P, Rutter M, George S. Temperamental characteristics as predictors of behavior in children. *Am J Orthopsychiatry.* 1973;43:328–339.

6. Graham P, Stevenson J. Temperament and psychiatric disorders: the genetic contribution to behavior in childhood. *Aust N Z J Psychiatry.* 1987;21:267–274.

7. Ferguson HD, Rapoport JL. Nosological issues and biological validation. In: Rutter M, ed. *Developmental Neuropsychiatry.* New York, NY: Guilford Press;1983:369–384.

8. Pfeffer J, Martin RP. Comparison of mothers' and fathers' temperament ratings of referred and nonreferred preschool children. *J Clin Psychol.* 1983;39:1013–1020.

9. Lambert NM. Temperament profiles of hyperactive children. *Am J Ortho-psychiatry.* 1982;52:458–467.

10. Klein PS, Tzuriel D. Preschoolers' type of temperament as predictor of potential difficulties in cognitive functioning. *Isr J Psychiatry Relat Sci.* 1986;23:49–61.

11. Keogh BK. Individual differences in temperament: A contribution to the personal, social, and educational competence of learning disabled children. In: McKinney JD, Feagans L, eds. *Current Topics in Learning Disabilities.* Norwood, NJ: Ablex Publishing Corp; 1983:33–55.

12. Gunn P, Berry P, Andrews RJ. The temperament of Down's syndrome infants: a research note. *J Child Psychol Psychiatry.* 1981;22:189–194.

13. Gunn P, Berry P. Down's syndrome temperament and maternal response to descriptions of child behavior. *Dev Psychol.* 1985;21:842–847.

14. Bender WN. Differences between learning disabled and non-learning disabled children in temperament and behavior. *Learning Disability Q.* 1985;8:11–18.

15. Kolvin I, Nicol AR, Garside RF, Day KA, Tweddle EG. Temperamental patterns in aggressive boys. *Ciba Found Symp.* 1982;89:252–268.

16. Goldsmith HH, Buss AH, Plomin R, Rothbart MK, Thomas A, Chess S, Hinde RA, McCall RB. Roundtable: what is temperament? four approaches. *Child Dev.* 1987;58:505–529.

17. Maziade M, Boudreault M, Thivierge J, Capéraà P, Côté R. Infant temperament: SES and gender differences and reliability of measurement in a large Quebec sample. *Merrill-Palmer Q.* 1984;30:213–216.

18. Maziade M. Côté R, Boudreault M, Thivierge J, Capéraà P. The New York longitudinal studies model of temperament: gender differences and demographic correlates in a French-speaking population. *J Am Acad Child Adolesc Psychiatry.* 1984;23:582–587.

19. Matheny AP, Wilson RS, Nuss SM. Toddler temperament: stability across settings and over ages. *Child Dev.* 1984;55:1200–1211.

20. Matheny AP, Wilson RW, Thoben AS. Home and mother: relations with infant temperament. *Dev Psychol.* 1987;23:323–331.

21. Goodyer IM, Kolvin I, Gatzani S. The impact of recent undesirable life events on psychiatric disorders in childhood and adolescence. *Br J Psychiatry.* 1987; 151:179–184.

22. Hollingshead AB. *Two-Factor Index of Social Position.* New Haven, Conn: Yale University Press; 1957.

23. Hegvik RL, McDevitt SC, Carey WB. The Middle Childhood Temperament Questionnaire. *Dev Behav Pediatrics.* 1982;3:197–200.

24. Maziade M, Boutin P, Côté R, Thivierge J. Empirical characteristics of NYLS temperament in middle childhood: congruities and incongruities with other studies. *Child Psychiatry Hum Dev.* 1986;17:38–52.

25. Rutter M. Epidemiology of psychiatric disorders. In: Rutter M, ed. *Education, Health and Behavior.* London, England: Longman Group Ltd; 1970:178–201.

26. Rutter M, Gould M. Classification. In: Rutter M, Hersov L, eds. *Child and Adolescent psychiatry: Modern Approaches.* Boston, Mass: Blackwell Scientific Publications Inc; 1985:304–321.

27. Guy W, ed. *ECDEU Assessment Manual for Psychopharmacology.* Revised. Rockville, Md: National Institute of Mental Health; 1976. US Dept of Health, Education, and Welfare publication (ADM) 76–338.

28. Thomas A, Chess S, eds. *Measurement and Rating of Temperament.* New York, NY: Brunner/Mazel Inc; 1977:118–131.

29. McDevitt SC, Carey WB. The measurement of temperament in 3–7 year old children. *J Child Psychol Psychiatry.* 1978;19:245–253.

30. Maziade M, Côté R, Boudreault M, Thivierge J, Boutin P. Family correlates of temperament continuity and change across middle childhood. *Am J Orthopsychiatry.* 1986;195–203.

31. Maziade M, Côté R, Thivierge J, Boutin P, Bernier H. Significance of extreme temperament in infancy for clinical status in preschool years, II: patterns of temperament change and implications for the appearance of disorders. *Br J Psychiatry.* 1989;154:544–551.

32. Maziade M. Should adverse temperament matter to the clinician? an empirically based answer. In: Kohnstamm GA, Bates JE, Rothbart MK, eds. *Temperament in Childhood.* New York, NY: John Wiley & Sons Inc. In press.

33. Kagan J, Reznick JS. Task involvement and cardiac response in young children. *Aust J Psychol.* 1984;36:135–147.

34. Reznick JS, Kagan J, Snidman N, Gersten M, Baak K, Rosenberg A. Inhibited and uninhibited children: a follow-up study. *Child Dev.* 1986;57:660–680.

35. Suomi SJ. Social development in rhesus monkeys: consideration of individual differences. In: Oliverio A, ed. *The Behavior of Human Infants.* New York, NY: Plenum Press; 1983:71–92.

36. Suomi SJ. Anxiety-like disorders in young nonhuman primates. In: Gittelman R, ed. *Anxiety Disorders of Childhood.* New York, NY: Guilford Press; 1986:1–23.

14

Psychiatric Correlates of Behavioral Inhibition in Young Children of Parents With and Without Psychiatric Disorders

Joseph Biederman, Jerrold F. Rosenbaum, Dina R. Hirshfeld,
Stephen V. Faraone, Elizabeth A. Bolduc, Michelle Gersten, and
Susan R. Meminger
Harvard Medical School, Boston
Jerome Kagan and Nancy Snidman
Harvard University, Cambridge
J. Steven Reznick
Yale University, New Haven

Behavioral inhibition is a laboratory-based temperamental category characterized by the tendency to constrict behavior in unfamiliar situations and assumed to reflect low thresholds of limbic arousal. We previously found behavioral inhibition prevalent in the offspring of parents with panic disorder and agoraphobia. In this report, we examined the psychiatric correlates of parents with panic disorder and agoraphobia, previously dichotomized as inhibited and not inhibited, and an existing epidemiologically derived sample of children, followed by Kagan and colleagues and originally identified at 21 months of age as inhibited or uninhibited. A third group of healthy children was added for comparison. Our findings indicate that inhibited children had increased risk for multiple anxiety, overanxious, and phobic disorders. It is suggested that behavioral inhibition may be associated with risk for anxiety disorders in children.

Reprinted with permission from *Archives of General Psychology*, 1990, Vol. 47, 21–26. Copyright © 1990 by the American Medical Association.

This research was supported in part by grant MH-40619 from the National Institute of Mental Health, Bethesda, MD, and by a grant from the John D. and Catherine T. MacArthur Foundation (J.K.).

The emergence and persistence of temperamental differences among children have been a focus of research in developmental psychology.[1-7] *Temperament* refers to stable, presumably inherited, response dispositions[8,9] that are evident early in life, are observable in a variety of situations, and probably influence personality development. Two of the better-known temperamental categories are based on responses or initial reactions to unfamiliar people and situations,[1-7] variably referred to as "shyness vs sociability," "introversion vs extroversion," or "withdrawal vs approach." In unfamiliar settings or with unfamiliar people, children characterized as "sociable," "uninhibited," or "extroverted" are not distressed, vocalize, smile, and spontaneously approach the unfamiliar object or setting. However, "shy," "inhibited," or "introverted" children typically interrupt ongoing behavior and show vocal restraint and withdrawal when confronted with novel stimuli. Data from the New York Longitudinal Study[10,11] indicate that the tendencies to approach or to withdraw from novelty are relatively enduring temperamental dimensions.

The most extensive research on behaviorally inhibited and uninhibited responses to the unfamiliar comes from ongoing longitudinal projects conducted by Kagan and colleagues[12-14] at the Harvard Infant Study Laboratory, Cambridge, Mass. This work suggests that approximately 10% to 15% of American white children are born predisposed to be irritable as infants, shy and fearful as toddlers, and cautious, quiet, and introverted when they reach school age; in contrast, about 15% of the population show the opposite profile. During a 7-year period, the Harvard group has followed two independent cohorts of white children, selected at either 21 or 31 months of age to be either behaviorally inhibited or uninhibited when exposed to unfamiliar rooms, people, and objects. In a laboratory setting, inhibited children manifested long latencies to interact when exposed to novelty, retreated from the unfamiliar, and ceased play and vocalizations while clinging to their mothers. The observed differences in behavioral inhibition were preserved to a notable degree from the original assessment in infancy to later assessments at 4, 5, and 7½ years of age, indicating that the tendency to approach or to withdraw from novelty is relatively enduring.[15]

The literature suggests that temperamental profiles in infancy may be associated with later difficulties. For example, Chess and Thomas[16,17] found that infants with preponderant withdrawal tendencies were at risk for developing avoidant or overanxious disorders in childhood. Carey et al[18] reported that infant temperament is a significant factor in predicting school adjustment in early grades. Gersten[19] showed that among the cohort followed up by Kagan and colleagues, inhibited and uninhibited behaviors could be observed in the school setting; many of the inhibited children during their first days of kindergarten and several months later continued to show severe social restraint and avoidance. These findings suggest that at least certain temperamental characteristics may be precursors to or risk factors for manifest psychopathology. However, the study of temperament as a predisposition to psychiatric disorders per se has received less attention. If a temperamental profile were a risk factor for the development of psychopathology, it should be found to be linked to manifest psychopathology in those with presumed high-risk temperamental traits. If such a link were established, the early recognition of young children with these temperamental traits would offer an opportunity for the development of preventive strategies such as behavioral interventions.

Our group hypothesized that behavioral inhibition may be one such high-risk temperamental category predictive of anxiety proneness. To date,[20] we have reported a high prevalence of behavioral inhibition in a group of 2- to 7-year old children born to adults in treatment for panic disorder and agoraphobia (high-risk children) compared with control children of parents without panic disorder. To investigate further the link between behavioral inhibition and anxiety disorders, it is necessary to examine whether this temperamental trait, reflecting the tendency to exhibit excessive arousal and withdrawal in the face of challenge or novelty, is already associated with manifest anxiety disorders in children. Because anxiety disorders are known to be familial,[21-26] it would be important in testing this hypothesis not only to evaluate high-risk children of parents with panic disorder and agoraphobia, but also to include those in which the assessment of behavioral inhibition would be unrelated to parental psychopathology. We had such an opportunity in the longitudinal cohort followed by Kagan and colleagues at Harvard University,[12] Cambridge, Mass, particularly since the assessments and determinations of behavioral inhibition in the high-risk children were done at the same laboratory (Harvard University Infant Study Laboratory) and by the same group of investigators (J.K., J.S.R., and N.S.) as that of the longitudinal cohort of Kagan et al. We report on the psychopathologic correlates of behavioral inhibition in two separate preexisting samples of children, one consisting of the high-risk offspring of parents with panic disorder and agoraphobia and a second sample of children followed longitudinally by Kagan and colleagues.

SUBJECTS AND METHODS

Rates of *DSM-III* psychiatric diagnoses were evaluated in two independently ascertained preexisting samples of children. One sample was cross-sectional and clinically derived (Massachusetts General Hospital [MGH], Boston, at-risk sample), and the other sample was epidemiologically derived and longitudinal (Kagan et al longitudinal cohort). Detailed methodology of the ascertainment of the groups is described in earlier reports.[12-15,20] All parents signed informed consent for participation in this study.

MGH Samples

MGH at-risk sample. The MGH at-risk group was a subset (30 of 32 [two refused to participate] of the older children (4 to 7 years old, mean = 5.4 ± 0.9 years) from the previously reported sample of 56 nonpatient children (2 to 7 years) with outpatient parents with panic disorder and agoraphobia treated at the Department of Psychiatry of MGH and children with relatives without disorders.[20] As described in the previous report, eligible children of outpatient parents treated for panic disorder and agoraphobia were matched for age, socioeconomic status (SES), and ordinal position with a control group of children with relatives having other psychiatric disorders before evaluation for behavioral inhibition at the Harvard University Infant Study Laboratory. The evaluation consisted of a series of age-appropriate cognitive tasks using protocols that had been developed and used in other studies on behavioral inhibition[12-15] and were designed to obtain an index of each child's behavior with an unfamiliar examiner under mild cognitive stress.[27] The observations of the protocol sessions were videotaped and scored by coders who had no knowledge of parental diagnosis. Based on these observations,[20] children were dichotomized into two mutually exclusive categories—inhibited and not inhibited. Assignments of children to the inhibited (N = 18) and not inhibited (N = 12) groups were done at the Harvard laboratory blindly to the assessment of psychopathology in the children and in their parents.

MGH healthy controls. Since the children who were not behaviorally inhibited had been ascertained by having a relative with a psychiatric disorder, they could not be considered a "normal" comparison group. Therefore, to contrast rates of psychiatric disorders with the MGH at-risk sample, an additional group of children without known medical or psychiatric disorders (healthy control) was deemed necessary. This healthy control group consisted of 20 nonadopted, white, non-Hispanic, healthy children with similar SES and geographic distribution to those of the MGH at-risk sample. This control group ranged in age from 4 to 10 years (mean = 7.8 ± 1.9 years) and was derived from pediatric primary care service referrals at MGH initially screened for the absence of known medical or psychiatric disorders. Although the temperamental characteristics of these children were not evaluated, on the basis of the findings of Kagan and colleagues,[12-15] it is expected that their rate of behavioral inhibition would not exceed 10% to 15%.

Kagan et al Longitudinal Cohort

The Kagan et al longitudinal cohort is a well-described[12-15] preexisting longitudinal cohort consisting of 41 children between the ages of 7 and 8 years (mean = 8.0 ± 0.2 years) at the time of psychopathologic assessment. These children had been originally screened by Kagan and colleagues at the age of 21 months from a larger group of 305 white children identified from birth registries, whose mothers, responding to questions in a telephone interview, had described their children as tending to be either inhibited or uninhibited. Based on these interviews, 117 children came to the Harvard laboratory of Kagan et al, where their behavior was observed and quantified in a variety of unfamiliar settings. The major behavioral signs of inhibition were long latencies before interaction with unfamiliar adults and the cessation of play or vocalization. The children who displayed these behaviors consistently, as well as those who consistently did not, were selected to form groups of most inhibited (inhibited) and most uninhibited (uninhibited) children. Each group represented about 10% of the original sample. These children had been followed longitudinally since their initial assessment and assignment to the inhibited (N = 22) and uninhibited (N = 19) groups at 21 months. Children without behavioral inhibition in this ascertainment site were called *uninhibited* to distinguish them from the not-inhibited children from the MGH at-risk sample. The uninhibited children from the Kagan et al cohort had been selected to be consistently bold and fearless in new situations (hence, uninhibited), while in the MGH at-risk sample, they consisted of children who were not behaviorally inhibited (hence, not inhibited).

Assessment of Psychopathology

This study of psychopathology consisted of systematic psychiatric assessment of all children 4 years of age and older at the time of evaluation based on interviews with mothers using the Diagnostic Interview for Children and Adolescents-Parent Version.[28-30] Rated *DSM-III* disorders were attention-deficit disorder (ADD), oppositional disorder, major depression, mania, separation anxiety disorder, overanxious disorder, avoidant disorder, phobic disorders, obsessive-compulsive disorder, enuresis, and encopresis. The Diagnostic Interview for Children and Adolescents does not distinguish between ADD with and without hyperactivity; therefore, the generic term *ADD* was used. In addition, the diagnosis of ADD was based on parental report alone and lacked external corroborating information such as a teacher's report.

Since meeting criteria for a single disorder in a structured interview that assesses multiple disorders may be too low a diagnostic threshold to be indicative of more serious psychopathology, we grouped those who met criteria for two or more anxiety disorders (multiple anxiety disorders) as reflective of severe anxiety and four or more disorders as indicative of more severe overall psychopathology (severe psychopathology).

All interviews were conducted by trained raters with graduate and undergraduate degrees in psychology with established interrater reliability (overall $\kappa = .88 \pm .04$). The training consisted of familiarization with the study design and objectives, psychiatric nosology (*DSM-III*), and the structured interview used. Raters in training first observed interviews carried out by experienced raters and clinicians and subsequently conducted at least two interviews while observed by senior raters before they started rating independently. Raters were supervised by the senior investigators (J.B. and J.F.R.) and doctorate-level psychologists (M.G. and S.R.M.). Interviews were audiotaped for random review and reliability assessments. Raters were "blinded" with respect to the temperamental classification of the children and final diagnostic assignment of the parents. Raters were not blinded to ascertainment site (MGH or Harvard). Before final diagnostic assignment, all diagnostic information was reviewed by the senior investigators (J.B. and J.F.R.), who also were blinded to the temperamental classification of the children. For every subject, all possible diagnoses were made. Diagnostic uncertainties were resolved by review of the available information following a best-estimate diagnostic approach proposed by Leckman et al.[31] Final diagnoses reflected the degree of certainty with which the diagnosis could be made (ie, definite, probable, or atypical). A definite diagnosis included subjects who clearly met all *DSM-III* diagnostic criteria; only definite diagnoses were used to determine rates of disorders. Rates of illness are reported as lifetime prevalences.

Analytic Approach

Statistical analyses were made between groups within each ascertainment site (MGH, inhibited vs not inhibited vs healthy controls; Harvard, inhibited vs uninhibited) without cross comparisons between the tow sites. For categorical data, pairwise comparisons between groups were made with Fisher's Exact Test (FET) unless otherwise specified. For continuous data, the nonparametric Kruskal-Wallis χ^2 (KWT) was used due to the distributional characteristics of the data. We had strong prior hypotheses about the plausible direction of departures from the null hypothesis for comparisons of anxiety disorders. Therefore, tests of statistical significance were one tailed for a priori hypotheses about anxiety disorders and two tailed for other analyses (all other disorders). For pairwise comparisons of disorders that were potentially confounded by age of SES, the Cochran-Mantel-Haenszel[32] measurement of general association was used to test pairwise comparisons of rates of disorders while controlling for potentially confounding third variables (age and SES). For these analyses, age was recoded into two categories based on a median split, and SES was recoded into three categories (SES $1 + 2 =$ high social class, SES $3 =$ middle social class, SES $4 + 5 =$ low social class). Results were called statistically significant ($P < .05$) or not statistically significant (NS).

RESULTS

MGH At-Risk Sample

No differences were seen in SES among inhibited, not inhibited, and healthy controls within the MGH ascertainment site (mean ± SD, 2.7 ± 1.4 vs 2.6 ± 1.1 vs 3.0 ± 0.8, respectively, by KWT; NS). However, age indicated statistically significant differences. Inhibited (mean ± SD = 5.9 ± 0.9 years) and not inhibited (4.9 ± 0.8 years) children were significantly younger than the healthy controls (7.8 ± 1.8 years) (P = .003 and .001, respectively), and children who were not inhibited were significantly younger than those who were (P = .02).

All evaluated disorders were higher in inhibited children than in the not-inhibited and healthy control children (Fig 1). Significant differences were detected in comparisons between inhibited children and the healthy controls in rates of four or more disorders per child (27.8% vs 0%, by FET, P = .02), two or more anxiety disorders per child (22.2% vs 0%, P = .04), and oppositional disorder (33.3% vs 5.0%, P = .04). Because of the differences in age, these analyses were repeated after statistically correcting for age and similar results were obtained (Cochran-Mantel-Haenszel test, P<.05). Although the rates in the not-inhibited and healthy control children were exactly the same for both four or more disorders (both 0%) and two or more anxiety disorders (both 0%) and were similar for oppositional disorder (8% and 5%, respectively), the comparisons between the inhibited and not-inhibited children failed to attain statistical significance, most likely due to the small numbers in these cells (Fig 1, at left). Although the rates of major depression (16.7% vs 0% vs 0%) and ADD (33.3% vs 16.7% vs 10.0%) were higher in inhibited children than in the not-inhibited children and healthy controls, these differences also failed to attain statistical significance.

Further examination of individual rates of anxiety disorders revealed that the rates of all evaluated anxiety disorders were higher in inhibited children than in the two comparison groups. However, statistical significance could only be established for overanxious disorder in comparisons between inhibited children and healthy controls (27.8% vs 0%, P = .02). This result remained statistically significant after controlling for age (CMH test, P<.05). In this analysis, again, although the rate of overanxious disorder was exactly the same in not-inhibited children (0%) as in the healthy controls, the comparison between the inhibited and not-inhibited children fell short of attaining statistical significance (P = .06). The rates of phobic disorders (11.1% vs 0% vs 0%), separation anxiety disorder (16.7% vs 8.3% vs 10%), and avoidant disorder (16.7% vs 0% vs 5%) were also higher in inhibited children than in not-inhibited children and healthy controls. However, these differences did not reach statistical significance (Fig 1, at right).

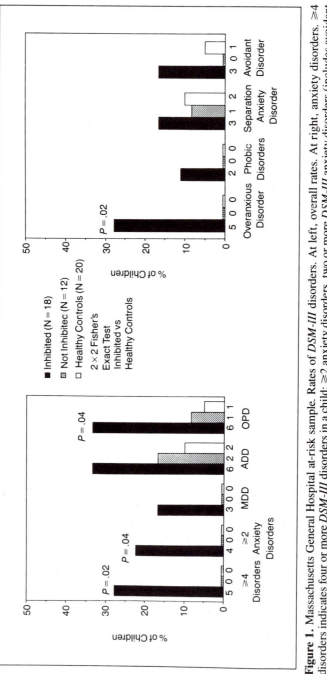
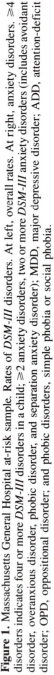

Figure 1. Massachusetts General Hospital at-risk sample. Rates of *DSM-III* disorders. At left, overall rates. At right, anxiety disorders. ≥4 disorders indicates four or more *DSM-III* disorders in a child; ≥2 anxiety disorders, two or more *DSM-III* anxiety disorders (includes avoidant disorder, overanxious disorder, phobic disorder, and separation anxiety disorder); MDD, major depressive disorder; ADD, attention-deficit disorder; OPD, oppositional disorder; and phobic disorders, simple phobia or social phobia.

Kagan et al Longitudinal Cohort

There were no differences in SES (mean ± SD = 1.8 ± 1.2 vs 2.1 ± 1.0, NS) or age (mean ± SD = 7.9 ± 0.2 years vs 8.0 ± 0.2 years, NS) between inhibited and uninhibited children within the ascertainment site of Kagan et al.

Although inhibited children had a substantially higher rate of two or more anxiety disorders (and of similar magnitude to that found in the MGH at-risk sample) when compared with uninhibited children, this difference fell short of attaining statistical significance (18.2% vs 0%, FET, P = .07). The rate of oppositional disorder, on the other hand, was significantly lower in inhibited children than in uninhibited children (0% vs 21.1%, P = .04). Although not statistically significant, the rate of four or more disorders was higher in inhibited than in uninhibited children (13.6% vs 10.5%), while the rates of major depression (0% vs 10.5%) and ADD (18.2% vs 31.6%) were lower (Fig 2, at left).

Examination of individual rates of anxiety disorders showed that also in this ascertainment site, the rates of all evaluated anxiety disorders were higher in inhibited children when compared with uninhibited children. However, statistical significance could only be established for phobic disorders (31.8% vs 5.3%, P = .04). Although more inhibited than uninhibited children had overanxious disorder (13.6% vs 10.5%), separation anxiety disorder (9.1% vs 5.3%), and avoidant disorder (9.1% vs 0%), these differences did not reach statistical significance (Fig 2, at right).

Exploratory Analyses

Since the structured interview used did not permit the assessment of adult-type anxiety disorders (ie, agoraphobia or social phobia), and to gain further understanding as to the characteristics of the phobic disorders, we examined the nature and frequency of the reported fears among the combined group of nine inhibited children who met the diagnostic criteria for a phobic disorder. The mean ± SD number of fears reported per child was 3.4 ± 2.1, with four children (44.4%) having five or more fears. The most frequently reported fears were fear of standing up and speaking in front of the class (N = 5, 55.5%), fear of animals or bugs (N = 5, 55.5%), fear of strangers (N = 4, 44.4%), fear of the dark (N = 4, 44.4%), fear of being called on in class (N = 3, 33.3%), fear of crowds (N = 3, 33.3%), fear of elevators (N = 2, 22.2%), and fear of physicians (N = 2, 22.2%).

COMMENT

This study investigated whether behavioral inhibition is associated with manifest anxiety syndromes in children, and if so, whether this association would be evident in the MGH high-risk sample (MGH at-risk group) and in the nonclinically derived

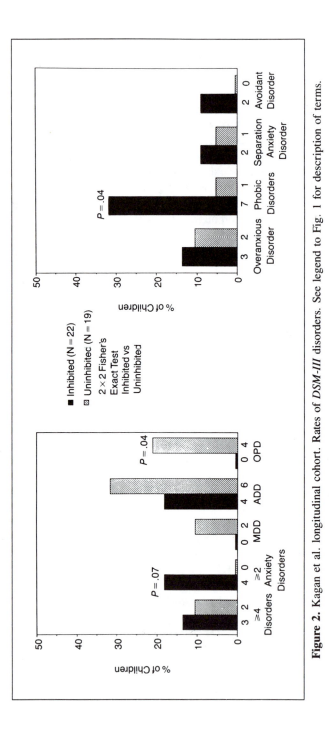

Figure 2. Kagan et al. longitudinal cohort. Rates of *DSM-III* disorders. See legend to Fig. 1 for description of terms.

longitudinal cohort followed by Kagan and colleagues (Kagan et al longitudinal cohort). Our findings indicate that inhibited children from both ascertainment sites had higher rates of multiple anxiety disorders (two or more anxiety disorders per child), accounted for by the high rate of over-anxious disorder (among MGH high-risk children) and phobic disorders (among the Kagan et al longitudinal cohort). These findings suggest an association between behavioral inhibition and childhood anxiety disorders. High rates of multiple anxiety disorders, thought to depict more severe or psychopathologic anxiety, were found only among inhibited children from both ascertainment sites (22.2% and 18.2%) and in none of the children from the other comparison groups.

The degree to which measurements of temperamental differences and psychopathology are distinct deserves attention; in particular, whether they represent different descriptions of the same phenomena or rest on concepts that are neither congruent nor tautological. Temperament and psychopathology are presumed to be different domains of human behavior. Temperament, conceptualized as a behavioral style, addresses the characteristic tempo, rhythmicity, and adaptability of behavior[33]; psychopathology, however, reflects abnormal behavior (symptoms) with associated distress and dysfunction. Moreover, the methods used in this study to assess temperament and psychopathology are dissimilar and without overlap. While the assessment and determination of behavioral inhibition was an objective laboratory-based observational assessment of the child's responses to an unfamiliar examiner and setting, the assessment of psychopathology was based on a criterion-based structured interview evaluating symptoms and behaviors of the child in the psychosocial domain. Moreover, not all inhibited children had anxiety disorders and vice versa, further indicating that behavioral inhibition and anxiety disorders are converging but not identical dimensions.

The assessment of psychopathology in the MGH at-risk children was retrospective, and the findings reflect lifetime rates of disorders. Thus, whether behavioral inhibition is a precursor of later psychopathology or simply another dimension of current or past psychopathology is unknown and requires further investigation. However, in the longitudinal cohort of Kagan et al, the assessment of psychopathology was done when the children were 7 to 8 years of age, while behavioral inhibition was first determined at 21 months, suggesting that this temperamental trait may precede the development of the anxiety disorders. Longitudinal follow-up of additional samples of young offspring of parents with anxiety disorders may help clarify the sequence of events from behavioral inhibition to manifest psychopathology.

The high rates of anxiety disorders found among inhibited children are consistent with school observations of inhibited children from the Kagan et al longitudinal cohort, who were observed to be more often shy, withdrawn, and restrained at the age of 5 years in their kindergarten classrooms compared with the uninhibited children.[19] School observations and teacher interviews suggest that approximately one third of these inhibited children already manifested symptoms of anxiety or social isolation at the age of 5 years. In many of these cases, the withdrawal from social contact was of sufficient intensity to interfere with everyday social functioning and the formation of peer relations, suggesting that children with behavioral inhibition may be at higher risk for school maladjustment, social dysfunction, and distress.

The high overall rates of anxiety disorders found in inhibited children from both ascertainment sites, even when restricted in this study to the presence of two or more disorders (multiple anxiety disorders) (Figs 1, at right, and 2, at right), is consistent with findings reported by several investigators in high-risk children of parents with panic disorder or agoraphobia.[34-36] The rate of separation anxiety disorder found in this study (16.7% and 9.1% in the MGH children and in the cohort of Kagan et al, respectively) was lower than rates reported by Weissman et al (37%)[34] in offspring of parents with major depression and panic disorder and by Turner et al (25%)[35] in high-risk children of parents with anxiety disorders. It is possible that this difference is due to methodologic differences between studies, particularly the much younger age of the children participating in our study compared with the other studies.

The MGH at-risk sample was largely derived from evaluations of offspring of parents with panic disorder and agoraphobia. In fact, 88% of children with behavioral inhibition were children with parents with panic disorder and agoraphobia (with or without comorbid MDD). Given that panic disorder and agoraphobia are familial illnesses,[21-26] our findings may be interpreted as suggesting that parental anxiety disorder confers a risk for a similar type of disorder in the child. However, a similarly high rate of two or more anxiety disorders was found in inhibited children from both the samples from the MGH (22%) and Kagan et al (18%). Since ascertainment of behavioral inhibition in the Kagan et al longitudinal cohort was not based on parental psychiatric illness, it is also possible to interpret our findings as suggesting that behavioral inhibition, or the tendency to exhibit excessive arousal in the face of novelty, presumed to underlie behavioral inhibition, may be a risk factor for childhood anxiety disorders or an added risk to parental psychopathology. This possibility could be evaluated by studying larger samples of children with and without behavioral inhibition whose parents do or do not have anxiety disorders.

Although no statistical comparisons were conducted between the two ascertainment sites (MGH and Harvard), it is of interest that inhibited children from the MGH at-risk site had higher rates of major depression and oppositional disorder than those of inhibited children from the ascertainment site of Kagan et al (Figs 1 and 2). These findings suggest that high rates of these disorders may be correlated with familial psychopathology and not with behavioral inhibition. The high rate of oppositional disorder among uninhibited children in the Kagan et al longitudinal cohort is not surprising, since these children were preselected as being particularly bold and outgoing.

Since the instrument used for ascertaining childhood psychopathology (Diagnostic Interview for Children and Adolescents-Parent Version) did not permit the evaluation of adult-type anxiety disorders, we do not know whether these children would have met diagnostic criteria for other anxiety disorders such as panic disorder, agoraphobia, or social phobia. However, many of the phobic children had fears resembling those of adult agoraphobics or social phobics (for example, fear of speaking in front of the class or being called on in class, fear of strangers, and fear of crowds), suggesting that they might have received the adult-type diagnoses had the instrument permitted such diagnoses. Since children can also develop adult-type anxiety disorders,[37] it will be important in future studies to use instruments capable of eliciting the full range of anxiety disorders to understand better the association between childhood and adult anxiety disorders.

The findings in this study should be viewed in light of their methodologic limitations. The two ascertainment samples were not symmetric. The MGH at-risk sample consisted of younger children from a generally lower social class background than the children from the Kagan et al ascertainment site. In addition, the definitions of the children without behavioral inhibition differed markedly between ascertainment sites. In the MGH at-risk group, the children did not meet study criteria for behavioral inhibition (not inhibited), while, in contrast, in the Kagan et al longitudinal cohort, they were selected for being uninhibited. However, similar definitions were used at both sites to characterize behavioral inhibition,[17] both groups of inhibited children were assessed and characterized by the same research team (Harvard Infant Study Laboratory) using similar protocols, and both groups had similar behavioral characteristics.

The assessment of psychopathology in the children was based on interviews with the mothers, which may have led to ascertainment bias and misrepresentation of psychopathology in the children. However, the same method was used to evaluate all groups of children. Some parents were known to have psychiatric disorders, and this may have affected the reported rates of childhood symptoms, since psychiatric patients may exaggerate symptoms in their children; or, alternatively, healthy mothers may have a tendency to underreport problem behaviors.[38] Nevertheless, high rates of anxiety disorders, similar to those found in the MGH at-risk sample, were found in the Kagan et al longitudinal cohort in which ascertainment of behavioral inhibition was not based on parental psychopathology.

While all children in the Kagan et al longitudinal cohort were 7 to 8 years of age, some children in the MGH at-risk sample were 4 to 6 years old. The assessment of psychopathology in children younger than 6 years may not be valid, since psychometric data are available for rating only children 6 years or older. However, we elected to include some children younger than 6 years, since the purpose of this pilot study was to obtain psychopathologic data on as many children as possible. Moreover, considering their younger age, the high lifetime rates of psychopathology found in the MGH at-risk sample are particularly striking, since these children are still within the age of risk for developing additional disorders.

Because of the multiple statistical comparisons performed, our findings may have been caused by chance. However, we had specific hypotheses on associations between behavioral inhibition and anxiety disorders. Because of the pilot nature of this study, we opted to present exploratory findings at the 5% level of significance without corrections for multiple comparisons.

Despite these limitations, the data suggest that behavioral inhibition to the unfamiliar, as defined in the previous work of Kagan and colleagues[12-15] and identified in children of agoraphobic parents,[20] may be one of multiple risk factors contributing to the development of preventive strategies. Longitudinal follow-up studies are needed to evaluate whether behavioral inhibition would be a risk factor for the development of anxiety disorders beyond childhood.

REFERENCES

1. Buss AH, Plomin R. *A Temperament Theory of Personality Development*. New York, NY: John Wiley & Sons Inc; 1975.
2. Bronson GW, Pankey. On the distinction between fear and wariness. *Child Dev.* 1977;48:1167–1187.
3. Carey WB, McDevitt SC. Stability and change in individual temperament diagnoses from infancy to early childhood. *J Am Acad Child Psychiatry.* 1978;17:331–337.
4. Hinde RA, Stevenson-Hinde J, Tamplin A. Characteristics of three-to-four year olds assessed at home and their interactions in preschool. *Dev Psychol.* 1985;21:130–140.
5. Plomin R, Rowe DC. Genetic and environmental etiology of social behavior in infancy. *Dev Psychol.* 1979;15:62–72.
6. Garcia-Coll C, Kagan J, Reznick JS. Behavioral inhibition in young children. *Child Dev.* 1984;55:1005–1019.
7. Goldsmith HH, Gottesman II. Origins of variation in behavioral style: a longitudinal study of temperament in young twins. *Child Dev.* 1981;52:91–103.
8. Goldsmith HH. Genetic influences on personality from infancy to adulthood. *Child Dev.* 1983;54:331–355.
9. Daniels D, Plomin R. Origins of individual differences in infant shyness. *Dev Psychol.* 1985;21:118–121.
10. Thomas A, Chess S. *Temperament and Development*. New York, NY: Brunner/Mazel Inc; 1977.
11. Thomas A, Chess S. Genesis and evolution of behavioral disorders: from infancy to early adult life. *Am J Psychiatry.* 1984;141:1–9.
12. Kagan J, Reznick JS, Snidman N. Biological bases of childhood shyness. *Science.* 1988;240:167–171.
13. Reznick JS, Kagan J, Snidman N, Gersten M, Baak K, Rosenberg A. Inhibited and uninhibited children: a follow-up study. *Child Dev.* 1986;51:660–680.

14. Kagan J, Reznick JS, Snidman, N. The physiology and psychology of behavioral inhibition in children. *Child Dev.* 1987;58:1459–1473.

15. Kagan J, Reznick JS, Snidman N, Gibbons J, Johnson MO. Childhood derivatives of inhibition and lack of inhibition to the unfamiliar. *Child Dev.* 1988;59:1580–1589.

16. Chess S, Thomas A. Temperamental individuality from childhood to adolescence. *J Am Acad Child Psychiatry.* 1977;16:218–226.

17. Chess S, Thomas A. *Origins and Evolution of Behavior Disorders.* New York, NY:Brunner/Mazel Inc.; 1984.

18. Carey WB, Fox M, McDevitt SC. Temperament as a factor in early school adjustment. *Pediatrics.* 1977;60:621–624.

19. Gersten M. *The Contribution of Temperament to Behavior in Natural Contexts.* Cambridge, Mass: Harvard Graduate School of Education; 1986. Doctoral dissertation.

20. Rosenbaum JF, Biederman J, Gersten M, Hirshfeld DR, Meminger SR, Herman JB, Kagan J, Reznick JS, Snidman N. Behavioral inhibition in children of parents with panic disorder and agoraphobia: a controlled study. *Arch Gen Psychiatry.* 1988;45:463–470.

21. Crowe RR, Noyes R, Pauls DL, Slymen D. A family study of panic disorder. *Arch Gen Psychiatry.* 1983;40:1065–1069.

22. Harris EL, Noyes R, Crowe RR, Chaudhry DR. Family study of agoraphobia. *Arch Gen Psychiatry.* 1983;40:1061–1064.

23. Crowe RR, Pauls DL, Slymen DJ, Noyes R. A family study of anxiety neurosis: morbidity risk in family of patients with and without mitral valve prolapse. *Arch Gen Psychiatry.* 1980;37:77–79.

24. Crowe RR. The genetics of panic disorder and agoraphobia. *Psychiatric Dev.* 1985;2:171–186.

25. Moran C, Andrews G. The familial occurrence of agoraphobia. *Br J Psychiatry.* 1985;146:262–267.

26. Torgeson S. Genetic factors in anxiety disorders. *Arch Gen Psychiatry.* 1983;40:1085–1089.

27. Kagan J, Reznick JS, Snidman N, Johnson MO, Gibbons J, Gersten M, Biederman J, Rosenbaum J. Origins of panic disorder. In Ballenger J, ed. *Clinical Aspects of Panic Disorder.* New York, NY: Alan R Liss Inc. In press.

28. Herjanic B, Reich W. Development of a structured psychiatric interview for children: agreement between child and parent. *J Abnorm Child Psychol.* 1982;10:307–324.

29. Orvaschel H, Sholomskas D, Weissman MM. Review of psychiatric interviews. In: Orvaschel H, Sholomskas D, Weissman MM, eds. *The Assessment of Psychopathology and Behavioral Problems in Children: A Review of Scales Suitable for Epidemiological and Clinical Research (1967-1979).* In: Mental Health Service System Reports series. Rockville, Md: US Dept of Health and Human Services, National Institute of Mental Health, Division of Biometry and Epidemiology; 1983:83–1037.

30. Orvaschel H. Psychiatric interviews suitable for use in research with children and adolescents. *Psychopharmacol Bull.* 1985;21:737–745.

31. Leckman JF, Sholomskas D, Thompson D, Belanger A, Weissman MM. Best estimate

of lifetime psychiatric diagnosis: a methodological study. *Arch Gen Psychiatry.* 1982;39:879–883.

32. Landis RJ, Heyman ER, Koch GG. Average partial association in three-way contingency tables: a review and discussion of alternative tests. *Int Stat Rev.* 1978;46:237–254.

33. Chess S, Hassibi M. Genesis and etiology. In: Chess S, Hassibi M, eds. *Principles and Practice of Child Psychiatry.* New York NY: Plenum Press; 1978:89–99.

34. Weissman MM, Leckman JF, Merikangas KR, Gammon GD, Prusoff BA. Depression and anxiety disorders in parents and children: results from the Yale family study. *Arch Gen Psychiatry.* 1984;41:845–852.

35. Turner SM, Beidel DC, Costello A. Psychopathology in the offspring of anxiety disorders patients. *J Consult Clin Psychol.* 1987;55:229–235.

36. Sylvester CE, Hyde TS, Reichler RJ. The Diagnostic Interview for Children and Personality Inventory for Children in studies of children at risk for anxiety disorders or depression. *J Am Acad Child Adolesc Psychiatry.* 1987;26:668–675.

37. Biederman J. Clonazepam in the treatment of prepubertal children with panic-like symptoms. *J Clin Psychiatry.* 1987;48(suppl):38–41.

38. John K, Gammon GD, Prusoff BA, Warner V. The Social Adjustment Inventory for Children and Adolescents (SAICA): testing of a new semistructured interview. *J Am Acad Child Adolesc Psychiatry.* 1987;26:898–911.

15

Temperament, Stress and Family Factors in Behavioural Adjustment of Three- Five-Year-Old Children

Michael Kyrios and Margot Prior

La Trobe University, Bundoora, Australia

In a longitudinal study, various aspects of the pre-schooler and his/her environment were assessed to delineate those factors most predictive of behavioural adjustment at 3–4 years of age, and again 12 months later. Factor analysis and a series of backwards stepwise multiple regression analyses facilitated the selection of variables to be included in a causal model. Path analysis suggested that temperamental characteristics were most strongly causally related to children's overall behavioural adjustment, and could protect children from the effects of maladjustment in the parental subsystem. According to the path model, the direct effect of parental maladjustment on pre-schoolers' behavioural adjustment was outweighed by its indirect effects, particularly at follow-up. The potential contaminating influence of parental maladjustment on their perceptions of children's temperament and behaviour, as well as the content and construct overlap between temperament and behavioural measures, was considered.

INTRODUCTION

Pre-school behavioural dysfunction is quite common (Earls, 1980; McFarlane, Allen, & Honzik, 1954; McGuire & Richman, 1986; Stevenson, & Graham, 1975, 1982), although prevalence estimates differ as a function of researchers' theoretical and methodological framework. Rates of around 15%–20% for general adjustment problems are typical of many epidemiological studies of pre-schoolers (Earls, 1980;

Reprinted with permission from *International Journal of Behavioral Development*, 1990, Vol. 13, No. 1, 67–93. Copyright © 1990 by The International Society for the Study of Behavioral Development.

This research was supported in part by grants from the National Health and Medical Research Council and the Royal Children's Hospital Research Fund.

Jenkins, Bart, & Hart, 1980; Richman et al., 1975), with boys generally reported to exhibit a higher prevalence in the areas of aggression, overactivity, and impulse control, particularly at day care or pre-school facilities (Crowther, Bond, & Rolf, 1981; McGuire & Richman, 1986). Longitudinal studies generally report that about 40%–50% of samples continue to exhibit some form of dysfunction over 2–5 year follow-up periods from around 3 years of age (Campbell, Ewing, Breaux, & Szumowski, 1986; Chazan & Jackson, 1974; Garrison & Earls, 1985; Richman et al., 1982). The research literature has been less conclusive on longer-term outcomes (Kohlberg, Ricks, & Snarey, 1984); however, a recent paper concluded that pre-schoolers exhibiting significant behavioural dysfunction were at least twice as likely to develop specific adult psychiatric disorders (Lerner, Inui, Trupin, & Douglas, 1985). Hence, it is not surprising to find clinical interest in the development of intervention and prevention programmes for pre-schoolers exhibiting problems in behavioural adjustment. However, to develop such programmes one needs to be aware of those variables which influence the development and maintenance of pre-school behavioural dysfunction.

The construct of "stress" is often related to the development of negative behavioural outcomes in children. Parent-rated indices of child, family, and social "stress" have been found consistently to be associated with increased risk for the development of both health and adjustment problems in children (Barron & Earls, 1984; Beautrais, Ferguson, & Shannon, 1982a,b; Coddington, 1972b; Earls, 1980; Heisel, Ream, Raitz, Rappoport, & Coddington, 1973; Johnson, 1982). Family and social stressors include: (1) problems in the parental subsystem such as marital dysfunction (Belsky, 1984; Emery, 1982; Goldberg & Easterbrooks, 1984; Johnson & Lobitz, 1974; Porter & O'Leary, 1980) and poor parental psychological functioning (Baldwin, Cole, & Baldwin, 1982; Billings & Moos, 1983; Ghodsian, Zajicek, & Wolkind, 1984; Panaccione, & Wahler, 1986; Seifer, Sameroff, & Jones, 1981); (2) problems in aspects of parent-child interactions and in particular, inadequate child-rearing practices (Anderson, Lytton, & Romney, 1986; Baumrind, 1967; Belsky, 1984; Dielman & Cattell, 1972; Dielman, Cattell, & Rhoades, 1972; Hinde & Tamplin, 1983; Susman, Trickett, Iannotti, Hollenbeck, & Zahn-Walker, 1985); (3) low social status or social disadvantage (Rutter, 1979); and (4) negative life events such as unemployment (Madge, 1983), or loss of a parent through death or divorce (Brown, Harris, & Bifulco, 1985; Hetherington, 1980; Wallerstein & Kelly, 1980). Rutter (1979) has indicated the multiplicative effect of stressors on each other and the disproportionate rise in risk associated with the presence of two or more stressors.

Individual contextual characteristics such as adequate social supports, satisfactory relationships, and adequate child-rearing practices have been found to mediate the effects of stress (Rutter, 1985). For instance, while children of a depressed parent have significantly more emotional, somatic, and behavioural problems than children of a non-depressed parent, the general family environment has been found to mediate the effects of parental depression on child adjustment (Billings & Moos, 1983). Parental depression has also been found to influence child-rearing practices (Susman et al., 1985), as has marital quality. In fact a major path of influence on children's behavioural development may be from marital quality, to parenting quality, to child outcomes (Goldberg & Easterbrooks, 1984).

Child characteristics such as sex, temperament, and competence may mediate the effects of environmental stressors such as marital discord (Garmezy, Master, & Tellegen, 1984; Porter & O'Leary, 1980; Rutter, 1979). Children who exhibit social and interpersonal competence and high intelligence have been found to overcome the effects of a stressed family and social environment (Garmezy et al., 1984). In particular, the concept of temperament has been proposed as a possible explanation of individual differences in susceptibility to stress.

Most researchers would agree that temperamental characteristics have a constitutional basis, and exhibit stability over time relative to other aspects of behaviour (Goldsmith et al., 1987; Goldsmith & Rieser-Danner, 1986). Certain temperamental characteristics have been associated with the development of adjustment problems (Barron & Earls, 1984; Cameron, 1978; Earls, 1981; Terestman, 1980; Thomas & Chess, 1977; Werner & Smith, 1982). Of particular relevance has been the concept of "difficult temperament", although there has been much debate concerning its definition, operationalisation, and measurement (Bates, 1980, 1983; Kagan, 1982; Plomin, 1982; Rothbart, 1982; Thomas, 1982; Thomas, Chess, & Korn, 1982).

In seeking to explain the influence of temperament and behavioural development, Thomas & Chess (1977) and Lerner (1983, 1984; Lerner & Lerner, 1983) have emphasised an interactionist approach with their "goodness of fit" model focusing on the degree of consonance or dissonance between children's temperamental characteristics and environmental contingencies. On the other hand, while acknowledging the potential influence of the environment on temperamental features, neo-Pavlovian conceptions of temperament focus on the psychobiological mechanisms underlying the individual's reactions to environmental demands (Strelau, 1983a, 1983b). This less interactionist approach is concordant with concepts of "stress resilience" which imply that certain individual characteristics can "protect" the individual from the influence of adverse environmental conditions. Temperament can influence the quality of interactions between the individual's reactions to the prevailing environment (Rutter, 1985).

However, such theoretical positions have been difficult to examine. While most researchers use parental reports of children's temperament, usually in the form of questionnaires or interviews, such reports have not been found to be independent or subjective factors such as parental personality and symptomatology, social class, or ethnicity (Bates & Bayles, 1984; Prior, Sanson, Carroll, & Oberklaid, 1989;

Prior, Kyrios, & Oberklaid, 1986; Sameroff, Seifer, & Elias, 1982; Vaughn, Bradley, Joffe, Seifer, & Barglow, 1987; Ventura & Stevens, 1986; Zeanah, Keener, & Anders, 1986). Although numerous studies have supported the relationship between measures of temperament and childhood behavioural outcomes (Barron & Earls, 1984; Cameron, 1978; Earls, 1981; Graham, Rutter, & George, 1973; Olweus, 1980; Terestman, 1980; Thomas & Chess, 1977, 1984), these results perhaps need to be interpreted with caution as temperament measures are probably not simply measures of constitutional temperament (Bates & Bayles, 1984; Crockenberg & Acredolo, 1983), but reflect behavioural style in the social context (Rothbart, 1981). Furthermore, few studies have examined the relationship of temperament and behavioural adjustment controlling for potentially influential factors such as parental psychological functioning and social class.

Many research limitations are related to the fact that, until recently, many studies of early childhood behavioural adjustment have been univariate in nature with little regard for the development of appropriate theoretical models to increase our understanding of dynamic developmental processes. However, the study of interactional processes and causal models has been greatly enhanced by the application of multivariate analytical techniques. For instance, Barron & Earls (1984) used path analysis to investigate a model that delineated the relationships between family stress, parent-child interactions, temperamental inflexibility, and pre-school behavioural adjustment. They concluded tentatively that temperamental flexibility and positive parent-child interactions could curtail the overall effect of high family stress on children's behavioural adjustment. However, such models are neither specific nor inclusive enough with regard to the possible range of environmental and child-related developmental influences.

The aim of this study was to construct and test a model containing a range of environmental and child factors hypothesised as influencing the development of pre-school behavioural dysfunction with a particular focus on temperament factors. A preliminary theoretical causal model for the behavioural adjustment of 3–5-year-old children suggested that adjustment in the parental subsystem (including personal and marital adjustment), child-rearing practices, temperament, childhood stressful life events, and developmental or ability measures (e.g. language abilities, developmental history, and motor coordination) would relate directly to pre-school children's behavioural adjustment, both concurrently and prospectively (see Fig. 1). The influence of temperament was considered through a "stress resistance" or "reactivity" perspective, where individual characteristics can affect reactions to a stressed environment. While temperament can exert a causal influence on behavioural adjustment, and while an individual's temperament may define what is stressful for that individual, the environment may itself exert a causal influence on the manifestation of temperament.

A number of paths of influence were expected to be salient: (1) from parental adjustment through child-rearing practices to childhood adjustment; (2) from parental adjustment through child-rearing practices to temperament and then through to childhood adjustment; (3) from parental adjustment through temperament to childhood adjustments; (4) from both child stress and health history to parental adjustment; (5) from developmental and ability measures through child-rearing practices to childhood adjustment.

As a wide range of environmental and child variables were assessed, data simplification techniques were used to develop a more parsimonious model, the implications of which were tested using path analysis based on least-squares methods (Blalock, 1971; Duncan, 1966; Kenny, 1979; Nie et al., 1975). While recent analytic advances (e.g. LISREL; see Joreskog & Sorbom, 1984) may be more powerful tools than ordinary least-squares regression techniques, their use is associated with additional restrictive assumptions about data (Biddle & Marlin, 1987). For this reason, many experts suggest the use of ordinary least-squares over maximum-likelihood methods, at least as a first step in the development of plausible causal models (Biddle & Marlin, 1987).

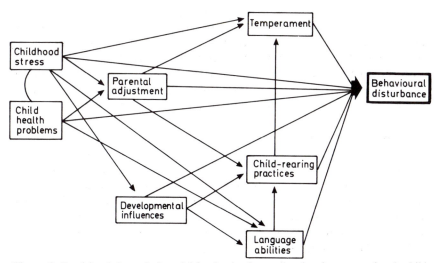

Figure 1. Provisional theoretical model for the development and maintenance of early childhood behavioural disturbance

METHOD

Subjects

Subjects were recruited through the Australian Temperament Project (ATP; see Oberklaid et al., 1984; Prior, Sanson, Oberklaid, & Northam, 1987). In Phase I, 120 mothers were interviewed about their child's behaviour and development, and completed questionnaires about various aspects of the child's environment. Environmental data, as rated by fathers, was also available for 109 subjects. In Phase II, one year later, mothers completed a further questionnaire on their children's current behavioural adjustment. Of the 112 children still available by Phase II, 102 attended a facility such as a kindergarten or family day-care centre, and a similar behavioural questionnaire was completed by the caretaker or pre-school teacher.

Mean age for the 120 children was 3 years 8 months (SD = 6.0 months), ranging from 34 to 50 months. Mean maternal age was 32.4 years (ranging from 22 to 44 years), while mean paternal age was 35.6 years (ranging from between 26 and 58 years). Of the 120 pre-schoolers, 49% were male, 47% were first-born, most were living with both biological parents (95%), and 96% of the parents were married. The remainder were living in households where parents were divorced, widowed, or living together. The number of people living in the household ranged from three to eight, with a median of four people.

Socioeconomic status (SES) was rated using an adaptation of Australian scales by Broom, Jones, & Zubrzycki (1976) for parental occupational status and educational attainment. Occupational status was rated on a 6-point scale, while highest educational attainment was rated on a 7-point scale. An index of SES was calculated by summing ratings for maternal and paternal education and occupation (alpha coefficient for SES index = 0.77) with higher scores indicating low SES. The distribution of occupational ratings were skewed towards the upper SES levels, with an underrepresentation of lower status occupations, particularly for mothers (see Table 1). However, educational attainment was evenly represented at all levels.

Measures and Procedures

Participation in the study involved structured interviews and administration of a word knowledge test in the subject's home and the completion of a number of questionnaires. Mothers constituted the major source of information about child characteristics, although a number of interviewer and teacher/caretaker ratings were included. Environmental information was gathered from mothers and, where possible, fathers. The measures used are summarised in Table 2.

Phase I. (i) The major outcome measure used in Phase I was the Behaviour screening questionnaire (BSQ; Richman & Graham, 1971) which assesses a range of behaviours via interviewer ratings of mothers' reports in a structured clinical interview. Behaviours assessed by the BSQ include: eating, sleeping, and toileting patterns; dependency; sibling and peer relations; worries; fears; tantrums; overactivity; concentration; mood; and ease of management. Ratings range from 1 to 3 on each of the 12 behavioural items depending on frequency and severity of symptoms. Interrater reliability coefficients for five different pairs of interviewers on the BSQ ranged from 0.89 to 0.98.

Validity checks on the BSQ, via maternal ratings on the Behaviour checklist (BCL; Richman, 1977) and teacher ratings on the Preschool behaviour questionnaire (PBQ; Behar & Stringfield, 1974), showed high agreement between concurrent BCL and BSQ ($r = 0.71$, $P < 0.01$), moderate agreement between BCL and BSQ separated by 6–12-month periods ($r = 0.48$, $P < 0.01$), and no significant agreement between concurrent PBQ and BSQ ($r = 0.15$, $n = 41$, n.s.).

(ii) From interviewer ratings of maternal reports, a number of indices were developed and alpha coefficients were calculated as a measure of internal consistency. Children's developmental milestones ($\alpha = 0.60$) assessed the age at which children first reached a number of developmental milestones such as walking unassisted, saying their first recognisable words, and being toilet trained; Children's level of motor coordination ($\alpha = 0.71$) comprised mother and interviewer ratings of children's fine and gross motor coordination; Children's health history ($\alpha = 0.73$) assessed children's health over the past year and the existence of chronic health problems;

TABLE 1
Subjects' Social Background Characteristics at Time of Phase I

1. Parental occupation:		
	Mothers' (%)	*Fathers'* (%)
Professional	30	29
Managerial: Proprietors	6	16
Clerical	45	27
Craftsmen; Foremen	8	21
Shop Assistants; Drivers	6	5
Rural Workers; Labourers	3	1
2. Parental education:		
	Mothers' (%)	*Fathers'* (%)
Some Tertiary, Graduate	23.7	31.9
Late Secondary, Technical	38.9	35.4
Early Secondary, Primary	37.3	32.8
3. Index of SES: Mean	12.48	
S.D.	4.41	
Range	4–23	

Children's attendance at a facility ($\alpha = 0.63$) assessed the intensity of current facility attendance and the length of time children had been attending a facility; Fathers' employment stability and status ($\alpha = 0.66$ and Mothers' employment stability and status ($\alpha = 0.84$) assessed current and past parental employment status, and the sta-

TABLE 2
Summary List of Instruments Used, Variables Measured, and Raters

Child variables	Instrument	Rater
1. Preschool Behavioural Adjustment	Behaviour screening questionnaire (BSQ) (Richman & Graham, 1971)	Mother reports, interviewer ratings
	Behaviour checklist (BCL) (Richman & Graham, 1971)	Mother
	Preschool behaviour questionaire (PBQ) (Behar & Stringfield, 1974)	Mother or teacher
2. Development history		
3. Fine and gross motor coordination	Structured interview	Mother reports, interviewer ratings
4. Health history		
5. Facility attendance		
6. Temperament	Short temperament scale for toddlers (STST)	Mother
7. Word knowledge	Peabody picture vocabulary test (PPVT) (Dùnn & Dunn, 1981)	Interviewer
8. Life events and stress	Life events schedule for preschoolers (CLER) (Coddington, 1972)	Mother, Father

Environmental variables	Instrument	Rater
1. Marital adjustment	Spanier dyadic adjustment scale (SDAS) (Spanier, 1976)	Mother, Father
2. Parental psychological functioning	General health questionnaire (GHQ) (Goldberg, 1978)	Mother, Father
3. Child-rearing practices	Child rearing practices questionnaire (CRPQ) (Barton, 1981)	Mother, Father
4. Parental employment	Structured interview	Mother reports, interviewer ratings
5. Social status		Interviewer ratings

bility of employment. Interrater reliability coefficients on the structured interview for the five pairs of interviewers ranged from 0.7 to 0.99.

(iii) After the structured interviews, the Peabody picture vocabulary test (PPVT; Dunn & Dunn, 1981) was administered to children in order to obtain a measure of verbal intelligence.

(iv) Two independent sets of questionnaires required individual completion by mothers and, where appropriate, fathers:

1. Total marital adjustment was measured with the Spanier dyadic adjustment scale (SDAS; Spanier, 1976), a 32-item self-administered questionnaire for which Australian normative data is available (Antill & Cotton, 1982). Alpha coefficients for the total adjustment score have been reported as ranging between 0.90 and 0.92 for various cohorts, while factor analysis has supported Spanier's (1976) original factor structure for the scale (Antill & Cotton, 1982).

2. The level of parental psychological functioning was assessed with the 28-item General health questionnaire (GHQ; Goldberg, 1978), a self-administered questionnaire based on factor analytic studies of the 60-item GHQ (see Goldberg & Hillier, 1979). Goldberg (1978) indicated high correlation (0.76) between GHQ total score and overall clinical assessment based on psychiatric interview.

3. The 60-item short version of the Child-rearing practices questionnaire (CRPQ; Barton, 1981) was used to assess child-rearing attitudes and practices. The CRPQ was developed from a factor analytic study of mothers' and fathers' ratings on a longer questionnaire based on the work of Sears, Maccoby, & Levin (1957), and is appropriate for use with both parents. Barton (1984) (Note 1) reported test–retest reliabilities ranging from 0.55 to 0.96. Pretesting had suggested that four CRPQ child-rearing dimensions were most appropriate for use with Australian parents: Use of rewards, Encouragement of independence, Use of rules and regulations, Use of punishment.

4. Childhood stress was assessed with the Coddington life events record (CLER; Coddington, 1972a, 1972b) completed by parents. This is a 30-item checklist of negative life events appropriate for use with pre-schoolers, and is based on the Holmes and Rahe (1967) stress scale. Each life event is associated with a standardised life stress score and the sum of life stress scores indicates the level of stress experienced over the past year. The CLER has acquired much evidence for its validity as a child stress measure (see Johnson, 1982), and is the only widely used stress scale that assesses negative life events as they effect the pre-school child.

5. A concurrent measure of temperament was obtained through a Short temperament scale for toddlers (STST; Prior, Sanson, & Oberklaid, in press). The STST consists of 30 items and measures 7 temperament factors (approach–

adaptability, irritability, persistence, rhythmicity, cooperation–manageability, distractibility–soothability, and activity–intensity). Alpha coefficients for the STST factors range from 0.56 to 0.85, with an overall test–retest reliability coefficient of 0.86 over an average 3.5-week period.

Phase II. The major outcome measure for the follow-up study was the PBQ (Behar & Stringfield, 1974), teacher (TPBQ and parent (MPBQ) versions), a 30-item questionnaire which yields a total score reflecting overall level of adjustment, as well as three subscale scores termed hostility–aggression, anxiety–fear, and hyperactivity–distractibility. The content of the PBQ and the Phase I BSQ was similar, and both was based on symptom-loading approaches (Links, 1983) to the measurement of behavioural adjustment. Sanson, Prior, Kyrios, & Oberklaid (1988) report alpha coefficients from Australian data ranging from 0.73 to 0.88 for the teacher version, and 0.69 to 0.84 for the parent version.

RESULTS

Data Reduction

Factor analyses were used as the major data reduction method to assist in the formulation of more specific causal models which would then be examined through path analyses (see Crano & Mendoza, 1987). As child and environmental data sets were thought to differ from a theoretical perspective, their respective factor structures were considered separately via oblique principal components factor analyses using the Kaiser normalisation method. The use of oblique factoring, rather than orthogonal, is considered preferable if interrelationships are required between the various emerging factors (Gorsuch, 1974), a desirable situation in light of the proposed path analysis which requires weak causal relations amongst variables.

Six factors emerged for the child data accounting for 65% of the variance, and five for the environmental data accounting for 57% of the variance (see Tables 3a, 3b). These were termed: (1) temperamental reactivity-low manageability—high scores characterised an unmanageable, irritable, highly active, and intense child temperament; (2) child stress and health problems—high scores indicated stressful life events and many health problems; (3) poor coordination-low approach—high scores were consistent with poorly developed motor coordination as rated by the mother and interviewer, and a non-approaching, non-adaptable child temperament; (4) temperamental self regulation—low scores signified an easily soothable, persistent, and regular child temperament; (5) word knowledge—high scores indicated high verbal intelligence; and (6) high rate of development—low scores were characteristic of late development, and a high intensity or long-standing attendance at a pre-school facility.

TABLE 3a
Factor Structure Matrix for Child Data ($N = 120$)

	I	II	III	IV	V	VI
High irritability (STST)	74	16	17	17	−10	−33
High activity–intensity (STST)	71	−05	−11	12	−03	−05
Low cooperation–manageability (STST)	65	17	09	38	33	−44
High stress (Mother CLER)	−04	87	−02	08	−03	00
High stress (Father CLER)	10	83	09	06	06	06
Poor health history (Int)	08	56	−24	−10	−05	−51
Poor coordination (Int)	−07	05	75	11	−14	−15
Low approach–low adaptability (STST)	45	01	63	−21	12	06
High distractibility (STST)	08	−17	17	71	−21	20
Low rhythmicity (STST)	16	19	−23	67	18	−06
Low persistence (STST)	28	22	16	60	24	−41
Word knowledge (PPVT)	−04	−05	−07	01	89	07
Poor developmental history (Int)	19	−05	09	01	−05	−73
High facility attendance (Int)	22	08	40	07	26	−48
Eigen value	2.54	1.77	1.39	1.17	1.14	1.03
% variance	18.1	12.7	9.9	8.4	8.2	7.3
Cumulative % variance	18.1	30.8	40.7	49.1	57.3	64.6

TABLE 3b
Factor Structure Matrix for Environmental Data

	I	II	III	IV	V
Mother marital adjustment (SDAS)	−80	03	13	−02	−07
Father marital adjustment (SDAS)	−79	00	21	03	10
Poor mother wellbeing (GHQ)	68	19	06	−06	13
Poor father wellbeing (GHQ)	67	15	−25	04	39
Father use of punishment (CRPQ)	25	72	01	−16	17
Mother use of punishment (CRPQ)	23	72	−23	06	04
Index of SES (Int)	−12	59	−07	−11	01
Mother use of rewards (CRPQ)	−10	−10	83	02	−11
Father use of rewards (CRPQ)	−14	−09	82	−05	03
Mother use of independence (CRPQ)	−05	07	07	−70	−08
Mother use of rules (CRPQ)	01	48	05	−66	−19
Father use of independence (CRPQ)	13	−24	−14	−63	27
Rather use of rules (CRPQ)	00	44	22	−55	−18
Mother employment history (Int)	03	06	04	06	77
Father employment history (Int)	22	03	−11	−03	64
Eigen value	2.71	2.03	1.47	1.28	1.13
% variance	18.1	13.5	9.8	8.5	7.5
Cumulative % variance	18.1	31.6	41.4	49.9	57.4

The five environmental factors were termed: (1) maladjustment in the parental subsystem—high scores indicated marital problems and a high degree of symptomatology in the mother and father; (2) high use of punishment in child-rearing—high scores were consistent with a high use of punishment by mother and father, and of low SES; (3) high use of rewards in child-rearing—high scores signified the high use of rewards by the mother and father; (4) encouragement of child autonomy and use of structure in child-rearing—high scores were indicative of parents who use rules and regulations in child-rearing, while encouraging age-appropriate independence in their child; and (5) parental employment status—high scores related to unstable employment history in mothers and fathers, and early re-employment in mothers after the child's birth.

Factor scales were constructed using only those factor loadings greater than equal to 0.40. Where cross-loadings occurred, variables were included in those factor scales on to which they loaded most highly. Correlations between factor scores and factor scales ranged between 0.84 and 0.98 with a mean of 0.92. In addition, as environmental factors include loadings from both mothers and fathers, it was necessary to exclude from all analyses using factor scales those subjects for whom father data was not available. While this would exclude from analyses those subjects in one-parent families, or those families with fathers who did not complete questionnaires, it was not thought appropriate for the factor scale computations to use the usual mean substitution methods that deal with missing data.

Correlational Analysis: Phases I & II

Correlational analysis of the eleven factors with the three major behavioural measures are presented in Table 4. General behavioural dysfunction at 3–4 years of age correlated significantly ($P < .01$) with measures of parental maladjustment, temperamental high reactivity–low manageability, and low temperamental self-regulation. General behavioural maladjustment at 4–5 years of age as rated by mothers again correlated significantly with parental maladjustment, high use of punishment, high reactivity–low manageability, and behavioural maladjustment at 3–4 years of age. Behavioural maladjustment at 4–5 years of age as rated by teachers did not correlate significantly with any of the predictors although there were some trends (with poor coordination-low approach, use of punishment, and reactivity—low manageability. Significant agreement between mothers and teachers on ratings of children's overall behavioural adjustment at age 4–5 years was found only for boys ($r = 0.38$, $P < 0.01$), although there was some mother–teacher congruence for the total sample on anxiety–fear and hyperactivity–distractibility scales of the PBQ ($r = 0.33$, $P < 0.01$ and $r = 0.73$, $P < 0.01$, respectively).

Sex Differences

No significant sex differences were found on the behavioural measures, nor on factor scales. Correlational analyses were repeated separately for boys and girls. Table 5 presents the results of these analyses, including results of tests of significance for differences between correlations and for the two sexes. For boys, total BSQ score correlated significantly ($P < 0.01$) only with reactivity–low manageability. For girls, total BSQ score correlated significantly with parental maladjustment, low use of rewards, reactivity–low manageability, and low self-regulation. However, significant differences were found between boys and girls only for correlations between total BSQ score and both high use of punishment and child stress and health problems.

The analyses were repeated for total MPBQ score. For boys, total MPBQ score correlated significantly only with reactivity–low manageability. For girls, total MPBQ score correlated significantly with parental maladjustment, high use of punishment, and reactivity–low manageability. Significant differences between correlations were found only for high use of rewards and self-regulation. No significant correlations were found between total TPBQ score and factor scales, for either boys

TABLE 4

Pearson Correlations: Behavioural Outcomes with Child and Environmental Factor Scales

Age of child 3–4 Years *Factor Scale*	*3–4 Years* *Total BSQ*	*4–5 Years* *Total MPBQ*	*4–5 Years* *Total TPBQ*
Parental maladjustment	0.35[c]	0.29[c]	−0.08
High use of punishment	0.10	0.28[b]	0.19
High use of rewards	−0.21[a]	0.06	0.03
Child structure and autonomy	−0.02	−0.13	−0.09
Parental employment history	0.00	0.13	−0.14
Reactivity–low manageability	0.40[c]	0.55[c]	0.17
Child stress/health problems	0.16	0.05	−0.09
Poor coordination–low approach	0.17	0.10	0.20
Low self-regulation	0.42[c]	0.14	−0.15
Word knowledge	0.00	0.04	−0.04
High rate of development	−0.19	0.08	−0.11
Sex	−0.01	−0.02	−0.16
Total BSQ score	—	0.39[c]	0.11

Two-tailed tests of significance.
[a] $P < 0.02$ (N.S.).
[b] $P < 0.01$.
[c] $P < 0.001$.

TABLE 5

Pearson Correlations Separately for Boys and Girls: Behavioural Outcomes with Child and Environmental Factors (Includes Test of Significance for Differences Between Correlation)

Age of child Factor scale	3–4 Years Total BSQ			4–5 Years Total MPBQ			4–5 Years Total TPBQ		
	Boys	Girls	Diff[c]	Boys	Girls	Diff[c]	Boys	Girls	Diff[c]
Parental maladjustment	24	42[a]	−1.02	24	35[a]	−0.59	−13	00	−0.57
High use of punishment	33	−04	1.90[b]	20	36	−0.84	23	10	0.58
High use of rewards	−06	−34[a]	1.49	32	−22	2.75[b]	09	−13	0.98
Chidl structure & autonomy	−13	07	−1.02	−24	−02	−1.11	−19	09	−1.25
Parental employment history	01	−09	0.53	−04	23	−1.38	−16	−15	−0.05
Reactivity–low manageability	38[a]	41[a]	−0.19	47[a]	57[a]	−0.70	19	02	0.78
Child stress/health problems	−05	29	−1.76[b]	−01	06	−0.35	−13	−03	−0.44
Poor coordination–low approach	32	04	1.54	22	−01	1.19	27	01	1.21
Low self-regulation	27	51[a]	−1.43	−03	29	−1.57[b]	−19	08	−1.24
Word knowledge	−11	19	−1.60	−05	14	−0.97	−13	−04	−0.41
High rate of development	−23	−09	−0.77	−02	16	−0.92	−11	−17	0.28

Pearson r: Two-tailed tests of significance [a]$P < 0.01$.

Significant differences between Pearson rs [b]$P < 0.05$.

[c]Ratio of r to z transformations (see Pearson & Hartley. 1962).

or girls although some trends were apparent for boys only. There were no significant sex differences for these correlations.

Although no meaningful sex differences emerged, because of the trend towards some statistically significant differences, sex was included in the subsequent multiple regression analyses as a potential child predictor of behavioural adjustment.

Multiple Regression Analysis: Phase I

Two backwards stepwise multiple regression analyses were performed separately for both Phases I and II, using child-centred and environmental variables as separate sets of potential predictors. From a backwards stepwise multiple regression of total BSQ score onto environmental factors, high parental maladjustment and low use of rewards emerged as significant contributing variables accounting for 13% of BSQ variance ($F = 8.93$, $P < 0.0003$). From a similar analysis using the child factors and sex as independent variables, high reactivity–low manageability and low self-regulation emerged as significant child variables accounting for 25% of BSQ variance) $F = 19.02$, $P < 0.0000$).

The significant child and environment predictors from the previous regression analyses were then entered simultaneously into a backwards stepwise multiple regression analysis to find the best overall predictors of children's behavioural adjustment, and to aid in the development of a specific path model. For Phase I, high parental maladjustment, high reactivity–low manageability, and low self-regulation were the best overall predictors of behavioural maladjustment, accounting for 28% of total BSQ score variance ($F = 11.42$, $P < 0.0000$).

Multiple Regression Analysis: Phase II

Similar backwards stepwise multiple regression analyses were performed for total MPBQ and TPBQ scores. Environmental variables remained the same as those for Phase I, while total BSQ score was added to the list of independent child variables, which also included the child factors and sex. Parental maladjustment and high use of punishment accounted for 12% of total MPBQ score variance ($F = 7.98$, $P < 0.0006$). Reactivity–low manageability, total BSQ score, and high rate of development remained after backwards regression of total MPBQ score onto child variables, accounting for 37% of MPBQ variance ($F = 21.11$, $P < 0.0000$). Backwards stepwise regression of total MPBQ score onto these remaining child and environmental predictors simultaneously revealed that high total BSQ score (i.e. low adjustment at 3–4 years of age), high rate of development, high use of punishment, and high reactivity–low manageability were the best predictors for maternal ratings of behavioural disturbance in the 4–5-year-olds, and accounted for 38% of total MPBQ score variance ($F = 16.90$, $P < 0.0000$).

No environmental variables were significantly predictive of behavioural disturbance as rated by teachers or caretakers in Phase II (i.e. total TPBQ score). Backwards regression of total TPBQ score onto child variables revealed that high reactivity–low manageability and high self-regulation were the best child-centred predictors, but accounted for only 5% of TPBQ variance ($F = 3.42, P <0.04$). As relatively little of total TPBQ score variance was accounted for using the current set of predictors, a path model for teacher ratings was not constructed.

Path Model: Phases I and II

On the basis of the reviewed literature and the initial series of correlational and multiple regression analyses, a theoretical model was proposed for examination with path analysis, the major implications of which are:

1. Stress, child-rearing practices, parental adjustment, rate of development, previous behavioural adjustment, and temperament all exhibit direct and/or indirect causal influences on maternal reports of early childhood behavioural adjustment.

2. Low self-regulation, high reactivity–low manageability, and high parental maladjustment exhibit direct causal relations with total BSQ score (i.e., low adjustment at 3–4 years of age).

3. High use of punishment, high parental maladjustment, high reactivity low manageability, high rate of development, and high total BSQ score (i.e. low adjustment at 3–4 years) directly predict behavioural maladjustment at 4–5 years as measured by total MPBQ score.

4. High use of punishment is causally linked to high reactivity–low manageability, while high use of rewards is linked to high self-regulation.

5. High parental maladjustment leads to the high use of punishment and the low use of rewards.

6. High rate of development is placed causally prior to low reactivity–high manageability and the high use of rewards.

7. Child health and stress problems directly relate to high parental maladjustment.

8. Self-regulation and reactivity–low manageability exhibit a completely spurious or non-causal covariance.

Hence, temperamental characteristics were seen to be influenced by environmental variables and were assumed to determine, to some extent, the influence that environmental variables have on behavioural adjustment. According to the model, positive temperamental characteristics could act to protect a child from the effects of an adverse environment. The conception of temperament on which the present path model is consistent with a stress resilience model of temperamental influence.

Path Analysis: Phases I and II

A trimmed path analytic model is presented in Fig. 2. Decomposition of direct and indirect effects is presented in Table 6. The large sample chi-square goodness-of-fit statistic (see Nie et al., 1975) calculated for the path model suggested an excellent fit (chi-square = 3.31, df = 9. *P* <0.99. From the model, it can be seen that:

1. Temperamental self-regulation and reactivity–low manageability exhibited the largest path coefficients with total BSQ score during Phase I, while reactivity–low manageability exhibited the largest relationship with total MPBQ score at Phase II. Hence, temperamental characteristics offered the greatest concurrent *and* predictive influence on behavioural adjustment at 3–4 and 4–5 years of age. While both high self-regulation and low reactivity–high manageability were related to behavioural adjustment at 3–4 years of age, only high reactivity–low manageability was causally linked to behaviour problems at 4–5 years of age.

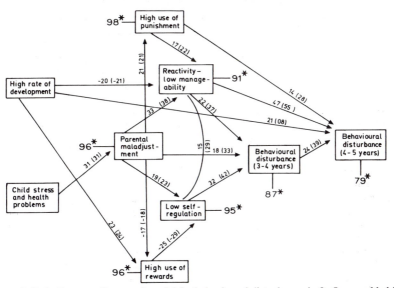

Figure 2. Path diagram of a causal model for behavioural disturbance in 3–5-year-old children. Note: Values above paths are path coefficients; values in parentheses are zero-order correlations. Decimal points have been omitted. *Unexplained variance $\sqrt{1 - R^2}$)

2. The concurrent direct influence of parental maladjustment on children's behavioural adjustment at 3–4 years of age was as notable as its indirect effects, but there was no direct path of influence from parental maladjustment (at age 3–4 years) to children's behavioural dysfunction 1 year later (i.e. total MPBQ score). The indirect influence of prior parental maladjustment on 4–5-year-olds' behavioural disturbance was through its causal influence on prior disturbance, temperamental reactivity–low manageability, and the high use of punishment in child-rearing. Generally, the influence of parental maladjustment could be curtailed by a non-highly reactive, manageable, and self-regulatory temperament, and to a lesser extent through the high use of rewards and low use of punishment in child-rearing.

3. Child-rearing factors did not exhibit significant direct causal paths with preschool behavioural adjustment, particularly when environmental and child-related predictors were considered simultaneously. The high use of rewards made a notable contribution to behavioural adjustment at 3–4 years of age through its causal link with temperamental self-regulation. However, the high use of punishment did not offer much direct predictive power in relation to either temperamental reactivity–low manageability or to behavioural dysfunction 1 year later.

TABLE 6
Decomposition of Effects for Path Model in Fig. 2

| Relationship | Total Covariance | Causal effects | | | Non-causal |
		Direct	Indirect	Total	
Behave 2–behave 1	39	24	none	24	15
Behave 2–react	55	47	07	54	01
Behave 2–punish	28	14	09	23	05
Behave 1–develop	08	21	−11	10	−02
Behave 1–react	37	22	none	22	15
Behave 1–self-reg.	42	32	none	32	10
Behave 1–parents	33	18	15	33	none
React–punish	22	17	none	17	05
React–develop	−21	−20	none	−20	−01
React–parents	38	33	04	37	01
Self-reg.–rewards	−29	−25	none	−25	−04
Self-reg.–parents	23	19	04	23	none
Punish–parents	21	21	none	21	none
Rewards	−18	−17	none	−17	−01
Rewards–develop	24	23	none	23	01
Parents–stress	31	31	none	31	none

Decimal points have been omitted.

4. High rate of development did not exhibit a significant zero order correlation with total MPBQ score, although it did exhibit a notable path coefficient. Hence, high early rates of development were associated with the development of behaviour problems at 4–5 years of age. However, a high rate of early development was also related to the high use of rewards in child-rearing, and to a non-highly reactive and manageable temperament, factors associated with optimal levels of behavioural adjustment in pre-school children. Thus, the low zero order correlation may be accounted for by the cancelling out of positive and negative effects on behavioural adjustment.

5. Childhood stress and health problems were causally and significantly related only to parental maladjustment. The influence of children's health problems and stressful life events on pre-school behavioural adjustment was seen to act via its effects on the parents.

DISCUSSION

These results suggest that temperamental characteristics exhibit the most predictive independent relationships with measures of early childhood behavioural adjustment, both concurrently and prospectively. In addition, maladjustment within the parental subsystem played an important role in childrens' behavioural adjustment, both directly and indirectly. Child-rearing practices and rate of development were limited in their prediction of children's adjustment, while children's stress and health problems, sex, and verbal intelligence did not directly relate to children's adjustment. Children's stress and health problems were, however, related to the level of parental maladjustment. Generally, temperamental characteristics (particularly, low reactivity–high manageability) appeared to curtail the influence of adverse family factors on children's adjustment. In addition, the strength of relationships between temperament and children's behavioural adjustment differed as a function of time, of the specific temperamental characteristic examined, and of the source of behavioural ratings.

Despite some significant (albeit unclear) sex differences, sex did not make a significant contribution to the present path model. The restricted range of the sex "dummy" variable used in regression analyses makes it difficult for sex to emerge as a strong predictor of behaviour, temperament, or child-rearing practices. It may be preferable to construct separate path models for boys and girls, or to analyse path models separately for boys and girls. In any case, these children may be too young for sex differences to emerge, especially as this was a normal not a clinical sample.

Teacher ratings of behaviour at pre-school facility were not strongly predicted by environmental or child variables. Behaviour at pre-school facilities may be dependent on an alternative range of predictors, such as teacher management strategies, group dynamics, and the potential for children in a "stressed" family to escape to a more adjusted or controlled environment such as that offered by the pre-school facility. While there was some agreement about children's behaviour at home (as rated by mothers) and at pre-school (as rated by teachers), it also appears that investigation of adjustment at pre-school may require identification and measurement of a different set of variables. Achenbach, McConaughy, & Howell (1987) have noted the variance in situations and informants which invariably limits the correlations obtained in assessment of childhood adjustment problems via different sources.

The major focus of the present study was to examine the influence of temperament on children's behavioural adjustment. The relationships between temperament ratings and other variables can be conceptualised in a number of alternative ways. Firstly, ratings of temperamental characteristics can be seen to have been shaped by environmental contingencies (i.e. how parents encourage or discourage particular behavioural patterns). Secondly, temperamental characteristics can be conceptualised as mediating the influence that environmental variables have on children's behavioural adjustment. Hence, positive temperamental characteristics can act to protect a child from the effects of an adverse environment, while a "difficult" temperament can predispose children to negative outcomes. Thirdly, temperament ratings can be seen to have been influenced by rater characteristics such as the level of parental adjustment. Fourthly, the high path coefficients between "difficult" temperament and behaviour problems may be due to problems of construct and content validity inherent potentially in the measures of temperament and/or pre-school behavioural adjustment.

Issues of measurement are pertinent to the clinical utility of the concept of temperament. Temperament ratings have not been found to be independent of rater characteristics such as level of adjustment (Vaughn et al., 1987). In the present study, once the effects of parental adjustment and child-rearing had been partialled out, the temperament factors remained significantly related to the early childhood behavioural adjustment measures. However, partialling out the effects of other variables does not deal with the potential problem of contamination between temperament and behavioural adjustment measures.

A recent study addressed the issue of contamination more directly. Sanson, Prior, & Kyrios (in press) asked a group of child psychologists to rate items taken from a temperament questionnaire, and from two pre-school behavioural adjustment instruments for their adequacy or "goodness" as measures of temperament and as measures of behavioural adjustment. Results indicated some general overlap between temperament and adjustment, although most contamination occurred for internalising behaviour problems (i.e. dependency, fears, worries). When items considered to be most contaminated were removed from particular temperament scales, weaker albeit still significant correlations were found between a few temperament scales and behaviour problem composites. This was particularly true of temperamental irritability and activity–intensity. However, rater conceptions of causal associations between temperament and behavioural adjustment were thought to influence these results. While the Sanson et al. (in press) study did not offer solutions to problems of contamination, it does point to the need to further develop conceptions and operationalisations of temperament and behavioural dysfunction.

The conception of temperament on which the present path model is based can be best seen within a "stress resilience" or "reactivity" paradigm. According to such a model, individual characteristics can influence one's reactions to a negative environmental context. In addition, the environment exerts an influence on the manifestation of those individual characteristics. For instance, a highly reactive temperament can intensify the influence of a stressful environment on children's behavioural adjustment. At the same time, negative environmental influences may change one's temperamental profile; for instance, by making a child more reactive or less self-regulatory. Any subsequent environmental stresses may promote behavioural dysfunction, despite an initially positive temperamental profile. While there is little doubt that children's temperamental characteristics also influence their environmental context (e.g. child-rearing practices, and probably to a lesser extent the level of parental adjustment), it was not possible to examine reciprocal influences with the present analytic approach. Rather, a follow-up cross-sectional methodology such as those evident in cross-lagged panel analysis might allow such reciprocity to be examined.

A more interactive approach allowing different weights to various temperamental and environmental contingencies, as well as reciprocal influences, and using nonrecursive path models could facilitate further model development. However, one of the greatest values of temperament concepts in developmental psychopathology may lie in the identification of those characteristics that offer protective, resilient, or mediating influences in behavioural development, particularly those that are stable in nature and "measureable".

Notwithstanding the limitations of the present exploratory path model, in particular the need for application to numerous samples to assess generalisability, it is argued that the concept of temperament can make an important contribution to our understanding of developmental and clinical concerns. Environmental stresses and, in particular, poor functioning within the parental subsystem do make major direct and indirect contributions to poor behavioural outcomes in early childhood. While the present path model supported the notion of temperament as a stress resilience factor, parental dysfunction was also seen as contributing to difficult temperament and early childhood behavioural dysfunction. On this basis, one could argue that intervention and preventative programmes for behaviourally maladjusted children should focus on parental well-being and marital adjustment (e.g. Dadds, Schwartz, & Sanders, 1987). Overall, this study reflects the recognition of temperament as a salient developmental factor, and illustrates the need to further develop current conceptions of temperamental influence on children's behavioural development.

REFERENCES

Achenbach, T. M., McConaughy, S. H., & Howell, C. T. (1987). Child/adolescent behavioral and emotional problems: Implications of cross-informant correlations for situational specificity. *Psychological Bulletin, 101(2),* 213–232.

Anderson, K. E., Lytton, H., & Romney, D. M. (1986). Mothers' interactions with normal and conduct-disordered boys: Who affects whom? *Developmental Psychology, 22,* 604–609.

Antill, J. K. & Cotton, S. (1982). Spanier's Dyadic Adjustment Scale: Some confirmatory analyses. *Australian Psychologist, 17,* 181–189.

Baldwin, A. L., Cole, R. E., & Baldwin, C. P. (1982). Parental pathology, family interaction, and the competence of the child at at school. *Monographs of the Society for Research in Child Development, 47* (5, Serial No. 197).

Barron, A P., & Earls, F. (1984). The relation of temperament and social factors to behaviour problems in three-year-old children. *Journal of Child Psychology & Psychiatry, 25,* 23–33.

Barton, K. (1981). Six child rearing dimensions common to both fathers and mothers. *Multivariate Experimental Clinical Research, 5,* 91–97.

Bates, J. E. (1980). The concept of difficult temperament. *Merrill-Palmer Quarterly, 26,* 299–319.

Bates, J. E. (1983). Issues in the assessment of difficult temperament. *Merrill-Palmer Quarterly, 29,* 89–97.

Bates, J. E. & Bayles, K. (1984). Objective and subjective components in mothers' perception of their children from age 6 months to 3 years. *Merrill-Palmer Quarterly, 30,* 111–130.

Baumrind, D. (1967). Child care practices anteceding three patterns of preschool behaviour. *Genetic Psychology Monographs, 75,* 43–88.

Beautrais, Al L., Ferguson, D. M., & Shannon, F. T. (1982a). Family life events and behavioral problems in preschool-aged children. *Pediatrics, 70,* 774–779.

Beautrais, A. L., Ferguson, D. M., & Shannon, F. T. (1982b). Life events and childhood morbidity: A prospective study. *Pediatrics, 70,* 935–940.

Behar, L., & Stringfield, S. (1974). A behavior rating scale for the preschool child. *Developmental Psychology, 10,* 601–610.

Belsky, J. (1984). The determinants of parenting: A process model. *Child Development, 55,* 83–96.

Biddle, B. J. & Marlin, M. M. (1987). Causality, confirmation, credulity, and structural equation modeling. *Child Development, 58,* 4–17.

Billings, A. G. & Moos, R. H. (1983). Comparisons of children of depressed and nondepressed parents: A social-environmental perspective. *Journal of Abnormal Child Psychology, 11,* 463–486.

Blalock, H. M. (1971). *Causal models in the social services.* Chicago: Aldine Publishing Co.

Broom, L., Jones, F. L., & Zubrzycki, J. (1976). *Opportunity and attainment in Australia,* Canberra: Australian National University Press.

Brown, G., Harris, T., & Bifulco, A. (1985). Long term effect of early loss of parent. In M. Rutter, C. Izard, & P. Read (Eds), *Depression in childhood: Developmental perspectives.* New York: Guilford Press.

Cameron, J. (1978). Parental treatment, children's temperament, and the risk of childhood behavioral problems. 2. Initial temperament, parental attitudes, and the incidence and form of behavior problems. *American Journal of Orthopsychiatry, 48,* 140–147.

Campbell, S. B., Ewing, L. J., Breaux, A. M., & Szumowski, A. M. (1986). Parent-referred problem three-year-olds: Follow-up at school entry. *Journal of Child Psychology & Psychiatry, 27,* 473–488.

Chazan, M. & Jackson, S. (1974). Behavioural problems in the infant school: Changes over two years. *Journal of Child Psychology & Psychiatry, 15,* 33–46.

Coddington, R. D. (1972a). The significance of life events as etiological factors in the diseases of children. 1. A survey of professional worker. *Journal of Psychosomatic Research, 16,* 205–213.

Coddington, R. D. (1972b). The significance of life events as etiological factors in the diseases of children. 2. A study of a normal population. *Journal of Psychosomatic Research, 16,* 205–213.

Crano, W. D. & Mendoza, J. L. (1987). Maternal factors that influence children's positive behavior: Demonstration of a structural equation analysis of selected data from the Berkeley Growth Study. *Child Development, 58,* 38–48.

Crockenberg, S. & Acredolo, C. (1983). Infant temperament ratings: A function of infants, of mothers, or both? *Infant Behaviour & Development, 6,* 61–72.

Crowther, J. H., Bond, L. A., & Rolf, J. E. (1981). The incidence, prevalence, and severity of behavior disorders among preschool-aged children in day care. *Journal of Abnormal Child Psychology, 9,* 23–42.

Dadds, M. R., Schwartz, S., & Sanders, M. R. (1987). Marital discord and treatment outcome in behavioral treatment of child behavior problems. *Journal of Consulting & Clinical Psychology, 55,* 396–403.

Dielman, T. E. & Cattell, R. B. (1972). The prediction of behavior problems in 6 to 8 year old children from mothers' reports of child-rearing practices. *Journal of Clinical Psychology, 28,* 13–17.

Dielman, T. E., Cattell, R. B., & Rhoades, P. (1972). Childrearing antecedents of early child personality factors. *Journal of Marriage and the Family, 2,* 431–436.

Duncan, O. D. (1966). Path analysis: Sociological examples. *American Journal of Sociology, 72,* 1–16.

Dunn, L. M. & Dunn, L. M. (1981). *Manual for the Peabody Picture Vocabulary Test– Revised,* Circle Pines, Minnesota: American Guidance Service.

Earls, F. (1980). Prevalence of behavior problems in 3 year old children: A cross-national replication. *Archives of General Psychiatry, 37,* 1153–1157.

Earls, F. (1981). Temperament characteristics and behavior problems in three-year-old children. *Journal of Nervous & Mental Disease, 169,* 367–373.

Emery, R. E. (1982). Interparental conflict and the children of discord and divorce. *Psychological Bulletin, 92,* 310–330.

Garmezy, N., Masten, A. S., & Tellegen, A. (1984). The study of stress and competence in children: A building block for developmental psychopathology. *Child Development, 55,* 97–111.

Garrison, W. & Earls, F. (1985). Change and continuity in behavior problems from the preschool period through school entry: An analysis of mothers' reports. In J. E. Stevenson (Ed.), *Recent research in developmental psychopathology.* New York: Pergamon Press. (Pp. 51–65.)

Ghodsian, M., Zajicek, E., & Wolkind, S. (1984). A longitudinal study of maternal depression and child behaviour problems. *Journal of Child Psychology & Psychiatry. 25,* 91–109.

Goldberg, D. P. (1978). *Manual of the General Health Questionnaire.* Great Britain: NFER Publishing Co.

Goldberg, D. P. & Hillier, V. F. (1979). A scaled version of the General Health Questionnaire. *Psychological Medicine, 9* 139–145.

Goldberg, W. A. & Easterbrooks, M. A. (1984). Role of marital quality in toddler development. *Developmental Psychology, 20,* 504–514.

Goldsmith, H. H., Buss, A. H., Plomin, R., Rothbart, M. K., Thomas, A., Chess, S., Hinde, R. A., & McCall, R. B. (1987). Roundtable: What is temperament? Four approaches. *Child Development, 58,* 505–529.

Goldsmith, H. H. & Reiser-Danner, L. A. (1986). Variation among temperament theories and validation studies of temperament assessment. In G. A. Kohnstamm (Ed.). *Temperament discussed: Temperament and development in infancy and childhood.* Lisse: Swets Publishing Service.

Gorsuch, R. L. (1974). *Factor analysis.* Hillsdale, N.J.: Lawrence Erlbaum Associates, Inc.

Graham, P., Rutter, M., & George, S. (1973). Temperamental characteristics as predictors of behavior disorder. *American Journal of Orthopsychiatry, 43,* 328–339.

Heisel, J. S., Ream, S., Raitz, R., Rappoport, M., & Coddington, R. D. (1973). The significance of life events as contributing factors in the disease of children. 3. A study of pediatric patients. *Journal of Pediatrics, 83,* 119–123.

Hetherington, E. M. (1980). Children and divorce. In R. Henderson (Ed.), *Parent-child interaction: theory, research, and prospect.* New York: Academic Press.

Hinde, R. A. & Tamplin, A. (1983). Relations between mother-child interaction and behaviour in preschool. *British Journal of Development Psychology. 1,* 231–257.

Holmes, T. H. & Rahe, R. H. (1967). The social readjustment rating scale. *Journal of Psychosomatic Research, 11,* 213–218.

Jenkins, S., Bart, M., & Hart, H. (1980). Behaviour problems in preschool children. *Journal of Child Psychology & Psychiatry, 21,* 5–17.

Johnson, J. H. (1982). Life events as stressors in childhood and adolescent. In B. B. Lahey & A. E. Kazdin (Eds), *Advances in Clinical Child Psychology,* Vol. 5. New York: Plenum Press.

Johnson, S. M. & Lobitz, G. K. (1974). The personal and marital adjustment of parents as related to observed child deviance and parenting behaviors. *Journal of Abnormal Child Psychology, 2*, 193–207.

Joreskog, K. G. & Sorbom, D. (1984). *LISREL VI: Analysis of linear structural relationships by the method of maximum likelihood, instrument variables, and least squares methods.* Moresville, In: Scientific Software.

Kagan, J. (1982). The construct of difficult temperament: A reply to Thomas, Chess, & Korn. *Merrill-Palmer Quarterly, 28*, 1–20.

Kenny, D. A. (1979). *Correlation and causality.* New York: Wiley & Sons.

Kohlberg, L., Ricks, D., & Snarey, J. (1984). Childhood development as a predictor of adaptation in adulthood. *Genetic Psychology Monographs, 110*, 91–172.

Lerner, J. A., Inui, T. S., Trupin, E. W., & Douglas, E. (1985). Preschool behavior can predict future psychiatric disorders. *Journal of the American Academy of Child Psychiatry, 24*, 42–48.

Lerner, J. V. (1983). The role of temperament in psychosocial adaptation in early adolescents: A test of a "goodness to fit" model. *Journal of Genetic Psychology, 143*, 149–157.

Lerner, J. V. (1984). The import of temperament for psychosocial functioning: Tests of a goodness-of-fit model. *Merrill-Palmer Quarterly, 30*, 177–188.

Lerner, J. V. & Lerner, R. M. (1983). Temperament and adaptation across life: Theoretical and empirical issues. In P. B. Baltes & O. G. Brim (Eds), *Life-span development and behavior (Vol. 5).* New York: Academic Press. (Pp. 197–231).

Links, P. S. (1983). Community surveys of the prevalence of childhood psychiatric disorders: A review. *Child Development, 54*, 531–548.

Madge, N. (1983). Unemployment and its effects on children. *Journal of Child Psychology & Psychiatry, 24*, 311–319.

McFarlane, J., Allen, L., & Honzik, M. (1954). *A development study of the behavior problems of normal children.* Berkeley: University of California Press.

McGuire, J. & Richman, N. (1986). The prevalence of behavioural problems in three types of preschool, *Journal of Child Psychology & Psychiatry, 27*, 455–472.

Nie, N. H., Hull, C. H., Jenkins, J. G., Steinbrenner, K., & Bent, D. H. (1975). *Statistical package for the social sciences.* New York: McGraw-Hill.

Oberklaid, F., Prior, M., Golvan, D., Clements, A., & Williamson, A. (1984). Temperament in Australian infants. *Australian Paediatric Journal, 20*, 181–184.

Olweus, D. (1980). Familial and temperamental determinants of aggressive behavior in adolescent boys: A causal analysis. *Developmental Psychology, 16*, 644–660.

Panaccione, V. F. & Wahler, R. G. (1986). Child behavior, maternal depression, and social coersion as factors in the quality of child care. *Journal of Abnormal Child Psychology, 14*, 263–278.

Pearson, E. S. & Hartley, H. O. (Eds) (1962). *Biometrical Tables for Statisticians,* Vol. 1. Cambridge University Press.

Plomin, R. (1982). The difficult concept of temperament: A response to Thomas, Chess, & Korn. *Merrill-Palmer Quarterly, 28*, 25–33.

Porter, B., & O'Leary, K. D. (1980). Marital discord and childhood behavior problems. *Journal of Abnormal Child Psychology, 8*, 287–295.

Prior, M., Kyrios, M., & Oberklaid, F. (1986). Temperament in Australian, American, Chinese and Greek infants: Some issues and directions for future research. *Journal of Cross-Cultural Psychology, 17*, 455–474.

Prior, M., Sanson, A., Carroll, R., & Oberklaid, F. (1989). Social class influences on temperament ratings of pre-school children. *Merrill-Palmer Quarterly, 35*, 239.

Prior, M., Sanson, A., & Oberklaid, F. The Australian Temperament Project. In G. A. Kohnstamm, J. E. Bates, & M. K. Rothbart (Eds), *Handbook of temperament in childhood*. Chichester, Sussex: Wiley (In press).

Prior, M., Sanson A., Oberklaid, F., & Northam, E. (1987). Measurement of temperament in one- to three-year-old children. *International Journal of Behavioral Development, 10*, 121–132.

Richman, N. (1977). Is a behaviour check-list for preschool children useful? In P. J. Graham (Ed.), *Epidemiological approaches in child psychiatry*. London: Academic Press.

Richman, N. & Graham, P. J. (1971). A behavioural screening questionnaire for use with three year old children: Preliminary findings. *Journal of Child Psychology & Psychiatry, 12*, 5–33.

Richman, N., Stevenson, J., & Graham, P. J. (1975). Prevalence of behaviour problems in 3 year old children: An epidemiological study in a London borough. *Journal of Child Psychology & Psychiatry, 16*, 277–287.

Richman, N., Stevenson, J., & Graham, P. J. (1982). *Preschool to school: A behavioural study*. London: Academic Press.

Rothbart, M. K. (1981). Measurement of temperament in infancy. *Child Development, 52*, 569–578.

Rothbart, M. K. (1982). The concept of difficult temperament: A critical analysis of Thomas, Chess, & Korn. *Merrill-Palmer Quarterly, 28*, 35–40.

Rutter, M. (1979). Protective factors in children's responses to stress and disadvantage. In M. W. Kent & J. E. Rolf (Eds), *Primary prevention of psychopathology* (Vol. 3): *Social competence in children*. Hanover, N. H.: University Press of New England.

Rutter, M. (1985). Resiliency in the face of adversity: Protective factors and resistance to psychiatric disorder. *British Journal of Psychiatry, 147*, 598–611.

Sameroff, A. J., Seifer, R., & Elias, P. K. (1982). Sociocultural variability in infant temperament ratings. *Child Development, 53*, 164–173.

Sanson, A., Prior, M., & Kyrios, M. (in press). The contamination of temperament and behaviour measures. *Merrill-Palmer Quarterly*.

Sanson, A., Prior, M., Kyrios, M., & Oberklaid. F. (1988). Australian normative data for parent and teacher versions of the Preschool Behaviour Questionnaire. Paper in preparation.

Sears, R. R., Maccoby, E. E., & Levin, H. (1957). *Patterns of child rearing*. Stanford, California: Stanford University Press.

Seifer, R., Sameroff, A. J., & Jones, F. (1981). Adaptive behaviour in young children of emotionally disturbed women. *Journal of Applied Developmental Psychology, 1*, 251–276.

Spanier, G. B. (1976). Measuring dyadic adjustment: New scales for assessing the quality of marriage and similar dyads. *Journal of Marriage and Family, 38*, 15–28.

Strelau, J. (1983a). A regulative theory of temperament. *Australian Journal of Psychology, 35,* 305–317.

Strelau, J. (1983b). *Temperament–Personality–Activity.* London: Academic Press.

Susman, E. J., Trickett, P. K., Iannotti, R. J., Hollenbeck, B. E., & Zahn-Walker, C. (1985). Child-rearing patterns in depressed, abusive, and normal mothers. *American Journal of Orthopsychiatry, 55,* 237–251.

Terestman, N. (1980). Mood quality and intensity in nursery school children as predictors of behavior disorder. *American Journal of Orthopsychiatry, 50,* 125–138.

Thomas, A. (1982). The study of difficult temperament: A reply to Kagan, Rothbart & Plomin. *Merrill-Palmer Quarterly, 28,* 313–315.

Thomas, A. & Chess, S. (1977). *Temperament and development.* New York: Brunner/Mazel.

Thomas, A. & Chess. S. (1984). *Origins and evolution of behavior disorders: From infancy to adult life.* New York: Brunner/Mazel.

Thomas, A., Chess, S., & Korn, S. J. (1982). The reality of difficult temperament. *Merrill-Palmer Quarterly, 28* 1–20.

Vaughn, B. E., Bradley, C. F., Joffe, L. S., Seifer, R., & Barglow, P. (1987). Maternal characteristics measured prenatally are predictive of ratings of temperamental "difficulty" on the Carey Infant Temperament Questionnaire. *Developmental Psychology, 23,* 152–161.

Ventura, J. N. & Stevens, M. B. (1986). Relations of mothers' and fathers' reports of infant temperament, parents psychological functioning, and family characteristics. *Merrill-Palmer Quarterly, 32,* 275–289.

Wallerstein, J. S. & Kelly, J. B. (1980). *Surviving the breakup: How children and parents cope with divorce.* New York: Basic Books.

Werner, E. E. & Smith, R. S. (1982). *Vulnerable, but invincible: A study of resilient children.* New York: McGraw-Hill.

Zeanah, C. H., Keener, M. A., & Anders, T. F. (1986). Developing perceptions of temperament and their relation to mother and infant behaviour. *Journal of Child Psychology & Psychiatry, 27,* 499–512.

REFERENCE NOTES

1. Barton, K. (1984). Personal communication.

16

Infant Proneness-to-Distress Temperament, Maternal Personality, and Mother-Infant Attachment: Associations and Goodness of Fit

Sarah Mangelsdorf
University of Michigan, Ann Arbor
Megan Gunnar, Roberta Kestenbaum,
Sarah Lang, and Debra Andreas
Institute of Child Development, University of Minnesota

Sixty-six mother-infant pairs were examined when the infants were 9 and 13 months. The purpose of this report was to examine relations between infant proneness-to-distress temperament, maternal personality characteristics, and mother-infant attachment. There were no main-effect relations between infant proneness-to-distress temperament as assessed at 9 months and infant attachment classification at 13 months. This was true whether security of attachment (A and C vs. B) or proposed temperament (A1-B2 vs. B3-C2) groupings of attachment classifications were examined. Infant proneness-to-distress temperament, however, was associated with maternal behavior and personality. Furthermore, security of attachment could be predicted by an interaction between maternal personality and proneness-to-distress. The importance of considering goodness-of-fit relations in predicting attachment security is discussed.

Reprinted with permission from *Child Development*, 1990, Vol. 61, 820–831. Copyright © 1990 by the Society for Research in Child Development, Inc.

This research was supported by NICHD grant HD-16494 to Megan Gunnar. The authors would like to thank all those who helped in this research including Joan Connors, Jill Isensee, Mary Larson, Louise Hertsgaard, Kay Gornick, and Linda Nelson. Special thanks are due to Auke Tellegen for his willingness to discuss results and interpretations.

Recently, there has been heated debate over the relative contributions of maternal sensitivity and infant temperament to the development of secure and insecure attachment (see Lamb, 1982, and Sroufe, 1985, for reviews). On one extreme, attachment theorists have argued that either temperament and attachment quality are orthogonal constructs (i.e., temperament variation may influence aspects of behavior but not the organization or security of attachment), or that relationship history totally transforms constitutional temperament variation such that it makes little or no contribution to the quality of attachment (Sroufe, 1985). On the other extreme, temperament theorists have argued either that infant temperament plays as important a role as maternal sensitivity in determining resistant behavior (see Goldsmith & Alansky, 1987), or that measures of attachment security are confounded with measures of temperament (Kagan, 1982).

Much of the temperament-attachment argument revolves around interpretation of attachment classifications derived from the Ainsworth and Wittag (1969) Strange Situation test. This assessment is used to classify infants into three molar categories: A, or Insecure Avoidant; B, or Secure; and C, or Insecure Resistant. Recently Main (Main, Kaplan, & Cassidy, 1985) has added a fourth category, D, or Disorganized, that will not be considered in this report. These molar categories are further divided into subcategories.

According to attachment theorists (Ainsworth, Blehar, Waters, & Wall, 1978), reunion behavior largely determines classification. Kagan (1982), has argued, however, that category placement is determined by the infant's proneness-to-distress temperament. Belsky and Rovine (1987) have recently offered an attempt at rapprochement between these positions. Based on initial work of Frodi and Thompson (1985), they argued that infants classified as A1's, A2's, B1's, and B2's do not cry much in the Strange Situation, while those classified as B3's, B4's, C1's, and C2's do cry, and this division of attachment classifications reflects proneness-to-distress temperament. Attachment security, however, determines whether the infant is classified as secure (B1–B4) or insecure (A or C). They support the temperament division of attachment categories with data showing consistency in classification category to mother and father when the temperament grouping is used (i.e., A1–B2 vs. B3–C2) but not when a security grouping (i.e., A and C vs. B) is used. Further, they reported differences on the Brazelton Neonatal Assessment Scale at birth and on Bates's (Bates, Freeland, & Lounsbury, 1979) Infant Characteristic Questionnaire at 3 months among infants later classified as A1–B2 versus B3–C2. Unfortunately, this attempt at rapprochement has not provided the final word in the temperament-attachment debate. Recently Goldsmith and Alansky (1987) published a review of the research on temperament and attachment concluding that proneness-to-distress temperament does predict resistant behavior as reliably as maternal sensitivity. And Connell and his colleagues (Connell & Goldsmith, 1982; Connell & Thompson, 1986; Thompson, Connell, & Bridges, 1988) have also recently argued that both temperamental and situational factors influence the amount of distress the infant expresses in the Strange Situation.

One reason the debate continues may be that most of the temperament assessment techniques used in these studies have serious methodological shortcomings. Most have involved parental report instruments with all their attendant problems, and when direct observations of proneness-to-distress temperament have been used they have involved assessments not initially designed to measure temperament (e.g., the Brazelton exam or observations of time crying during brief home observations), often with poor test-retest reliability. One purpose of the following study was to examine the relations between proneness-to-distress temperament and attachment classifications using an observational instrument designed to assess emotional temperament. The one chosen was the Louisville Temperament Assessment (Matheny & Wilson, 1981). This is an hour-long laboratory assessment involving two long (19 and 30 min) maternal separations and a number of tasks or vignettes. The central measure is a scale, Emotional Tone, scored every 2 min. Although the scale ranges from distress to high positive affect, in practice scores typically reflect negative affect or distress. The Louisville research group has reported remarkable stability in emotional tone across the first 2 years of life (Matheny, 1984; Matheny, Riese, & Wilson, 1985; Riese, 1987). In addition, emotional tone from the assessment has been shown to correlate significantly with maternal reports of infant emotional temperament (Wilson & Matheny, 1986). Finally, emotional tone as scored from this assessment shows evidence of stability, generalizability, and heritability supports the use of their procedures to assess proneness-to-distress temperament.

A second purpose of the study was to examine the relations between maternal personality, infant proneness-to-distress temperament, and quality of attachment. Despite its potential relevance, there have been few studies examining associations between normal variations in maternal personality and either infant behavior, maternal behavior, and/or the security of the mother-infant attachment relationship. The studies that do exist clearly indicate that mothers who are more introverted and who have difficulty adapting to new situations and people have infants who are more easily distressed by separation and strangers (Daniels & Plomin, 1985; Weber, Levitt, & Clark, 1986). These mothers also tend not to expose their babies to as much novel stimulation, and this, perhaps in addition to genetic similarities between mother and child, appears to be one mechanism relating maternal introversion or shyness to the infant's proneness-to-distress in response to strange places and people (Daniels & Plomin, 1985). Beyond maternal introversion/extroversion, few other relations between maternal personality and infant behavior have been explored.

Regarding mother-infant attachment quality, the associations with maternal personality are not clear. Maternal psychopathology does appear to be related to insecure attachment, especially A (avoidant) and D (disorganized) classifications (Gaensbauer, Harmon, Cytryn, & McKnew, 1984; Radke-Yarrow, Cummings,

Kuczynski, & Chapman, 1985). Few relations, however, have been found with non-pathological variations in maternal personality. Among a large number of measures, Egeland and Farber (1984) found only that maternal maturity and complexity of thinking predicted security of attachment at 12 months. Similarly, Belsky and Isabella (1988), again using a large battery of measures, found only that mothers of secure (B) infants scored better on interpersonal affection than did mothers of insecure (A and C) infants. In addition, mothers of avoidant (A) infants displayed significantly poorer levels of ego strength than did mothers of either secure (B) or resistant (C) infants. Finally, using only the five dimensions on the Dimensions of Temperament Scale (DOTS), Weber and colleagues (1986) found that reactivity distinguished mothers of A's (more reactive) from mothers of B1 and B2 infants but did not distinguish them from mothers of B3, B4, or C infants. In fact, mothers of C's did not differ from mothers of B infants on any of the DOTS dimensions.

In part, failure to obtain many significant associations between maternal personality and quality of attachment may indicate that these associations are not direct. This may also contribute to the conflicting evidence regarding emotional temperament and attachment classifications. It has been argued that measures of attachment quality reflect characteristics of the relationship rather than characteristics of only one or the other member of the dyad (Ainsworth et al., 1978). Of course, extremely deviant characteristics of either the mother or infant might dictate the course of their relationship. Nonetheless, within the normal range one would expect that characteristics of both infant and mother would contribute to relationship quality. This argument has been made repeatedly with regard to infant temperament. Most researchers expect that if infant temperament influences attachment quality it does so through affecting how the mother responds to the infant. This influence may operate through interaction with characteristics of the mother or her situation (Campos, Barrett, Lamb, Goldsmith, & Stenberg, 1983; Sroufe, 1985). A classic example of this type of transactional or goodness-of-fit model (Thomas & Chess, 1977) is Crockenberg's (1981) evidence that newborn irritable temperament is predictive of insecure attachment only if coupled with low maternal social support. One important goodness-of-fit consideration may be the fit between the mother's personality and the infant's temperament. This possibility was the third question addressed in the following report.

The data were drawn from a short-term longitudinal study of infants between the ages of 9 and 13 months. The primary purpose of the study was to examine infant physiological stress reactivity assessed through activity of the adrenocortical system and its relation to proneness-to-distress temperament and quality of attachment. These analyses were reported in Gunnar, Mangelsdorf, Larson, and Hertsgaard (1989). Briefly, increases in cortisol, the hormonal product of the adrenocortical system, were positively correlated with proneness-to-distress temperament as assessed using the Louisville Temperament Assessment. Proneness-to-distress at 9 months in the Louisville Assessment predicted distress in the Strange Situation and maternal reports of emotional temperament at 13 months. Changes in cortisol at both 9 and 13 months were unrelated to quality of attachment. The data on adreno-cortical activity will not be considered further in the present report.

METHOD

Subjects

The subjects were 75 mothers and their infants. The infants were 9 months (± 2 weeks) at first testing. Testing was also conducted at 13 months (± 2 weeks), and the 35 mother-daughter and 31 mother-son pairs that completed both assessments constituted the sample analyzed in this report. All families were intact. Average maternal education was 15.4 years (range 10–20 years); average paternal education was 15.5 years (range 12–20 years). While the range was wide for maternal educa-tion, 87% of the mothers had at least some college. Analyses also indicated that maternal education was not significantly associated with any of the variables dis-cussed in this report. Approximately half of the families (56%) had only one child when first tested. Fifty-four of the mothers were not working outside the home even part time by the time the infant was 9 months, while seven were working less than 20 and five more than 20 hours a week.

Procedures

Procedures described in detail in other reports will be mentioned only briefly here. The mothers were contacted by phone, procedures were described, and an appointment was made for the initial home visit.

Nine-month home visit. Home visits (60–75 min) were scheduled in the morning hours at the parents' discretion with the restriction that we observe a normal feeding. The purpose of the visit was to teach the mother to obtain saliva for cortisol determi-nation and to observe mother-infant feeding and play interaction. The Egeland Feeding and Play Scales were completed (Egeland, Deinard, Taraldson, & Brunnquell, 1975). In most cases one observer visited the family; for 15 families, two observers were present to obtain estimates of agreement. Based on previous reports (Vaughn, Taraldson, Crichton, & Egeland, 1980), seven infant and nine maternal scales were chosen for analysis. Observer agreement within 1 scale point for the infant scales ranged from Cohen's kappa of 0.50 to 0.92 (low value was for Look Mother, and often one observer could not see the infant's face). Agreement within 1 scale point for the maternal scales ranged from Cohen's kappa of 0.75 to 1.00.

The key infant variable was a nine-point scale labeled Baby's Positive

Temperament, a scale of the infant's emotional tone during the home observations. The infant scales were combined into one measure of Home Emotional Temperament by weighting each measure according to its correlation coefficient with the Baby Temperament measure (see Gunnar et al., 1989, for details). The Home Temperament measure was then reverse scored so that higher values would reflect emotional distress. The nine maternal scales were: Quality of Vocalization, Maternal Expressivity, Positive Regard during Feeding, Attitude toward Feeding, Sensitivity, Delight, Supportiveness during Play, Patience during Play, and Attitude toward Play. These scales were factor analyzed. One primary factor was identified, accounting for 59.3% of the variance. Because the factor weights indicated a roughly equal weighting of the scales and because we had no strong theoretical reason for emphasizing some scales over others, all nine scales were standardized and averaged to yield one score for Maternal Home Behavior.

Nine-month Louisville Assessment. Within 1 week of the home observation, the mother and infant came to the University for the Louisville Temperament Assessment. The assessment (Matheny & Wilson, 1981) consisted of a 6-min Warm-up period with mother, infant, and the first experimenter; a 19-min Separation during which the infant was with the first experimenter, who attempted to engage the infant in a variety of tasks or vignettes (Vignette 1); a 5-min Reunion with the mother, during which time the infant was introduced to the second experimenter; and a 30-min separation with the second experimenter during which this experimenter also attempted to get the infant interested in a series of tasks (Vignette 2). The two Vignette segments were terminated early and behavior scores prorated if the infant became too upset (Gunnar et al., 1989). The sessions were videotaped and scored for Emotional Tone, the principal emotional state during each 2-min scoring period: (1) extremely upset, wailing, or protesting to (9) highly excited, gleeful, or animated (Cohen's kappa $= 0.85$). (Note that scores were then reversed so that higher values would reflect proneness-to-distress behavior.) Three Emotional Tone scores were computed: Warm-up, Separation (mean of Vignettes 1 and 2), and Reunion. Infant Home Emotional Temperament was correlated modestly ($r = .23$, $p < .10$) with Warm-up Emotional Tone; therefore these measures were standardized and averaged to yield a measure of Nonseparation Emotional Tone. Nonseparation, Separation, and Reunion Emotional Tone scores were then factor analyzed and one Nine-Month Emotional Temperament score was computed using the factor weights (see Gunnar et al., 1989).

Nine-month maternal laboratory behavior. In order to augment the home measures of maternal behavior, during the 6-min Warm-up period of the Louisville Assessment maternal behavior was scored using two scales. One scale, Maternal Expressivity, was adapted from a similar nine-point Egeland Feeding and Play Scale. The two end descriptors were: (1) no emotion is communicated to the baby (the child is handled in a completely impersonal way and ignored even when it is handled or cared for), and (9) very much emotion is communicated through continual use of expressive means (she is almost constantly involved in expression of her feelings toward baby). The second scale, Maternal Supportiveness, was a nine-point scale designed to assess the mother's ability to read the baby's signals and her sensitivity in supporting her baby's attempts to achieve goals. This scale was adapted from maternal measures described in Ainsworth et al. (1978) with descriptors made applicable to our laboratory setting. The two end descriptors were: (1) the mother is extremely unsupportive either because she seems constantly to misread signals or is unwilling to help the child achieve goals. She may appear to have her own agenda and be trying to force the baby to conform. She may also appear to be much more interested in interacting with the experimenter than in "mothering" the baby. And (9) exceptional supportiveness: the mother is so in tune with her baby that she never misses a cue in helping the baby negotiate the social and physical environment. Appears to anticipate the baby's needs, including the need to act independently.

Each scale was scored every 2 min, and the resulting three scores on each scale for the 6-min Warm-up period were averaged. Observer agreement within 1 scale point using Cohen's kappa were 0.76 for Maternal Expressiveness and 0.86 for Maternal Supportiveness. In order to reduce the data, the two laboratory measures and one home measure of maternal behavior were intercorrelated: correlations ranged from 0.25 to 0.44. From their descriptors, the Maternal Home Behavior and Laboratory expressivity scales appeared to reflect maternal warmth, while the Laboratory Supportiveness scale was designed to assess sensitivity. In order to equally weight warmth and supportiveness, the scales were standardized and then summed, first multiplying the Laboratory Supportiveness scale by 2 to yield one measure: Maternal Warmth and Support. A missing value was recorded for one mother for whom no data from the 6-min Warm-up period were available because of equipment problems. The Maternal Warmth and Support scale was used in analyses with infant temperament and maternal personality in order to capitalize on the statistical association between the subscales. However, in analyses with Attachment Quality only, the Laboratory Supportiveness scale was used because sensitivity, and not expressivity, has been predicted to be related to attachment security (Ainsworth et al., 1978).

Multidimensional Personality Questionnaire. Maternal personality was assessed using Tellegen's (1982) Multidimensional Personality Questionnaire (MPQ). This assessment was chosen because it was designed to assess normal variations in personality and has been shown to have good reliability and validity. Our analyses were based on the three higher-order factors derived from the MPQ. These were chosen because Tellegen has argued that the first two factors reflect temperamental characteristics (Tellegen, 1982). The first factor, Positive Affectivity, has been described as an introversion-extroversion factor (Tellegen et al., 1988). The second factor, Negative Affectivity, has been described as an anxiety or neuroticism factor. Finally, interpretation of the third factor, Constraint, is not as clear. Based on its high-loading subscales, it reflects rigidity, traditionalism, and low risk taking.

The mothers were given the MPQ to complete during the two vignette segments of the Louisville Assessment. Some mothers did not complete the questionnaire during the laboratory visit. They were given a stamped, addressed envelope and completed the questionnaires at home. Five of the 66 mothers failed to provide completed questionnaires. Questionnaire data were computer scored, validity scales were reviewed (no questionnaires were rejected), and T scores for the 11 primary scales and three higher-order factors were retained for analysis.

Thirteen-month infant assessments. When the infants were 13 months ($\pm$ 2 weeks) the mothers were mailed the Fullard, McDevitt, and Carey (1984) Toddler Temperament Scale. Proneness-to-distress temperament was reassessed at 13 months using three scales (Approach/Withdrawal, Adaptability, and Mood) from this questionnaire. These scales were used because they had been shown to correlate highly with emotional temperament measured using the Louisville Assessment (Matheny, 1984). Because these scales were significantly intercorrelated (r's 0.33–0.53) they were standardized and averaged to yield one Questionnaire Temperament measure (Gunnar et al., 1989). One week later the mother-infant relationship was assessed using the Strange Situation (Ainsworth & Wittig, 1969). Standard procedures were used such that separations were shortened for infants who became highly distressed. Videotapes of the sessions were coded according to procedures described in Ainsworth et al. (1978) by two coders trained by L. A. Sroufe. Intercoder agreement was 90% for subclassifications. Disagreements were resolved through conferencing. When coders could not agree or the behavior was ambiguous, L. A. Sroufe was brought in for consultation. Three infants were unclassifiable and possibly "D" relationships because the infants showed a combination of avoidant and resistant behavior. Because of the small number, these infants were not included in subsequent quality-of-attachment analyses. Of the remaining 63, 16% ($n = 10$) were Avoidant (A), 58% were Secure (B) (16 were B1 or B2 and 21 were B3 or B4), and 25% were Resistant ($n = 16$). Others have reported similar distributions for comparable samples (e.g., Belsky & Rovine, 1987).

In addition to quality-of-attachment coding, another coder, blind to classifications, scored all the tapes using the Emotional Tone Scale. Emotional Tone was scored every minute and averaged within each 3-min Strange Situation episode. (Again, the scale was reversed so that higher scores would reflect proneness-to-distress.) Agreement estimates (Cohen's kappa = 0.81) were obtained with the coder who scored the 9-month Louisville videotapes. Three summary Emotional Tone scores were computed: Preseparation (average of episodes 2 and 3), Separation (average of episodes 4, 6, and 7), and Reunion (average of episodes 5 and 8). These data were used to determine whether the division in emotional tone between A1–B2 and B3–B4 infants would be obtained and to determine whether this division held across preseparation, separation, and reunion phases of the Strange Situation.

Independence of coders/experimenters. All assessments were completed by coders and experimenters blind to infant and mother behavior in other assessments.

Salivary cortisol. Saliva was sampled for cortisol determination at both ages. The methods and results for salivary cortisol are reported in Gunnar et al. (1989).

RESULTS

Quality of attachment and emotional temperament. In order to assess both the security and the proposed temperament divisions of attachment classifications simultaneously, the classifications were organized into two dimensions. The security dimension had two levels of insecure versus secure (A and C vs. B) and the proposed temperament dimension had two levels of low versus high criers (A1–B2 vs. B3–C2). The 9-Month Temperament scores and the 13-Month Questionnaire Temperament scores were then analyzed using 2 (Insecure/Secure) × 2 (low/high criers) × 2 (age) analysis of variance with age as the repeated measure. The results revealed no significant main or interaction effects for security or for the low/high criers dimension (all F's <1.0).

A follow-up analysis was performed to determine that the A1–B2 versus B3–C2 infants were expressing the expected differences in emotional tone in the Strange Situation. A multivariate analysis of variance was computed using Preseparation, Separation, and Reunion measures of emotional tone in the Strange Situation. The low/high crier factor was highly significant, Hotellings $F(3,51) = 22.5$, $p < .001$. Univariate tests indicated that B3–C2 infants were more negative than A1–B2 infants for Preseparation, Separation, and Reunion measures of emotional tone, F's >4.0, p's $<.05$.

Maternal personality and maternal behavior. The T scores for the three higher-order factors on the MPQ exhibited means and standard deviations within the bounds expected for a normal sample. To examine the relations between these personality factors and maternal behavior, a stepwise multiple regression was performed with Maternal Warmth and Support as the dependent measure. The results showed that only Maternal Positive Affectivity contributed to the prediction of Maternal Warmth and Support with mothers who scored higher on positive affectivity also being warmer and more supportive of the baby (see Table 1).

Relations between maternal measures and infant emotional temperament. Because we had no strong prediction about the order of entry for the predictor variables, stepwise regressions were performed for both the 9-Month Emotional Tone and 13-Month Questionnaire measures of proneness-to-distress temperament. For the 9-month measure, the three higher-order maternal personality factors and Maternal Warmth and Support were entered as predictors. For the 13-Month Questionnaire measure, Emotional Temperament at 9 months was first entered to

TABLE 1

Regression Analyses for Relations Between Maternal Personality, Maternal Behavior, and Infant Temperament

DEPENDENT VARIABLES	BETAS FOR PREDICTORS					Multiple R	F	df
	Positive Affectivity	Negative Affectivity	Con- straint	Warmth/ Support	9-Month Temperament			
Maternal Warmth and Support ...	.30	N.S.[a]	N.S.	X[b]	X	.30	5.06*	1,58
9-month Temperament[c]	.30	N.S.	N.S.	-0.27	X	.46	6.82**	2,51
13-month Questionnaire[d]	N.S.	.31	N.S.	N.S.	-.38	.52	9.99**	2,55

[a] Nonsignificant, variable not in final equation.
[b] Variable not considered in the regression analysis.
[c] Louisville Assessment.
[d] Toddler Temperament Scale.
* $p < .05$.
** $p < .01$.

control for what was already known about the baby's emotional temperament, and then the maternal measures were entered as predictors. The results of both regression analyses are shown in Table 1. Proneness-to-distress at 9 months was predicted by lower scores on both Maternal Positive Affectivity and Maternal Warmth and Support. At 13 months, once the variance associated with the objective measure of infant proneness-to-distress temperament at 9 months was removed, mothers who reported their infants to exhibit more negative emotionality scored higher on Negative Affectivity.

Analyses were performed to further examine the relations between maternal variables and infant proneness-to-distress temperament at 9 months. Of the scales loading most highly on the Positive Affectivity factor, only Social Closeness was significantly correlated with infant proneness to-distress, $r(58) = -0.30, p < .05$. Of the three measures used to compute Maternal Warmth and Support, only the laboratory measure of Maternal Supportiveness was significantly associated with proneness-to-distress at 9 months, $r(64) = -0.37, p < .01$. Similar analyses were performed examining the scales loading most highly on Maternal Negative Affectivity and their relations with Questionnaire Temperament at 9 months. Only the scale of Stress Reactivity was significantly correlated with maternal reports of infant negative emotionality, $r(57) = 0.44, p < .01$.

Maternal measures and emotional tone in the Strange Situation. Preseparation, Separation, and Reunion emotional tone variables were examined controlling first for the two measures of proneness-to-distress temperament, the 9-Month Louisville Assessment measure and the 13-Month Toddler Temperament Questionnaire measure. The results of the three regression analyses yielded significant Multiple R's using the two temperament measures as predictors (Preseparation $= 0.34$, Separation $= 0.60$, and Reunion $= 0.38$) as expected from previous analyses (see Gunnar et al., 1989). Once temperament was controlled, the maternal measures did not add uniquely to the prediction of Strange Situation infant emotionality.

Maternal measures and security of attachment. Relations between security of attachment and the four major maternal measures were first analyzed using one-way Anovas and the molar A/B/C attachment classifications. The means and F values are shown in Table 2. None of the analyses were significant.

The possibility that 13-month attachment security could be predicted by the interaction of maternal and infant measures obtained earlier in development was explored next using the four maternal measures and the infant emotional temperament measure obtained at 9 months. The scores for emotional temperament at 9 months were divided at the mean to yield two groups: low proneness-to-distress (below the mean on the reverse-scored Louisville Emotional Temperament measure) and high proneness-to-distress (above the mean on the same measure). To provide a sufficient number of subjects in each cell, attachment classifications were regrouped into Secure (B) and Insecure (A and C) groups.

Neither Positive Affectivity, Negative Affectivity, nor Maternal Warmth and Support yielded significant interactions, p's $>.20$. However, a significant proneness-to-distress $\times$ security interaction was noted for constraint, $F(1,52) = 4.74$, p $<.05$. Newman-Keuls post-hoc tests using the harmonic n indicated that Maternal Constraint was not associated with attachment security for infants low on proneness-to-distress, but for infants high on proneness-to-distress, low maternal constraint was associated with secure attachment.

While the use of parametric analyses preserved statistical power, they placed security of attachment as an independent variable when, in fact, it was conceptually the dependent measure. For clarity, the significant interaction described above was reanalyzed nonparametrically. Chi-square tests were computed separately for low and high proneness-to-distress groups, examining the number of secure and insecure infants who had mothers scoring high (above the mean) or low (below the mean) on maternal constraint. The less powerful chi-square analysis produced results in the same direction as the more powerful parametric analysis (see Table 3).

DISCUSSION

Proneness-to-distress temperament at 9 months did not predict attachment classifications 4 months later. Despite strong evidence that the Louisville assessment provided a good measure of proneness-to-distress, it did not predict either the proposed temperament division of attachment categories (i.e., A1–B2 vs. B3–C2) or the security division (A and C vs. B). These null results did not appear to be due to developmental changes in proneness-to-distress temperament between 9 and 13 months because the Questionnaire Temperament measure obtained at 13 months also failed to differentiate A1–B2 from B3–C2 infants. In all, these data provided no support for the Belsky and Rovine (1987) argument that A1–B2 infants are less temperamentally prone to distress than are B3–C2 infants, nor for arguments that proneness-to-

TABLE 2

Relations Between Maternal Measures and Security of Infant Attachment

MATERNAL MEASURE	MEANS BY MOLAR ATTACHMENT CLASSIFICATIONS			F	p
	(A) Avoidant	(B) Secure	(C) Resistant		
Positive Affectivity	45.70	48.30	45.43	.58	N.S.
Negative Affectivity ...	45.20	47.24	45.93	.22	N.S.
Constraint	60.20	54.94	56.64	1.67	N.S.
Warmth/Support	.40	.04	$-.56$	.30	N.S.

NOTE.—N's for personality measures were 10, 33, 14 for A, B, and C, respectively; for Warmth and Support they were 10, 36, and 15 for A, B, and C, respectively.

distress temperament plays a significant, direct role in determining the security division of attachment classifications. Similar null relations were reported earlier between measures of adrenocortical stress reactivity and attachment classifications (Gunnar et al., in press).

The present results provided good evidence, however, for a link between maternal personality, maternal behavior, and infant emotional temperament. Mothers who expressed more warmth and provided more sensitive support of the baby at 9 months scored higher concurrently on the Positive Affectivity factor of the MPQ. Tellegen (Tellegen, 1985) has reported that the personality traits summarized by Positive Affectivity are those conducive to joy, excitement, and positive engagement. Low scores on this dimension should reflect depressive tendencies. The results were consistent, therefore, with those data indicating that maternal depression is associated with flat affect and poor sensitivity (Gaensbauer et al., 1984).

The results also indicated that both maternal Positive Affectivity and Warmth and Support were associated with the baby's emotional temperament at 9 months. Indeed, although correlated with one another, these variables contributed uniquely to the variance in proneness-to-distress. The aspect of maternal Warmth and Support most highly correlated with proneness-to-distress temperament was Maternal Supportiveness, a variable associated with emotional security in other studies (e.g., Ainsworth et al., 1978). The aspect of Positive Affectivity most strongly associated with 9-month proneness-to-distress was Social Closeness, suggesting that mothers who enjoy the company of others more have infants who are less prone to distress when being played with and left with new people. This is consistent with evidence that infants of extroverted mothers are less distressed by strange people and places (Daniels & Plomin, 1985; Weber et al, 1986). The similarity between mother and infant, as noted earlier, may reflect both genetic influence and the possibility that more extroverted mothers expose their infants to more new people and more stimulation.

TABLE 3

Relations Between Maternal Constraint, Infant Proneness-to-Distress Temperament, and Attachment Security

	Secure	Insecure
High proneness-to-distress:		
Low constraint	12	3
High constraint	7	8
		$\chi^2(1, N = 30) = 3.59, p < .10$
Low proneness-to-distress:		
Low constraint	7	8
High constraint	7	6
		$\chi^2(1, N = 28) = 0.36$, N.S.

Emotional temperament at 13 months was assessed using maternal report. As in the Matheny, Wilson, and Thobin (1987) study, the objective measure of infant temperament obtained from the Louisville assessment accounted for a significant proportion of variance in the maternal report measure, despite the fact that in our study the objective measure was obtained 4 months before the questionnaire measure. Interestingly, after removing the variance associated with the observational measure, maternal Negative Affectivity still contributed to the mother's report of her infant's temperament. Specifically, mothers scoring high on Negative Affectivity, possibly reflecting anger and anxiety (Tellegen, 1985), reported that their infants were more prone to distress than the objective, observational measure obtained earlier would have indicated. We cannot tell from these data whether this association reflects genetic or experiential factors, or merely the influence of maternal personality on maternal perceptions of the infant. This last possibility, however, is consistent with earlier findings by Matheny and his colleagues (1987).

The third issue was whether there were direct relations between maternal characteristics and infant emotionality in the Strange Situation. The results indicated that none of the maternal measures contributed to the prediction of emotionality in the Strange Situation once infant temperament at 9 months was controlled. Thus any influence of earlier maternal characteristics on later Strange Situation emotionality appears to operate through effects on infant proneness-to-distress temperament emerging earlier in development. In addition, none of the maternal measures was directly related to the molar attachment security classifications. This was somewhat surprising with regard to the Maternal Supportiveness measure as attachment theorists have argued that this aspect of maternal behavior determines the security of the relationship. Perhaps despite the fact that we observed the mother and infant long enough to obtain relations between maternal sensitivity/support and infant emotional temperament, our observation period was not long enough to detect relations with later attachment security. Attachment researchers (e.g., Vaughn et al., 1980) have suggested that one needs to observe for a number of hours to obtain measures of maternal sensitivity that are reliable enough to predict the course of the mother-infant relationship.

As noted earlier, however, the failure to find strong or reliable direct links between either infant or maternal characteristics and relationship security may also reflect the inadequacy of models assigning the development of attachment security solely or primarily to the characteristics of only one member of the relationship. As described by goodness-of-fit models, attachment security as well as other aspects of interpersonal relationships are most likely emergent qualities of the interplay between the characteristics of both members of a dyad (see Crockenberg, 1981). Our results are consistent with this view; an insecure relationship was more probable when infants who were prone to distress had mothers who were high on the MPQ Constraint factor. The fact that maternal characteristics appeared more crucial for infants high rather than low on proneness-to-distress temperament was similar to Crockenberg's (1981) finding that maternal social support predicted attachment quality only for the more difficult, irritable infants, and to her (Crockenberg, 1987) finding that relations between maternal anger/punitiveness and toddler anger/noncompliance were stronger if the infant had been high rather than low on irritability at 3 months of age. Taken together, these data suggest that while a prone-to-distress temperament does not cause an insecure or difficult mother-child relationship, it may narrow the range of caregiver environments in which the relationship can develop securely. The prone-to-distress infant most likely taxes the caregiver more, requiring that the caregiver has better emotional supports and a personality better suited for taking care of a demanding child. In addition, the prone-to-distress infant may also be more vulnerable to nonoptimal care.

We can only speculate on what the interaction patterns are like that might lead to insecurity for mothers and infants with a combination of high constraint and high proneness-to-distress. Certainly, Heinicke (1988) has reported that maternal sensitivity in dealing with infant proneness to separation distress is related to later positive socioemotional development. Furthermore, it would seem likely that mothers high on the two Constraint scales of traditionalism and control (i.e., low on impulsiveness) might be especially likely to respond rigidly and insensitively to their infants' distress in response to strangers and separation. These mothers both might be more concerned that, if reinforced, the distressed behavior might lead to later dependency, and they might also have more difficulty spontaneously altering their plans when their babies express a need for their presence. Mothers with similar high scores on Constraint, however, might have little difficulty providing adequate support to a baby who is less prone to distress and has less trouble with stressors.

To summarize, infant proneness-to-distress temperament appears to be related to both maternal personality and maternal behavior. In addition, maternal personality appears to influence maternal reports of infant temperament once objective indices of infant emotional temperament are controlled. No evidence was found, however, directly linking either infant proneness-to-distress temperament or maternal personality and behavior to attachment classifications deprived from the Strange Situation. Instead, attachment security could be predicted from an interaction between infant and mother characteristics, with maternal personality being a more crucial factor for infants high on temperamental proneness-to-distress. These data support the need to consider goodness-of-fit models in relating maternal and infant characteristics to attachment security. They also point to the need to consider both maternal personality and behavior in examining the correlates of infant temperament.

REFERENCES

Ainsworth, M., Blehar, M., Waters, E., & Wall, S. (1978). *Patterns of attachment.* Hillsdale, NJ: Erlbaum.

Ainsworth, M., & Wittig, B. (1969). Attachment and exploratory behavior of one-year-olds in a strange situation. In B. Foss (Ed.), *Determinants of infant behavior* (Vol.4, pp. 111–136). New York: Barnes & Noble.

Bates, J. E., Freeland, C.A.B., & Lounsbury, M. L. (1979). Measurement of infant difficultness. *Child Development, 50,* 794–803.

Belsky, J., & Isabella, R. (1988). Maternal, infant, and social-contextual determinants of attachment security. In J. Belsky & T. Nezworski (Eds.), *Clinical implications of attachment* (pp. 41–94). Hillsdale, NJ: Erlbaum.

Belsky, J., & Rovine, M. (1987) Temperament and attachment security in the strange situation: An empirical rapproachment. *Child Development, 58,* 787–795.

Campos, J. J., Barrett, K. C., Lamb, M. E., Goldsmith, H. H., & Stenberg, C. (1983). Socioemotional development. In M. M. Haith & J. J. Campos (Eds.), P. H. Mussen (Series Ed.) *Handbook of child psychology: Vol. 2. Cognitive development* (pp. 781–915). New York: Wiley.

Connell, J. P., & Goldsmith, H. H. (1982). A structural modeling approach to the study of attachment and Strange Situation behaviors. In R. N. Emde & R. J. Harmon (Eds.), *The development of attachment and affiliative systems* (pp. 213–242). New York: Plenum.

Connell, J. P., & Thompson, R. A. (1986). Emotion and social interaction in the Strange Situation: Consistencies and asymmetric influences in the second year. *Child Development, 57,* 733–745.

Crockenberg, S. (1981). Infant irritability, mother responsiveness and social support influences on the security of infant attachment. *Child Development, 52,* 857–865.

Crockenberg, S. (1987). Predictors and correlates of anger towards and punitive control of toddlers by adolescent mothers. *Child Development, 58,* 964–975.

Daniels, D., & Plomin, R. (1985). Origins of individual differences in human shyness. *Developmental Psychology, 21,* 118–121.

Egeland, B., Deinard, A., Taraldson, B., & Brunnquell, D. (1975). *Manual for feeding and play observation scales.* Minneapolis: University of Minnesota.

Egeland, B., & Farber, E. A. (1984). Infant-mother attachment: Factors related to its development and expression over time. *Child Development, 55,* 753–771.

Frodi, A., & Thompson, R. (1985). Infants' affective responses in the Strange Situation: Effects on prematurity and quality of attachment. *Child Development, 56,* 1280–1291.

Fullard, W., McDevitt, S.C., & Carey, W. B. (1984). Assessing temperament in one- to three-year-old children. *Journal of Pediatric Psychology, 9,* 205–216.

Gaensbauer, T. J., Harmon, R. J., Cytryn, L., & McKnew, D. H. (1984). Social and affective development in children with manic-depressive parents. *American Journal of Psychiatry, 141,* 223–229.

Goldsmith, H. H., & Alansky, J. A. (1987). Maternal and infant temperamental predictors of attachment: A meta-analytic review. *Journal of Consulting and Clinical Psychology,* **55,** 805–816.

Gunnar, M., Mangelsdorf, S., Larson, M., & Hertsgaard, L. (1989). Attachment, temperament and adrenocortical activity in infancy: A study of psychoendocrine regulation. *Developmental Psychology,* **25,** 355–363.

Heinicke, C. M. (1988, April). *Factors influencing the continuity of positive parent-infant mutuality.* Paper presented at the Sixth International Conference on Infant Studies, Washington, DC.

Kagan, J. (1982). *Psychological research on the human infant: An evaluative summary.* New York: William T. Grant Foundation.

Lamb, M. E. (1982). Parent-infant interaction, attachment and socioemotional development in infancy. In R. N. Emde & R. J. Harmon (Eds.), *The development of attachment and affiliative systems* (pp. 195–209). New York. Plenum.

Main, M., Kaplan, N., & Cassidy, M. (1985). Security in infancy, childhood, and adulthood: A move to the level of representation. In I. Bretherton & E. Waters (Eds.), Growing points in attachment theory and research. *Monographs of the Society for Research in Child Development,* **50**(Serial No. 209).

Matheny, A. P. (1984). Twin similarity in the developmental transformations of infant temperament as measured in a multi-method, longitudinal study. *Acta Geneticae Medicae Gemellologiae,* **33,** 181–189.

Matheny, A. P., Riese, M. L., & Wilson, R. S. (1985). Rudiments of infant temperament: Newborn to nine months. *Developmental Psychology,* **21,** 486–494.

Matheny, A. P., & Wilson, R. S. (1981). Developmental tasks and rating scales for laboratory assessment of infant temperament. *JSAS Catalog of Selected Documents in Psychology,* **11** (Ms. No. 2367).

Matheny, A. P., Wilson, R. S, & Thobin, A. S. (1987). Home and mother: Relationships with infant temperament. *Developmental Psychology,* **23,** 323–331.

Radke-Yarrow, M., Cummings, M., Kuczynski, L., & Chapman, M. (1985). Patterns of attachment in two- and three-year-olds in normal families with parental depression. *Child Development,* **56,** 884–893.

Riese, M. (1987). Longitudinal assessment of temperament from birth to 2 years: A comparison of full-term and preterm infant. *Infant Behavior and Development,* **10,** 347–363.

Sroufe, L. A. (1985). Attachment classification from the perspective of infant-caregiver relationships and infant temperament. *Child Development,* **56,** 1–14.

Tellegen, A. (1982). *Brief Manual for the Differential Personality Questionnaire.* Unpublished manuscript, University of Minnesota, Department of Psychology, Minneapolis.

Tellegen, A. (1985). Structures of mood and personality and their relevance to assessing anxiety, with an emphasis on self-report. In A. H. Tuma & J. D. Master (Eds.), *Anxiety and the anxiety disorders* (pp. 681–716). Hillsdale, NJ: Erlbaum.

Tellegen, A., Lykken, D., Bouchard, T., Wilcox, I., Segal, N., & Rich, S. (1988). Personality similarity in twins reared apart and together. *Journal of Personality and Social Psychology,* **54,** 1031–1039.

Thomas, A., & Chess, S. (1977). *Temperament and development.* New York: Brunner/Mazel

Thompsom, R. A., Connell, J. P., & Bridges, L. J. (1988). Temperament, emotion, and social interactive behavior in the Strange Situation: A component process analysis of attachment system functioning. *Child Development,* **59,** 1102–1111.

Vaughn, B., Taraldson, B., Crichton, L., & Egeland, B. (1980). Relationships between neonatal behavioral organization and infant behavior during the first year of life. *Infant Behavior and Development,* **3,** 47–66.

Weber, R. A., Levitt, M. J., & Clark, M. C. (1986). Individual variation in attachment security and strange situation behavior: The role of maternal and infant temperament. *Child Development,* **57,** 56–65.

Wilson, R. S., & Matheny, A. P. (1986). Behaviorgenetics research in infant temperament: The Louisville Twin Study. In R. Plomin & J. Dunn (Eds.), *The study of temperament: Changes, continuities and challenges* (pp. 81–98). Hillsdale, NJ: Erlbaum.

Part V
CLINICAL SYNDROMES

Diagnostic and statistical manuals describe disorders, whereas child psychiatrists and psychologists are, of course, concerned with children. In the first paper in this section—an overview of borderline disorders of childhood—attention is focused on a group of children whose patterns of behavioral disturbance do not fit comfortably into well-established diagnostic categories. Clinical accounts of children whose behavior is characterized by rapidly alternating symptoms; severe, often overwhelming anxiety; disproportionate outburst of anger; impulsivity; intermittent impairment of reality testing; magical and grandiose thinking; fantasies of omnipotence; and disturbed interpersonal relations, encompassing both aloof withdrawal and intense overinvolvement have regularly appeared since the early 1940s.

In their review of this literature, Petti and Vella suggest that children who have been designated by clinicians as "borderline" can be divided into two broad categories: borderline personality disorder/borderline spectrum and schizotypal personality disorder/autism/schizophrenia spectrum classifications. Clinical descriptions, biological correlates, delimitation from other disorders, outcome, family studies, hypothesized etiologies, therapeutic considerations, and responses to treatment are presented for each.

This summary of the phenomenology and metapsychology of these children who are difficult to characterize, diagnose, and treat, provides a needed orientation to what are becoming increasingly heated diagnostic debates. Petti and Vella urge that premature closure of classifications of children who fail to meet current diagnostic criteria be avoided. Tasks for future research include the development of reliable, valid rating scales and trait markers, as well as the further delineation of subtypes with attention devoted to their clinical, neurophysiological, and neuropsychological features, etiologies, and specific therapeutic interventions.

The diagnosis of personality disorders during childhood and adolescence is an aspect of child psychiatry that is currently in a state of flux and marked by controversy. In view of generally modest associations between childhood behavioral and personality attributes and adult psychiatric disorder, many clinicians and investigators are reluctant to make a diagnosis of personality disorder during a period of rapid developmental change. Progress in this area, too, has been hampered by a lack of personality assessment instruments with established reliability for adolescents.

Brent, Zelenak, Bukstein, and Brown's examination of the reliability and validity of the Structured Interview for the *DSM-III* Diagnosis of Personality Disorder (SIDP) is a step toward remedying this gap. Subjects were 23 affectively ill adolescents and their parents. Interviews were videotaped and rerated. All but three subjects (87 percent) met criteria for at least one personality trait or disorder. Overall reliability, as calculated by a weighted $_k$ coefficient, was modest (mean $_k$ = 0.49) ranging from $_k$ = 0.24 for borderline personality disorder to $_k$ = 1.00 for schizoid disorder. Some support for the validity of Cluster II personality disorders (borderline, histrionic, narcissistic) was found. Cluster II patients tended to have higher rates of attention deficit disorder and bipolar disorder and higher rates of suicidal gestures among second-degree relatives. The authors reported some difficulty differentiating symptoms of affective illness from those of personality disorder and deciding when personality traits were impairing enough to call them disorders. Nevertheless, the findings are promising. A methodology is at hand to investigate the stability of personality disorder diagnoses during the adolescent period, not only among those with affective disorders, but with other Axis I conditions as well.

The stability over time of yet another clinical condition—obsessive-compulsive disorder (OCD)—is the subject of the report by Flament, Koby, Rapoport, Berg, Zahn, Cox, Denckla, and Lenane. Twenty-five of 27 patients (93 percent) who had participated in a study of severe primary OCD with onset in childhood or adolescence, were seen two to seven years after initial study and compared with a group of normal controls who were matched for age, sex, and IQ and followed up for the same period.

The findings are striking. Only seven (28 percent) of the subjects received no psychiatric diagnosis at follow-up. Of the remaining 18 subjects, 17 still had OCD: five were diagnosed with OCD only; and 12 patients also received another psychiatric diagnosis, most commonly anxiety and/or depression. The one patient who no longer had OCD but had another form of major psychopathology was a 17-year-old boy with atypical psychosis. At the time of initial assessment, this boy had been considered atypical because of the lack of egodystonicity of his straightening rituals and defective communication skills. Neither initial response to clomipramine nor any other baseline variable predicted outcome. The stability of the diagnosis of OCD in this clinically referred sample was remarkable. The authors point out that none of the children had received drug treatment or sufficiently intense behavioral treatment to satisfy current criteria of adequacy. Whether more effective interventions will serve to modify what these data suggest is the chronic character of childhood onset OCD is a subject for much-needed future research.

Studies of depressive disorders in childhood and adolescence abound, yet less attention has been directed toward a consideration of manic symptomatology. Carlson's review provides the reader with an overview of the current state of knowledge regarding the diagnosis of child and adolescent mania. The clusters and variation of symptoms of classical mania have deviated little from Kraepelin's description. Although the characteristics of the disorder are clear, involving expansive and volatile mood that reflects itself in grandiosity, overcommitment, recklessness, and displeasure at being thwarted; and tireless energy that is manifested by hyperactivity, pressured speech, racing thoughts, inability to maintain attention, and feeling that sleep is unnecessary, the range of severity has been considerably less clear.

Carlson points out that distinctions among normality, hypomania, and mania reflect differences in degree of disorder, whereas differences among mania, psychotic mania, schizoaffective mania, and schizophrenia raise questions about different kinds of disorders. Furthermore, there is still no unequivocal way to make the distinctions. Time-honored criteria such as degree of thought disorder or presence of first-rank symptoms and mood incongruence of psychotic symptoms have not been reliable in distinguishing a manic course from a schizophrenic course. Similar problems have bedeviled the recognition of mania in children and adolescents. Although Kraepelin recognized the condition in about 3 percent of patients by age 15 and almost 20 percent by age 20, the boundaries between mania and schizophrenia, disruptive behavior disorders, and adjustment reactions during the developmental period have been difficult to assess. This is partly due to strongly held, prevailing biases of clinicians. Carlson's review is an important step in dispelling these biases and in pointing out the need for longitudinal studies to discover the extent to which illness manifestations are age related or state or trait dependent.

As Benjamin, Costello, and Warren point out, the expression of anxiety as a symptom, a syndrome, and a disorder of childhood has been known to the psychiatric community since the 19th century, yet a belief that childhood anxiety symptoms are transient and innocuous, as well as a lack of agreed diagnostic criteria have inhibited systematic epidemiological investigation. This report of anxiety disorders in a pediatric sample addresses this gap in knowledge. The subjects were 300 children aged seven to 11, selected from a sequential sample of 789 children enrolled in a health maintenance organization. Psychiatric interviews with children and parents using the Diagnostic Interview Schedule for Children (DISC) yielded a one-year weighted prevalence for one or more *DSM-III* anxiety disorders of 15.4 percent, combining diagnoses based on either child or parent interviews. Consistent with findings of other studies indicating that children are better reporters of subjective symptoms like anxiety and depression than their parents, the prevalence rate for anxiety disorders based on parent interviews alone was only half as high (6.6 percent) as the rate based on child interviews alone (10.5 percent).

Different informants also provided different pictures of the degree of functional impairment in children with anxiety disorders. Parents judged them to have good social functioning but high levels of psychiatric symptoms, whereas teachers judged anxious children to have no more psychopathology than normal children but to show impaired social and academic functioning. The study raises important methodologic questions that are thoughtfully discussed. In addition, the findings underscore the amount of distress and impaired functioning caused by anxiety that is experienced by children in the community.

The final paper in this section is a comprehensive review of the effects of chronic disease during childhood and adolescence. Eiser focuses on the impact of illness on the individual child and on the family. Her careful summary provides a sound basis for concluding that the field has undergone significant change in recent years. A traditional deficit-centered model increasingly is being replaced by approaches that take account of coping resources and individual competence. Rather than focus on the identification of psychopathology, professionals are beginning to see children and families dealing with chronic illness as ordinary people in exceptional circumstances rather than as deviant. Nevertheless, chronically ill children remain vulnerable in terms of physical health and behavioral, social, and emotional maladjustment. Along with their families, they continue to require tangible help and guidance.

17

Borderline Disorders of Childhood: An Overview

Theodore A. Petti
University of Pittsburgh School of Medicine
Ricardo M. Vela
Albert Einstein College of Medicine, New York City

This selected review considers children classified as "borderline" and focuses on two broad categories: Borderline personality disorder/ borderline spectrum and schizotypal personality disorder/autism/ schizophrenia spectrum classifications. Clinical descriptions, biological correlates, delimitation from other disorders, outcome, family studies, hypothesized etiologies, therapeutic considerations, and response to treatment are presented for each. Data support the subclassification of the heterogeneous groupings of borderline children into at least the two categories, and their differentiation from each other and from other clinical disorders in the population. Overlap across the borderline categories exists for individual children. The nature and shortcomings of relevant studies are described, the need for scientifically based research championed, and a differential approach to directive treatment of borderline children advocated. Further subclassification of borderline disorders should result in more cost-effective diagnosis and treatment.

A body of literature describing severely disturbed children whose clinical pictures cross over several diagnostic categories has developed. Rich clinical descriptions in terms of individual cases and large groups of borderline children have abounded (Mahler, et al., 1949; Weil, 1953; Ekstein and Wallerstein, 1954; Geleerd, 1958;

Reprinted with permission from *Journal of the American Academy of Child and Adolescent Psychiatry,* 1990, Vol. 29, No. 3, 327–337. Copyright ©1990 by the American Academy of Child and Adolescent Psychiatry.

Marcus, 1963; Rosenfeld and Sprince, 1963; Frijling-Schreuder, 1969; Pine, 1974, 1986; Chethik, 1979, 1986; Morales, 1981; Kernberg, 1983a; Robson, 1983; Bemporad, et al., 1987). There appear to be two major streams of classification. First, psychoanalytic and psychodynamic authors have created a rich, descriptive literature which contributes a psychodynamic perspective for classification and treatment. In the 1950s, child psychoanalysts began describing a group of children who were distinguishable from frankly psychotic children, yet more severely disturbed than "psychoneurotic" children. These children exhibited serious ego development disturbances, were prone to overwhelming anxiety, and manifested ego fragmentation and regression when exposed to everyday stresses. Upon removal of the stress, they were noted to regain their reality testing ability, as contrasted to the less reversible nature of the psychosis in psychotic children. Magical and grandiose thinking, responses to fantasy as real, and very disturbed relationships with others were more frequently observed in the borderline child, as compared to normal or neurotic children by the analysts (Mack, 1975).

The second stream is more descriptive and has concentrated on youngsters bordering on the schizotypal/autistic/schizophrenic spectrum of childhood disorders. Wolff and Chick (1980) comment on the similar descriptions of "borderline" youngsters from both streams: abnormal psychological defenses, intrusion of primary process thinking into their waking life, omnipotence perceived in interactions with others, a long duration of symptomatology, and poor response to interpretive psychotherapy.

This review has arbitrarily divided those severely disturbed children into two sets of disorders: (1) the borderline personality disorder (BPD) (APA, 1980; 1987)/borderline spectrum; and (2) the schizotypal personality disorder (SPD) (APA, 1980; 1987)/autistic/schizophrenic spectrum. The overview will consider the historical antecedents of these categories and their overlap; discuss issues of controversy, including clinical descriptions, posited etiologic mechanisms, biological correlates, and outcome; and consider therapeutic interventions. A major effort will be made to demonstrate that the general area of borderline disorders can be divided into more distinct categories which correspond to BPD/type/borderline spectrum and SPD/autism/schizophrenia spectrum disorders.

CLINICAL DESCRIPTION

The clinical description is meant to delineate the association of specific clinical features in characterizing a particular disorder. Though many clinicians seem to find the concept of borderline children useful, its validity has not been established. The heterogeneity of borderline disorders has resulted in varied clinical descriptions depending on the group under discussion and the orientation of the clinical researcher.

Borderline Personality Disorder/Borderline Spectrum

Freud's 1918 description of the Wolfman may have been the first retrospective psychoanalytic description of a borderline child/adolescent (Anthony, 1983). Mahler and associates (1949) considered a variety of more "benign" cases of childhood psychosis "in which larger parts of the personality remained intact," as compared to those with frank psychosis due to their ability to employ "neurosis-like defense mechanisms." Weil (1953, 1956) described "certain severe disturbances of ego development" which evolved around the areas of social adaptation, manageability, and "neurotic-like" behavior. In 1954, Ekstein and Wallerstein used the term "borderline" to describe children, analogous to the "borderline" adults depicted by Knight (1953). These children were notable for their alternation of neurotic and psychotic ego organization and fluctuations in functioning during the therapy hour. A number of psychoanalytically oriented papers followed describing characteristics and dynamics (Geleerd, 1958; Marcus, 1963; Rosenfeld and Sprince, 1963; Frijling-Schreuder, 1969; Pine, 1974; Morales, 1981; Bemporad et al., 1987). An edited work (Robson, 1983) provides a comprehensive overview.

In an attempt to obtain a consensus on the diagnosis of borderline disorder in children, Vela et al. (1983) analyzed the text of seven key psychoanalytically oriented works addressing this topic and "translated" the psychoanalytic terminology into descriptive terms. Reported behaviors were clustered together into groups of symptoms. Six symptoms were agreed upon by six or more of the authors: (1) disturbed (intense) interpersonal relationships, (2) disturbances in the sense of reality, (3) excessive intense anxiety, (4) impulsive behavior, (5) fleeting "neurotic-like" symptoms, and (6) uneven or distorted development. High agreement on this core group of symptoms may indicate that the authorities were describing a similar psychiatric disorder.

Other schema outside *DSM-III-R* (APA, 1987) have been proposed. Bemporad and associates (1982) have developed a set of diagnostic criteria based on a literature review and consideration of 24 hospitalized, latency-aged children. The characteristics areas of general pathology may be summarized as follows: (1) relationships to others; (2) thought content and processes; (3) nature and extent of anxiety; (4) lack of control; (5) fluctuations in functioning; and (6) associated features which are said to include poor social functioning, inability to learn from experience or adapt to novel situations, and poor hygiene. As can be seen, the first four symptoms correspond with Vela's consensus criteria (with fluctuations in functioning implicit throughout), especially in the manifestation of disturbance in interpersonal relationships.

Developmental, instinctual, ego, and object relations deficits are also frequently considered major features of borderline children (Chethik, 1986). Other subclassifications have been suggested for such borderline children, including "fluid" (Gilpin, 1981) and "highly functioning" borderline children (Chethik, 1986).

Morales (1981) has tried to integrate the psychoanalytic oriented literature to define a borderline spectrum which runs from the psychotic end to the narcissistic personality disorder end. Though these sub-categories have not been validated by research, their range illustrates the heterogeneity of the clinical presentation of borderline children.

Borderline disorders of childhood are not included in the section of "Disorders Usually First Evident in Infancy, Childhood or Adolescence," but the *DSM-III-R* specifies that the BPD "should be diagnosed in children and adolescents, rather than the corresponding children disorders, if the Personality Disorder criteria are met, the disturbance is pervasive and persistent, and it is unlikely that it will be limited to a developmental stage. The other Personality Disorder categories (e.g., Schizotypal Personality Disorder) may be applied to children or adolescents in those unusual instances in which particular maladaptive personality traits appear to be stable" (p. 335).

In the most stinging indictment of the concept, Gualtieri et al. (1983) report that none of the 16 children, 6 to 13 years of age, referred as "borderline" for inpatient care or comprehensive evaluation, met *DSM-III* criteria for BPD (APA, 1980). The authors conclude that child psychiatrists seemed to use the term "more to denote a disorder characterized by disorganized cognitive faculties, but less severe or pervasive than childhood psychoses" (p. 70). No mention was made as to whether the children met criteria for SPD, though nine were diagnosed as attention deficit disorder with hyperactivity, two with adjustment reaction, and one each with "Conduct Disorder," "Conduct Disorder and ADD + H," "Childhood schizophrenia," "Adjustment reaction and ADD + H," and separation anxiety disorder.

Schizotypal Personality Disorder/Autism/Schizophrenia Spectrum

In 1944, Asperger described a psychiatric syndrome which he named "Autistic Psychopathy of Childhood" (AP). These children were characterized by abnormalities of gaze, poverty of expression and gesture, as well as unusual voice production. Those with high intelligence would become specialists in the natural sciences, mathematics, engineering and art, while those with low intelligence would function as "automata," and when of intermediate intellect as eccentrics (Wolff and Barlow, 1979). Resembling many children labeled as "borderline" or "schizotypal" today, they often displayed learning disabilities and difficulties in concentration or of being distracted from within. Similar to children with infantile autism, their social adaptation was impaired and they were unable to experience empathy, or conform to social conventions.

Wolff and Barlow (1979) list the clinical features of "schizoid personality in childhood" (SPC) as: emotional detachment and being solitary; lack of adaptability or rigidity assuming obsessional proportions; sensitivity (easily hurt, touchy) marked by periodic suspiciousness and paranoid ideation; lack of empathic feelings towards others; and "odd ideation often with metaphorical use of language" (p. 30). These children with SPC were differentiated from autistic children by the presence of language, emotional responsiveness toward others, and lack of involvement in ritualistic and compulsive behavior. The clinical features were considered to be almost identical to those described by Asperger. Classification as a personality disorder was justified by the nature of its lifelong and unchanging patterns of deviate functioning, and persistence of the disorder into adulthood (Wolff and Chick, 1980).

Asperger's (AP) description of SPD type children has been repeatedly supported by the literature except that AP includes impaired nonverbal communication, while SPD of *DSM-III* includes abnormal perceptual experiences and ideas of reference as symptoms. Nagy and Szatmari (1986) reviewed 20 charts of children identified by pediatricians and psychiatrists as having at least one symptom related to disordered thinking and one to social isolation or oddities of behavior. Many of the 18 boys and two girls had a number of chart diagnoses including borderline autism, BPD, borderline psychosis, schizoaffective disorder, and childhood neuroses. All met three or more SPD criteria (with 18 meeting four or more) and had documented magical thinking/bizarre preoccupations, social isolation, and social anxiety; all were considered by their parents as abnormal before age 5 years but able to relate better to adults. None could establish or maintain friendships with peers. Rarely found were ideas of reference, paranoid thinking, or illusions. However, several workers considered children meeting criteria for AP to be experiencing a variant of autism or pervasive developmental disorder (PDD) (Wing, 1981; Rutter, 1985; Pomeroy and Friedman, 1987; Bowman, 1988); while others consider SPD to be on the schizophrenic disorder spectrum (Russell et al., 1987). Pomeroy and Freidman (1987), in a retrospective chart review, selected children with chronic socialization problems (not secondary to shyness or anxiety), hallucinations, delusions and/or obsessive/compulsive symptoms, but not meeting criteria for the diagnosis of infantile autism or severe brain injury. Separating the group into early (before age 3 years) and late (after 5 to 7 years), they found the early group could be subdivided into an autistic and schizoid spectrum; while the latter group seemed to be comprised of children resembling Asperger's and the *DSM-III* schizoid disorder diagnoses. The neuropsychological profile of the children diagnosed as AP showed little evidence of gross deficits in language and was characterized by lateralizing features indicative of nondominant hemisphere dysfunction.

Pine (1983), in his broad use of the concept "borderline," considers "schizoid personality" of childhood to be part of the borderline group of children. However, the nature of the interpersonal relationships differentiate borderline children from those under the schizoid/schizotypal spectrum. Borderline children are considered overdependent, possessive, overdemanding, and socially disinhibited (Vela et al.,

1983), while schizoid children are considered solitary, emotionally detached, and unempathic (Wolff and Chick, 1980).

BIOLOGICAL CORRELATES

As child psychiatry begins to employ techniques useful in understanding the neurophysiological and neuropsychological correlates of psychiatric disorders, we can expect marked advances regarding the borderline disorders. To date, several rich paths to investigate childhood borderline disorders have begun to be defined.

BPD/Borderline Spectrum

The association of organic brain pathology and children diagnosed as "borderline" appears repeatedly in the literature. Rosenfeld and Sprince (1963) were the first to note the finding of "organicity" in some borderline children. In a follow-up of 29 subjects with infantile borderline psychosis, Wergeland (1979) found neurological signs of brain damage and pathological EEGs in 10 of them. Aarkrog (1981) reports evidence of organicity manifested by abnormal EEGs, physical signs of brain damage, or signs of brain damage in psychological testing in nine out of 29 borderline adolescents who had been evaluated in childhood. Bemporad and associates (1982) reported evidence of "organic involvement" in 22 of 24 borderline children. This was manifested by a variety of findings including abnormal (nondiagnostic) EEGs, visual-motor problems, history of early seizures, attentional disorder and hyperactivity, poor fine and gross motor coordination, speech articulation problems, reading and mathematical disability, petit mal seizures, and others. However, a preliminary study revealed no significant differences in signs of minimal brain damage in children meeting borderline personality organization criteria compared to a clinic group not meeting the criteria (Liebowitz, 1984).

Rogeness and associates (1984) have investigated dopamine-beta-hydroxylase (DBH) in disturbed children. The deficiency of this enzyme can result in either excess dopamine or deficient norepinephrine and could be related to the dopamine hypothesis of schizophrenia or the norepinephrine hypothesis of depression. Lowered DBH levels have been found in autistic children, children who are psychotic, and children with conduct disorder, undersocialized (UCD). Twenty emotionally disturbed boys whose DBH values were less than or equal to 2μ/min/L plasma were compared to 20 emotionally disturbed boys with DBH values greater than 15μ/min/L. All had required psychiatric hospitalization. Most of the boys with the lower levels had values of zero (the zero DBH group). Forty percent of the zero DBH group were diagnosed as BPD.

In a larger study, the UCD group of boys with near-zero DBH demonstrated more schizotypal, schizophrenic, and borderline symptoms, particularly, brief psychotic episodes, than did the conduct disorder, socialized boys with DBH levels greater than six (Rogeness et al., 1986). However, the wide range of activity in normal populations for the DBH enzyme makes it unreliable as a marker or indicator of underlying neurophysiological disorder (Cohen et al., 1983).

It is evident that there is no pathognomic finding or any one-to-one correlation between a specific organic pathology and the development of borderline disorders in children. However, the high incidence of "organicity" in these children raises various possibilities: (1) that the presence of organic involvement (broadly defined) predisposes to the development of borderline disorder in children; (2) there is a subgroup of borderline children with an organic etiology (which raises the question of the important differential diagnosis between borderline disorder and organic personality syndrome); and (3) the combination of organic and environmental factors (see section on etiology) contributes to the development of borderline disorder. Additional research is needed to elucidate this issue.

SPD/Autism/Schizophrenia Spectrum

Significantly higher platelet levels of monoamine oxidase activity were demonstrated in boys under 13 years with SPD and schizophrenia than matched controls or boys with major depressive disorder (MDD). Whole blood serotonin levels were also significantly higher for SPD and schizophrenia groups as compared to the MDD group, but not significantly different from the control group (Rogeness et al., 1985).

Nagy and Szatmari (1986) report a high frequency in SPD children of various neurodevelopmental markers of brain dysfunction, e.g., clumsiness, EEG abnormalities, and psychometric test deficits. Such nonspecific findings have been reported in most studies of borderline and conduct disordered children and, hence, add little to validity though they may be more frequent in SPD than BPD children (Petti and Law, 1982).

DELIMITATION FROM OTHER DISORDERS

Exclusionary criteria are considered by Feighner and associates (1972) as the major factor in differentiating a particular diagnosis. This has been a particular problem with the borderline diagnoses. However, studies do support the borderline classification as having unique characteristics and allowing differentiation from other disorders.

Leichtman and Nathan (1983) have described the highly atypical and distinctive manner in which such children function in response to differing aspects of the testing situation. In contrast to other children, borderline children openly demonstrate their conflicts and problems during testing, without the need for specific test instruments, and in a manner which compels the examiner's attention. "They tend to be anxious, impulsive, and intolerant of frustration; they exhibit pronounced character-ological and interpersonal problems; they are subject to abrupt mood swings and sharp regression; and they are apt to interpret the world around them and to interact with others in idiosyncratic ways" (p. 124).

BPD/Borderline Spectrum

Borderline disorders in children have been differentiated from neurotic, schizotypal, psychotic, and other severe childhood disorders using different diagnostic criteria and methodologies. Petti and Law (1982) reviewed the charts of 10 children, ages 6 to 12 years of age, who were hospitalized for severe psychopathology and manifested borderline psychotic features. The symptoms described in the hospital record were matched to the *DSM-III* criteria for BPD, SPD, and PDD. An eleventh child was dropped from the study because he met criteria for all three disorders. Five of the children met criteria for BPD and five for SPD. Criteria for PDD were met by two children in both the BPD and SPD groups. Significant differences were found between the groups regarding symptoms comprising the criteria for each (with children meeting BPD criteria demonstrating greater impulsivity, unstable relationships, problems with anger, affective instability, self-damaging acts) and for the total of BPD symptom ratings. They suggest that the retrospective analysis of hospital-records methodology did not allow for an even greater differentiation in symptoms between the groups.

The overlap of SPD and BPD diagnoses in the child excluded from the analysis is consistent with the 20% overlap found in adults (Spitzer et al., 1979). In contrast to this, a recent study of children with SPD reports no overlap at all, although it does not appear that the BPD criteria were a specific focus of the data collection (Russell et al., 1987).

Liebowitz (1984), in a preliminary report, employed modified structural criteria of Kernberg (1977) in diagnosing borderline personality organization. Of the 65 children and adolescents, ages 6 to 17, seen for comprehensive outpatient evaluation, 17 met criteria for borderline personality organization; when these youngsters were compared to the other 48, they demonstrated a statistically significant increase in frequency of all BPD symptoms except for intolerance of being alone. the borderline personality organization group also had significantly greater amounts of intense anxiety, depression and low self-esteem, omnipotent-grandiose fantasies, lack of empathy, no lasting peer-group relationships, and disorganization.

Bentivegna and associates (1985) applied Bemporad's criteria in a chart review study and were able to significantly differentiate 70 borderline children from two other control groups.

Adult criteria for differentiating individuals with a borderline personality disorder (Gunderson and Singer, 1975) have also been employed in children (Bradley, 1979;

Greenman et al., 1986). In a retrospective study of 86 hospitalized 6- to 12-year-olds, Greenman and associates used a modified adult scale, the Diagnostic Interview for Borderlines (DIB-R)(Gunderson et al., 1981), to identify borderline children and to demonstrate the extent to which the youngsters manifested features described in the literature (i.e., the Bemporad criteria). Moderate concordance between the Bemporad criteria and modified adult criteria was documented. They concluded that the validity and utility of the term to describe youngsters meeting that set of adult (Gunderson) and Bemporad criteria are in question, since they found few significant differences between identified borderline and none-borderline children serving as controls. However, the methodology is flawed. The selection criteria lack specificity (Gualtieri and Van Bourgondien, 1987). Over 30% of the children were diagnosed as borderline using the DIB-R, of which only two (7%) were diagnosed as BDP and 15% "other personality disorder." In contrast, 5% were diagnosed as BPD in the non-borderline control group!

Employing broad criteria for borderline diagnoses, Rubin and associates (1984) statistically differentiated borderline from neurotic children, with the former having more severe behavioral pathology, disturbances in ego functions and modulation of affect, as well as difficulties in directing attention. However, selection criteria overlapped considerably with the Degree of Disturbance Scale employed.

Verhulst (1984) obtained 28 items from the literature, said to distinguish borderline from other children, and asked Dutch child psychiatrists to endorse those that were specific to a borderline, neurotic, and psychotic child in their practice. Scoring highest were "social isolation" (97%), "micropsychotic episodes" (93%), "high level of anxiety" (91%), and "predominantly primitive defense mechanisms" (91%). Of the 28 characteristics described for borderline children, only the presence of marked separation anxiety, feelings of loneliness, and hyperactivity failed to be significantly different between borderline and "neurotic" children. Likewise, a psychotic child was described as having significantly less "demanding, clinging, and unpredictable relationships," "predominantly primitive defense mechanisms," shifting levels of ego functioning, and feelings of loneliness than a borderline child. Characteristics reported significantly more often in psychotic, compared to borderline children, included "withdrawn, aloof in contact with others," need fulfilling relationships, language and speech peculiarities, special interest or talent in one area, and resistance to change in the environment. Methodological flaws in the study include a potentially biased sample.

SPD/Autism/Schizophrenia Spectrum

The two studies employing *DSM-III* criteria support the differentiation of SPD children from others in the same clinical setting. Compared to BPD children, those with SPD demonstrated increased symptoms of magical thinking, odd speech, inadequate rapport, suspiciousness/paranoia, and total of SPD ratings (Petti and law, 1982)). Likewise, in comparing schizotypal personality traits in the borderlines, compared to the others, significant differences were found in distrust, suspiciousness and paranoid ideation, hypersensitivity with a trend toward significance in peculiar thoughts and bizarre fantasies, and average total number of SPD traits (Liebowitz, 1984).

In a carefully controlled study comparing children from 4.5 to 14.0 years of age (mean = 9.5), diagnosed as either SPD (*DSM-III*) or schizophrenia, Russell and associates (1987) report that 20 met SPD and 35 schizophrenia criteria. One SPD child did not meet the *DSM-III-R* revised criteria calling for five rather than four associated symptoms. Full criteria for SPD were met by 69% of the children with a schizophrenic disorder. Only social anxiety/sensitivity to criticism was found to be statistically significant more frequently in the SPD group. Significantly less hallucinations, delusions, and thought disorder were found in the SPD compared to the schizophrenia controls. Additional *DSM-III* diagnoses, but not BPD, were found in 80% of the SPD children. The authors assert that SPD should be reclassified as schizotypal disorder and added to the Axis I of the DSM, given its phenomenological close relationship to the diagnosis of schizophrenia; or the diagnosis and criteria should be listed in the childhood disorders section. This is much in line with Meehl's (1962) suggestion that borderline disorders exist on a continuum of "schizotypy" with schizophrenia (Shapiro, 1983). SPD children do manifest symptoms of both schizophrenia and PDD (Nagy and Szatmari, 1986).

Wolff and Barlow (1979) compared children labeled SPC with well-functioning autistic and normal children on tests of cognitive processes, language, memory, and intelligence. They report that the SPC group cooperated less on tests of memory, cognition, and language and were less motivated to succeed than the other two groups; inner preoccupation seemed to hamper performance. The SPC group was intermediate in scatter in subtest scores between the normal and autistic control groups. On the Illinois Test of Psycholinguistic Abilities, the autistic and SPC groups had mainly negative, while the normal controls had positive subtest scores on most items. Schizoid children were clearly higher functioning and showed less repetitive behavior on tests of perseveration and pattern impositions than autistic children, and could not be differentiated from normal controls. Overall, the SPC children functioned intermediately between the control groups, sharing the stereotypy and tendency to impose patterns, some linguistic handicaps, and lack of perceptiveness for meaning with the autistic controls.

OUTCOME

Determining the course of a disorder assists in ruling out whether the disorder could be attributed to another disorder or illness, and the extent to which the original diagnosis describes a homogeneous group. Available studies provide some interesting information concerning the course of the disorder. Most studies, however, are poorly controlled, employ loose definitions of children defined as borderline, and consider the psychodynamically defined borderline child.

BPD/Borderline Spectrum

No systematic studies have been reported on the course of children diagnosed as BPD. However, a number of studies have examined groups of children falling within the spectrum. Kestenbaum (1983), employing the consensus criteria (Vela et al., 1983), reviewed seven cases, retrospectively diagnosed as borderline, which had been in treatment. After 14 to 30 years, one of the seven was diagnosed as BPD, one as SPD, one as schizoid, two as schizophrenia, one as bipolar disorder, and one as anxiety disorder. These results suggest that the consensus criteria, as a reflection of early "lumping" efforts of nosologists, may lack predictive validity except to predict extensive psychopathology.

Etemad and Szurek (1973) reviewed the charts of 84 children, 27 diagnosed as "borderline," using Ekstein and Wallerstein's definition of the disorder. The follow-up period extended from 5 to 23 years, and the age range of the patients at the time of the last follow-up was from 10 to 34 years. Outcome was limited to the need for rehospitalization and no data were provided about the diagnosis at follow-up. About 41% of the sample was not hospitalized after discharge, while the rest required different degrees of continued hospitalization. No conclusion about outcome can be made from this study except that the majority of the cases appeared to have a serious disturbance requiring prolonged intensive treatment.

In another study, Wergeland (1979) followed up 29 "borderline psychotic" children who had been hospitalized for observation in a psychiatric unit. The children were diagnosed using Ekstein and Wallerstein's, Pine's, and Brask's definitions of borderline children. The follow-up period was 4 to 19 years and the age range at follow-up was 12 to 30 years. About one-third of the patients were still borderline or "manifest psychotic" at the time of follow-up, regardless of whether they received treatment or not. The rest were either symptom free or had varying degrees of neurotic symptomology. This study points toward a better prognosis for these children than would be expected. However, there was a selection bias in the study: the more disturbed children were the ones who were assigned for treatment.

Aarkrog (1981) studied 50 borderline adolescents referred for adolescent psychiatric ward hospitalization. She used the Danish classification for borderline states, comprising three main types: infantile borderline psychosis (with four subtypes), pseudoneurotic, and pseudopsychopathic borderline states. The study consisted of two parts: a follow-back study and a 5-year real time prospective study. Of the 50 adolescents, 29 had been evaluated in childhood, 11 of them diagnosed as "infantile borderline psychosis" following the Danish classification. At the time of the follow-up, 70% of the borderline adolescents were still borderline. The 11 children diagnosed as "borderline infantile psychosis" in childhood continued to be borderline through adolescence and early adulthood (Aarkrog, 1981; personal communication).

In conclusion, even though most clinicians seem to assume that borderline children grow into borderline adults and that borderline psychopathology has its developmental roots in early childhood, there is some *supportive* but no *conclusive* evidence that this is the case. Additional research involving controlled follow-up studies, with adequate samples, definite, inclusive diagnostic criteria, and standardized methods of measuring outcome into adulthood are needed in order to establish predictive validity. Possible guides for future studies are available from those with young adults (McGlashan, 1986a, b).

SPD/Autism/Schizophrenia Spectrum

Asperger reported that only one of the 200 boys he identified later developed a schizophrenic disorder. Wolff and Chick (1980) carefully followed the schizoid borderlines and have confirmed the earlier findings of Asperger. Matched to a control group of children with other psychiatric disorders referred to the same child psychiatric department, 22 boys with schizoid disorder were followed about 10 years later. Schizoid disorder was diagnosed in 18 of the SPC boys and one control. On follow-up, the schizoids were "clearly deficient in their interpersonal relationships"; with most showing impaired empathy and odd style of communication. In a related work, Cull et al. (1984) report a 12-year follow-up of 23 SPC boys demonstrating significant correlation and continuity of the SPC disorder over time. Preliminary results of a later study with schizoid and control subjects at a mean age of 28 years, confirms that a majority of the schizoid children are indistinguishable from SPD adults, with 19 of 25 schizoid children diagnosed as SPD; four controls were later diagnosed as SPD. Three "schizoids" and no controls were identified as borderline using a scaled score of 7 or greater on the DIB. In addition, only one definite and one doubtful case of schizophrenia were identified at the follow-ups of the SPC youngsters at mean ages of 22 and 28 years, respectively (Wolff, 1989).

FAMILY STUDIES

No controlled family or genetic studies have been conducted for the borderline disorders of childhood. Asperger's early description noted that some of the boys had mothers with the disorder. He later reported a family member with features of the disorder for all the boys that he studied (Nagy and Szatmari, 1986). Bowman (1988) described a father and his four sons who present symptoms along the autism/

Asperger spectrum in terms of clinical psychological and psycholinguistic profiles. Separating familial from genetic factors is of critical importance, since familial contributions have been strongly suggested as a major factor in adolescent (Shapiro, 1978) and adult (Gunderson et al., 1980) borderlines and BPD (Torgersen, 1984), while genetic factors seem to influence the development of SPD diagnosed in adults (Torgersen, 1984).

ETIOLOGIES PROPOSED FOR THE BORDERLINE DISORDERS

A panoply of etiologies have been proposed for the development and maintenance of the borderline child. Psychoanalysts have posited irregularities in the early mother-child relationship and disturbances in ego development (Geleerd, 1958; Rosenfeld and Sprince, 1963; Mahler, 1971; Masterson, 1972; Masterson and Rinsley, 1975; Rinsley, 1980; Chethik, 1986). Support for the theoretical role of disruption of the early infant–mother bond in borderline pathology has been provided by the findings of Bradley (1979). History of maternal separation before the age of 5 years was statistically greater in a group of 14 children and adolescent borderline patients than in control groups of psychotic, nonpsychotic, and delinquent children. Minimal brain dysfunction, severe developmental or sensory deficits (e.g., deafness or blindness), or developmental lags possibly interacting with psychodynamic factors (Kernberge, 1983a) may be considered causal or associated conditions.

Bemporad and associates (1982), besides notion the increasing frequency of organic impairment in their borderline sample when compared to siblings or to children with other forms of psychopathology, report histories of abuse, neglect, and inconsistent care. Mothers were noted to be frequently unstable, easily frustrated, and unable to sustain empathic relationships; the fathers showed difficulty in self-control and instability in relationships. One or both parents often participate in or encouraged the unrealistic fantasies of the child. Pine (1986) offers an integrative psychoanalytic model that assumes neurophysiological handicaps and/or toxic environmental conditions that impact on failure to develop core aspects of higher functioning and result in maladaptive coping mechanisms, thus leading to the development of the borderline child.

THERAPEUTIC CONSIDERATIONS

Given the heterogeneous nature of borderline children, therapeutic treatment becomes a major challenge. The entire armament of child psychiatry has been focused and advocated for borderline children, including education and appropriate behavioral management (Wing, 1981), psychoanalytically oriented psychotherapy (Rinsley, 1980; Gilpin, 1981; Kernberg, 1983b), collaborative therapy (Weger et al., 1981), partial hospitalization (Stambler and Mutter, 1981; Hanson et al., 1983), intensive residential treatment (Lewis and Brown, 1979, 1980; Masterson and Rinsley, 1975), family interventions (Weger et al., 1981; Combrinck-Graham, 1986) and psychopharmacology (Petti and Unis, 1981; Petti, 1983).

The differential diagnosis is critical in treatment planning for this group of children. As Kernberg (1983b) notes, the organic and psychological factors must be assessed in borderline children in order to appropriately plan for and implement effective treatment.

BPD/Borderline Spectrum

Psychotherapy for borderline children evolved from the classical psychoanalytic principles used with reported success in the treatment of neurotic adults and children. In recent years, the trend has been to emphasize modifications in psychotherapeutic technique required to divert psychotic functioning and strengthen defense mechanisms.

Ekstein and Wallerstein (1956) examined the technical problems of the use of psychoanalytic interpretations in therapy and recommended the use of "interpretation within the regression," thus supporting the therapist's primary aim of maintaining the relationship and preventing the disruption of contact. Interpretations aiming at insight were to be made only after lessening regressive tendencies. Communication was to remain within primary process fantasy and modes of expression, until the child had acquired the "strength" to move to a more mature position. Examples used to illustrate this technique reveal that the therapist would not confront the child with cognitive distortions and maladaptive psychotic thinking, but rather would agree with the child's false beliefs during what would appear to be mini-psychotic episodes.

Rosenfeld and Sprince (1965) later proposed modifications to facilitate repression and displacement rather than making unconscious material conscious. They emphasized that children had to be helped to build up defenses, and that therapists should provide a function similar to the "auxiliary ego," help the child become aware that tension can be contained, and facilitate the use of displacement as a defense mechanism. They asserted that the affect, tone, or facial expression of the therapist is of greater importance than the verbal content of an interpretation, and questioned the usefulness of interpreting aggressive impulses. Gilpin (1976) reviewed the literature that emphasizes the critical importance in developing stable introjects and details an illustrative case wherein the therapist serves as an auxiliary ego in assisting with verbalizations over making decisions, in sorting out complexities, and in differentiating causal relationships. The pivotal role of interpreting transference is stressed.

In contrast to this, Lewis and Brown (1979) emphasize fostering the development of reality testing through helping the child recognize and understand his/her reactions to various events occurring in daily life, and clarifying distinctions between reality and fantasy. Providing a consistent object (interpersonal) relationship and helping the child to develop mastery mechanisms and to maintain control during the therapy hour, in order to limit regressive, sexualized, and aggressive behavior to manageable levels, were considered to be critical. Chethik (1979) similarly suggests that interpretations in therapy with borderline children should be ego supportive, helping the child to build up defenses and to strengthen and develop coping skills.

Smith et al. (1982) advocate the use of four major modalities: psychotherapy, medication, family therapy, and environmental support. They divide the treatment of borderline children into three stages: (1) allaying anxiety and making an alliance, (2) promoting ego development, and (3) internalization. Anxiety is seen as an obstacle in the formation of a therapeutic alliance. During the first phase of treatment, exploration of anxiety is avoided as this may escalate into panic. The therapist curtails the elaboration of sexual and aggressive fantasy material, avoids dynamic exploration and may need to restrain the child physically if he or she becomes aggressive. During the second stage, the therapist helps strengthen every area of the child's development and defensive structure. The dangers of regression, panic, and loss of control are monitored and the therapist talks with the child about events occurring in his/her real life in order to avoid isolation from the therapist. The last phase is seen as somewhat open-ended, analogous to therapy with neurotic children, and frequently extending into young adulthood.

The importance of resolving separation-individuation issues in borderline children is stressed by Kernberg (1983b), as she enumerates the associated "mirroring" functions and their relevance to the therapist in helping to resolve the pathological clinging, shadowing, and darting. For the young borderline child, she advocates working with the mother-child dyad in making manifest the anxieties and fears of abandonment, total loss, or annihilation. She presents a set of 12 considerations for the psychodynamic therapist to address.

Vela and Petti (1988) have suggested a more directive model of therapy for borderline disorders of childhood. Nondirective therapy is seen as counterproductive in the treatment of borderline children. Vela (1988) argues that psychotherapy for borderline children must involve the clarification of limits from the beginning, monitoring the expression of feelings, providing structure when necessary, clarifying the difference between reality and fantasy, discouraging regressed, withdrawn and psychotic behavior, and directly confronting maladaptive behavior. Cognitive misperceptions should be modified and corrected.

SPD/Autism/Schizophrenia Spectrum

In speaking of Asperger's syndrome, Wing (1981) asserts that the handicaps can be addressed through appropriate management and education. She cites the importance for both parents and teachers in recognizing the difficulties, sometimes subtle, in comprehension of abstract language which can make communication difficult. Wing suggests that the repetitive speech and motor habits cannot be extinguished, but can be modified to make them more socially useful and acceptable over time. The goal of education is to develop the child's special interests and general competence to the extent that will allow independence in later life.

Most descriptions of psychodynamically oriented therapeutic interventions focus on the BPD spectrum child where the techniques are consonant with the theoretical and etiologic constructs. Bauer and Modarressi (1977) provide a theoretical basis for working with SPD spectrum children from object relationship theory and developmental ego psychology perspectives. The strategies to allow "joining" therapist and child are nicely illustrated.

PSYCHOPHARMACOTHERAPY

Psychopharmacological interventions are being used with increasing frequency in controlling the symptoms of the borderline disorders, particularly those associated with BPD (Petti, 1983; Petti and Law, 1982; Rogeness et al., 1984). Rinsley (1980) has suggested that psychotropic medications for borderline children be targeted to specific symptoms, e.g., stimulations for hyperactivity an imipramine for depression. A biological mechanism has been posited by Rogeness and associates (1984) who noted that significantly more of their zero DBH boys were treated with psychotropics than the comparison group. They report that 25% required a combination of neuroleptic drugs and methylphenidate, which allowed successful placement outside the hospital setting, and suggest that the combination may redress neurotransmitter imbalances through multiple channels, as may imipramine.

The work of Schulz and associates (1988) highlights the heterogeneous responses of borderline patients to psychotropic agents as earlier described by Klein (1975) for adults and Petti (1983) for children. Diverse groups of medications, ranging from anxiolytic agents, tricyclic antidepressants, psychomotor stimulants, neuroleptics, and lithium have been described as helping ameliorate symptoms in borderline disordered children. Select anticonvulsants (e.g., carbamazepine and valproic acid) may assume an even greater role in the future as children with an organic component are better delineated.

The psychopharmacological treatment of borderline patients may call for greater clinical skill than for any other childhood disorder or syndrome as related to expectations, fears, fantasies, conflicts, etc., of children and their families regarding medication (Petti and Sallee, 1986). Psychotherapeutic support is often vital in successful pharmacotherapy of childhood borderline conditions (Petti, 1989). Specific guidelines for medication of children with the borderline disorders have not developed.

RESPONSE TO TREATMENT

Cantwell (1985) suggested that response to treatment is a critical component of the validation process. The "medical model" holds that outcome with regard to course or response to therapeutic intervention is really the test of the diagnosis as an hypothesis. Unfortunately, no well-controlled group studies exist to which we can turn. Of 62 treated borderline cases reviewed by Bentivegna and associates (1985), 32 improved, 25 showed no change, and five became worse. The better treatment outcome correlated with the length of treatment and with receiving some residential treatment. A case study (Petti and Unis, 1981) and anecdotal case reports suggest that BPD borderline children respond to imipramine treatment. If researchers in the field would accept operational definitions of the disorder, e.g., those for SPD and BPD, develop rating scales, and use them in sound single case design or, optimally, in multisite collaborative studies, then we should be able to better support the existence of subgroups of "borderline" children and their differential response to treatment.

DISCUSSION

Issues related to borderline disorders for both children and adults continue to engender much discussion. BPD has been used as a descriptor of a clinical picture of an unstable personality and psychodynamically as both a descriptor of personality organization and as an indicator of severity or degree of impairment. The question of whether the diagnostic criteria should include a history of transient, but self-limited, deficits in reality testing persists (Widiger et al., 1988). The same may be said for the BPD diagnosis in children and adolescents. Alternatively, transient psychotic episodes may indicate degree of severity of even a unique subgroup of both BPD and SPD spectrum children.

Likewise, SPD/SPC and schizoid personality disorders (APA, 1987) have been considered as separate disorders, as well as either variants along a schizophrenia spectrum of a single personality disorder in adults (Widiger et al., 1988). The recent report and review by Wolff (1989) offers further support for this view. The modification of *DSM-III-R* allowing SPD and schizoid personality disorder to be diagnosed in the same person and not to be exclusionary, redefine Wolff's group even more into the SPD classification. This in turn suggests that the major differential for this group will be SPD, PDD, and schizophrenic disorder and that such youngsters can be removed from the classification of borderline disorders.

Current wisdom suggests that the amount of space required to present a topic area is inversely proportional to the degree of scientific certainty associated with it. The borderline disorders of childhood support this rule. This review has attempted to present material representative of the literature. At this point an attempt will be made to summarize the current state of the field:

1. The generic term "borderline" when applied to children can reasonably be divided into two broad syndromes: the BPD/borderline spectrum and SPD/ schizotypal spectrum syndromes with some overlap in individual cases. Children meeting criteria for either cluster can be differentiated from children from general or clinical populations.

2. The BPD group remains a heterogeneous amalgam of wide ranging psychopathology with repeated efforts by clinicians to classify and subclassify the very disturbed children falling within its purview. However, there is a core group of psychopathological symptoms with which most clinicians seem to agree.

   (a) The co-morbidity with other psychiatric disorders (e.g., UCD, ADHD, specific and mixed developmental disabilities) obscures the group's definition.

   (b) Continuity with the adult forms of BPD spectrum disorders has been demonstrated in some studies. Poor outcome and persistent psychopathology is expected for most children falling within this spectrum of disorders. Retrospective studies suggest that the related adult disorders begin during childhood.

   (c) Familial loading for the disorder is probably the result of a neurodevelopmental predisposition interacting with inadequate, insufficiently nurturing parenting figures in a conflictual or abusive environment.

   (d) Psychotropic agents do have a beneficial effect on ameliorating distressing associated symptoms and seem to assist these children to better organize their thinking and to increase aspects of self-control, while decreasing the disabling panic experienced during conflict. Well controlled, double-blind group studies for this group have not been reported.

   (e) Dynamic, structured, long-term psychotherapies can be very effective in assisting BPD spectrum children to develop the requisite skills, controls, and interrelatedness with peers required to function in the mainstream. Educational and/or residential programs (when needed) play a critical role in the overall care for such children as do education and supportive work with the families. The traditional role of intensive psychoanalytic psychotherapy and psychotherapeutic intervention has been questioned. Controlled studies have not been conducted.

3. The SPD group appears to be more homogeneous in the clinical presentation of children so diagnosed; but the range and severity of psychopathology is extensive. However, the following conclusions can be drawn:

   (a) Predictive validity has been demonstrated for the non-*DSM-III-R* SPC (equivalent to SPD of the *DSM-III-R*) subgroup. The children who fit into this classification should be treated and studied as a syndrome, distinct from the general classification of borderline children and comprised of specific disorders.

(b) The SPD group falls within the less severe pathology region of the schizophrenia spectrum, but the evolution of the clinical picture into full schizophrenic or autistic disorders is infrequent. The finding by Russell and associates (1987) of significantly more sensitivity to criticism in SPD, as compared to children with a schizophrenia disorder, also suggests a higher level of relatedness in the SPD group.

(c) The reported familial loading for SPD is probably genetically based and manifested through the differential expression of biochemical and neuropsychological mechanisms.

(d) Currently available psychotropic agents do not serve a major role in SPD spectrum children except possibly to ameliorate targeted symptoms, e.g., hyperactivity, depression, anxiety, or transient psychotic decompensation. Educationally oriented and directive psychotherapeutic interventions with emphasis on learning theory based therapies offer the greatest benefit to SPD spectrum children at this time.

CONCLUSION

In conclusion, we must avoid premature closure of classifications of children who fail to meet our current diagnostic categories. There appear to be a number of borderline disorders with differing etiologies, phenomenology, associated features, and required treatments. Assuming the premise of this overview that borderline conditions in children can be roughly divided into BPD and SPD spectrum classifications with little overlap, then the task for present and future research involves (1) development of reliable, valid rating scales, and trait markers and; (2) the further delineation of the subtypes, with attention devoted to their clinical, neurophysiological, and neuropsychological features, etiologies, and specific therapeutic interventions. We must accept the fact that our classification of disorders affecting children is still early in its development and that "borderline" represents a syndrome about which we have a number of paths to explore, subtypes to delineate, and intervention strategies to test. Thus, we must build upon the existing rich data base and insights which astute clinicians and researchers have provided.

REFERENCES

Aakrog, T. (1981), The borderline concept in childhood, adolescence and adulthood. *Acta Psychiatr. Scand.*, (Suppl. 392).

American Psychiatric Association. (1987), *Diagnostic and Statistical Manual of Mental Disorders, (Third Edition-Revised)*, Washington, DC: American Psychiatric Association.

———(1980), *Diagnostic and Statistical Manual of Mental Disorders (Third Edition)*, Washington, DC: American Psychiatric Association.

Anthony, E.J. (1983), The borderline child in an overall perspective. In: *The Borderline Child*, ed. K.S. Robson. New York: McGraw-Hill, pp. 11–29.

Asperger, H. (1944), Die autistischen psychopathen im kindesalter. *Archiv fuer Psychiatrie und Nervenkrankheiten*, 177:76–137.

Bauer, R. & Modarressi, T. (1977), Strategies of therapeutic contact: working with children with severe object relationship disturbance. *Am. J. Psychother.* 31:605–617.

Bemporad, J.R., Smith, H.F., & Hanson, G. (1987), The borderline child. In: *Basic Handbook of Child Psychiatry, (Vol. 5)*, ed. J. Noshpitz, New York: Basic Books, Inc., pp. 305–311.

————————————& Cicchetti, D. (1982), Borderline syndromes in childhood: criteria for diagnosis. *Am. J. Psychiatry*, 139:596–601.

Bentivegna, S.W., Ward, L.B. & Bentivegna, N.P. (1985), Study of a diagnostic profile of the borderline syndrome in childhood and trends in treatment outcome. *Child Psychiatry Hum. Dev.*, 15:198–205.

Bowman, E.P. (1988), Asperger's syndrome and autism: the case for a connection. *Br. J. Psychiatry*, 152:377–382.

Bradley, S.J. (1979), The relationship of early maternal separation to borderline personality in children and adolescents: a pilot study. *Am. J. Psychiatry*, 136:424–426.

Cantwell, D. (1985), Depressive disorders in children, validation of clinical syndromes. *Psychiatr Clin North Am.* 8:779–791.

Chethik, M. (1986), Levels of borderline functioning in children: etiological and treatment considerations. *Am. J. Orthopsychiatry*, 56:109–119.

————(1979), The borderline child. In: *The Basic Handbook of Child Psychiatry, (Vol. II)*. ed. J. Noshpitz, New York: Basic Books, Inc., pp. 304–321.

Cohen, D.J., Shaywitz, S.E., Young, J.G. & Shaywitz, B.A. (1983), Borderline syndromes and attention deficit disorders of childhood: clinical and neurochemical perspectives. In: *The Borderline Child*, ed. K.S. Robson, New York: McGraw-Hill, pp. 197–221.

Combrinck-Graham, L. (1986, March), *The borderline syndrome in childhood: the family systems approach*. Presented at Borderline Syndrome in Children, Minneapolis, MN.

Cull, A., Chick, J., & Wolff, S. (1984). A consensual validation of schizoid personality in childhood and adult life. *Br. J. Psychiatry*. 144:646–648.

Ekstein, R. & Wallerstein, J. (1956), Observations on the psychotherapy of borderline and psychotic children. *Psychoanal. Study Child*. 11:303–311.

————————(1954), Observations on the psychology of borderline and psychotic children. *Psychoanal. Study Child*, 9:344–369.

Etemad, J.G. & Szurek, S.A. (1973), A modified follow-up study of a group of psychotic children. In: *Clinical Studies in Childhood Psychoses*, eds. S.A. Szurek & I.N. Berlin. New York: Brunner/Mazel, pp. 348–371.

Feighner, J.P., Robins, E., Guze, S.B., Woodruff, R.A., Winokur, G. & Munoz, R. (1972), Diagnostic criteria for use in psychiatric research. *Arch. Gen. Psychiatry*, 26:57–63.

Freud, S. (1918), From the history of an infantile neurosis. In: *Collected Papers, (Vo. 3)*. New York: Basic Books, pp. 473–605, 1959.

Frijling-Schreuder, E. (1969), Borderline states in children. *Psychoanal. Study Child*, 24:307–327.

Geleerd, E. (1958), Borderline states in childhood and adolescence. *Psychoanal. Study Child*, 13:279–295.

Gilpin, D.C. (1981), The true fluid borderline child in psychotherapy. In:*Three Further Faces of Childhood*, eds. E.J. Anthony & D.C. Gilpin. New York: Spectrum Publications, pp. 257–267.

————(1976), Psychotherapy of borderline psychotic children. *Am. J. Psychother.* 30:483–496.

Greenman, D.A., Gunderson, J.G., Cane, M. & Saltzman, P.R. (1986). An examination of the borderline diagnosis in children. *Am. J. Psychiatry*, 143:998–1003.

Gualtieri, C.T. & Van Bourgondien, M.E. (1987), So-called borderline children. *Am. J. Psychiatry*, 144:832.

————Koriath, J. & Van Bourgondien, M.E. (1983), "Borderline" children. *J. Autism Dev. Disord.*, 13:67–62.

Gunderson, J.G. & Singer, M.T. (1975), Defining borderline patients: an overview. *Am. J. Psychiatry*, 132:1–10.

————Kolb, J.E. & Austin, W. (1981), The diagnostic interview for borderline patients. *Am. J. Psychiatry*, 138:896–903.

————Kerr, J. & Englund, D.W., (1980), The families of borderlines. *Arch. Gen. Psychiatry*, 37:27–33.

Hanson, G., Bemporad, J.R. & Smith, H.F. (1983). The day and residential treatment of the borderline child. In: *The Borderline Child*, ed. K.S. Robson. New York: McGraw-Hill, pp. 257–276.

Kernberg, O. (1977), The structural diagnosis of borderline personality of organization. In: *Borderline Personality Disorders: The Concept, the Syndrome, the Patient*, ed. P. Hartocollis. New York: International Universities Press, pp. 87–121.

Kernberg, P.F. (1983a), Borderline conditions: childhood and adolescent aspects. In: *The Borderline Child*, ed. K.S. Robson. New York:McGraw-Hill, pp. 101–109.

————(1983b), Issues in the psychotherapy of borderline conditions in children. In: *The Borderline Child, ed. K.S. Robson. New York: McGraw-Hill*, pp. 223–256.

Kestenbaum, C.J. (1983), The borderline child at risk for major psychiatric disorder in adult life. In: *The Borderline Child*, ed. K.S. Robson. New York: McGraw-Hill, pp. 49–81.

Klein, D.F. (1975), Psychopharmacology and the borderline patient. In: *Borderline States in Psychiatry*, ed. J.E. Mack. New York: Grune and Stratton, pp. 75–91.

Knight, R. (1953), Borderline states, *Bull, Menninger Clin.* 17:1–12.

Leichtman, M. & Nathan, S. (1983), A clinical approach to the psychological testing of borderline children. In: *The Borderline Child*, ed. K.S. Robson. New York: McGraw-Hill, pp. 121–170.

Lewis, M. & Brown, T.E. (1980), Child care in the residential treatment of the borderline child. *Child Care Quarterly*, 9:41–50.

————————(1979), Psychotherapy in the residential treatment of the borderline child. *Child Psychiatry Hum. Dev.* 9:181–188.

Liebowitz, J.M. (1984; October), *Personality traits of borderline children and adolescents: an empirical study*. Presented at the Annual Meeting of the American Academy of Child Psychiatry, Toronto, Canada.

Mack, J.E. (1975), Psychopharmacology and the borderline patient. In: *Borderline States in Psychiatry*, New York: Grune & Stratton.

Mahler, M.S. (1981), "A study of the separation—individuation process: and its possible application to borderline phenomena in the psychoanalytic situation." *Psychoanal. Study Child*, 26:403–424.

————Ross, J.R., Jr. & DeFries, Z. (1949), Clinical studies in benign and malignant cases of childhood psychosis. *Am. J. Orthopsychiatry*, 19:295–305.

Marcus, J. (1963), Borderline states in childhood. *J. Child Psychol. Psychiatry.* 4:208–218.

Masterson, J.R. (1972), Treatment of the borderline adolescent: a development approach. In: *The Borderline Syndrome*, eds. J.F. Masterson & D.B. Rinsley. New York: Wiley.

————& Rinsley, D.B. (1975), The borderline syndrome: The role of the mother in the genesis and psychic structure of the borderline personality. *Int. J. Psychoanal.*, 56: 163–177.

McGlashan, T.H. (1986a), The Chestnut Lodge follow-up study: III. long term outcome of borderline personalities. *Arch. Gen. Psychiatry*, 43:20–30.

————(1986b), Schizotypal personality disorder. *Arch. Gen. Psychiatry*, 43:329–334.

Meehl, P.E. (1962), Schizotaxia, schizotypy, schizophrenia. *American Psychologist*, 17:827–838.

Morales, J. (1983), The borderline spectrum in children. In: *Three Further Faces of Childhood*, eds. E.J. Anthony & D.C. Gilpin. New York: Spectrum Publications, pp. 221–230.

Nagy, & Szatmari, P. (1986), A chart review of schizotypal personality disorders in children. *J. Autism Dev. Disord.* 16:351–367.

Petti, T.A. (1989), Individual psychotherapy in children. In: *The Comprehensive Textbook of Psychiatry (Fifth Edition)*, eds. H.I. Kaplan & B.J. Sadock, Baltimore: Williams & Wilkins, pp. 1910–1926.

————(1983), Psychopharmacologic treatment of borderline children. In: *The Borderline Child*, ed. K.S. Robson. New York: McGraw-Hill, pp. 235–256.

————& Sallee, F.R. (1986), Issues in childhood and adolescent psychopharmacology. In: *Advances in Learning and Behavioral Disabilities, (suppl. 1)* eds. K.D. Gadow & A.D. Poling. Greenwich, CT:JAI Press, Inc., pp. 281–311.

————& Law, W. (1982), Borderline psychotic behavior in hospitalized children: approaches to assessment and treatment. *J. Am. Acad. Child Psychiatry*, 21:197–202.

————& Unis, A. (1981), Imipramine treatment of borderline children: case reports with a controlled study. *Am. J. Psychiatry*, 138:515–518.

Pine, F. (1986), On the development of the "Borderline-Child-To-Be." *Am J Orthopsychiatry*, 56:450–457.

————(1983), A working nosology of borderline syndromes in children. In: *The Borderline Child*, ed. K.S. Robson. New York: McGraw-Hill, pp. 83–100.

————(1974), On the concept "Borderline" in children. *Psychoanal. Study Child*, 29:341–368.

Pomeroy, J.C. & Friedman, C. (1987), *Asperger Syndrome— a clinical sub-type of PDD: the neuropsychological evidence.* Presented at the Annual Meeting of the Academy of Child and Adolescent Psychiatry, Washington, D.C.

Rinsley, D.B. (1980) Diagnosis and treatment of borderline and narcissistic children and adolescents. *Bull. Menninger Clin.*, 44:147–170.

Robson, K.S. (1983), *The Borderline Child: Approaches to Etiology, Diagnosis, and Treatment.* New York: McGraw-Hill.

Rogeness, G.A., Hernandez, J.M., Macedo, C.A., Amrung, S.A. & Hoppe, S.K. (1986), Near-zero plasma dopamine-B-hydroxylase and conduct disorder in emotionally disturbed boys. *J. Am. Acad. Child Psychiatry*, 25:251–527.

———Mitchell, E.L., Custer, G.J. & Harris, W.R. (1985), Comparison of whole blood serotonin and platelet MAO in children with schizophrenia and major depressive disorder. *Biol. Psychiatry*, 20:270–275.

———Hernandez, J.M., Macedo, C.A., Mitchell, E.L., Amrung, S.A. & Harris, W.R. (1984), Clinical characteristics of emotionally disturbed boys with very low activities of dopamine-B-hydroxylase. *J. Am. Acad. Child Psychiatry*, 23:203–208.

Rosenfeld, S, & Sprince, M. (1965), Some thoughts on the technical handling of borderline children. *Psychoanal. Study Child*, 20:495–517.

————(1963), An attempt to formulate the meaning of the concept "borderline." *Psychoanal. Study Child*, 18:603–635.

Rubin, S. S., Lippman, J. & Goldberg-Hier, M. (1984), Borderline and neurotic children: what's the difference anyhow? *Child Psychiatry Hum. Dev.*, 15:4–20.

Russell, A.T., Bott, L. & Sammons, C. (1987), *The phenomenology of schizotypal disorder of childhood: A schizophrenia spectrum disorder?* Presented at the Annual Meeting of the American Academy of Child and Adolescent Psychiatry, Los Angeles, CA.

Rutter, M. (1985), Infantile autism and other pervasive developmental disorders. In: *Child and Adolescent Psychiatry: Modern Approaches (Second Edition)*, eds. M. Rutter & L. Hersov. Oxford: Blackwell Scientific Publications, pp. 545–566.

Schultz, S.C., Cornelius, J., Schulz, P.M. & Soloff, P.H. (1988), The amphetamine challenge test in patients with borderline disorder. *Am. J. Psychiatry*, 145:809–814.

Shapiro, E. (1978), Research on family dynamics: clinical implications for the family of the borderline adolescent. *Adoles. Psychiatry*, 6:36–376.

Shapiro, T. (1983), The borderline syndrome in children: a critique. In: *The Borderline Child*, ed. K.S. Robson, New York: McGraw-Hill, pp. 12–29.

Smith, H.F., Bemporad, J.R. & Hanson, G. (1982), Aspects of the treatment of borderline children. *Am. J. Psychother.*, 36:181–199.

Spitzer, R.L., Endicott, J. & Gibbon, M. (1979), Crossing the border into borderline personality and borderline schizophrenia: the development of criteria. *Arch. Gen. Psychiatry*, 36:17–24.

Stambler, M. & Mutter A.Z. (1981), The institution as family: creating a "holding environment" for treating disorders of the self in children and parents from multiproblem families. *Psychiatr. Clin. North Am.* 4:549–560.

Torgersen, S. (19844), Genetics and Nosological aspects of schizotypal and borderline personality disorders. *Arch. Gen. Psychiatry*, 41:546–554.

Vela, R.M. (1988, September), *Psychotherapy of borderline children*. Paper presented at Bronx-Lebanon Hospital Center, NY.

———& Petti, T.A. (1988, May), *Borderline disorder of childhood: theory and practice*. Presented at 141st Annual Meeting of the APA, Montreal, Quebec, Canada.

———Gottlieb, E.H. & Gottlieb, H.P. (1983), Borderline syndromes in childhood: a critical review. In: *The Borderline Child*, ed. K.S. Robson, New York: McGraw-Hill, pp. 31–48.

Verhulst F.C. (1984), Diagnosing borderline children. *Acta Paedopsychiatrica*, 50:161–173.

Weger, L., Gilpin, D. & Morales, J. (1981), The borderline child in the Jones family: collaborative therapy with a borderline child. In: *Three Further Faces of Childhood*, eds. E.J. Anthony, & D.C. Gilpin. New York: Spectrum Publications, pp. 243–255.

Weil, A.P. (1956), Some evidence of deviational development in infancy and early childhood. *Psychoanal. Study Child*, 11:292–299.

———(1953), Certain severe disturbances of ego development in childhood. *Psychoanal. Study Child*, 8:271–286.

Wergeland, H. (1979), A follow-up study of 29 borderline psychotic children 5 to 20 years after discharge. *Acta Psychiatr. Scand.*, 60:465–476.

Widiger, T.A., Frances, A., Spitzer, R.L. & Williams, J.B. (1988), The *DSM-III-R* personality disorders: an overview. *Am. J. Psychiatry*, 145:786–795.

Wing, L. (1981), Asperger's Syndrome: a clinical account. *Psychol. Med.*, 11:115–129.

Wolff, S. (1989, March), *Schizoid disorders of childhood*, Paper presented at The Sheppard and Enoch Pratt Hospital, Baltimore, MD.

———& Barlow, A. (1979), Schizoid personality in childhood: a comparative study of schizoid, autistic and normal children. *J. Child Psychol. Psychiatry*, 20:29–46.

———& Chick, J. (1980), Schizoid personality in childhood: a controlled follow-up study. *Psychol. Med.* 10:85–100.

18

Reliability and Validity of the Structured Interview for Personality Disorders in Adolescents

David A. Brent

Western Psychiatric Institute and Clinic, Pittsburgh

Janice P. Zelenak

St. Francis Health System, Pittsburgh

Oscar Bukstein and Robert V. Brown

Western Psychiatric Institute and Clinic, Pittsburgh

The Structured Interview for the DSM-III *Personality Disorders was administered to 23 currently affectively ill adolescents and their parents. Interviews were videotaped and recreated; interrater agreement was moderate (weighted* κ =0.49; *unweighted* κ = 0.59). *Moreover, there was evidence of convergent validity for Cluster II traits and disorders (borderline, histrionic, narcissistic), insofar as these diagnoses were associated with higher scores on the novelty-seeking subscale of the Tridimensional Personality Questionnaire as predicted. Cluster II patients tended to have higher rates of attention deficit disorder and bipolar disorder, and higher rates of suicidal gestures among second-degree relatives. Some difficulty was encountered differentiating symptoms of affective illness from those of personality disorder and in deciding when personality traits were impairing enough to call using*

Reprinted with permission from *Journal of the American Academy of Child and Adolescent Psychiatry,* 1990, Vol. 29, No. 3, 349–354. Copyright © 1990 by the American Academy of Child and Adolescent Psychiatry.

This project was supported in part by seed proposal #144 from MHCRC as well as the W.T. Grant Foundation, and NIMH KO8 MH00581-01 Clinical Investigator Award to the first author. The expert administrative assistance of Karen Rhinaman is gratefully acknowledged, as well as the helpful advice of Dr. Bruce Pfohl and Ms. Dalene Stangl. This paper is dedicated to the memory of Joaquim Puig-Antich, M.D., 1944–1989.

*standardized functional impairment criteria for differentiating person-
ality style from disorder. Additional work is advocated to learn if personality disorders are precursors, epiphenomena, or the consequences
of affective disorder.*

Personality disorders have recently been subjected to increased scrutiny. This
renewed interest coincides in part with the formalization of diagnostic criteria
(American Psychiatric Association, 1980, 1987; Gunderson et al., 1981) and the
correspondent development of instruments for the assessment of personality disorder (e.g., Diagnostic Interview for Borderlines, Personality Disorders
Examination, Structured Interview for *DSM-III* Personality Disorders, and
Structured Clinical Interview for *DSM-III* Disorders). In additional, there is
increased evidence validating the existence of these diagnostic constructs, which
are reported most frequently in the literature as comorbid conditions in adult,
affectively ill patients. Such validation consists primarily of a consistent natural
history characterized by refractoriness to and poor compliance with treatment,
poor social adjustment, and a high risk for suicide and suicidal behavior
(Weissman et al., 1978; Nace et al., 1983; Tyrer et al., 1983; Pfohl et al, 1974;
Stone et al., 1987). Additional evidence to support the validity of these diagnostic
constructed includes the persistence of dysfunctional personality traits in
eutyhymic patients with affective illness (Akiskal et al., 1983; Hirschfeld et al.,
1983a), distinct patterns of familial aggregation (Lorganger et al., 1982; Pope
et al., 1983; Soloff and Millward, 1983; Pfohl et al., 1984), and correlation of
aggressive/impulsive personality disorders with low CSF 5-hydroxyindoleactic
acid (Brown and Goodwin, 1986; Traskman-Bendz et al., 1986; Coccaro et al.,
1989). Because comorbid personality disorders have such deleterious effects on
the prognosis of affectively ill patients, an improved understanding of the
interrelationship between personality and affective illness is likely to lead to progress in the treatment of affectively ill patients.

With regard to the comorbidity of affective illness and personality disorder,
it is unclear if personality disorder predisposes to affective illness, is an epiphenomena of depressive disorder, or is a consequence of chronic affective impairment (Akiskal et al., 1983; 1985). However, it is difficult to disentangle the
etiological web of personality and affective disorder in the patient who presents
with both. Anamnestic approaches, particularly in adults, are likely to be unreliable. In order to study the origin and evolution of personality disorder in affectively disordered patients, it is optimal to target patients who are just at the initial
stages of an "affective career," e.g., children and adolescents with recent onset
of affective disorder.

In contrast to the plethora of investigations on the association of affective and
personality disorders in adults, there has been a paucity of similar studies in ado-

lescents. This is due in part to the clinical concern about whether "personality disorder" can be reasonably diagnosed in adolescent-aged patients, for whom personality may still be in a state of flux. However, in answer to this concern, a longitudinal study of adolescents showed that certain dysfunctional personality traits do endure into adulthood (Parnas et al., 1982). Moreover, studies of personality disorder in adolescents have been convergent with the above-noted studies in adult patients, insofar as adolescent personality disorder had been associated with suicide attempts, affective disorder, social impairment, and a family history of affective disorder (Crumley, 1979; Friedman et al., 1982; McManus et al., 1984; Marton et al., 1989).

Progress in this area has until recently been hampered by the lack of personality assessment instruments with established reliability for adolescents. To date, reliability in adolescent samples has been established for: the Diagnostic Interview for Borderlines (DIB) (Gunderson et al., 1981) on inpatients (McManus et al., 1984); the Structured Clinical Interview for *DSM-III* Personality Disorder (SCID) (Spitzer et al., 1984, New York State Psychiatric Institute, Unpublished manuscript) in eating disordered patients (Wonderlich et all, 1987); and the Personality Diagnostic Examination (PDE) (Loranger et al., 1984, New York Hospital-Cornell Medical Center, Unpublished manuscript) in affectively ill adolescents (Marton et al., 1989). Concurrent validity of personality diagnosis was assessed in only one of these studies of adolescents (Marton et al., 1989), and in that particular study, reliability was reported as percent agreement rather than with the more conservative κ coefficient. Moreover, in only one of these three studies (Marton et al. 1989) were additional parental informants interviewed as is recommended by Zimmerman et al. (1986). In summary, while preliminary work is promising, the reliability and validity of personality disorder diagnoses has not yet been firmly established in adolescent samples.

Therefore, to prepare for more detailed investigations of the interrelationships of affective and personality disorders among youth, the authors examined the reliability and validity of the Structured Interview for the *DSM-III* Diagnosis of Personality Disorder (SIDP) (Pfohl et al., 1983, University of Iowa, Unpublished manuscript) in affectively disordered adolescent patients. The SIDP was chosen because of its complete coverage of all *DSM-III* personality disorders (as compared to the DIB), more modest length (compared to the PDE), and the availability of published reliability and validity studies in adults at the time the present investigation (Stangl et al., 1985) was begun. Specifically, three sets of questions were addressed in this preliminary study: (1) can personality disorder be diagnosed reliably in affectively ill adolescents; (2) do certain Axis I and family history diagnoses correlate with specific personality disorders; and (3) do self-report measures of personality traits distinguish between those with and without specific personality disorders as diagnosed by the SIDP?

METHOD

Sample

The sample consisted of 23 adolescent patients referred to Western Psychiatric Institute and Clinic. Of the total, nine (39%) were inpatients, and 14 (61%) were outpatients. The media age of the group was 16 years, and the majority were female (65%) and white (87%). Diagnostically, almost all had a diagnosis of major depressive disorder (96%), either unipolar (66%), recurrent unipolar (4%), or bipolar (22%). The remaining subjects had primary diagnoses of bipolar disorder, mixed state (4%). In almost half the cases (48%), affective disorder was accompanied by nonaffective comorbidity. Fourteen of the group 61%) had suicidal behavior as part of their presentation, five (22%) presented with suicidal ideation with a plan or a suicidal threat, and the remainder (17%) were nonsuicidal.

Assessment Procedure

All participants were recruited to be subjects in this study in accordance with the guidelines of the Psychosocial Institutional Review Board of the University of Pittsburgh. Subjects were interviewed within 1 month of clinical intake, and all were in the midst of an episode of affective psychiatric disorder at the time of the interview. While it might be argued that it would be preferable to interview subjects when they had remitted from an affective episode, the authors elected to follow a procedure similar to the initial report on the reliability and validity of the SIDP in adult inpatients, in which subjects were interviewed in episode (Stangl et al., 1985). Current and lifetime psychiatric diagnoses using *DSM-III* criteria were obtained by semi-structured interviews with child and parent using the K-SADS-E and P (Orvaschel et al., 1982; Chambers et al., 1985). The severity of depressive symptoms in the subjects was assessed by using the Beck Depression Inventory (BDI) (Beck et al., 1961). Family history of psychiatric disorder was obtained from the parent by an interviewer blind to the proband diagnosis using the Family History-Research Diagnostic Criteria method (Andreasen et al., 1977) with diagnostic criteria modified to *DSM-III*.

Personality disorders were assessed by use of the SIDP. Approximately 20% of the items were modified slightly for use with adolescents (e.g., less emphasis on occupation, more on school). This modification was approved by one of the SIDP co-developers before being used in this project (Stangle, personal communication, 1987). The SIDP consists of 160 items divided into 16 topical sections of 10 items each (e.g., self-esteem, dependency). The items in these topical sections are used to determine whether the patient met a specific criteria for a given personality disorder. There are several points for the interviewer to exercise judgment in the use of the

SIDP: (1) the interviewer must decide if a particular personality descriptor (e.g., dependency) is attributable to an Axis I disorder or is truly a trait-phenomenon independent of Axis I state; (2) if the interviewer decides that a particular symptom is a trait-phenomenon, then it must be rated as to its clinical significance; and (3) the interviewer must decide if the traits elicited translate to clinically significant criteria for the diagnoses of specific personality disorders.

Each subject was classified according to *DSM-III* criteria into one of three categories: (1) disorder (met all criteria); (2) trait (met all but one criteria); or (3) no disorder. Furthermore, given the overlap in criteria of different personality disorders (Pfohl et al., 1984), subjects were classified into clusters of related personality traits and disorders (Stangl et al., 1985). Cluster I consists of paranoid, schizotypal, and schizoid personality; Cluster II of borderline, narcissistic, and histrionic personality, and Cluster II of compulsive, passive-aggressive, avoidant, and dependent personality traits and disorders.

The SIDP was chosen for this initial investigation because adequate test-retest reliability has been demonstrated in adult inpatients (κs ranged from 0.45 to 0.90; Stangl et al., 1985). Moreover, convergent validity between categorical diagnoses on the SIDP with appropriate subscales on the Minnesota Multiphasic Personality Inventory (MMPI) was demonstrated (Stangl et al., 1985). At the time this investigation was being planned, this instrument was the only one of several available interviews for which published reports supported both reliability and validity for a broad coverage of all possible personality disorders.

The SIDP was administered to the adolescent, and a parental informant was interviewed as well. For the interviews with the parental informant, the "informant" version of the instrument was employed consisting of a subset (N–65) of the items (Zimmerman et al., 1986), and information from both sources was combined into a summary diagnosis. The interviewer who administered the SIDP was separate from the one who administered the K-SADS-E/P, but the SIDP interviewer reviewed the information on Axis I disorders prior to the conduct of the SIDP. This was done in order to enable the SIDP interviewers to ascertain if specific responses to items were truly trait phenomena or were secondary to Axis I disorder. In 17 cases (74%), the SIDP interviews were videotaped and reviewed by a second interviewer trained in the use of the SIDP, in order to establish interrater agreement.

Additionally, the parents and subjects were each administered two self-report inventories, the MMPI and Tridimensional Personality Questionnaire (TPQ), aimed at tapping the parent's perception about the subject or the subject's self-perception, respectively. Both the MMPI and TPQ have been designed to assess personality traits, and as such, allowed for the testing of convergent validity with the SIDP.

The version of the MMPI used was the 168-item version of Overall et al. (1976). While an extensive literature exists on this instrument, the MMPI has been criticized on the grounds that the items conform to much earlier diagnostic systems than

DSM-III (Widiger et al., 1985). Therefore, the authors elected to use one additional measure, the TPQ (Cloninger, 1987). This instrument has 80 items, and as the name suggests, the TPQ yields scores on three orthogonal axes: harm-avoidance, reward-dependence, and novelty-seeking. Preliminary data in a sample of sophomore medical students demonstrated adequate test-retest reliability, internal consistency, orthogonality of the three dimensions and convergence with other self-report measures of personality (Cloninger, 1987).

Data Analysis

Interrater reliability was assessed by use of Cohen's κ (Fleiss, 1981). Both unweighted (no disorder vs. either trait or disorder) and weighted κs (no disorder vs. trait vs. disorder) as well as standard errors for these κ coefficients were calculated. Subsequent data analyses on personality diagnoses used the diagnoses rendered by the primary interviewer, although analyses based on the diagnoses of the secondary interviewers yielded essentially the same results.

The relationship between severity of depression on the BDI and specific personality clusters was assessed by use of the Student's *t*-test. The association between personality clusters and dichotomous variables such as comorbid diagnoses or family history of psychiatric disorder was evaluated by use of the χ^2 statistic or Fisher's exact test. The interrelationship of the various personality disorders and their tendency to actually fall within these three clusters was assessed by a nonparametric correlation coefficient, Spearman's ρ (Hays, 1981).

The convergent validity of three personality clusters with either the MMPI or TPQ subscales was tested by comparing those with and without a given cluster trait or diagnosis, using multivariate analysis of variance (MANOVA). Additional statistical tests using individual analyses of variance were performed only if the MANOVA indicated an overall omnibus effect.

RESULTS

Reliability

The frequency with which a given trait or disorder was diagnosed ranged from 60% for histrionic disorder to 0% for schizoid disorder (Table 1). All but three subjects (87%) met criteria for at least one personality trait or disorder. The median number of disorders and traits per subject were two and three, respectively. Reliability, as calculated by a weighted κ coefficient, ranged from κ = 0.24 for borderline personality disorder to 1.00 for schizoid disorder, with a mean κ = 0.49 (Table 2). For unweighted κs, the mean was κ = 0.59, with a range of 0.32 for narcissistic personality disorder to 1.00 for schizoid and schizotypal disorders (Table 2).

Verification of the Three Major Personality Clusters

The intercorrelations between different personality traits and disorders were examined by use of Spearman's ρ (Table 3). This made it possible to learn to what extent previously reported clusters could be empirically validated. In fact, Table 3 provides modest support for this classification scheme: within Cluster I, paranoid and schizotypal disorder were highly intercorrelated ρ = 0.47, $p<0.05$). Within Cluster II, narcissistic, borderline, and histrionic disorders were all intercorrelated (ρs = 0.32 to 0.36, $ps<0.05$). However, avoidant disorder appeared most closely tied to Cluster I disorders, namely paranoid (ρ = 0.41, $p<0.05$) and schizotypal disorders (ρ = 0.43, $p<0.05$). Passive-aggressive disorder was significantly correlated with two out of three Cluster II disorders (ρs = 0.34 to 0.57, $p<0.05$). The interrelationships of various personality disorders will require further investigation before any definitive conclusions can be drawn.

Axis I Diagnostic Correlates of Personality Traits and Disorder

There was no relationship between self-rated depression, as measured by the BDI, and the presence of any of the diagnostic clusters (which refer to presence of either trait or disorder). Also, no relationship was detected between any Axis I psychiatric disorder and the presence of either Cluster I or Cluster III. However, patients with Cluster II disorders (borderline, narcissistic, histrionic) were not significantly more

TABLE 1

Frequency (%) of Personality Traits [a]* and *DSM-III* Disorders as Diagnosed by the SIDI[b]*

	None		Trait		Disorder	
	N	%	N	%	N	%
Cluster I	16	70	6	26	1	4
Paranoid	16	70	7	30	0	0
Schizoid	23	100	0	0	0	0
Schizotypal	21	91	1	4	1	4
Cluster II	7	30	8	35	8	35
Histrionic	9	39	10	43	4	17
Narcissistic	16	70	6	26	1	4
Borderline	12	52	6	26	5	22
Cluster III	7	30	6	26	10	43
Passive-aggressive	11	48	3	13	9	39
Avoidant	16	70	6	26	1	4
Compulsive	21	91	2	9	0	0
Dependent	21	91	2	9	0	0

[a]A trait is defined as one criteria shy of a *DSM-III* disorder.
[b]Diagnosed by the primary interviewer.

TABLE 2
Weighted and Unweighted Interrater Agreement κ for SIDP-diagnosed Personality Traits and Disorders in Adolescents

Diagnosis	Number		Weighted		Unweighted	
	Trait	Disorder	κ	Se	κ	Se
Paranoid	5	1	0.58[a]	0.23	0.58[a]	0.20
Schizoid	0	0	1.00	–	1.00	–
Schizotypal	1	1	0.45[a]	0.17	1.00	–
Histrionic	9	2	0.61[a]	0.16	0.62[a]	0.19
Narcissistic	5	1	0.46[a]	0.13	0.32	0.21
Borderline	4	4	0.24	0.19	0.40[a]	0.21
Passive-aggressive	1	8	0.42[a]	0.15	0.53[a]	0.18
Avoidant	5	1	0.36	0.23	0.34	0.24
Compulsive	2	0	0.32	0.17	0.69[a]	0.33
Dependent	2	0	0.43	0.24	0.43	0.33
Overall κ			0.49[a]	0.17	0.59[a]	0.19

[a] $p < 0.05$.

TABLE 3
Intercorrelation[a] Among Personality Disorder Diagnoses and Clusters

	1	2	3	4	5	6	7	8	9	10
1. Paranoid	—									
2. Schizoid	0.00	—								
3. Schizotypal	0.47[a]	0.00	—							
4. Histrionic	0.19	0.00	-0.10	—						
5. Narcissistic	0.15	0.00	0.13	0.33[a]	—					
6. Borderline	0.36[a]	0.00	0.11	0.44[a]	0.38[a]	—				
7. Passive-aggressive	0.27	0.00	0.36[a]	0.34[a]	0.57[a]	0.24	—			
8. Avoidant	0.41[a]	0.00	0.43[a]	-0.33[a]	-0.25	-0.12	-0.07	—		
9. Compulsive	0.13	0.00	0.48[a]	0.30	0.43[a]	0.09	0.36[a]	0.12	—	
10. Dependent	0.47[a]	0.00	-0.10	0.13	0.43[a]	0.32	0.36[a]	0.12	-0.10	—

Cluster I · Cluster II · Cluster III

[a] Spearman's ρ, $p < 0.05$.

likely than those without Cluster II disorders to have diagnoses of attention deficit disorder (31% vs. 0%), and bipolar disorder (either bipolar I or II, 31% vs. 0%).

Family History Correlates of Personality Disorder

There were no differences in the rates of disorder in the first-degree or second-degree relatives of Cluster I vs. non-Cluster I or Cluster II vs. non-Cluster III patients. For the relatives of Cluster II patients, there were no differences in the rates of disorder for first-degree relatives, although second-degree relatives of Cluster II patients showed a much higher rate of suicidal gestures, compared to the relatives of non-Cluster II patients (38% vs. 18%, $\chi^2 = 6.92$, $df = 1$, $p = 0.009$).

Concurrent Validity of Personality Disorder Diagnoses

None of the MANOVAs comparing MMPI factors or clinical scale scores differentiated between clusters. Similarly, none of the MANOVAs on the harm-avoidance nor the reward-dependence subscales of the TPQ indicated a significant effect with regard to specific clusters. Furthermore, for novelty-seeking, no significant omnibus effects for MANOVAs emerged for either Clusters I or III. However, there was a significant overall effect with regard to novelty-seeking (as reported by the subjects' parents) for Cluster II, $F(12,3) = 20.94$, $p = 0.01$, as well as for follow-up analyses of variance. Several subscales within novelty-seeking differentiated the Cluster II from non-Cluster II subjects: "disorderly," 4.0(1.6)vs. 1.3(1.0),$F(1,17) = 14.05$, $p = 0.002$, "exploratory" 5.1(1.0) vs. 2.0(0.9), $F(1,17) = 44.28$ $p<0.004$. Finally, Cluster II subjects scored significantly higher on total novelty-seeking than did non-Cluster II patients, 23.8(7.20) vs. 13.0 (4.3), $F(1,17) = 12.41$, $p = 0.003$.

DISCUSSION

Before focusing on the implications of this study, it is important to consider the limitations of this project. The main limitation stems from the small sample size, which prevented more molecular analyses. A second limitation is that most subjects were only interviewed once so that interactions between affective symptomatology and personality disorder could not be disentangled. since subjects were interviewed while they were in the midst of a current affective disorder, they may have presented a distorted picture of their "typical" personality, which made it difficult for interviewers to disentangle state from trait phenomena (Coppen and Metcalfe, 1965; Kerr et al., 1970; Hirschfeld et al., 1983b). However, the authors followed the procedure of Stangl et al. (1985) in their original report on the reliability and validity of the SIDP of interviewing subjects while in the midst of a psychiatric episode. Also, the authors relied heavily on the report of parents, who could be more objective about their child's personality traits, current affective disorder notwithstanding.

This report adds to other investigations supporting the reliability and validity of personality disorder diagnoses in adolescence. Interrater agreement using the SCID-II in eating disordered patients was reported to range from $\kappa = 0.56$ to 0.77 (Wonderlich et al., 1987), agreement using the DIB was $\kappa = 0.72$ to 0.85 (McManus et al., 1984), and percent agreement using the PDE, ranged from 80 to 100% (Marton et al., 1989).

Stangle et al. (1985), reported on the reliability of the SIDP in adult inpatients and found an interrater agreement of $\kappa = 0.70$, and a test-retest reliability of $\kappa = 0.66$, compared to our interrater agreement of $\kappa = 0.49$ to 0.59. Criteria for "agreement" in the present study were more stringent, insofar as "agreement" was defined by Stangl et al. (1985) as concordance on 50% or more of personality diagnoses in a given subject. Nevertheless, one may be justified in asking why reliability in this study was not higher than $\kappa = 0.49$ to 0.59, especially when the second rater's activities were primarily rerating videotaped interviews. It is felt that the source of variance stemmed primarily from interrater differences of opinion as to whether: (1) a given trait was attributable to an affective disorder or not, and; (2) a given trait was present to a clinically significant degree. The first problem can be overcome by both relying on informants and reinterviewing subjects once they have experienced a remission. The second issue can be addressed by providing anchor points for functional impairment in the interview, as would be required by *DSM-III-R* (American Psychiatric Association, 1987).

This study provides modest support for previously described clusters of personality disorders. As has been reported by others, there is a high degree of overlap between disorders, such as histrionic and borderline disorders, that seems to be attributable to overlap in the criteria themselves (Pfohl et al., 1984). Also, avoidant disorder, putatively a Cluster III disorder, was more closely related to Cluster I than to Cluster III.

The present study also provides some convergent validation of personality diagnoses. Specifically, Cluster II traits and diagnoses (borderline, histrionic, narcissistic), were related to the novelty-seeking scale on the TPQ, as was predicted by Cloninger (1987). In fact, it is unclear if the scores on the TPQ were reflective of true Axis II pathology, or instead were attributable to the contribution of such Axis II pathology, or instead were attributable to the contribution of such Axis I disorders as attention deficit disorder and bipolar illness. One might have expected Cluster II to also show lower "harm-avoidance" (Cloninger, 1987), but the high proportion of patients in this sample who either attempted, threatened, or seriously contemplated suicide (76%) may have precluded detection of subgroup differences on this dimension.

It was of further interest that Cluster II patients were also those who showed a trend toward being more likely to have concomitant comorbid diagnoses of bipolar and attention deficit disorders. Many of the criteria for borderline personality disorder are virtually indistinguishable from bipolar or cyclothymic disorder (Wetzel et al., 1980; Akiskal, 1981; Akiskal et al., 1985): e.g., affective liability, impulsivity, self-destructive and risk-taking behavior, physically self-damaging acts, and inappropriate displays of anger (American Psychiatric Association, 1980). Moreover, the poor response of borderline patients to amitriptyline and their superior response to neuroleptics (Soloff et al., 1986a, b) is also consistent with an overlap between borderline personality disorder and bipolarity. As such, the overlap between Cluster II and bipolarity can be taken as support of Akiskal's view that such disorders may represent either epiphenomena or consequences of affective disorders (Akiskal, 1981; Akiskal's et al., 1983, 1985). The significance of an increased prevalence of attention deficit disorder among Cluster II patients is unclear. This may represent an early manifestation of bipolar illness, or it may simply be related to ongoing problems with regulation of impulse control. Only longitudinal studies will enable investigators to disentangle the relationships between specific Axis I and Axis II disorders.

The findings regarding differences in family history between the relatives of Cluster II and non-Cluster II probands merit comment. The association between familial suicide gestures and Cluster II personality disorders suggest a common etiology to impulsive suicidal behavior and personality disorder as has been observed in recent adoption (Wonder et al., 1986), and biological studies (Coccaro et al., 1989). Naturally, this observation must be replicated in a larger sample. The authors are currently conducting a family study to learn if there is indeed an association between familial suicidality and personality disorders.

In summary, this study demonstrates modest reliability for personality disorder diagnoses in adolescent patients. There is also support for the validity of Cluster II personality disorders specifically. Additional studies are recommended in which affectively disordered adolescents are interviewed while ill and then followed up and reinterviewed during remission. Such prospective studies will make it possible to determine if the personality traits and disorders diagnosed cross-sectionally in time persist, and if the persistence of personality disorder is independent or interactive with the course of affective illness.

REFERENCES

Akiskal, H.S. (1981), Subaffective disorders: dysthymic, cyclothymic and bipolar II disorders in the "borderline realm." *Psychiatr. Clin. North Am.,* 4:25–47.

———Hirschfeld, R.M. A. & Yerevanian, B.I. (1983), The relationships of personality to affective disorders. A critical review. *Arch. Gen. Psychiatry,* 40:801–810.

———Chen, S.E., Davis, G.C., Puzantian, V.R., Kashgarian, M. & Bolinger, J.M. (1985), Borderline: an adjective in search of a noun. *J. Clin. Psychiatry,* 46:41–48.

American Psychiatric Association (1980), *Diagnostic and Statistical Manual DSM-III (Third edition)*. Washington, DC: American Psychiatric Association.

————(1987), *Diagnostic and Statistical Manual DSM-III (Third edition-Revised)*, Washington, DC: American Psychiatric Association.

Andreasen, N., Endicott, J., Spitzer, R. & Winokur, G. (1977), The family history method using research diagnostic criteria: reliability and validity, *Arch. Gen. Psychiatry*, 34:1229–1235.

Beck, A., Ward, C., Mendelson, M. et al. (1961), An inventory for measuring depression. *Arch. Gen. Psychiatry*, 4:53–63.

Brown, G.L. & Goodwin, F.K. (1986), Cerebrospinal fluid correlates of suicide attempts and aggression. In: *Psychobiology of Suicidal Behavior*, Vol. 487, ed. J.J. Mann & N. Stanley. New York: Annals of the New York Academy of Sciences, pp. 175–188.

Chambers, W., Puig-Antich, J., Hirsch, M. et al. (1985), The assessment of affective disorders in children and adolescents by semi-structured interview: test-retest reliability of the K-SADS-P. *Arch. Gen. Psychiatry*, 42:669–674.

Cloninger, C.R. (1987), A systematic method for clinical description and classification of personality variant. *Arch. Gen. Psychiatry*, 44:573–588.

Coccaro, E.F., Siever, L.J., Klar, H.M. et al. (1989), Serotonergic studies in patients with affective and personality disorders: correlates with suicidal and impulsive aggressive behavior. *Arch. Gen. Psychiatry*, 46:587–599.

Coppen, A., & Metcalfe, M. (1965), Effect of depressive illness on MPI scores. *Br. J. Psychiatry*, 41:236–239.

Crumley, F.E. (1979), Adolescent suicide attempts. *JAMA*, 22:2404–2407.

Fleiss, J.L. (1981), *Statistical Methods for Rates and Proportions (Second edition)*. New York: Wiley, pp. 211–237.

Friedman, R.C., Clarkin, J.F., Corn, R., Aronoff, M.S., Hurt, S. W. & Murphy, M.C. (1982), *DSM-III* and affective pathology in hospitalized adolescents. *J. Nerv. Ment. Dis.*, 170:511–521.

Gunderson, J.G., Kolb, J.E. & Austin, V. (1981), The diagnostic interview for borderline patients. *Am. J. Psychiatry*, 138:896–903.

Hays, W.L. (1981), *Statistics (Third edition)*. New York: Holt, Rinehart & Winston, Inc., pp. 435–437.

Hirschfeld, R.M.A., Klerman, G.L., Clayton, P.J. & Keller, M. B. (1983a), Personality and depression: empirical findings. *Arch. Gen. Psychiatry*, 40:993–998.

————————————————McDonald-Scott, P. & Larkin, B.H. (1983b), Assessing personality: effects of depressive state on trait measurement *Am. J. Psychiatry*, 140:695–699.

Kerr, T.A., Schapira, K., Roth, M. & Garside, R.F. (1970), The relationships between the Maudsley Personality Inventory and the course of affective disorders. *Br. J. Psychiatry*, 116:11–19.

Loranger, A.W., Oldham, J.M. & Tulis, E.H. (1982), Familial transmission of borderline personality disorder. *Arch. Gen. Psychiatry*, 39:795–802.

Marton, P., Korenblum, M., Kutcher, S., Stein, B., Kennedy, B. & Pakes, J. (1989), Personality dysfunction in depressed adolescents. *Can. J. Psychiatry* 34:810–813.

McManus, M., Lerner, H., Robbins, D. & Barbour, C. (1984), Assessment of borderline symptomatology in hospitalized adolescents. *J. Am. Acad. Child Psychiatry,* 23:685–695.

Nace, E.P., Saxon, J.J. & Shore, N. (1983), A comparison of borderline and nonborderline alcoholic patients. *Arch. Gen. Psychiatry,* 40:54–56.

Orvaschel, H., Puig-Antich, J., Chambers, W. et al. (1982), Retrospective assessment of prepubertal major depressive episode with the Kiddie-SADS-E. *J. Am. Acad. Child Psychiatry,* 21:392–397.

Overall, J.E., Higgins, W. & DeSchweinitz, A. (1976), Comparison of differential diagnostic discrimination for abbreviated and standard MMPI. *J. Clin. Psychol.,* 32:237–245.

Parnas, J., Teasdale, T.W. & Schulsinger, H. (1982), Continuity of character neurosis from childhood to adulthood. a prospective longitudinal study. *Acta Psychiatr. Scand.,* 66:491–498.

Pfohl, B., Stangl, D. & Zimmerman, M. (1984), The implication of *DSM-III* personality disorders for patients with major depression. *J. Affective Disord.,* 7:309–318.

Pope, H.G., Jonas, J.M., Hudson, J.I., Cohen, B. & Gunderson, J.G. (1983), The validity of *DSM-III* borderline personality disorder. *Arch. Gen. Psychiatry,* 40:54–56

Soloff, P.H. & Millward, J.W. (1983), Psychiatric disorders in the families of borderline patients. *Arch. Gen. Psychiatry,* 40:37–44.

———George, A., Nathan, R.S., Schulz, P.M. & Perel, J.M. (1986a), Paradoxical effects of amitriptyline on borderline patients. *Am. J. Psychiatry,* 143:1603–1605.

————————————Ulrich, R.F. & Perel, J.M. (1986b), Progress in pharmacotherapy of borderline disorders. A double-blind study of amitriptyline haloperiodol, and placebo. *Arch. Gen. Psychiatry,* 43:691–697.

Stangl, D., Pfohl, B., Zimmerman, M., Bowers, W. & Corenthal, CC. (1985), A structured interview for *DSM-III* personality disorders: a preliminary report. *Arch. Gen. Psychiatry,* 42:591–596.

Stone, M.H., Hurt, S.W. & Stone, D.K. (1987), The PI 500: longterm follow-up of borderline inpatients meeting *DSM-III* criteria I: global outcome. *J. Pers. Assess.,* 1:291–298.

Traskman-Bendz, L., Asberg, M. & Schaling, D. (1986), Serotonergic function and suicidal behavior in personality disorders. In: *Psychobiology of Suicidal Behavior,* Vol. 487, ed. J.J. Mann & M. Stanley. New York: Annals of the New York Academy of Sciences, pp. 168–174.

Tyrer, P., Casey, P. & Gail, J. (1983), Relationship between neurosis and personality disorder. *Br. J. Psychiatry,* 142:404–408.

Weissman, M.M., Prusoff, B.A. & Klerman, G.L. (1978), Personality and the prediction of long-term outcome of depression. *Am. J. Psychiatry,* 135:797–800.

Wender, P.H., Kety, S.S., Rosenthal, D., Schulsinger, F., Ortmann, J. & Lunde, I. (1986), Psychiatric disorders in the biological and adoptive families of adopted individuals with affective disorders. *Arch. Gen. Psychiatry,* 43:923–929.

Wetzel, R.D., Cloninger, C.R., Horg, B. & Reich, T. (1980), Personality as a subclinical expression of the affective disorder. *Compr. Psychiatry*, 21:197–205.

Widiger, T.A., Williamss, J.B.W., Spitzer, R.L. & Frances, A. (1985), The MCMI as a measure of *DSM-III*. *J. Pers. Assess.*, 49:366–507.

Wonderlich, S.A., Swift, W.J. & Goodman, S. (1987, October), *Eating disorders and personality disorders*. Presented at the Annual Meeting of the American Academy of Child and Adolescent Psychiatry, Washington, DC.

Zimmerman, M., Pfohl, B., Stangl, D. & Corenthal, C. (1986), Assessment of *DSM-III* Personalities: the importance of interviewing as informant. *J. Clin. Psychiatry*, 47:261–263.

19

Childhood Obsessive–Compulsive Disorder: A Prospective Follow-up Study

Martine F. Flament
Hôpital International de l'Université de Paris

Elisabeth Koby, Judith L. Rapoport, Carol J. Berg, Theodore Zahn, and Christine Cox
National Institute of Mental Health, Bethesda

Martha Denckla
Johns Hopkins University School of Medicine, Baltimore

Marge Lenane
National Institute of Mental Health, Bethesda

Twenty-five of 27 patients (93%) who had participated in a study of severe primary obsessive–compulsive disorder with onset in childhood or adolescence, were seen 2–7 yrs after initial examination (mean, 4.4 yrs). They were compared to a group of normal controls matched for age, sex and IQ and followed up for the same period. Continued psycho-pathology was striking for the patients, with only seven (28%), three males and four females, receiving no psychiatric diagnosis at follow-up. Seventeen subjects (68%) still had obsessive–compulsive disorder, 12 patients (48%) had another psychiatric disorder, most commonly anxiety and/or depression; neither initial response to clomipramine or any other baseline variable predicted outcome.

INTRODUCTION

Because of its relative rarity in clinical settings (Berman, 1942; Judd, 1965; Hollingsworth, Tanguay, Grossman & Pabst, 1980), childhood obsessive-

Reprinted with permission from *Journal of Child Psychology and Psychiatry*, 1990, Vol. 31, No. 3, 363–380. Copyright © 1990 by the Association for Child Psychology and Psychiatry.

compulsive disorder (OCD) has not been as carefully studied as its adult counterpart. However, it has been long recognized that this disorder, in contrast to other emotional disorders, has a frequent onset in childhood or adolescence (Black, 1974; Rapoport, 1986), with presentation in virtually identical form to that seen in adults (Flament & Rapoport, 1984). A recent epidemiological study by Flament *et al.* (1988) has shown that, during adolescence, the true prevalence of OCD is much higher than expected from clinical estimates: in an unselected adolescent population of over 5500 subjects the weighted lifetime prevalence rate of the disorder was found to be 1.9%, supporting current estimates for OCD in the general adult population (Anthony *et al.*, 1985; Karno, Golding, Sorenson & Burnam, 1988).

Follow-up studies of adult patients with OCD (Lewis, 1936; Langfeldt, 1938; Rudin, 1953; Muller, 1953; Pollitt, 1957; Balsev-Olesen & Geert-Jorgensen, 1959; Ingram, 1961; Kringlen, 1965; Grimshaw, 1965; Lo, 1967) have stressed the chronic course and relative "purity" of outcome of the disorder. In these studies, the prognosis of obsessional states was considered even more severe than that of other neurotic disorders (Ingram, 1961; Kringlen, 1965); complete recovery was rare (from 12% of the subjects in Rudin's study to 32% in Lewis's) but spontaneous improvement was reported in 14% (Lewis's study) to 50% (Lo's study) of the patients. Complete disability was seen in only a minority of cases (Ingram, 1961; Kringlen, 1965), with all but the most severe continuing to work (Lewis, 1936; Rudin, 1953). However, social isolation, celibacy and/or marital maladjustment were common (Ingram, 1961; Kringlen, 1965; Lo, 1967). Depression was the most common complication (Rosenberg, 1968; Goodwin, Guze & Robins, 1969) and the largest single cause of hospitalization for patients with OCD (Welner, Reich, Robins, Fishman & Van Doren, 1976) but suicidal risk was low (Pollitt, 1957; Kringlen, 1965). Development into psychosis was rare in typical cases (Pollitt, 1957; Lo, 1967) but occurred for some initially "doubtful" or "atypical" obsessions (Rudin, 1953; Muller, 1953; Ingram, 1961; Kringlen, 1965).

Most of the studies cited above are old, and, although some of them concern large numbers of patients (up to 130 subjects in Rudin's study), the length of the follow-up varies greatly, and the number of patients lost for follow-up was as much as 35%. Furthermore, the samples followed were probably heterogeneous, as no common diagnostic definition for the "obsessional neurotics" was employed. In addition, there was little mention of treatment received, if any, except for leucotomy which was performed on substantial numbers of patients in some studies. Follow-up contact varied between and within studies, from short mailed questionnaires to personal re-examination by the investigators, and structured interviews were not employed.

One adult follow-up study (Ingram, 1961) has reported that symptomatology in childhood was a poor prognostic indicator; however, direct prospective data from juvenile population is meager.

Berman (1942) reported on six clear-cut cases of OCD in 11- and 12-yr-old children hospitalized in two different institutions. He found good prognosis for any one episode but long-term outcome was less favorable: 6–18 months after discharge, two cases were considered well, except for occasional anxiety, but two others had chronic OCD while two subjects, followed for 6 and 7 yrs, respectively, developed "trends suggestive of schizophrenia".

Warren (1960) followed up 15 adolescents admitted to the Maudsley Hospital with obsessive–compulsive states, aged between 12 and 17 yrs, and re-examined them when aged 19–24 yrs. No treatment was specified except for one patient who was leucotomized. Only two subjects (13%) were considered completely recovered, four (27%) had a tendency to mild obsessive–compulsive symptoms under stress, four (27%) were somewhat handicapped by obsessional symptoms and the remaining five (33%) still had severe obsessional pathology, one being hospitalized.

Hollingsworth *et al.*(1980) identified 17 cases of severe obsessive–compulsive neurosis from a retrospective chart review of all children treated as in- or out-patients at the UCLA Neuropsychiatric Institute for a 16-yr period. All obsessive–compulsive children had been treated with intensive psychotherapy (for an average of 17.7 months), and one of them also received behavior therapy. The authors interviewed 10 of these cases (59%), 1.5–14 yrs after their first admission. At follow-up, the mean age for the 10 subjects was 19.9 yrs (range, 12–30 yrs). Only three of the 10 (30%) denied any obsessive thoughts or compulsions, while seven (70%) reported that obsessive–compulsive behavior still continued to some degree but was less than pretreatment level. One of the 10 had decompensated during adolescence in an acute schizophrenic reaction which had resolved without recurrence; one had been hospitalized for suicidal ideation and depression but none had ever made a suicidal attempt. On follow-up, all 10 subjects reported problems with social life and peer relationships, none were married; their areas of greatest strength were the pursuit of a higher education, and employment in jobs in which compulsiveness could be utilized or was socially acceptable. Bolton, Collins and Steinberg (1983) followed 15 obsessive–compulsive adolescents who had been treated with behavior therapy. At follow-up 1–4 yrs later all but two remained improved.

Finally, Zeitlin (1986) noted continuation of obsessional symptoms in 10 children who had received a diagnosis of obsessive–compulsive neurosis and who were later seen at the Maudsley Hospital as adults. Four received a diagnosis of OCD, while five were considered to have another neurotic disorder, mainly depression. However, several of the five diagnosed as depressed also had obsessive–compulsive symptoms, and might have met criteria for OCD if multiple diagnoses were employed.

Since 1975, a sample of children and adolescents with severe primary OCD has been studied at the National Institute of Mental Health (NIMH) as part of a clinical trial of clomipramine treatment of this disorder (Rapoport *et al.*, 1981; Behar *et al.*, 1984; Flament *et al.*, 1985; Rapoport, in press).

The NIMH study of childhood OCD utilized structured psychiatric interviews of probands and all first-degree relatives, as well as neurological, neuropsychological, electroencephalographic and electrophysiologic examinations. Briefly, the sample impressed the raters with the relative normality of many of the families, the presence of "soft" neurological signs, including subtle choreiform movements, and deficits on perceptuo–spatial tasks relative to a matched control group. Depression was rare in the group at baseline and sleep EEG laboratory studies revealed no difference from controls.

Because of the wide range of behavioral and biological measures, and the relatively large number of cases, several questions could be addressed by a prospective follow-up of such a group. One major question was whether clinical prognosis for childhood obsessive–compulsive disorder resembles that for adults. In addition, we were interested in whether age of onset, ratings of clinical symptomatology or personality, the presence/absence of depression, family psychopathology, any baseline biological measure and/or response to clomipramine predicted follow-up outcome. Finally, as depression was infrequent at initial presentation for our pediatric group, but is a common complication of OCD, the presence of, and predictors of depression at follow-up were of interest.

The present study is of the 27 children seen at the NIMH between 1977 and 1983 and followed up 2–7 yrs later. All had been evaluated for this study as in-patients at the NIMH, and 19 had participated in a clomipramine treatment trial. This is the first prospective follow-up of children and adolescents with severe primary OCD.

SUBJECTS AND METHODS

Subjects

Twenty-seven children, seen consecutively for severe primary obsessive–compulsive disorder, were admitted between September 1977 and June 1983 (Rapoport *et al.*, 1981; Behar, *et al.*, 1984; Flament *et al.*, 1985).

Inclusion criteria were: an age of 6–18 yrs; diagnosis of OCD by DSM-III criteria (American Psychiatric Association, 1980) with at least 1 yr duration of the symptoms; full-scale IQ of 80 or more; and absence of physical illness, organic mental disorder, psychotic disorder or primary affective disorder (i.e. a depressive disorder prior to the onset of the obsessive–compulsive symptoms). Subjects with other psychiatric disorders associated with OCD (including a mood disorder postdating the onset of OCD) were admitted into the study. All 27 patients were hospitalized for a 1-week baseline evaluation, followed, for 19 of them, by a controlled trial of clomipramine (Flament *et al.*, 1985). After evaluation and/or the drug trial, patients were referred to community practitioners for follow-up treatment, the nature of which depended on the outcome of the medication trial, family needs and/or preferences, and local treatment opportunities.

Twenty-nine, age-, sex-, and IQ-matched, healthy volunteers were recruited from the local community between 1977 and 1983, within 6 months of each patient and studied as in-patients for a 3–5 day period. All were free of current or past psychiatric diagnosis by structured diagnostic interview.

Follow-up design

Seven years after the beginning of the initial study, patients and controls were contacted and asked to return for 3–5 days of in-patient evaluation; the controls were seen as out-patients. Subjects were offered financial compensation for their participation according to NIH volunteer guidelines; subjects, and their families when appropriate, gave informed consent for the investigation. Follow-up evaluations were carried out between September 1984 and July 1986.

Methods

The diagnostic and testing procedures used at first admission and at follow-up for patients and controls are summarized in Table 1.

Clinical evaluation

At baseline, patients and controls were administered the Diagnostic Interview for Children and Adolescents (DICA) (Herjanic & Campbell, 1977; Welner, Reich, Herjanic, Jung & Amado, 1987); at follow-up, subjects under 18 yrs of age received the DICA and those aged 18 or above, the NIMH Diagnostic Interview Schedule (Robins, Helzer, Croughan & Ratcliff, 1981). Based on these interviews, lifetime DSM-III diagnoses were made by one of the authors (MFF) and then compared to clinical diagnoses given by another author (JLR) after traditional clinical interview.

At baseline and at follow-up, all subjects were given the card-sort form Leyton Obsessional Inventory—Child Version (LOI—CV) (Berg, Rapoport & Flament, 1986). Patients received additional clinical ratings including the Obsessive Compulsive Rating Scale, the Comprehensive Psychopathological Scale (Asberg, Montgomery, Perris, Schalling & Sedwall, 1978), the NIMH Self-Rating Scale (Post, Kopin & Goodwin, 1973) and its Subscale for Depression (Flament *et al.*, 1985), and the NIMH Global Scales for Depression, Anxiety, OCD and Global Impairment (Murphy, Pickar & Alterman, 1982). At follow-up, diagnostic validity was established in the patient group: for the two independent raters giving multiple diagnoses, the kappa statistic was 0.67 ($p < 0.01$).

Family History

At first admission family history had been obtained for each patient regarding all first-degree relatives with, whenever possible, a structured diagnostic interview, a modification of the Schedule for Affective Disorders and Schizophrenia—Lifetime Version (SADS—L) (Mazure & Gershon, 1979) for parents and siblings over 18 yrs of age and the DICA (Herjanic & Campbell, 1977; Welner *et al.*, 1987) for siblings under 18, or at least one structured telephone interview. At follow-up, interim family history was obtained.

Interim History and Patient's Self-report

At follow-up, in addition to an interim history taken by the clinician, patients were asked about their earliest memories of the disorder, how they coped when at

TABLE 1

Assessment Measures for Obsessive–Compulsive Patients and Controls at First Admission and at 2–7 Yrs Follow-up

Measures[a]	OCD Patients		Controls	
	Baseline	Follow-up	Baseline	Follow-up
Diagnostic interview (DICA under 18 yrs, DIS at and above 18 yrs)	X	X	X	X
Leyton Obsessional Inventory—Child Version	X	X	X	X
Clinical ratings for obsessive–compulsive symptoms, depression, anxiety and global functioning	X	X		
Family history	X	X		
Interim history (patient's self-report essay)		X		
Neurological examination (PANESS)	X	X		
Neurological testing	X	X	X	X
Psychological measures	X	X	X	X
Electroencephalogram	X	X		
CT scan of the brain	X	X		
Dexamethasone suppression test	X	X		

[a]DICA indicates the Diagnostic Interview for Children and Adolescents; DIS, the NIMH Diagnostic Interview Schedule; PANESS, Physical and Neurological Examination for Soft Signs; CT, Computed Tomography.

their worst, how their families were affected, what had helped them and what had made the problem worse. Their more adult views on the disorder and advice to younger patients first dealing with the problem were particularly solicited.

Neurological Examination

At follow-up, as at baseline, the patients were examined by one of the authors (MBD) with an extended development-oriented neurological examination, the Physical and Neurological Examination for Soft Signs (PANESS) (Denckla, 1973, 1974, 1985a, b).

Neuropsychological Examination

At follow-up, all subjects received a battery of neuropsychological tests which included those tests which at baseline had discriminated subjects and controls (Behar *et al.*, 1984): The Money Road Map Test of Directional Sense (Money, Alexander & Walker, 1965), the Stylus Maze Learning (Butters, Soeldner & Fedio, 1972) and Rey-Osterrieth Complex Figure Test (Rey, 1941; Osterrieth, 1944). Complete neuropsychological data are reported separately (Cox, Brouwers, Berg, Rapoport & Fedio, in press); only results from the Money Road Map and the Stylus Maze are presented here.

Psychophysiological Measures

For patients and controls, skin conductance (SC) and heart rate (HR) were recorded during an initial rest period, a series of 10 non-signal tones, and a simple reaction time (RT) task (Zahn, Rapoport & Thompson, 1980). Some details of the procedure differed at baseline, the rest period was 3 minutes and tones were 75 dB, 500 Hz presented at 20–30 second intervals, while at follow-up the rest period was 5 minutes and tones were 85 dB, 1000 Hz, presented at 30–50 second intervals. The indices of autonomic activity examined were the frequency of spontaneous SC responses (SCR/minute), the mean SC level, the mean HR during the rest and tone periods, and the number of SCRs elicited by the tones (1–4 second onset latency). In addition, mean RT was measured as an index of attention.

EEG and CT Scan

EEG and X-ray computed tomography (CT) of the brain were performed for each patient at first admission and at follow-up; CT scans from age- and sex-matched normal controls obtained from a community hospital were used for comparison with the patients' scans. Detailed procedures and results of these examinations have been reported separately (Behar *et al.*, 1984; Luxenberg *et al.*, 1988).

Dexamethasone Suppression Test

For patients only, the standard test was used with a 1 mg dose of dexamethasone given orally at 11 pm, and blood samples obtained at 4 pm and 11 pm the following day for determination of cortisol concentration. A value of 5 μ/dl or greater at either the 4 pm or 11 pm sample was considered a positive test (Carroll *et al.*, 1981).

Statistical Analysis

For all measures, Student's *t*-tests were computed between patients and controls at follow-up. Within each group, comparisons were made between first admission and follow-up score using paired *t*-tests. In addition, subgroups of patients were considered according to diagnosis at follow-up, current treatment, etc. as appropriate. Follow-up parameters were examined with linear regression analysis, using outcome measures alone and together with baseline scores.

RESULTS

Completion Rate

All 27 patients who participated in the initial NIMH childhood OCD study (or their families) could be contacted, but two refused further participation. Twenty-five agreed to some form of follow-up examination: 18 were seen as in-patients, three as out-patients, and two were interviewed during home visits; two more subjects did not want to participate personally in the study but agreed to let their current psychiatrists (one was a NIH psychiatrist, the other was a local practitioner working in close collaboration with the NIH) complete all of the clinical examination.

Thus, completion rate for follow-up clinical examination in the patient group was 25 out of 27 (93%, see Table 2). Whenever possible, the neuropsychological tests and Leyton Inventory were administered even to patients seen in their home. Laboratory procedures such as psychophysiological testing, CT scan, could only be completed for the 21 patients seen at the NIH (78% of the sample).

All 29 controls were contacted for follow-up: 23 (79%) agreed to come back and participate in the study; two could not return because they lived out of the area and one because of medical illness; three refused.

Demographic Characteristics of the Patients and Controls

Descriptive statistics of patient and control groups at first admission and at follow-up are summarized in Table 2.

In the patient group, there was a 2:1 male/female ratio; age of onset of OCD ranged from 3 to 16 yrs. At first admission, patients (and controls) were 10–18 yrs old (mean age ($\pm$ SD), 14.4 ($\pm$ 2.1) yrs) and psychological testing showed average to high average IQ scores, homogenous for verbal and performance subscales. The follow-up study took place 2–7 yrs later with a mean ($\pm$ SD) follow-up period of 4.4 ($\pm$ 1.7) yrs; patients and controls were 13–24 yrs old.

TABLE 2

Sample Characteristics at First Admission and at Follow-up for
Obsessive-Compulsive Subjects and Controls

	OCD Patients	Controls
First admission		
N	27	29
Males	18	21
Females	9	8
Age at first admission		
mean $\pm$ SD		
range	10 – 18	10 – 17
IQ (mean $\pm$ SD)		
Verbal	105.9 $\pm$ 11.8	110.6 $\pm$ 8.4
Performance	104.7 $\pm$ 14.0	111.6 $\pm$ 10.7
Full scale	105.9 $\pm$ 12.9	112.3 $\pm$ 8.5
Age of onset OCD		
mean $\pm$ SD	10.3 $\pm$ 3.7	–
range	3 – 16	
Duration of illness		
mean $\pm$ SD	4.1 $\pm$ 2.9	–
range	1 – 10	
Follow-up		
N (% of initial sample)	25 (93%)	23 (79%)
Males	16	16
Females	9	7
Age of follow-up		
mean $\pm$ SD	18.8 $\pm$ 2.6	18.5 $\pm$ 2.1
range	13 – 24	14 – 22
Follow-up period (yrs)		
mean $\pm$ SD	4.4 $\pm$ 1.7	4.7 $\pm$ 1.6
range	2 – 7	2 – 7

Diagnoses at First Admission

At baseline, in addition of course to a DSM-III diagnosis of OCD, 40% of patients had one or more associated psychiatric disorder(s), as summarized in Table 3.

As shown, 16 subjects (59% of the sample) had OCD as their only current diagnosis. Six (22%) presented a major depressive episode at the time of admission and five more (19%) had history of such an episode in the past; there were more boys than girls among the depressed patients. Three girls (11% of the sample) had a current diagnosis of anxiety disorder (two had separation anxiety disorder; one had overanxious disorder) and one boy had a water phobia when younger. Three subjects (11%) were diagnosed as conduct disordered and 2 (7%) were abusing alcohol.

No subject was considered psychotic at baseline (this would have been an exclusion criterion), but it is of interest for follow-up to note that several patients had atypical symptoms: three had bizarre ritualistic behaviors, two reported "hearing" voices telling them what to do ("check the door," "touch this electric socket") and one was obsessed with the idea of someone controlling his mind.

Interim Treatment History

During the follow-up period, all but two patients had received some form(s) of treatment; however, these treatments had often been only briefly or irregularly administered.

Following the controlled drug trial, seven patients were maintained on clomipramine ranging in duration from a few moths to 3 yrs. Five received other tri-

TABLE 3
Children with Obsessive-Compulsive Disorder Associated Psychopathology at
First Admission

Associated diagnosis	Males (N = 18) N	Females (N = 9) N	Total (N = 27) N (%)
No other current diagnosis	11	5	16 (59%)
No other lifetime diagnosis	6	5	11 (41%)
Major depression (current episode)	5	1	6 (22%)
Major depression (past episode)	4	1	5 (19%)
Separation anxiety disorder (current)	0	2	2 (7%)
Overanxious disorder (current)	0	1	1 (4%)
Simple phobia (past)	1	0	1 (4%)
Alcohol abuse (current)	1	1	2 (7%)
Conduct disorder (current)	2	1	3 (11%)

cyclic antidepressant medications, most often imipramine, and three had (unsuccessful) trials of monoamine oxidase inhibitors. Five patients received neuroleptics, usually for short periods of time except for one girl who was maintained symptom-free with prolonged treatment with haloperidol. Four patients received anxiolytics. Lithium was thought to be helpful for three others, and tryptophan, megavitamins and dilantin had each been tried briefly. A number of psychological treatments were administered by private practitioners or treatment centers, in the patients' local communities. Sixteen children received psychotherapy or counselling from a few weeks to 3 yrs; supportive psychotherapy, with or without the administration of medications, was considered essential for many of them. Three patients had group therapy, and family therapy was used in two cases. Three subjects had had 2–3 yrs of residential treatment. Three received behavior therapy, and hypnosis was considered helpful for one adolescent boy.

Results of Follow-up Evaluation

Sociofamilial status. Family status and school or professional activities at the time of follow-up for subjects from the patient and control groups are shown on Table 4.

At the same age, more patients (74%) than controls (57%) were still living with their families. Although no patient was hospitalized at the time of follow-up, one was at home under close supervision of his father, who had retired early in order to take care of him, and eight patients (30%), but no controls, had been hospitalized at some time since study at the NIH.

TABLE 4
Sociofamilial Status at Follow-up for Obsessive-Compulsive Subjects and Controls

	Obsessive–compulsive subjects ($N = 27$) N (%)	Controls ($N = 28$) N (%)
Living with family	20[a] (74%)	16 (57%)
Living on their own	7 (26%)	12 (43%)
Hospitalized during follow-up period	8 (30%)	0 (0%)
In school	16[b] (59%)	24 (86%)
Employed	7 (26%)	4 (14%)
Unemployed	3 (11%)	0 (0%)
Professional status unknown	1 (4%)	0 (0%)
Married	1[c] (4%)	0 (0%)

[a]One under care of father.
[b]One in special education, one in professional school.
[c]Separated, one child.

More controls (86%) than patients (59%) were still at school, while more patients (26%) had already started to work; three patients (11%) had no current school or work activity. Only one patient had been married; she was currently separated, with one young child.

Clinical status. Tables 5 and 6 show current and lifetime diagnoses of subjects in both the patient and the control samples. The most striking findings were the continued psychopathology for the patient group and the mixed diagnostic picture.

Current Diagnoses

At the time of follow-up (see Table 5), only seven patients (28%), four females and three males, received no current psychiatric diagnosis and were considered completely well. Of the 17 patients (68%) who still qualified for a diagnosis of OCD, only five (20% of the sample) had OCD as their only disorder while 12 (48%) received one or more additional current diagnoses. The only patient who no longer had OCD but had another form of major psychopathology was a 17-yr old boy with atypical psychosis. He had had catatonic symptoms for months and, when seen for follow-up, presented marked negative symptoms and severe functional impairment. At the time of his first admission, this boy was considered atypical because of the lack of egodystonicity of his straightening rituals and defective communication skills.

In the control group, as expected, psychopathology was less prominent and followed a different pattern. Eight subjects (35%) had one or more current psychiatric diagnoses at the time of the follow-up, most often alcohol or drug abuse, none had OCD.

Lifetime Diagnoses

The lifetime diagnoses for patients and controls are shown in Table 6.

As seen, depressive, anxiety and psychotic disorders were more frequent in the patient than in the control group. More than half of the patients had major unipolar, often recurrent, depression, and 44% suffered or had suffered from some form(s) of anxiety disorder. Males and females were equally affected. Besides the one patient considered psychotic at follow-up, another, a 15-yr old girl, had been hospitalized 1 yr earlier for a short (2 week) episode of schizophreniform disorder with agitation, auditory hallucinations and thoughts of being possessed. This episode had resolved and at follow-up, the girl met criteria for OCD (severe), and marked separation anxiety.

Among the controls, none had a depressive disorder, one had had a single manic episode, one social phobia, and one a simple phobia; there was no case of psychosis.

TABLE 5
Clinical Evaluation at Follow-up for Obsessive–Compulsive Subjects and Controls:
Current Diagnosis

Current diagnosis	Obsessive–compulsive subjects (N = 25) N (%)	Controls (N = 23) N (%)
No diagnosis	7 (28%)	15 (65%)
OCD only	5 (20%)	0 (0%)
OCD + other disorder(s)	12[a] (48%)	0 (0%)
No OCD, other disorder(s)	1[b] (4%)	8[c] (35%)

[a]Eight had an anxiety disorder, three major depression, five obsessive compulsive personality disorder, one antisocial personality disorder, one immature personality disorder, one borderline intellectual functioning.
[b]Atypical psychosis.
[c]Five had alcohol abuse, two drug abuse, one conduct disorder, one oppositional disorder, one simple phobia, one antisocial personality disorder.

TABLE 6
Clinical Evaluation at Follow-up: Lifetime Diagnosis

Lifetime diagnosis[a]	Obsessive–compulsive subjects (N = 25) N (%)	Controls (N = 23) N (%)
OCD	25 (100%)	0 (0%)
Mood disorder	13[b] (52%)	1[e] (4%)
Anxiety disorder	11[c] (44%)	2[f] (9%)
Psychotic disorder	2[d] (8%)	0 (0%)
Conduct disorder	2 (8%)	3 (13%)
Oppositional defiant disorder	0 (0%)	1 (4%)
Alcohol abuse	2 (8%)	5 (22%)
Drug abuse	0 (0%)	5 (22%)
Obsessive–compulsive personality	5[g] (20%)	0 (0%)
Antisocial personality disorder	1 (4%)	1 (4%)
Immature personality disorder	1 (4%)	0 (4%)
Suicide attempts	5[g] (20%)	1 (4%)

[a]Multiple diagnoses given.
[b]Major depression.
[c]Four had generalized anxiety, two social phobia, two separation anxiety, one panic disorder, one overanxious disorder, one simple phobia.
[d]One had atypical psychosis, one transient schizophreniform disorder.
[e]Manic episode.
[f]One had social phobia, one simple phobia.
[g]All males.

More frequent among controls than among patients was alcohol and/or drug abuse (eight controls but only two patients), conduct and oppositional disorder.

Five patients, all males, and no controls, were considered to have an obsessive–compulsive personality disorder. Other personality disorders were rare in both groups.

Suicide attempts had been frequent in the patient group: five male patients had made one or several suicide attempts during the follow-up period. For three of them, these gestures appeared secondary to the frustration and despair of severe obsessive–compulsive symptoms during adolescence; one tried to choke himself with a belt, one took an overdose of clomipramine and one cut his wrist. Another boy had taken two large impulsive overdoses with clomipramine at age 20 during depressive episodes. The last case, a 19-yr old boy with antisocial personality disorder, had taken several overdoses of various medications during angry outbursts.

In the control group, only one girl reported a suicide gesture, slashing her wrist at age 14; she received no psychiatric diagnostics at follow-up.

Symptom Evaluation and Change

Clinical rating scale scores at first admission, after 5 weeks of clomipramine treatment and at follow-up, are shown in Table 7.

Compared to first admission, mean scores for obsessive–compulsive symptoms (Obsessive–Compulsive Rating Scale, NIMH Global Scale for OCD, Leyton Obsessional Inventory—Child Version) were significantly lower ($p < 0.05$) both at 5 weeks of clomipramine treatment and at follow-up. (Mean scores on scales measuring depression, anxiety or global impairment were relatively low at baseline and unchanged under any condition.)

Thus, for the sample as a whole, the initial improvement in obsessive–compulsive symptoms after treatment was maintained at follow-up. However, individual scores after 5 weeks of clomipramine treatment and at follow-up were not significantly correlated and similarly none of the measures of long-term outcome were predicted from initial treatment response. That is, for some individuals, greatest response to medication occurred months after initial treatment. For a few others an initial good response had seemed to "wear off".

At follow-up, the severity of obsessive–compulsive symptoms varied. Among those with OC symptoms, four (16%) had only mild obsessions and/or compulsions, nine (36%) had moderate to marked symptoms, and four (16%) had severe symptoms as defined by the Comprehensive Psychopathological Rating Scale. For most, the type of ritual or content of the obsession changed over the years. At first admission, the most frequent clinical picture was fear of contamination with the associated rituals of washing, cleaning and avoiding touching. At follow-up, the most common compulsions included checking (50% of the subjects), repeating (27%) or performing odd gestures (27%), washing or cleaning (22%), touching, arranging or counting; four subjects (18%) had obsessional thoughts without rituals.

While only five boys (20% of the sample) had a diagnosis of obsessive–compulsive personality disorder at follow-up, some obsessive–compulsive traits were common: 50% reported being excessively perfectionist and 41% complained of indecisiveness.

Twelve subjects (48%) had had a fluctuating course without complete remission. The disorder had been truly episodic for eight other patients (32%), with periods of remission of 6 months–9 yrs. Three subjects (9%) had only had one episode, one patient had maintained a constant level of OCD, while one other had gradually and steadily worsened.

Patients' Self-report

Certain themes emerged across the patients' essays when they were read as a group. The history of their disorder, while essentially unchanged had different emphases, perhaps due to their more mature perspective. Retrospectively, eight male subjects were more certain than brief episodes (less than 6 months) of obsessive–compulsive behavior had occurred when they had been between 2 and 6 yrs of age.

TABLE 7
Symptomatic Changes for 25 Obsessive-Compulsion Patients from First Admission to 2-7 Yrs. Follow-up

Measure	First admission $\bar{x} \pm$ SD	After 5 weeks of clomipramine treatment $\bar{x} \pm$ SD	2–7 yrs follow-up $\bar{x} \pm$ SD
Leyton Obsessional Inventory—Child Version:			
Yes	20.2 ± 8.3	11.6 ± 7.1[a]	12.7 ± 7.5
Resistance	31.4 ± 18.7	19.6 ± 18.9[a]	19.2 ± 15.0
Interference	28.9 ± 19.3	15.4 ± 18.3[a]	15.5 ± 14.7
Obsessive–compulsive rating	13.1 ± 3.2	9.6 ± 3.6[a]	9.2 ± 3.7
NIMH Self-rated depresssion scale	7.7 ± 7.4	7.2 ± 7.8	7.8 ± 8.1
NIMH Global scales for:			
OCD	7.4 ± 2.7	5.2 ± 3.3[a]	5.2 ± 2.5[a]
Depression	3.5 ± 2.3	3.2 ± 2.4	3.0 ± 2.3
Anxiety	4.6 ± 2.6	3.7 ± 2.1	4.4 ± 2.1
Global impairment	6.6 ± 3.2	5.2 ± 3.5	4.4 ± 2.4

[a]Significantly lower than at first admission (paired t-test < 0.05).

Five male subjects felt that their counting rituals in grade school had been the precursors to the sexual preoccupations in adolescence although they could not verbalize more precisely how these "felt" continuous.

The patients' retrospective recall of months to years of hiding the disorder from families and friends were particularly poignant; they had only turned to their families in desperation, and recall their dismay about their families' helplessness as one of the most painful memories.

Common themes emerged concerning treatment and self-help. Keeping extremely busy was always seen as helpful; almost any activity, if mandated by outside schedule or organization, could help keep the rituals away. Exercise seemed also particularly helpful. Psychotherapy was seen as useful for family problems and for shyness, but not for the disorder.

Several patients reported inventing a "do-it-yourself" behavior therapy; they were helped by their determination to "brave it out" and to expose themselves to the feared or "trigger" stimulus while preventing themselves from ritualizing. Slowly (over weeks and months) this had seemed helpful. Other "tricks" were to make others "take the responsibility" for their actions so that it was "ok" to pass the door, stove, etc. Their major advice to younger patients was to keep up hope as they had learned to live with or overcome their disorder more than they had expected to do when younger.

CT Scans

CT scans of the patients at follow-up were compared with scans of sex- and age-matched normal controls using a volumetric analysis not used in the baseline study. These data are reported separately (Luxenberg *et al.*, 1988).

Dexamethasone Suppression Test

Eighty-eight per cent of the patients at baseline and 93% at follow-up had a negative dexamethasone suppression test. It is noteworthy that even OC patients seen during a clinical depressive episode at either time of examination did not have a positive test.

Neuropsychological Testing

At baseline, compared to their age- and IQ-matched normal controls, OCD patients showed impairment in spatial orientation and judgment (Behar *et al.*, 1984; Cox *et al.*, in press). Results from the two tests with the most striking patient–control differences, the Road Map and Stylus Maze test, are presented in Table 8. These deficits were selective in that scores on other tests measuring attention, memory and perception, judged to be of equal difficulty, did not differ between groups. On the Money's Road Map of Directional Sense, patients committed more left–right errors, particularly in the rotated or inverted position; on the Stylus Maze Learning Task, obsessive–compulsive subjects had higher error rates and more frequent rule breakings.

At follow-up (see Table 8), patients and controls had naturally improved with age, as reflected in their significantly decreased error scores on retest, but the relative discrepancy between groups persisted. The patients' deficits were still specific in the entire test battery; they were not simply a reflection of current clinical functioning when multiple comparisons were performed.

Neuropsychological impairment did not correlate with any measure of disorder severity at baseline or at follow-up.

Prediction of Outcome

Correlational analysis was performed among the different outcome variables described above, and between outcome and baseline measures.

TABLE 8
Leyton Obsessional Inventory and Neuropsychological Test Scores for OCD Patients and Controls at First Admission and at 2–7 Yrs. Follow-up

Measure	First admission		Follow-up	
	OCD Patients $\bar{x} \pm$ SD $N = 27$	Controls $\bar{x} \pm$ SD $N = 29$	OCD Patients $\bar{x} \pm$ SD $N = 21$	Controls $\bar{x} \pm$ SD $N = 23$
LOI—CV Yes	20.2 ± 8.3[a]	12.5 ± 6.1	12.7 ± 7.5[ce]	11.3 ± 7.1
Resistance	31.4 ± 18.7[a]	11.5 ± 8.2	19.2 ± 15.0[bce]	10.6 ± 7.4
Interference	28.9 ± 19.3[a]	10.3 ± 8.5	15.5 ± 14.7[bce]	7.7 ± 6.3
Street Map (No. of errors)				
away	1.9 ± 2.3[a]	0.6 ± 1.2	1.4 ± 2.1[bc]	0.3 ± 0.8
toward	4.2 ± 3.7[a]	1.2 ± 1.4	2.3 ± 2.8[bc]	0.7 ± 1.0
combined	6.1 ± 5.7[a]	1.8 ± 1.9	3.8 ± 4.1[bc]	1.0 ± 1.6
Maze (No. of errors)				
errors	87.1 ± 35.8[a]	59.6 ± 23.9	69.6 ± 38.4[bc]	44.9 ± 11.4[d]
crossovers	5.8 ± 4.8[a]	3.5 ± 2.9	4.2 ± 7.6	0.9 ± 1.6[d]
combined	92.9 ± 38.4[a]	63.1 ± 25.1	73.8 ± 42.3[bc]	45.9 ± 10.9[d]

Unpaired Student's *t*-tests:
[a]Significantly different than controls at baseline.
[b]Higher than controls at follow-up.
[c]Significantly lower than baseline for patients.
[d]Significantly lower than baseline for controls.
[e]Group × time interaction significant at $p < 0.05$.

There was difficulty in prediction of outcome as so few subjects were considered well at follow-up. What was most striking, however, was that an initial good response to clomipramine treatment conveyed no prognostic benefit: some of the initial non-responders had done well, while some former "good responders" had continued OCD that no longer could be adequately controlled by drug and/or they had developed other disorders. Because treatment during the follow-up period was sparse and uncontrolled, it was not possible to relate any particular therapy to long-term outcome. It is clear, however, that initial drug treatment had not drastically changed long-term outcome.

Severity of the symptoms at baseline, and presence or absence of neurological or neuropsychological impairment, were not significant predictors of outcome. Similarly, a family history of depression and/or anxiety disorder had no predictive value in determining later clinical state.

DISCUSSION

The most striking finding is the continued psychopathology for this group of children. Not only was OCD still prevalent, but the depression and anxiety which frequently accompanies the disorder in adult samples was more widely prevalent in middle and late adolescence. As in other studies, however, the diagnosis "bred true", that is, the major disorder in most cases remained OCD, and most specifically, the diagnosis of psychosis was only considered for two cases.

The results are in keeping with those of Zeitlin (1986) and of Warren (1960) in showing continuity of symptoms of obsessions between childhood and adult life.

Neuropsychological, neurological and CT scan differences from controls were seen. Possibly, because of the widespread continued psychopathology, and therefore the lack of a "well" contrast group, it was not possible to make meaningful predictions about the relationship between severity of current psychopathology and these neurobiological features.

The relationship between OCD, depression and anxiety is provocative. Most, if not all studies, find a relationship between these disorders (Welner *et al.*, 1976). A number of interpretations are possible, of course, including a basic tie between disorders representing a common etiology, whether biological or other, or alternately that depression and anxiety are understandable sequelae of prolonged handicap from OCD. None of the explanations are entirely satisfactory. As depression often predates OCD (Welner *et al.*, 1976), it is too simplistic to see these disorders as secondary to OCD. On the other hand, the differential response to clomipramine over DMI (Leonard, Swedo, Rapoport, Coffey & Cheslow, 1988), the normal dexamethasone suppression test, and male preponderance of childhood cases suggest a different underlying pathophysiology.

While this is the largest and only prospective study of childhood OCD to date, a number of limitations are evident. First, the study is of a clinically referred sample. While certain characteristics are similar to that seen in a community based sample (Flament *et al.*, 1988), a number of unknown factors may contribute to the poor outcome of this population. However, we believe these data reflect the malignant nature of the disorder, as a similar outcome was obtained in the 2-yr follow-up study of the adolescent non-referred sample studied by Flament *et al.* (Berg, Rapoport, Whitaker & Davies, 1989). Finally, the follow-up term ranged from only 2 to 7 yrs, so the study must be viewed as an intermediate step in their development. It would be interesting to look at a longer follow-up period.

Psychiatric diagnoses were made in each case by two psychiatrists for whom reliability had been established in previous studies; however, diagnoses were not made blind. There was no practical way to overcome these methodological problems. The scoring of most of the measures, however, including DIS, neuropsychological tests, autonomic tests, CT scan and DST permits some external validation.

It is clear that the treatment of this population of children with OCD was unsatisfactory. None of the group had had drug treatment and/or sufficiently intense behavioral treatment to satisfy the criteria of those working most intensely with the population (Marks, 1979; Bolton *et al.*, 1983). Geographic diversity and our own staff limitations precluded a controlled treatment phase. A larger outcome study with more strenuous interim consultations and treatment monitoring is now ongoing.

REFERENCES

American Psychiatric Association, Committee on Nomenclature and Statistics (1980). *Diagnostic and statistical manual of mental disorders* (3rd edn). Washington, DC: American Psychiatric Association.

Anthony, J. C., Folstein, M., Romanoski, A. J., Von Korff, M. R., Nestadt, G. R., Chahal, R., Merchant, A., Brown, C. H., Shapiro, S., Kramer, M. & Gruenberg, E. M. (1985). Comparison of the lay diagnostic interview and a standardized psychiatric diagnosis. *Archives of General Psychiatry,* **42,** 667–675.

Asberg, M., Montgomery, S., Perris, C., Schalling, D. & Sedvall, G. (1978). A comprehensive psychopathological rating scale. *Acta Psychiatrica Scandinavica,* **271,** 5–27.

Balslev-Olesen, T. & Geert-Jorgensen, E. (1959). The prognosis of obsessive compulsive neurosis. *Acta Psychiatrica Scandinavica* Supplement, 136, 232–241.

Behar, D., Berg, C., Rapoport, J. L., Denckla, M., Mann, L., Cox, C., Fedio, P., Zahn, T. & Wolfman, M. (1984). Computerized tomography and neuropsychological test measures in children with obsessive compulsive disorder. *American Journal of Psychiatry,* **14,** 363–368.

Bolton, D., Collins, S. & Steinberg, D. (1983). The treatment of obsessive-compulsive disorder in adolescence: a report of fifteen cases. *British Journal of Psychiatry,* **142,** 456–464.

Berg, C. J., Rapoport, J. L. & Flament, M. F. (1986). The Leyton Obsessional Inventory—Child Version. *Journal of the American Academy of Child Psychiatry*, **25**, 84–91.

Berg, C. J., Rapoport, J. L., Whitaker, A. & Davies, M. (1989). Childhood obsessive compulsive disorder: a two-year prospective follow-up of a community sample. *Journal of the American Academy of Child Adolescence Psychiatry*, **28**, 528–533.

Berman, L. (1942). The obsessive-compulsive neurosis in children. *Journal of Nervous and Mental Diseases*, **95**, 26–39.

Black, A. (1974). The natural history of obsessional neurosis. In H. R. Beech (Ed.), *Obsessional states* (pp. 19–54.) London: Methuen.

Butters, N., Soeldner, C. & Fedio, P. (1972). Comparison of parietal and frontal lobe spatial deficits in man: extrapersonal vs personal (egocentric). *Perceptual Motor Skills*, **34**, 27–34.

Carroll, B. J., Feinberg, M., Greden, J., Tarika, J., Albala, A. A., Haskett, R. F., James, N. M., Kronfol, Z., Lohr, N., Steiner, M., de Vigne, J. P. & Young, E. (1981). A specific laboratory test for the diagnosis of melancholia. *Archives of General Psychiatry*, **38**, 15–22.

Cox, C., Brouwers, P., Berg, C., Rapoport, J. L. & Fedio, P. (1990). Neuropsychological correlates of obsessive compulsive disorder in adolescents. In J. Rapoport (Ed.), *Obsessive compulsive disorder in children and adolescents*. Washington, DC: American Psychiatric Press (in press).

Denckla, M. B. (1973). Development of speed in repetitive and successive finger movements in normal children. *Developmental Medicine and Child Neurology*, **15**, 635–645.

Denckla, M. B. (1974). Development of coordination in normal children. *Developmental Medicine and Child Neurology*, **16**, 729–741.

Denckla, M. B. (1985a). Revised physical and neurological examination for soft signs. *Psychopharmacology Bulletin*, **21**, 773–779.

Denckla, M. A. (1985b). Scoring the revised physical and neurological examination for subtle signs. *Psychopharmacology Bulletin*, **21**, 780–792.

Flament, M. & Rapoport, J. L. (1984). Childhood obsessive compulsive disorder. In T. R. Insel (Ed.), New findings in obsessive compulsive disorder (pp. 24–43). Washington, DC: American Press.

Flament, M., Rapoport, J. L., Berg, C. J., Sceery, W., Kilts, C., Mellstrom, B. & Linnoila, M. (1985). Clomipramine treatment of childhood obsessive compulsive disorder; a double-blind controlled study. *Archives of General Psychiatry*, **42**, 977–983.

Flament, M., Whitaker, A., Rapoport, J. L., Davies, M., Zeremba-Berg, C., Kalikow, K., Sceery, W. & Shaffer, D. (1988). Obsessive compulsive disorder in adolescence: an epidemiological study. *Journal of the American Academy of Child Psychiatry*, **27**, 764–771.

Goodwin, D. W., Guze, S. B. & Robins, E. (1969). Follow-up studies in obsessional neurosis. *Archives of General Psychiatry*, **20**, 182–187.

Grimshaw, L. (1965). The outcome of obsessional disorder: a follow-up study of 100 cases. *British Journal of Psychiatry*, **111**, 1051–1056.

Herjanic, B. & Campbell, J. W. (1977). Differentiating psychiatrically disturbed children on the basis of a structured interview. *Journal of Abnormal Child Psychology*, **5**, 127–135.

Hollingsworth, C. E., Tanguay, P. E., Grossman, L. & Pabst, P. (1980). Long-term outcome of obsessive compulsive disorder in childhood. *Journal of the American Academy of Child Psychiatry*, **19**, 134–144.

Ingram, I. M. (1961). Obsessional illness in mental hospital patients. *Journal of Mental Science*, **107**, 382–402.

Judd, L. L. (1965). Obsessive compulsive neurosis in children. *Archives of General Psychiatry*, **12**, 136–143.

Karno, M., Golding, J., Sorenson,S. & Burnam, M. (1988). The epidemiology of obsessive compulsive disorder in five U.S. communities. *Archives of General Psychiatry*, **45**, 1094–1099.

Kringlen, E. (1965). Obsessional neurotics: a long-term follow-up. *British Journal of Psychiatry*, **111**, 709–722.

Langfeldt, G. (1938). Studiet av tvangsfenomenenes forekomst, genese, klinikk og prognose. *Tidsskrift for den Norske laegeforening*, **13**, 16.

Leonard, H., Swedo, S., Rapoport, J., Coffey, M. & Cheslow, D. (1988). Treatment of obsessive compulsive disorder with clomipramine and desmethylimipramine: a double blind crossover comparison. *Psychopharmacology Bulletin*, **24**, 252–266.

Lewis, A. (1936). Problems of obsessional illness. *Proceedings of the Royal Society of Medicine*, **29**, 325–336.

Lo, W. H. (1967). A follow-up study of obsessional neurotics in Hong-Kong Chinese. *British Journal of Psychiatry*, **113**, 823–832.

Luxenberg, J. S., Flament, M. F., Swedo, S. E., Friedland, R. P., Rapoport, J. L. & Rapoport, S.I. (1988). Neuroanatomic abnormalities in obsessive compulsive disorder detected with quantitative X-ray computed tomography. *American Journal of Psychiatry*, **145**, 1089–1093.

Marks, I. (1979). Cure and care of neurosis. *Psychological Medicine*, **9**, 629–660.

Mazure, G. & Gershon, E. (1979). Blindness and reliability in lifetime psychiatric diagnosis. *Psychiatry*, **36**, 21–525.

Money, J., Alexander, D. & Walker, H. (1965). *A standardized roadmap test of directional sense*. Baltimore: Johns Hopkins University Press.

Muller, C. (1953). Der Übergang von Zwangsneurose in Schizophrenie im Lichte der Zwangskrankheit. *Schweizer Archiv für Neurologie und Psychiatrie*, **72**, 218–225.

Murphy, D. L., Pickar, D. & Alterman, I. S. (1982). Methods for the quantitative assessment of depressive and manic behavior. In E. I. Burdock, A. Sudilovsky & S. Gershon (Eds), *The behavior of psychiatric patients* (pp. 355–392). New York: Marcel Dekker.

Osterrieth, P. L. (1944). Le test de copie d'une figure complexe. *Archives de Psychologie*, **10**, 206–356.

Pollitt, J. (1957). Natural history of obsessional states: a study of 150 cases. *British Medical Journal*, **26**, 194–198.

Post, R. M., Kopin, J. & Goodwin, F. K. (1973). Tetrahydrocanabinol in depressed patients. *Archives of General Psychiatry*, **28**, 345–352.

Rapoport, J. L., Elkins, R., Langer, D., Sceery, W., Buchsbaum, M., Gillin, J., Murphy, D.,

Zahn, T., Lake, R., Ludlow, W. & Mendelson, W. (1981). Childhood obsessive compulsive disorder. *American Journal of Psychiatry,* **138,** 1545–1554.

Rapoport, J. L. (1986). Childhood obsessive compulsive disorder. *Journal of Child Psychology and Psychiatry,* **27,** 289–295.

Rapoport, J. L. (Ed.) (1990). *Obsessive compulsive disorder in children and adolescents.* Washington, DC: American Psychiatric Press (in press).

Rey, A. (1941). Examen clinique en psychologie dans les cas d'encephalapathie traumatique. *Archives de Psychologie,* **28,** 286–340.

Robins, L., Helzer, J., Croughan,J. & Ratcliff, K. (1981). National Institute of Mental Health diagnostic interview schedule: its history, characteristics and validity. *Archives of General Psychiatry,* **38,** 381–391.

Rosenberg, C. M. (1968). Complications of obsessional neurosis. *British Journal of Psychiatry,* **114,** 477–478.

Rudin, E. (1953). Ein Beitrag zur Frage der Zwangskrankheit, insbesondere ihrer hereditaren Beziehungen. *Archiv für Psychiatrie und Zeitschrift gesamter neurologisher Psychiatrie,* **191,** 14–54.

Warren, W. (1960). Some relationships between the psychiatry of children and of adults. *Journal of Mental Science,* **106,** 815–826.

Welner, A., Reich, T., Robins, E., Fishman, R. & Van Doren, T. (1976). Obsessive compulsive neurosis: record, follow-up and family studies. I. Inpatient record study. *Comprehensive Psychiatry,* **17,** 527–539.

Welner, Z., Reich, W., Herjanic, B., Jung, K. & Amado, H. (1987). Reliability, validity and parent-child agreement studies of the diagnostic interview for children and adolescents (DICA). *Journal of the American Academy of Child and Adolescent Psychiatry,* **26,** 649–653.

Zahn, T. P., Rapoport, J. L. & Thompson, C. L. (1980). Autonomic and behavioral effects of dextroamphetamine and placebo in normal and hyperactive prepubertal boys. *Journal of Abnormal Child Psychology,* **8,** 145–160.

Zeitlin, H. (1986). *The natural history of psychiatric disorder in children.* Oxford: Oxford University Press.

20

Annotation: Child and Adolescent Mania— Diagnostic Considerations

Gabrielle A. Carlson
State University of New York at Stony Brook

INTRODUCTION

The history of mania in children and adolescents extends back to Kraepelin, who recognized the condition in about 3% of his patients by age 15 and almost 20% by age 20 (Kraepelin, 1921). Little attention was paid to his observations, however, so the existence and putative significance of juvenile mania remained controversial for the next 40 yrs. Anthony and Scott (1960) took the first definitive steps to resolve the controversy regarding the nature and frequency of mania and manic depressive insanity in young people with a study that was a landmark for three reasons: (1) they defined childhood as being prior to puberty, thus separating issues of childhood and adolescent disorder; (2) they delineated specific criteria to define juvenile manic depression well before this was the established way to proceed in psychiatry; and (3) they demonstrated the continuity of prepubertal manic depression with the adult disorder by describing a 12-yr old boy whose episodes continued into adulthood.

Anthony and Scott (1960) never described manic symptomatology *per se* but required that a child's clinical picture conform to that established by Kraepelin, among others. Since then, the emergence of operational symptom criteria has made a great impact on the consistent delineation of psychiatric syndromes. Significantly, there has always been general concordance regarding specific symptoms of mania. Thus, the condition as we know it has deviated little from Kraepelin's description (Kendall, 1985). While the clusters and variations of symptoms that characterize classical mania have been relatively clear (e.g. expansive and volatile mood which reflects itself in grandiosity, overcommitment, recklessness, and displeasure at being thwarted; tireless energy that is manifested by hyperactivity, pressured speech, racing thoughts, inability to maintain attention and feeling that sleep is unnecessary), the range of severity of mania has been considerably less clear. This is true for adults and is evidenced by the varied attempts to classify the spectrum of mania with such diagnostic terms as cyclothymia, bipolar II disorder, bipolar I disorder, and schizoaffective mania.

ISSUES OF SEVERITY

Cyclothymia was initially considered a personality disorder, though its possible relationship as a harbinger of manic depression was recognized early on (Kraepelin, 1921). It has been upgraded to the status of a clinical "disorder" in the current *DSM III, DSM III-R* [American Psychiatric Association (APA), 1980, 1987] classification and although its chronicity (duration of 1–2 yrs in youths and adults, respectively) is defined, its severity is not. *DSM III-R* notes that, by definition, there is "no *marked* (italics mine) impairment in social and occupational functioning" as there is in mania and that the hypomanic phase may be either productive or produce occupational and social difficulty. Thus there is a blurring both at the boundaries between cyclothymia and normality, where there is no impairment, and cyclothymia and mania where there is.

In trying to operationalize the severity of mania more clearly, investigators (e.g. Dunner, 1983; Perris, 1966) have defined bipolar I disorder by a manic episode that required hospitalization and bipolar II disorder by hypomania that produces impairment but not hospitalization. (The difference between cyclothymia and bipolar II is in the severity of the depressive episode.) This distinction, however, has not been included either in the Research Diagnostic Criteria (RDC; Spitzer, Endicott & Robins, 1978) or the American Psychiatric Disorder classifications (*DSM III, DSM III-R;* APA, 1980, 1987).

While the distinctions between normality, hypomania and mania reflect differences of degree of disorder, differences between mania, psychotic mania, schizoaffective mania and schizophrenia raise questions of different kinds of disorders. Moreover, there is still no unequivocal way to make the distinctions. Such time-honored criteria of degree of thought disorder, or presence of Schneiderian first rank symptoms and mood incongruence of psychotic symptoms, at least during the manic episode, have not been reliable in distinguishing a manic course from a schizophrenic course (see Kendall, 1985, for a review).

SEVERITY ISSUES IN CHILDREN AND ADOLESCENTS

The above diagnostic deliberations have considerable significance for children and adolescents. For instance, the lifetime prevalence of mania in a non-referred sample of 14–16 yr olds, systematically evaluated with the Diagnostic Interview for Children and Adolescents, Parent and Child versions (DICA/DICA-P) (Herjanic

& Reich, 1982) varied from 0.6% using RDC criteria and including duration and severity criteria to 13.3% using DSM III-R and ignoring both degree of severity and duration of episode (Carlson & Kashani, 1988). In addition, as for adults, the area of greatest clinical significance has been distinguishing between adolescent mania and schizophrenia.

Recognition of mania in adolescents and older children and not misdiagnosing it as schizophrenia has been particularly hampered because of the strongly held and prevailing bias that schizophrenia is more frequent in young people. A similar, erroneously-held notion, in spite of Kraepelin's data, and that of Wertham (1929), Perris (1966) and Winokur, Clayton and Reich (1969), has been that mania did not occur in adolescents. Since then, two large studies, one in the United States (Loranger & Levine, 1978) and one in New Zealand (Joyce, 1984), have not only replicated Kraepelin's observation but have demonstrated unequivocally that bipolar disorder frequently begins in adolescence and young adulthood. Furthermore, although a number of older studies of adolescent manic depression had described manic episodes as "wild" (Campbell, 1952; Kasanin, 1931), or as having "schizophrenic coloring" (Landolt, 1957) and schizophreniform features (Olsen, 1961), most of the case and series reports of the 1970s (Berg, Hullin, Allsopp, O'Brien & MacDonald, 1974; White & O'Shanick, 1977; van Krevelen & van Voorst, 1969; Engstrom, Robbins & May, 1978; Horowitz, 1977) were noteworthy only for their identification of classic and identifiable mania and bipolar manic depression in teenagers.

Carlson and Goodwin (1973) had previously examined the diagnostic confusion between mania and schizophrenia which occurred in a population of adult manic patients at the National Institutes of Mental Health who had their entire manic episodes unfold often to very psychotic proportions (Carlson & Goodwin, 1973). With that in mind, Carlson and Strober (1978) reviewed records of six clearly bipolar (by then) late adolescents. They found all had been earlier misdiagnosed as having had schizophrenia. This was usually because the affective episodes were psychotic, the youngsters manifested a thought disorder, and the staff overlooked or misinterpreted the euphoria, depression and irritability.

This observation has been made repeatedly since (Bashir, Russell & Johnson, 1987; Hassanyeh & Davison, 1980; Joyce, 1984; Hsu & Starzynski, 1986) and raises the question of whether young people are particularly predisposed to developing psychotic symptoms. Three studies suggest this may be the case (Ballenger, Reus & Post, 1982; Joyce, 1984; Rosen, Rosenthal, Van Dusen, Dunner & Fieve, 1983). While Brockington, Wainwright and Kendall (1980) report that the presence of auditory hallucinations and passivity feelings have a more grave consequence for outcome than delusions of reference or persecution, a review of their data does not strongly support that conclusion. This observation, however, has not been examined specifically in adolescents. It is worth noting that the adolescent onset of bipolar disorder does not worsen the prognosis of the disorder (Carlson, Davenport & Jamison, 1977; McGlashan, 1988) nor does adolescence *per se* diminish lithium response (Strober, Hanna & McCracken, in press; Strober, Morrell, Lampert & Burroughs, in press).

ISSUES OF SUBSYNDROMAL MANIA

There is a growing body of research examining the boundary between mania and subsyndromal forms of the disorder. This research is especially relevant to adolescents for two reasons. Firstly, as noted earlier, bipolar disorder may, and cyclothymia does begin in adolescence (Akiskal, Downs, Jordan, Watson, Daugherty & Pruitt, 1985; Klein, Depue & Slater, 1986). Secondly, just as there has been a bias that severe, psychotic psychopathology must be schizophrenic in nature, milder disorders have been considered to be either "adolescent turmoil' or adjustment reactions (see Carlson & Strober, 1978, for a review). While some adolescents undoubtedly experience emotional lability, especially in the years around puberty (Rutter, Graham, Chadwick & Yule, 1976), the consensus is that psychiatric symptoms producing functional impairment should not be dismissed as a normal or a necessary part of adolescent development (Graham & Rutter, 1985). It is obvious, however, that the duration and intensity of hypomanic symptoms will be critical to distinguishing hypomania from more short-lived, non-pathological emotional lability that may be part of the adolescence.

The distinction between lability and cyclothymia is important because the predictive validity of cyclothymia and hypomania for an ultimate bipolar course has been amply demonstrated (Akiskal, Dzenveredjian, Rosenthal & Khani, 1977; Klein & Depue, 1984). The familial aggregation of bipolar relatives of cyclothymes has also confirmed its position in the bipolar spectrum (Akiskal *et al.*, 1977, 1985; Klein, Depue & Slater, 1985; Endicott, Nee, Andreasen, Clayton, Keller & Coryell, 1985). Depue *et al.* (1981) have constructed a self-report measure called the General Behavior Inventory (GBI) which delineates the range of symptoms felt to be part of hypomania (and dysthymia). Built into the measure are ratings of duration, intensity and frequency of symptoms. This instrument has shown both reliability and impressive sensitivity and specificity in the populations tested so far. For instance, the defined cut-off score selected 24% of 41 15–21-yr old offspring of bipolar parents and none of the 22 matched offspring of a psychiatrically disordered control group (Klein, Depue & Slater, 1986). These young people also met independent interview criteria for bipolar II disorder and cyclothymia. Although the samples were relatively small, the dimensional approach that the GBI provides may be the best way of quantifying levels of severity and duration for subsyndromal mania and depression. Unfortunately, it may not be possible to use this instrument in subjects much younger than 15 because of the complexity of the questions, yet it is the peripubertal population on whom such distinctions would be most enlightening.

ISSUES OF CO-MORBIDITY

Another boundary problem occurs because of the symptom similarities between childhood disruptive or externalizing disorders [attention deficit/hyperactivity disorder (ADHD) and conduct disorder (CD)] and non-psychotic mania. [For this discussion I am combining ADHD and CD both because both disorders are reported and because criteria have changed over time such that conventional wisdom now suggests that many hyperactive children described before *DSM III* had combined ADHD and CD (Hinshaw, 1987; Taylor, 1986; Prior & Sanson, 1986; Taylor, 1986).] In both disorders, hyperactivity, distractibility, intrusiveness, poor judgment, volatile and irritable behavior especially when thwarted, impulsive risk taking, poor sleep habits and denial of problems prevail. Hyperactive, conduct-disordered children may brag and tell "tall stories" making them appear grandiose as well. One cannot even depend on eliciting a history of euphoria since its absence does not rule mania out and its presence is very difficult to elicit from children and their parents (Carlson, 1984). The major symptomatic difference is that ADHD/CD is largely chronic with an age of onset usually before age 6 or 7 whereas mania is episodic. In fact, I have made the point elsewhere that the further one gets from requiring clear-cut episodes of disorder, as part of the definition, the more muddied these waters become (Carlson, 1983, 1984).

The symptom overlap between hyperactivity and mania has prompted a number of investigators to explore the possibility that some hyperactive children are "masked" manics. Examination of relatives of hyperactive children for bipolar disorder (Biederman *et al.*, 1986; Cantwell, 1972; Lahey *et al.*, 1988; Morrison & Stewart, 1971; Stewart, DeBlois & Cummings, 1980), treatment of hyperactive children with lithium (Whitehead & Clark, 1970; Greenhill, Reider, Wender, Buchsbaum & Zahn, 1973) and follow-up of hyperactive children into adulthood (Gittelman, Mannuzza, Shenker & Bonagura, 1985; Weiss, Hechtman & Lily, 1986) have not confirmed that hypothesis. Interestingly, however, the converse is not true. A significant minority of bipolar children and adolescents have been described as having past histories compatible with hyperactivity and/or conduct disorder (see Carlson, 1983, 1984, and Casat, 1982, for reviews, also Akiskal *et al.*, 1985; Endicott *et al.*, 1985; Koehler-Troy, Strober & Malenbaum, 1986; Reiss, 1985). Positive family histories of mania and depression have been prominent in the case history descriptions and psychopathology has either remitted completely or been attenuated with lithium carbonate treatment.

Although for the most part there has been a relationship between the disruptive behavior disorders and mania/bipolar disorder only in families with a bipolar or major depressive relative, the question arises as to what if any relationship exists between the two disorders. There are several possibilities, which can be summarized as follows:

(1) ADHD/CD is a prodrome or subsyndromal form of mania which has been developmentally modified and will look more obvious with puberty. This is probably the most frequent interpretation and has been discussed elsewhere (see Carlson, 1983, 1984, for reviews, also Akiskal, Khani & Scott-Strauss, 1979; Akiskal *et al.*, 1985).

(2) Children with prepubertal bipolar disorder (which is manifested by ADHD/CD) have a particularly virulent form of bipolar disorder as exemplified by its early age of onset. Several investigators (Rice *et al.*, 1987; Smeraldi, Gasperini, Macciardi, Bussoleni & Morabito, 1983) have observed especially high morbidity risks of affective disorder among relatives of early onset bipolars. Specifically, Strober *et al.* (1988) report that adolescent bipolar patients with prepubertal ADHD/CD psychopathology had even higher rates of affective disorder (44.1% vs 23.5%) and bipolar disorder (29.4% vs 8.6%) in relatives than adolescent-onset bipolars. Further indication of the greater severity of prepubertal-onset patients' disorder is their relatively poor response to lithium. Only 40% had responded (and then only partially) to the drug after 6 weeks in contrast to an 80% response in the adolescent-onset group.

(3) The ADHD/CD represents one of many non-specific early responses to family psychopathology (e.g. Gershon *et al.*, 1985).

(4) Mania occurring after the onset of ADHD/CD is a condition known in the adult literature as secondary affective disorder, a concept articulated originally by Monro (1966) and Woodruff, Murphy and Herjanic (1967). In this instance, secondary means that another psychiatric disorder temporally precedes the affective disorder and suggests that both disorders coexist (co-morbidity) without necessarily causal implications. However, the outcome is usually worse than that for either disorder alone. Alcoholism and substance abuse are the non-effective disorders most often cited in conjunction with bipolar disorder (e.g. Akiskal *et al.*, 1985; Andreasen, Grove, Coryell, Endicott & Clayton, 1988; Black, Winokur, Bell, Nasrallah & Hulbert, 1988). Andreasen *et al.* (1988), however, report that the primary–secondary nosology contributes little to our understanding of bipolar disorder since factors like age of onset, number of episodes and family history of psychopathology are similar in bipolars with and without previous other psychiatric disorders. Unfortunately, they do not describe treatment response for their primary and secondary bipolars which would be additionally helpful in determining the validity of the distinction. Black *et al.* (1988) on the other hand, call mania with pre-existing other disorders "complicated mania" and note that those with prior psychopathology (usually alcohol, substance abuse or antisocial personality) had significantly earlier age of onset, more suicidal behavior, lower rates of recovery, less adequate lithium

trails but probably poorer response to lithium than a matched group of bipolar-only patients.

(5) Children with ADHD/CD who develop mania have "secondary mania" as originally described by Krauthammer and Klerman (1978), that is, a manic syndrome which occurs following and is probably precipitated by such organic factors as metabolic disturbances, specific drugs, seizures, central nervous system infections, tumors, and other CNS pathology (Stasiek & Zetin, 1985). The relationship between "brain damage" and mania has been mentioned by different investigators with remarkably similar observations. In the study cited above, Black *et al.* (1988) reported that "complicated" manics with prior medical disorders had more organic psychopathology, later age of onset of mania and a much higher death rate at follow-up than either uncomplicated or psychiatrically complicated manics. In a series of papers, Cook, Shukla & Hoff (1986), Cook, Shukla, Hoff and Aronson (1987) and Shukla, Cook, Hoff and Aronson (1988) documented that patients with *DSM III* diagnosed mania and "brain damage" as attested by abnormal EEGs, encephalitis, tumor, stroke and head trauma had significantly lower rates of affective and other psychopathology in family members, more irritability and less psychosis in episodes, and both poorer response to lithium and better response to carbamazepine. This is very similar to findings reported by Himmelhoch and Garfinkel (1986) who enlarge upon Kraepelin's description of "mixed" mania. While their focus is on patients with high rates of concurrent depressive and manic symptomatology (hence the mix), they report high rates of alcohol and sedative abuse, high rates of abnormal EEGs, migraine, head injury, hyperactivity and learning disabilities, low rates of psychosis, and poor treatment response to lithium. Finally, Endicott *et al.* (1985) noted that compared to bipolar I patients, RDC-diagnosed bipolar II patients were more likely to have prior histories of other mental disorder (especially alcoholism and antisocial personality) and of migraine and migraine equivalents. Although Andreasen *et al.* (1988) do not perform the specific analysis (both the Andreasen and Endicott studies are part of the NIMH collaborative study and describe the same population), it appeared that bipolar II patients and secondary bipolar I patients had similar and poorer 6-month outcomes than primary bipolar I patients.

We might deduce from these data that mania and bipolar disorder occurring secondary to specific or even non-specific CNS pathology have a different and usually worse outcome than primary bipolar I disorder. Himmelhoch and Garfinkel (1986) conclude this as well. It is possible that patients with concurrent substance and/or alcohol abuse and mania, the most frequently cited co-morbid conditions, have additional liability either because they have two serious psychiatric disorders or because the neurotoxic effects of alcohol or drugs changes the phenomenology and course of the manic episode.

It is unlikely that one explanation will suffice to clarify the relationship between ADHD/CD and mania in children and adolescents. For instance, in youngsters with acute onsets of symptoms of ADHD or CD after age 10, a manic episode should be considered, especially if there are first- or second-degree relatives with major depression or bipolar disorder. However, in youngsters with long-standing behavior disorders, in whom discrete episodes are difficult to discern and in whom lithium does not terminate symptoms, a subsequent manic episode may have a course similar to a secondary affective disorder. There are other precedents in child psychiatry. For instance, mania and bipolar disorder have been documented in both moderate to severe mental retardation (Carlson, 1979; Reid, 1972; Sovner & Hurley, 1983) including Down's Syndrome (McLaughlin, 1987) and autism (Kerbeshian, Burd & Fisher, 1987; Komoto & Hirata, 1984; Steingard & Biederman, 1987). In these cases, there has been amelioration of the affective symptoms by antimanic pharmacotherapy without remission, not surprisingly, of the primary disorder. It may be more difficult to disentangle response when the behavioral overlaps of inattention, impulsivity, defiance and aggression of the primary ADHD/CD are intermingled with the manic episode. One may either invoke this hypothesis to explain the data of Strober *et al*. (1988) and Himmelhoch and Garfinkel (1986), many of whose mixed manic patients were adolescents, or speculate that non-specific organic factors are occurring to produce the ADHD/CD symptomatology and causing a "secondary mania" with its attendant treatment refractoriness.

It is also possible that bipolar adults with alcohol/substance abuse and/or antisocial personality are manifesting the ultimate outcome of their earlier ADHD/CD. Gittelman *et al*. (1985) have found that about 20% of 100 hyperactive boys developed conduct disorder/antisocial personality and substance abuse by late adolescence and young adulthood. None had developed bipolar disorder or cyclothymia suggesting that an additional risk factor is probably necessary for that outcome to supervene.

CONCLUSION

In conclusion, while acute mania and episodic bipolar disorder are unambiguous in persons of any age without other psychopathology, the boundaries at both the mild and serious ends of the spectrum of these disorders are cloudier. Concurrent or prior other psychopathology should not necessarily be swept under the same diagnostic "rug". The diagnostic issues are surprisingly similar in children, adolescents and adults. Strategies of systematically exploring familial psychopathology, treatment response and long-term outcome have been helpful in defining and refining syndromes. It would seem propitious for future research to explore the existence of childhood disorders like ADHD/CD in probands and family members of bipolar patients more thoroughly and to obtain more consistent evaluations of organic brain pathology in manic and bipolar patients. In addition, it will be necessary to explore pharmacological interventions that might work differentially on both disorders if indeed co-morbidity is occurring with behavior disorders and bipolar disorder. Finally, it will be important to follow symptom pictures longitudinally to discover the extent to which illness manifestations like psychosis are age-related or state-or trait-dependent.

REFERENCES

Akiskal, H. S., Downs,J., Jordan, P., Watson, S., Daugherty, D. & Pruitt, D. B. (1985). Affective disorders in referred children and younger siblings of manic depressives. *Archives of General Psychiatry,* **42,** 996–1004.

Akiskal, H. S., Dzenderedjian, A. H., Rosenthal, R. H. & Khani, M. (1977). Cyclothymic disorder: validating criteria for inclusion in the bipolar affective group. *American Journal of Psychiatry,* **134,** 1227–1233.

Akiskal, H. S., Khani, M. K. & Scott-Strauss, A. (1979). Cyclothymic temperamental disorders. *Psychiatric Clinics of North America,* **2,** 527–554.

American Psychiatric Association (1980). *Diagnostic and statistical manual of mental disorders.* Washington, D.C.: American Psychiatric Association.

American Psychiatric Association (1987). *Diagnostic and statistical manual of mental disorders (revised).* Washington, D.C.: American Psychiatric Association.

Andreasen, N. C.,Grove, W. M., Coryell, W.H., Endicott, J. & Clayton, P. J. (1988). Bipolar versus unipolar and primary versus secondary affective disorder: which diagnosis takes precedence? *Journal of Affective Disorders,* **15,** 69–80.

Anthony, E. J. & Scott, P. (1960). Manic depressive psychosis in childhood. *Journal of Child Psychology and Psychiatry,* **1,** 53–72.

Ballenger, J. C., Reus, V.I. & Post, R. M. (1982). The "atypical" presentation of adolescent mania. *American Journal of Psychiatry,* **139,** 602–606.

Bashir, M., Russell, J. & Johnson, G. (1987). Bipolar affective disorder in adolescence: a 10-year study. *Australian and New Zealand Journal of Psychiatry,* **21,** 36–43.

Berg, I., Hullin, R., Allsopp, M., O'Brien, P. & MacDonald, R. (1974). Bipolar manic-depressive psychosis in early adolescence—a case report. *British Journal of Psychiatry,* **125,** 416–417.

Biederman, J., Munir, K., Knee, D., Habelov, W., Armentano, M., Autor, S., Hoge, S. K. & Waternaux, C. (1986). A family study of patients with attention deficit disorder and normal controls. *Journal of Psychiatric Research,* **20,** 263–274.

Black, D. W., Winokur, G., Bell, S., Nasrallah, A. & Hulbert, J. (1988). Complicated mania—comorbidity and immediate outcome in the treatment of mania. *Archives of General Psychiatry,* **45,** 232–236.

Brockington, I. F., Wainwright, S. & Kendall, R. E. (1980). Manic patients with schizophrenic or paranoid symptoms. *Psychological Medicine,* **10,** 73–83.

Campbell, J. D. (1952). Manic depressive psychosis in children—report of 18 cases. *Journal of Nervous and Mental Disease,* **116,** 424–439.

Cantwell, D. P. (1972). Psychiatric illness in the families of hyperactive children. *Archives of General Psychiatry,* **27,** 414–417.

Carlson, G. A. (1979). Affective psychoses in mental retardates. *Psychiatric Clinics of North America,* **2,** 499–510.

Carlson, G. A. (1983). Bipolar affective disorders in childhood and adolescence. In D. P. Cantwell & G. A. Carlson (Eds), *Affective disorders in childhood and adolescence—an update* (pp. 61–88). New York: Spectrum Productions.

Carlson, G. A. (1984). Classification issues of bipolar disorders in childhood. *Psychiatric Developments,* **4,** 273–285.

Carlson, G. A., Davenport, Y. B. & Jamison, K. (1977). A comparison of outcome in adolescent and late onset bipolar manic depressive illness. *American Journal of Psychiatry,* **134,** 919–922.

Carlson, G. A. & Goodwin, F. K. (1973). The stages of mania. *Archives of General Psychiatry,* **28,** 221–228.

Carlson, G. A. & Kashani, J. H. (1988). Manic symptoms in non-referred adolescent population. *Journal of Affective Disorders,* **15,** 219–226.

Carlson, G. A. & Strober, M. (1978). Manic depressive illness in early adolescence: a study of clinical and diagnostic characteristics in six cases. *Journal of American Academy of Child Psychiatry,* **17,** 138–153.

Casat, C. D. (1982). The under- and over-diagnosis of mania in children and adolescents. *Comprehensive Psychiatry,* **23,** 552–559.

Cook, B. L., Shukla, S. & Hoff, A. L. (1986). EEG abnormalities in bipolar affective disorder. *Journal of Affective Disorders,* **11,** 147–149.

Cook, B. L., Shukla, S., Hoff, A. L. & Aronson, T. A. (1987). Mania with associated organic factors. *Acta Psychiatrica Scandinavica,* **76,** 674–677.

Depue, R. A., Slater, J. F., Wolfstetter-Kausch, H., Klein, D., Goplerud, E. & Farr, D. (1981). A behavioral paradigm for identifying persons at risk for bipolar depressive disorder: a conceptual framework and five validation studies. *Journal of Abnormal Psychology,* **90,** 381–437.

Dunner, D. L. (1983). Sub-types of bipolar affective disorder with particular regard to bipolar II. *Psychiatric Developments,* **1,** 75–86.

Endicott, J., Nee, J., Andreasen, N., Clayton, P., Keller, M. & Coryell, W. (1985). Bipolar II: combine or keep separate? *Journal of Affective Disorders,* **8,** 17–28.

Engstrom, F. W., Robbins, D. W. & May, J. G. (1978). Manic depressive disease in adolescence: a case report. *Journal of the American Academy of Child Psychiatry,* **17,** 514–520.

Gershon, E. S., McKnew, D., Cytryn, L., Hamovit, J., Schreiber, J., Hibbs, E. & Pellegrini, D. (1985). Diagnoses in school-age children of bipolar affective disorder patients and normal controls. *Journal of Affective Disorder,* **8,** 283–291.

Gittelman, R., Mannuzza, S., Shenker, R. & Bonagura, N. (1985). Hyperactive boys almost grown up. I. Psychiatric status. *Archives of General Psychiatry,* **42,** 937–947.

Graham, P. & Rutter, M. (1985). Adolescent disorders. In M. Rutter & L. Herzov (Eds), *Child and adolescent psychiatry: Modern approaches.* Oxford and London: Blackwell Scientific Publications.

Greenhill, L. L., Reider, R. O., Wender, P. H. Buchsbaum, H. & Zahn, P. (1973). Lithium carbonate treatment of hyperactive children. *Archives of General Psychiatry, 28,* 636–640.

Hassanyeh, F. & Davison, K. (1980). Bipolar affective psychosis with onset with age 16. Report of 10 cases. *British Journal of Psychiatry, 137,* 530–539.

Herjanic, B. & Reich, W. (1982). Development of a structured psychiatric interview for children: agreement between child and parent on individual symptoms. *Journal of Abnormal Child Psychology, 10,* 307–324.

Himmelhoch, J. M. & Garfinkel, M. E. (1986). Sources of lithium resistance in mixed mania. *Psychopharmacology Bulletin, 22,* 613–620.

Hinshaw, S. P. (1987). On the distinction between attentional deficits/hyperactivity and conduct problems/aggression in child psychopathology. *Psychological Bulletin, 101,* 443–463.

Horowitz, H. A. (1977). Lithium and the treatment of adolescent manic depressive illness. *Diseases of the Nervous System, 6,* 480–483.

Hsu, L. K. G. & Starzynski, M. S. W. (1986). Mania in adolescence. *Journal of Clinical Psychiatry, 47,* 596–599.

Joyce, P. R. (1984). Age of onset in bipolar affective disorder and misdiagnosis as schizophrenia. *Psychological Medicine, 14,* 145–149.

Kasanin, J. (1931). The affective psychoses in children. *American Journal of Psychiatry, 6,* 897–926.

Kendall, R. E.(1985). The diagnosis of mania. *Journal of Affective Disorders, 8,* 207–213.

Kerbeshian, J., Burd, L. M. S. & Fisher, W. (1987). Lithium carbonate in the treatment of two patients with infantile autism and atypical bipolar symptomatology. *Journal of Clinical Psychopharmacology, 7,* 401–405.

Klein, D. N. & Depue, R. A. (1984). Continued impairment in persons at risk for bipolar affective disorder: results of a 19 month follow-up study. *Journal of Abnormal Psychology, 93,* 345–347.

Klein, D. N., Depue, R. A. & Slater, J. F. (1985). Cyclothymia in the adolescent offspring of parents with bipolar affective disorder. *Journal of Abnormal Psychology, 94,* 115–127.

Klein, D. N., Depue, R. A. & Slater, J. F. (1986). Inventory identification of cyclothymia. IX. Validation in offspring of bipolar I patients. *Archives of General Psychiatry, 43,* 441–445.

Koehler-Troy, C., Strober, M. & Malenbaum, R. (1986). Methylphenidate-induced mania in a prepubertal child: a case report. *Journal of Clinical Psychiatry, 47,* 566–567.

Komoto, J. & Hirata, J. (1984). Infantile autism and affective disorder. *Journal of Autism and Developmental Disabilities, 14,* 81–84.

Kraepelin, E. (1921). *Manic depressive insanity and paranore.* Edinburgh: Livingstone.

Krauthammer, C. & Klerman, G. L. (1978). Secondary mania. *Archives of General Psychiatry, 35,* 1333–1339.

van Krevelen, D. & van Voorst, J. (1969). Lithium in the treatment of a cryptogenic psychosis of a juvenile. *Acta Paedopsychiatrica,* **26,** 148–152.

Lahey, B. B., Piacentini, J. C., McBurnett, K., Stone, P., Hartdagen, S. & Hynd, G. (1988). Psychopathology in the parents of children with conduct disorder and hyperactivity. *Journal of the American Academy of Child and Adolescent Psychiatry,* **27,** 163–170.

Landolt, A. D. (1957). Follow-up studies on circular manic depressive reactions occurring in the young. *Bulletin of the New York Academy of Medicine,* **33,** 65–73.

Loranger, A. P. W. & Levine, P. M. (1978). Age of onset of bipolar affective illness. *Archives of General Psychiatry,* **35,** 1345–1348.

McGlashan, T. H. (1988). Adolescent versus adult onset of mania. *American Journal of Psychiatry,* **145,** 221–224.

McLaughlin, M. (1987). Bipolar affective disorder in Down's Syndrome. *British Journal of Psychiatry,* **151,** 116–117.

Monro, A. (1966). Some familial and social factors in depressive illness. *British Journal of Psychiatry,* **112,** 429–441.

Morrison, J. R. & Stewart, M. A. (1971). A family study of the hyperactive child syndrome. *Biological Psychiatry,* **3,** 189–195.

Olsen, T. (1961). Follow-up study of manic-depressive patients whose first attack occurred before the age of 19. *Acta Psychiatrica Scandinavica* Supplement, 162, 45–51.

Perris, C. (1966). A study of bipolar (manic-depressive) and unipolar recurrent depressive psychoses. *Acta Psychiatrica Scandinavica,* **42** (Supplement 194).

Prior, M. & Sanson, A. (1986). Attention deficit disorder with hyperactivity: a critique. *Journal of Child Psychology and Psychiatry,* **27,** 307–319.

Reid, A. H. (1972). Psychosis in adult mental defectives. I. Manic depressive psychosis. *British Journal of Psychiatry,* **120,** 205–212.

Reiss, A. L. (1985). Bipolar disorder. *Journal of Clinical Psychiatry,* **46,** 441–443.

Rice, J., Reich, T., Andreasen, N. C., Endicott, J., Van Eerdewegh, M., Fishman, R., Hirschfeld, R. M. A. & Klerman, G. L. (1987). The familial transmission of bipolar illness. *Archives of General Psychiatry,* **44,** 441–450.

Rosen, L. N., Rosenthal, N. E., Van Dusen, P. H., Dunner, D. L. & Fieve, R. R. (1983). Age at onset and number of psychotic symptoms in bipolar I and schizoaffective disorder. *American Journal of Psychiatry,* **140,** 1523–1524.

Rutter, M., Graham, P., Chadwick, O. & Yule, W. (1976). Adolescent turmoil: fact or fiction? *Journal of Child Psychology and Psychiatry,* **17,** 35–56.

Shukla, S., Cook, B. L., Hoff, A. L. & Aronson, T. A. (1988). Failure to detect organic factors in mania. *Journal of Affective Disorders,* **15,** 17–20.

Shukla, S., Hoff, A., Aronson, T. A. & Cook, B. (1990). Treatment outcome in manics with associated neurologic factors. *American Journal of Psychiatry* (in press).

Smeraldi, G., Gasperini, M., Macciardi, F., Bussoleni, C. & Morabito, A. (1983). Factors affecting the distribution of age of onset in affective parents. *Journal of Psychiatric Research,* **17,** 309–317.

Sovner, R. & Hurley, A. (1983). Do the mentally retarded suffer from affective illness? *Archives of General Psychiatry,* **40,** 61–67.

Spitzer, R. L., Endicott, J. & Robins, E. (1978). Research Diagnostic Criteria, New York Biometrics Research, Evaluation Section, New York State Psychiatric Institute.

Stasiek, C. & Zetin, M. (1985). Organic manic disorders. *Psychosomatics, 26,* 394–402.

Steingard, R. & Biederman, J. (1987). Case report: lithium responsive manic-like symptoms in two individuals with autism and mental retardation. *Journal of the American Academy of Child and Adolescence Psychiatry, 26,* 932–935.

Stewart, M. A.,DeBlois, S. & Cummings, C. (1980). Psychiatric disorder in the parents of hyperactive boys and those with conduct disorder. *Journal of Child Psychology and Psychiatry, 21,* 283–292.

Strober, M., Hanna, G. & McCracken, J. (1990a). Affective disorders in adolescence. In L. K. Hsu and M. Herson (Eds), *Recent developments in adolescent psychiatry.* New York: Wiley (in press).

Strober, M., Morrell, W., Burroughs, J., Lampert, C., Danforth, H. & Freeman, R. (1988). A family study of bipolar I disorder in adolescence. *Journal of Affective Disorders, 15,* 255–268.

Strober, M., Morrell,N., Lampert, C. & Burroughs, J. (1990b). Lithium carbonate in prophylactic treatment of bipolar I illness in adolescents: a naturalistic study. *American Journal of Psychiatry* (in press).

Taylor, E. A. (1986). Childhood hyperactivity. *British Journal of Psychiatry, 149,* 562–573.

Weiss, G., Hechtman, L. T. & Lily, T. (1986). *Hyperactive children grown up—empirical findings and theoretical considerations.* New York & London: The Guilford Press.

Wertham, T. L. (1929). A group of benign, chronic psychoses: prolonged manic excitements: with a statistical study of age, duration and frequency in 2000 manic attacks. *American Journal of Psychiatry, 9,* 17–78.

White, J. H. & O'Shanick, G. (1977). Juvenile manic-depressive illness. *American Journal of Psychiatry, 134,* 1035–1036.

Whitehead, P. L. & Clark, L. D. (1970). Effect of lithium carbonate, placebo, and thioridazine on hyperactive children. *American Journal of Psychiatry, 127,* 824–825.

Winokur, G., Clayton, P. J. & Reich, T. (1969). *Manic depressive illness.* St. Louis: C. V. Mosby.

Woodruff, R. A., Murphy, G. E. & Herjanic, M. (1967). The natural history of affective disorders. I. Symptoms of 72 patients at the time of index hospital admission. *Journal of Psychiatric Research, 5,* 255–263.

21

Anxiety Disorders in a Pediatric Sample

Richardean S. Benjamin
Old Dominion University, Norfolk, Virginia

Elizabeth J. Costello
Duke University, Durham, North Carolina

Marcia Warren
Western Psychiatric Institute and Clinic, Pittsburgh, Pennsylvania

Three hundred children aged 7 to 11, selected from a sequential sample of 789 children enrolled in a health maintenance organization (HMO), were the subjects of this study of the prevalence and correlates of anxiety disorders. Psychiatric interviews with 300 children and parents, using the Diagnostic Interview Schedule for Children (DISC), yielded a one-year weighted prevalence for one or more DSM-III views. The prevalence rate for anxiety disorders based on parent interviews alone was only half as high (6.6%) as the rate based on child interviews alone (10.5%). Ratings of psychiatric symptomatology and functional impairment in children with anxiety disorders relative to other children differed as a function of the source of the information. Parents of children with anxiety disorders judged them to have good social function but high levels of psychiatric symptoms, relative to parents of children with no disorder. Teachers judged anxious children to have no more psychopathology than normal children, but to show impaired social and academic functioning. Factors associated with an increased likelihood of anxiety disorders, based on both parent and child interviews, were school failure, stressful life events, maternal anxiety or depression, and being female. Physical illness and high levels of pediatric service utilization were not associated with increased anxiety. The findings are discussed in light of other community studies of anxiety disorders in children.

Reprinted with permission from *Journal of Anxiety Disorders*, 1990, Vol. 4, 293–316. Copyright © 1990 by Pergamon Press plc.

This work was supported by contract 278-83-00006 from the National Institute of Mental Health, and by a William T. Grant Faculty Scholar Award to the second author.

The expression of anxiety as a symptom, a syndrome, and a disorder of childhood has been known to the psychiatric community since the 19th century, yet there continues to be a lack of systematic epidemiological study of its characteristics (Weissman & Orvaschel, 1986). Two factors have contributed to what may seem like a deliberate attempt to ignore in children a condition that affects anywhere from 4% to 8% of the adult population (Marks, 1986; Reich, 1986; Weissman, 1985): the belief that childhood anxiety symptoms are transient and innocuous, and the lack of agreed diagnostic criteria.

Lapouse and Monk (1959) found that fears and worries were a relatively common feature of childhood, and not necessarily disabling, supporting the widely held view that children's fears were transient and would eventually disappear with developmental changes. On the other hand, several investigators have noted that fears and shyness, a form of early social anxiety, are relatively stable phenomena in children (Eme & Schmidt, 1978; MacFarlane, Allen & Honzik, 1954). In a general population study, Richman and her colleagues (1982) found that fears at age three were associated with the development of "neurotic" disorders five years later. In the classic epidemiologic study of the Isle of Wight by Rutter, Tizard, & Whitmore (1970) children with "emotional" disorder at age 11 were twice as likely to have psychiatric problems in adolescence as other youngsters. Nor was the outcome random: children with emotional disorders had the same type of disturbance later (Rutter, 1980). Thus, it appears that fears and anxieties in early childhood are not necessarily innocuous events.

The second factor associated with a lack of information on anxiety disorders in children is the absence of agreed diagnostic criteria (Weissman & Orvaschel, 1986). Before the more recent editions of the International Classification of Diseases, and the American Psychiatric Association's third diagnostic classification system, the study of childhood psychiatric disorders focused primarily on reporting behavior problems, fears, and worries. However, with ICD-9 (World Health Organization, 1979), and *DSM-III* (America Psychiatric Association, 1980), the opportunity arose to incorporate more systematic methodological practices into the study of childhood anxiety disorders. Recently, a few studies using clinical samples have been published, reporting familial patterns of disorder and patterns of comorbidity (Hoehn-Strauss, 1987; Mattison & Bagnato, 1987; Strauss, Last, Hersen, & Kazdin, 1988). It is not possible, however, to generalize from clinical samples to the general population, because factors associated with familial disorder or comorbidity may influence treatment seeking (Weissman, 1985). In order to study prevalence rates and the effect on these putative risk factors, nonreferred samples are needed.

This paper presents data from a community-based study to address five questions related to anxiety disorders in children:

(1) What is the prevalence of anxiety disorders in a prepubertal community sample of children?

(2) How does information source (parent versus child report of symptoms) influence the identification of anxiety disorder?

(3) What are the patterns of comorbidity associated with anxiety disorders in a community sample?

(4) What risk factors for anxiety disorders can be identified?

(5) Are children with anxiety disorders more impaired in level of functioning than children with no psychiatric disorder, or less impaired than other disturbed children?

METHODS

Sample

A sequential sample of 789 children aged 7 to 11 was recruited from a healthcare maintenance organization (HMO) in Southwest Pennsylvania from November 1984 to October 1985. The HMO provides comprehensive inpatient and outpatient services in exchange for a fixed monthly payment. Mental health services are provided by the HMO's staff of psychiatrists, psychologists, counselors, and social workers; in rare cases a child may be referred to a child psychiatrist or child psychiatric hospital department outside the HMO. There is a restriction on the number of hospital days or treatment sessions covered by the subscription, but in general, cost is not a barrier to referral or treatment for psychiatric problems. All children must, however, be assessed by a pediatrician before being referred for psychiatric evaluation.

The HMO is a large and rapidly growing organization serving some 72,000 people at six sites in and around Pittsburgh, an industrial city of over 2 million inhabitants. Two of the six medical centers run by the HMO were used for the study. The "urban" site was close both to two large universities and to an area of the city inhabited mainly by a poor, black community, and drew its subscribers from both affluent and poor sectors of society. The "suburban" site drew its subscribers from a wide geographical area; most of them were white and worked in the steel mills or in the growing range of manufacturing and service industries that are replacing steel as Pittsburgh's livelihood. Each site had approximately 1400 children aged 7 to 11 years enrolled. Every child visiting the two pediatric clinics between November 1984 and October 1985 was eligible for the first stage of the study, subject to the following criteria: (1) only one child aged 7 to 11 per household was screened; (2) children not accompanied by an English-speaking adult were not screened; (3) any child who had made three visits during the study period without being screened was excluded from the sample, to avoid oversampling children with multiple visits; (4) 40 participants in an earlier pilot study were excluded. Of 1349 children aged 7 to 11 visiting the clinics once or more during the study period, 208 were siblings of screened children, 18 were not accompanied by an English-speaking adult, 40 were pilot subjects, 7 made three unscreened visits, the parents of 64 (5%) refused to sign the consent forms, and 29 were missed because of pressures of time and "patient flow'" in the clinic. This left 987 parents who consented to the screening. Of these, 631 (64%) completed the screening questionnaire in the clinic, and the rest took it home to complete; 158 (16%) returned it completed but 198 (20%) did not, despite telephone calls and letters asking them to do so.

We compared the 198 families who did not complete screening questionnaires with the 789 who did on age, sex, the child's presenting complaint, the study site, and the pediatricians' judgment of family psychiatric history, major family stressors, and current emotional or behavioral problems in the child. There was only one significant difference: 83% of the nonreturned forms belonged to families from the urban site $\chi^2 = 11.6$ $p.001$).

The characteristics of the final screened sample are shown in Table 1. The racial and social status characteristics of the sample as a whole were not significantly different from those of the same aged population of the city of Pittsburgh.

Procedures and Measures

A two-stage procedure was used to derive the sample. At stage one, parents of 789 children completed the child Behavior Checklist (CBCL: Achenbach & Edelbrock, 1983). Twenty-four percent of children were give scores in the clinical range, that is, at or above the level reached by 77% of children referred for mental health services but only 10% of nonreferred children in Achenbach & Edelbrock's standardization sample.

At stage two of the study, 300 children were selected for detailed psychiatric interviews. Every child scoring in the clinical range ("high risk group") was asked to participate in the second stage of the study. Each week, an equivalent number of children scoring in the normal range ("low risk group"), selected using a random number table, were also asked to take part. The overall refusal rate was 26%; refusal rates from the high-risk and low-risk groups were not significantly different. The Diagnostic Interview Schedule for Children (DISC) was used to make diagnoses. The DISC is a fully structured psychiatric interview for parents and children that uses computer algorithms based on DSM-III criteria to derive diagnoses (Costello, Edelbrock, Kalas, Kessler, & Klaric, 1982). Because of its highly structured nature, the inter-rater reliability of the DISC interviews is high (Edelbrock, Costello, Dulcan, Kalas, & Conover, 1985; Anderson, Williams, McGee & Silva, 1987). Interviewers were trained to achieve at least 98% inter-rater reliability at the level of item responses. The quality of interviewing was maintained through-

TABLE 1
Characteristics of Screened Sample ($N = 789$)

Sex	No.	(%)
F	406	(51.5)
M	383	(48.5)
Age,years		
7	168	(21.3)
8	155	(19.6)
9	151	(19.1)
10	154	(19.5)
11	161	(20.4)
Race		
W	618	(78.3)
B	146	(18.5)
Missing	25	(3.2)
Social status*		
Low (0-30)	143	(18.1)
Middle (40-60)	316	(40.1)
High (70+)	307	(38.9)
Missing	23	(2.9)
Site		
Urban	331	(42.0)
Suburban	458	(58.0)
Primary diagnosis by pediatrician		
1. Prophylactic procedures and well care	160	(20.6)
2. Infective and parasitic	64	(8.2)
3. Endocrine, nutritional, and metabolic	10	(1.3)
4. Nervous system and sense organs	133	(17.1)
5. Respiratory system	166	(21.3)
6. Digestive system	12	(1.5)
7. Genitourinary system	9	(1.2)
8. Skin and cellular tissue	41	(5.3)
9. Musculoskeletal system	14	(1.8)
10. Congenital anomalies	4	(0.5)
11. Accidents, poisoning, violence	63	(8.1)
12. Symptoms, signs, and ill-defined conditions	26	(3.3)
13. All other medical	5	(0.6)
14. Mental disorder	26	(3.3)
15. None	45	(5.8)
Missing	11	(1.4)

* Hollingshead (1975)

out the study by means of spot checks on the tape-recorded interviews and repeated inter-rater reliability tests. Inter-rater reliability for anxiety symptoms was equal to that for symptoms in other areas. Because diagnoses are made by computer, the inter-rater reliability level for diagnoses is by definition as high as that for symptoms.

Parents and children were interviewed separately, at home, by experienced psychiatric social workers trained to use the DISC. Each parent living in the child's home completed the General Health Questionnaire (Goldberg, 1970), a self-report measure of psychological distress, on which scores of five or over have been found in several studies to be highly correlated with psychiatric disorder. The Global Assessment Scale for Children (CGAS) (Shaffer, Gould, Brasic et al., 1983) was also completed after each diagnostic interview with the parent or the child. The CGAS was developed to provide a single, unidimensional, global measure of the severity of disturbance and adequacy of functioning. Subjects are rated on a 100 point scale, of which every decile is anchored by descriptions of levels of functioning. Stressful events in the life of parent and child were assessed using scales developed by Pilkonis, Anker, and Rubinsky (1984), for a multi-site collaborative study of psychotherapy outcome. Respondents indicate on a check list the occurrence, during the past six months, of any of 98 life events affecting health, finances, education, and relationships. They next indicate, for the three most important events (if any), the level of stress they experienced, using a three-point scale (0, 1, 2). Total stress score used in these analyses is the sum of stress ratings for the three events listed. The scale was chosen because of its predictive power in the study for which it was developed (Pilkonis et al., 1984), and its inclusion of a measure of the subjective impact of life events. For our study, the scale for adults was augmented by a set of items taken from Coddington's (1972) measure of children's life events. It should be noted that the parent, not the child, was asked to complete the life events measure as it related to the child's life during the past six months. Family psychiatric history was obtained from the parent, using a brief questionnaire noting, for all the child's first-degree relatives, any history of psychiatric treatment, or problems with drugs or alcohol. At the screening session parents were asked for permission for the child's teacher to be requested to complete the Teacher Report Form (TRF: Achenbach & Edelbrock, 1986), the teacher version of the CBCL. Three telephone interviews at monthly intervals after the baseline collected information on medical and psychiatric service use at the HMO and elsewhere. Finally, a review of the children's medical records provided information on medical history from age three or date of joining the HMO, whichever came first.

Data Analysis

To obtain prevalence estimates for the whole sample of 789 children, the data from the "high risk" and "low risk" children were weighted by their sampling frequency (Rutter et al., 1970). The use of a two-stage design with weighting permitted estimates to be made for a much larger sample than could feasibly have been interviewed in detail, at only a modest cost in terms of wider confidence limits around the estimates (Shrout, Skodol, & Dohrenwend, 1986). Thus, although the interview stage oversampled children with high scores on the CBCL, the prevalence data reflect rates for the *unselected* sample of 789 children screened. The between-group comparisons of risk factors and impairment, on the other hand, are based on unweighted data since they reflect within-sample variability. For analysis and discussion purposes, three groups were formed based on DISC diagnoses for the past year: (1) No diagnosis (NO DIAG) (2) Anxiety Disorders only (ANX) and (3) Behavioral Disorders only (BHVR). The ANX grouping included the following diagnoses: separation anxiety, simple phobia, overanxious disorder, avoidant disorder, agoraphobia, and social phobia. There were no other cases of panic disorder or obsessive-compulsive disorder. The BHVR group included the following disorders: all forms of conduct disorder, oppositional disorder, and attention deficit disorder with or without hyperactivity. Children with a diagnosis of enuresis *only* were placed in the "No Diagnosis" group. Three children with *only* a self-reported diagnosis of depression or dysthymia were omitted from these three groups: we discuss them briefly below.

The data are reported here for diagnoses based on (a) the parent DISC; (b) the child DISC; (c) the result of combining into one group children with one or more anxiety diagnosis based on the parent's or the child's report separately. The SAS General Linear Model (GLM) procedure was used to analyze differences between groups on continuously distributed variables, using Duncan's wide range tests for significance of between-group differences. The increased risk of other disorders in the presence of an anxiety disorder was calculated using the Mantel-Haenszel method, controlling for sex.

RESULTS

Prevalence of Anxiety Disorders

One-year prevalence rates for four broad diagnostic groups are presented in Table 2. Anxiety disorders were the most common diagnoses according to both parents and children. They occurred almost four times as often as behavioral disorders according to the children (9.9% vs 2.6%), whereas parents reported them only a little more commonly than they reported conduct problems (5.6% vs. 4.1%). It is clear from Table 2 that there was very little overlap between parents' and children's reports, a finding that has been replicated in many recent studies using structured interviews of parents and children separately (Angold, 1989; Costello, 1989). Anxiety and behavioral disorders co-occurred in 12% of diagnosed cases according to parents, and 6% according to the children.

Table 3 examines the prevalence of specific anxiety disorders, by informant and sex of subject. Simple phobias were the most commonly reported disorders among both boys and girls, according to both informants. Parents also reported several cases of overanxious disorder in both sexes, whereas boys rarely reported this about themselves. There were no significant sex differences in parent-reported diagnoses, or in child-reported separation anxiety or agoraphobia, but girls reported significantly more overanxious disorder and social and simple phobia. Both boys and girls reported much higher levels of separation anxiety than their parents reported

TABLE 2
One Year % Prevalence of Psychiatric Disorders by Diagnostic Group and Source of Information (Weighted Estimates Based on $N = 789$)

	Parent		Informant Child		Parent and/or Child	
	%	(S.E.)	%	(S.E.)	%	(S.E.)
Anxiety disorders only	5.6	(0.9)	9.9	(1.4)	15.4	(1.5)
Behavioral disorders only	4.1	(0.6)	2.6	(0.6)	5.2	(0.8)
Depressive disorders only	0.4	(0.3)	0.4	(0.1)	0.8	(0.4)
Both anxiety and behavioral disorders	1.4	(1.8)	0.8	(0.4)	2.2	(0.5)

SE = Standard error

TABLE 3
One Year % Prevalence of Specific Anxiety Disorders, From Parent and Child Reports (Weighted Estimates Based on $N = 789$)[a]

	Parent report			Child Report			Parent or Child report		
	Boys	Girls	Both	Boys	Girls	Both	Boys	Girls	Both
Simple Phobia	1.7	4.2	3.0	5.0	8.1	6.7	5.9	11.9	9.1
Separation Anxiety	0.4	0.4	0.4	3.1	5.0	6.1	3.0	5.0	4.1
Agoraphobia	0	0	0	0.8	1.5	1.2	0.8	1.5	1.2
Social Phobia	0	0	0	0	2.0*	1.0	0	2.0	1.0
Avoidant disorder	0.4	1.4	1.0	0.4	0.7	0.6	0.8	2.1	1.6
Overanxious Disorder	1.7	3.7	3.0	0.8	3.0*	2.0	2.5	6.4	4.6
One or more Anxiety disorders	4.3	8.6	6.6	7.2	13.5	10.5	10.1	19.8	15.4
Two or more Anxiety disorders	0	0.8	0.4	2.1	3.0	2.6	2.1	4.5	3.4

[a]Standard errors available from the first author.

about them. This was particularly true of younger children: self-reported separation anxiety dropped significantly between 7 and 11, whereas parent-reported symptom rates were lower, but constant across the age range.

The other point of note in Table 3 is the high rate of co-occurrence of anxiety disorders as reported by the children. One in four of children reporting any anxiety disorder met criteria for two or more, whereas multiple diagnoses occurred in only 6% of diagnosed cases according to parents.

Correlations between symptom scores for the various anxiety disorders are shown in Table 4. The scales used were standardized to have a range of 50 points. There was a much higher level of agreement in some areas than others; from $r = .43$ for overanxious symptoms in girls to $\cdot01$ for avoidant symptoms in girls. These levels of agreement can be compared with an overall correlation of $r = .43$ for total symptom score on the DISC-P and DISC-C. There were no significant sex differences in the parent-child correlations.

Patterns of Comorbidity

Tables 5a and 5b provide data on comorbidity of anxiety disorders (since these are within sample comparison, they are based on the unweighted samples data). Children with every type of anxiety disorder except avoidant disorder were likely to report one or more simple phobias (last row of Table 5a). However, simple phobia was also reported on its own very frequently (last column of Tables 5a and 5b). The significance of simple phobia as diagnosed by the DISC is discussed below.

Other psychiatric comorbidity associated with an anxiety diagnosis is shown in Table 6. The patterns of comorbidity were the same for parent-and child-reported diagnoses, so the data are combined here. Behavioral disorders (conduct disorder,

TABLE 4

Mean Anxiety Symptom Score by Informant and Sex of Subject, and Parent-Child Correlation

	Boys		Girls			
Informant:	Parent	Child	Parent	Child	Parent-Child Correlation	
					Pearson r.	$P<$
Simple Phobia	3.7	5.0	5.2	7.0	.30	.0001
Separation Anxiety	3.7	11.0	5.4	11.0	.18	.01
Agorphobia	1.1	3.6	1.6	3.9	.13	.05
Social Phobia	7.3	6.3	8.9	8.7	.21	.001
Avoidant Disorder	7.0	14.7	9.1	15.3	-.04	NS
Overanxious Disorder	13.5	13.1	16.8	15.4	.38	.0001

TABLE 5a
Co-Occurrence of Anxiety Disorders, Based on Child Report (N = 300)

	Overanxious Disorder (N=8)	Separation Anxiety (N=15)	Agoraphobia (N=5)	Social Phobia (N=3)	Avoidant Disorder (N=3)	Simple Phobia (N=21)
Overanxious Disorder	-	4/15	1/5	2/3	0/4	4/21
Separation Anxiety	4/8	-	4/5	1/3	0/3	7/21
Agoraphobia	1/8	4/15	-	1/3	0/3	3/21
Social Phobia	2/8	1/15	1/5	-	0/3	2/21
Avoidant Disorder	0/8	0/15	0/5	0/3	-	0
Simple Phobia	4/8	7/15	3/5	2/3	0/3	-

TABLE 5b
Co-Occurrence of Anxiety Disorders, Based on Parent Report (N = 300)

	Overanxious Disorder (N=13)	Separation Anxiety (N=2)	Avoidant Disorder (N=5)	Simple Phobia (N=12)
Overanxious disorder	0/2	2/5	-	1/12
Separation anxiety	0/13	-	0/5	0/12
Avoidant disorder	2/13	0/2	-	1/12
Simple phobia	1/13	0/2	1/5	-

TABLE 6
Psychiatric Comorbidity Associated with Anxiety Disorder

	Boys		Girls		Mantel-Haenszel estimate of relative risk controlling for sex
	Anxiety disorder Present (N=19)	Anxiety disorder Absent (N=121)	Anxiety disorder Present (N=39)	Anxiety disorder Absent (N=118)	
	N (%)	N (%)	N (%)	N (%)	
Behavioral Disorder Present	6 (31.5)	18 (14.9)	7 (17.9)	8 (6.7)	RR = 2.3 95% C.I. 1.2-4.3 X^2 7.7, p.= .007
Fisher's Exact Test	p=.07		p=.04		
Depressive Disorder Present	2 (10.5)	1 (0.8)	1 (2.5)	1 (0.8)	RR = 6.45 95% C.I. 1.4-28.2 X^2 6.12, p.= .013
Fisher's Exact Test:	p=.04		p=0.4		

oppositional disorder, and attention deficit disorder) were twice as common in children with anxiety disorders as in those without. The increased risk of behavioral problems in children with anxiety disorder was significant at $p<.05$. for girls, but not for boys. In the case of depressive disorders an increased risk was also found, which in this case seems to have been stronger in boys than girls. However, the numbers of comorbid cases were small: there were only five children with depressive disorders (mainly self-reported dysthymia), of whom three also had anxiety disorders. The risk of depression was over six times as high in children with anxiety disorders as in children without.

Because we were particularly interested in the relationship between anxiety and depression, we examined the data further by comparing the symptom scores across diagnostic groups for four types of depressive symptoms: cognitive, affective, neurovegetative and suicidal, using multivariate analysis of variance with planned between-group contrasts. Although none of the children in the ANX group had received a diagnosis of depression, their scores on the parent- and child-reported depression scales were higher than those of the NO DIAG children (see Figure 1), significantly so on all scales according to the children, and on the affective and suicidal scales according to the parents. The three children with only depressive diagnoses (all based on self-report) had mean depression scores in the same range as those of the ANX group. However, the depression scale scores of the anxious

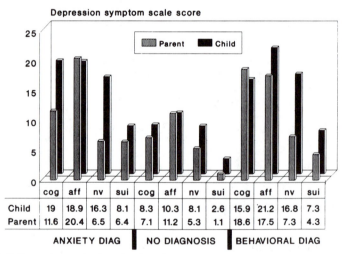

Figure 1. Informant reports at pretreatment

children were very similar to those of the children with behavioral disorders, so the association was not specific to "internalizing" disorders. In general, boys and girls in each diagnostic group had very similar depression scores; the single exception was in the parent-reported BHVR group, where girls had twice the total depression score of boys: 74.0 vs. 38.2

Correlates and Risk Factors

Table 7 summarizes the data on ways in which children with anxiety disorders differed from children with no disorder on the one hand, and on the other hand from children with behavioral disorders. The number of children with mixed disorders was too small to be reliably compared with others; in general, it resembled the behaviorally disordered group, as others have also found (Anderson et al., 1987; Rutter et al., 1970).

Multivariate analyses were run for each group of correlates or risk factors, separately for parent and child-based diagnoses, by sex. Results were consistently in the same direction, and so are reported here for both sexes together, based on cases reported by parent and/or child. Where results for a subgroup diverged from the trend, this is reported in the text.

The first group of analyses combines factors assessed that did not rely on the judgment of an informant. It includes age, sex, SES (based on the occupation of the head of the household), IQ, and medical service utilization. Multivariate anova showed a significant but small different among the groups ($F(24,570)$ 2.9, $p<.001$; Wilks's lambda .88). Table 7 indicates which of the comparisons between the ANX group and either of the other groups was significant in planned contrasts. On only one of these measures did the anxious children differ from those with no diagnosis: girls (but not boys) were much more likely to have repeated a grade in school (30% vs. 6%), despite having the same mean IQ. The same excess of anxious girls who had failed a grade was found on the basis of parent and child reports separately.

The second section of Table 7 contains measures that relied on the judgment of the index child's main caretaker, usually the mother. The multivariate anova was significant ($F(12,582)$ 11.0, $p<.0001$) and Wilks's lambda was .69, indicating a considerable effect of diagnostic group on mothers' judgments about correlates and risk factors. On each of these measures the mothers of the ANX group reported more problems than mothers of the NO DIAG group. However, when parent and child reports were analyzed separately, the pattern was not so consistent. Mothers of ANX children had worse scores in all areas except family psychiatric history, where 31% of both the ANX and NO DIAG groups had a family history of mental illness. Children who received ANX diagnoses on the basis of self-report were also seen by their mothers as having more externalizing problems on the CBCL and more stressful events in their own and their parents' lives, but their mothers did

TABLE 7
Correlates of and Risk Factors for ANX Compared with NO DIAG and BHVR Based on Parent and/or Child Reports

	ANX	NO DIAG	BHVR
Source of information			
I. Independent ratings			
Sex: % female	66	51	33.0*
Race: % white	83	83	67
SES: % low	12	12	35
No father in home %	19	13	18
In special class %	27	20	14
Repeated grade %	20	8.0**	38.0*
Serious chronic illnes %	5	3	3
Mean no. of pediatric follow-up visits	1.8	1.2	1.0
Mean annual non-psychiatric pediatric visits before interview	4.9	3.3	2.6*
Family adversity	0.8	0.5	1.0
IQ (PPVT) mean score	106	106	99.0*
Age, mean	8.7	9.0	9.0
II. Parent ratings			
CBCL Total Behavior Problem Score	47.7	30.0***	60.8*
Internalizing scale	19.5	12.5**	20.0
Externalizing scale	26.0	14.4*	35.4**
Stressful events in parents' life	1.8	0.9**	0.8*
Stressful events in child's life	0.9	0.4*	0.5
Subjective distress (mother)	3.8	2.6*	2.7
Family history of psychiatric problems	41.0	31.0***	53.0
III. Teacher ratings			
TRF Total Behavior Problem Score	26.5	19.2	45.3**
Internalizing problems	6.7	4.8	7.1
Externalizing problems	18.5	13.8	35.4**

Significance of difference between ANX and either NO DIAG or BHVR groups, by Duncan's wide range tests of planned contrasts:

* $p.<.05$
** $p.<.01$
*** $p.<.001$

not rate them as having more behavioral problems on the CBCL, or more internalizing problems than the NO DIAG group.

Section III shows teachers' assessments of ANX children overall, and on the internalizing and externalizing subscales of the TRF. Teachers judged ANX children to have no more problems than the NO DIAG group; the mean score of the ANX group for the total TRF scale fell well within the normal range.

When comparing children having a psychiatric diagnosis with "normal" children, it is important to check whether the differences observed are specific to the particular diagnosis, or whether they are common to all diagnostic groups. Comprising the ANX with the BHVR group gave us the opportunity to examine this. On the "independent" measures (section I of Table 7) the ANX group differed from the BHVR group in being more likely to be female (66% vs. 33%), less likely to have repeated a grade (20% vs. 38%), having a higher IQ score, and having made more non-psychiatric visits to their pediatricians in the years before the interview (4.9 vs. 2.6). The only difference by informant was that the parent-reported BHVR group were more likely to be in the lowest SES strata (0–30 on the Hollingshead scale) than other groups; this was not true of the child-reported BHVR group.

Of the section II measures, mothers of the BHVR group reported more externalizing problems than mothers of the ANX group. Stressful life events were reported as more severe by ANX than by BHVR parents. In general, however, the ANX group and the NO DIAG group showed greater differences than did the two groups with a diagnosis.

Section III shows that teachers of ANX children saw them as having significantly fewer externalizing problems than the BHVR group, but having internalizing problems in the same range.

According to these analyses, the judgment that anxious children have more stressful lives and a worse family history is supported by information from the mother, but not by independent correlates such as the father's absence from home or a measure of family adversity. Unlike mothers, teachers saw no more pathology in anxious children than in those with no diagnosis.

Level of Functioning in Children with Anxiety Disorders

Table 8 provides a summary of various measures of social functioning. These too are grouped by the source of the information: parent, teacher, or clinician. Based on multivariate analysis of variance with planned contrasts, *parents* judged the ANX group to be no more impaired than the NO DIAG group in social functioning (getting on with family and friends), level of social activities (hobbies, clubs, part-time work), or performance at school. Judgments made by parents of the ANX group were more favorable than those made by parents of the BHVR group about their children. This suggests that whereas parents of BHVR children perceived their children to show somewhat impaired social functioning, relative to "normal" children, parents of ANX children did not. This contrasts with the ANX parents' judgments about correlates and risk factors (Table 7), where the latter *did* report more symptoms of emotional and behavioral problems in their children, and greater exposure to risk factors, than did parents of children with no diagnosis.

Teachers, on the other hand, clearly saw the anxious children as more impaired than the NO DIAG group, and furthermore judged them to be as impaired as the BHVR children. This pattern can be seen in the global competence score on the TRF and in all five specific areas: academic performance, hard work, appropriate behavior, the extent to which the child is learning at the same rate as other pupils, and a rating of "happiness." Table 7, however, showed that teachers did not rate ANX children as having more psychopathology than the NO DIAG group. Thus teachers and parents disagreed about the relative functional competence of anxious children, teachers judging them to be impaired to the same extent as behavioral

TABLE 8
Impairment in Social Functioning and Anxiety Disorders

	ANX	NO DIAG	BHVR
Parent Ratings			
Social functioning	7.7	7.7	7.0
Activities	6.2	6.2	4.6**
School performance	4.4	4.9	3.9**
Social Competence Total	18.4	19.3	15.5*
Teacher Ratings			
Academic performance	2.8	3.3*	2.8
Work	3.4	4.5**	3.4
Behavior	3.8	4.6*	3.2
Learning	3.6	4.6*	3.6
Happiness	3.6	4.5*	4.0
Social Competence Total	14.5	18.2***	14.4
Clinical Ratings			
Global Assessment Scale			
(from interview with parent)	68.0	79.8***	57.9**
Global Assessment Scale			
(from interview with child)	72.2	81.1***	65.7*

Significance of difference between ANX and either NO DIAG or BHVR groups, by Duncan's wide range tests of planned contrasts:

* $p < .05$

** $p < .01$

*** $p < .001$

disturbed children, and more so than the NO DIAG group, while parents judged them to be as competent as "normal" children, and less impaired than the BHVR group in most areas.

Finally, the *clinicians* who made a global rating of current functioning, using the CGAS, judged the ANX group to be significantly *more* impaired than the NO DIAG group, on the one hand, but significantly *less* impaired than the BHVR group on the other. Comparisons on the basis of the functioning measures were the same whether the judgment was based on child or parent reports.

DISCUSSION

Analyses were undertaken to answer questions about the prevalence and correlates of anxiety as far as this could be done from a community sample of 7 to 11-year-olds. In this section we discuss the results of the analyses for each question in light of other research, as well as the limitations of this sample.

1. Prevalence of Anxiety Disorders in Children

The one year prevalence of anxiety disorders found in this sample is high (15.4% ±1.5%). Before reviewing our results in the light of other research, we need to consider two aspects that might limit its generalizability: the high rate of simple phobias, and the use of a pediatric clinic sample.

The effect of simple phobia on prevalence rates. The prevalence of simple phobias in this sample was 9.1%. This is higher than reported by other recent community studies using similar diagnostic methods (see Table 9). As Table 5a shows, 50% or more of children with overanxious disorder, separation anxiety, agoraphobia, or social phobia or overanxious disorder also reported one or more simple phobias. Parents, however, seldom noted this co-occurrence (Table 5b). Since simple phobias accounted both for a large proportion of the total rate of anxiety disorders and for much of the comorbidity, we explored the possibility that problems such as unreasonable fear of dogs, elevators, snakes, and so on, were trivial in the sense that children with *only* such a problem were less disturbed or impaired in other ways than children with other types of anxiety disorder. There were nine children (15% of all anxious children) who had only a simple phobia. This group of nine had levels of CBCL internalizing and externalizing problems identical with those of the other anxious children. The teachers judged those children with only a simple phobia to have *worse* problems than other anxious children on both the internalizing scale (7.2 vs. 6.6) and the externalizing scale (26.5 vs. 17.6) on the TRF, but the differences did not reach statistical significance. The social competence scales showed no differences between the children with only simple phobia and other anxious children. Although the size of the sample makes it difficult to test for the null hypothesis with confidence, these findings make it unlikely that the rate of anxiety disorders found in this study was artificially swelled by a group of otherwise "normal" children who just happened to be afraid of dogs or snakes. This subgroup shared the levels of impairment found in other anxious children—levels which, as the analyses reported earlier showed, distinguished them in many ways from children with no psychiatric disorders.

The effect of sample characteristics on prevalence rates. It is possible that the rate of anxiety disorders seen in this sample is higher than would be seen in the general community because the children were recruited when visiting their primary care practitioner. We tested this possibility in several ways. First, we examined the possibility that children with serious chronic medical illness, or those with a history of high levels of pediatric service use, would be more anxious. As Table 7 shows, none of these measures of exposure to the medical setting was significantly increased in the presence of an anxiety disorder. Children with anxiety disorders were also just as likely as the NO DIAG group to have come to the pediatric clinic

TABLE 9
Studies Reporting Prevalence of *DSM-III* Anxiety Disorders in Children

Study	Anderson et al. 1987	Bird et al. 1985	Velez et al. 1989	Costello et al. 1988	Kashani et al. 1987	Offord et al. 1987
Location	New Zealand	Puerto Rico	United States	United States	United States	Ontario
Sample Source	Community	Community	Community	Community (Pediatric Clinic)	Community	Community
Sample Size	782	777	776	789	150	2,679
Age	11	4-16	11-20	7-11	14-16	4-16
Informants	Child (I) Parent (Q)	Child (I) Parent (I)	Child (I) Parent (I)	Child (I) Parent (I)	Parent (I) Parent (Q)	Child (12-16)(Q) Parent (Q) Teacher (4-11) (Q)
RESULTS						
Any anxiety disorder	7.5%			15.4%	8.7%	9.9% ("Emotional Disorder")
Separation Anxiety		3.5%	4.8%	5.4%	4.1%	
Overanxious Disorder	2.9%		2.7%	4.6%		
Simple Phobia	2.4%	2.3%			9.1%	

for a well-child visit, and to have no current medical condition. The chance that physical illness contributed to the rate of anxiety was further reduced by the fact that the psychiatric interviews with parents and children took place in the child's home two to four weeks after the pediatric visit, and were not associated either temporarily or geographically with the pediatric clinic visit.

For all these reasons, we believe that the rate of anxiety disorders found in this community sample of prepubertal children is reasonably representative of the rate to be expected in the population. It is also consistent with pre-DSM studies of the prevalence of emotional or neurotic problems, which included the fears and worries characteristic of anxiety disorders. (Agras, Sylvester, & Oliveau, 1969; Eme & Schmidt, 1978; Glidewell, Mensh, & Gilea; 1957, Lapouse & Monk, 1959; MacFarlane et al., 1954; Shepherd, Oppenheim, & Mitchell, 1971). Table 9 shows the rates of anxiety disorders found in some recent studies, with details of how the information was collected. (A review of the pre-DSM-III literature can be found in Weissman and Orvaschel, 1986). Rates for separation anxiety and overanxious disorder are not dissimilar, but this study found much higher rates of simple phobia than are reported elsewhere, particularly from the girls' self-report (8.1%). The relative rates of anxious, behavioral, depressive, and mixed disorders found in this study are also consistent with those reported elsewhere (see Costello, 1989, for a review of recent studies). Taken together, these observations suggest that the study in general produced results consistent with those expected on the basis of other work, and that the high rate of anxiety disorders should not be dismissed as simply the result of methodological factors.

Very little information is available about the population prevalence of specific anxiety disorders in children (Weissman and Orvaschel, 1986). For this reason, we have provided details by sex and informant in Table 3, with due caution about their generalizability given the low number of cases in any given category. There were no cases of panic disorder or of obsessive-compulsive disorder diagnosed, and other categories contain only one or two cases. On the other hand, the excess of child-reported over parent-reported cases, and of girls over boys, is consistent with the community studies reviewed in Table 9, and with clinical experience (Angold, 1990a; Hersov, 1985; Last et al., 1987; Werry, Reeves, & Elkind, 1987).

2. The Influence of Source of Information on the Identification of Anxiety Disorders

The results of many studies of childhood psychopathology are published in a form that makes it difficult or impossible to examine the rates of diagnosis or risk factors separately by source of information. Yet perhaps the main point to emerge from the analyses presented here is the interaction of informant with information in the anxiety disorders. First, the children who reported disorders were in the main not the children whose parents reported anxiety disorders in their children (Table 3). Second, the correlation between parent-and child-reported symptoms varied by anxiety diagnosis, from $r = \cdot 04$ to $r = .38$ (Table 4). Third, even among adult informants, parents, teachers, and clinicians perceived very different patterns of symptomatology, and of associations between symptoms and other characteristics (Table 7).

A study that used the same assessment method provides an opportunity to compare parent-child agreement in our sample with that found in a clinical sample. A.J. Costello and colleagues (Edelbrock, Costello, Dulcan, Kalas & Conover, 1985) administered the DISC to 299 parent-and-child pairs in a tertiary care child psychiatric clinic. They reported parent-child agreement separately for ages 6 to 9, 10 to 13 and 14 to 18, finding increasing agreement with age in most areas. In general the level of agreement on anxiety symptoms was lower in the clinic sample than in this nonreferred group for the two lower age groups, which encompass the 7-to-11 year-old range of our sample. For the 6 to 9 and 10 to 13 groups respectively, the parent-child correlations were: separation anxiety .06, .03 (HMO group, .18); overanxious .10, .21 (HMO group, .38); simple fears .13, .31 (HMO group, .30); social phobias .11, .26 (HMO group, .21). For the children in the clinic sample whose ages matched those in the HMO group, the parent-child correlation for anxiety symptoms in general was .11, compared with .41 for the HMO group. Herjanic and Reich (1982) reported kappas of .08 to .36 for parent-child agreement on anxiety symptoms, from a sample of 307 pairs, of whom all but 50 children were psychiatric referrals. Achenbach and colleagues' meta-analysis (Achenbach, McConaughy & Howell, 1987) found few studies reporting parent-child comparisons of "overcontrolled" symptoms, but those they found reported correlations of .28 to .40.

Apart from presenting difficulties to the writer and reader, this lack of unanimity has important implications for research, diagnosis, and treatment. We believe that results should be analyzed separately by informant and sex, and only presented as grouped data if no differences emerge in the analysis. Of course, this means that studies run the risk of multiple analyses and small sample sizes. In the data presented here, for example, some of the between-sex or between-informant differences may not have appeared to be significant because of small samples. Researchers working on several studies using similar data-collection methods are currently planning analyses of pooled data that may help to clarify some of these issues (Cohen, 1990).

For clinical purposes, however, it is not possible to maintain such an agnostic attitude; a decision has to be made as a basis for treatment. The results of this study suggest that to diagnose an anxiety disorder only in cases where both parent and child independently report the symptomatology will lead to a serious underdiagnosis of children with significant functional impairment. But a cross-sectional study of the kind reported here cannot answer critical questions about the long-term consequences of child- and parent-reported anxiety. A follow-up study is currently in progress, and together with others (e.g., McGee & Williams, 1989; Velez, Johnson & Cohen, 1989) will help to clarify this issue. We would also emphasize the importance of community was well as clinical samples for answering questions like this; because children rarely refer themselves for treatment, problems of referral bias (especially when the referrer is the parent) bedevil the informant-information problem in clinical samples.

3. Patterns of Comorbidity

Clinical and epidemiological studies using detailed, structured psychiatric interviews have begun to change the way childhood psychopathology is viewed; in particular, they have illuminated the extent to which troubled children have symptoms in a wide range of areas. The DSM taxonomy used in most such studies was developed with the primary goal of "clinical usefulness for making treatment and management decisions in varied clinical settings" (American Psychiatric Association, 1987), and incorporates a hierarchical decision-making structure "organized on the assumption that a more pervasive disorder high in the hierarchy. . . . might present with symptoms found in less pervasive disorders lower in the hierarchy. . . . but not the reverse" (American Psychiatric Association, 1987). It is our view that the evidence of a hierarchical organization of psychiatric disorders in children is not strong enough to permit an uncritical application of such a diagnostic decision rule, especially to data from a nonclinical sample. We therefore used algorithms that made any diagnosis for which the child had the necessary symptoms and met the criteria for onset, duration, and impairment. Other studies applying similar rules have also found high rates of comorbidity in the community (Anderson et al., 1987; Angold, 1990; Velez et al., 1989) and in clinical studies (Strauss et al., 1988). This study both replicates and extends other findings. Like others, we found that children tend to have multiple diagnoses within the broad categories of "internalizing" or "externalizing" disorders, rather than across those categories. However, the presence of an anxiety disorder increased the likelihood of behavioral disorders as well as depression. Numbers were not large enough to examine the issue of whether anxiety disorder was differentially associated with specific types of externalizing disorder, as Angold (1990) suggests.

The issue of co-occurrence of different childhood anxiety disorders has not been addressed elsewhere using population-based data, and once again the small size of specific comorbid groups makes the findings tentative rather than conclusive. However, the patterns of comorbidity shown in Table 5a are, we believe, worthy of replication and further study; in particular the high rate of comorbidity associated with child-reported overanxious disorder.

4. Risk Factors for Anxiety Disorders

Given the differences in diagnostic rates as a function of informant, we have to suspect that correlations between diagnosis and putative risk factors may also be a function of informant. For example, we have found this to be the case for symptoms of hyperactivity, inattention, and impulsiveness (HIA syndrome) on the one hand and measures of social functioning and conduct problems on the other (Costello, Loeber, & Stouthamer-Loeber, 1990). Parent-based diagnoses of anxiety disorders were highly associated with parent reports of other psychiatric symptoms, with stress in the life of parent and child, and with mental health problems of the mother and other family members (Table 7, section II), all information coming from the mother. Thus, although the association with family psychiatric history and mother's mental state replicates findings from other studies (Last et al., 1987; Shepherd et al., 1971; Weissman, Leckman, Merikangas, Gammon & Prusoff, 1984), we believe that these data should be treated with caution.

Stress in the child's life, reported by *parents*, was associated with an increased rate of diagnoses based on *children's* reports of symptoms, which suggests that the stress-anxiety link found in many studies of adults (Holmes & Masuda, 1974; Monroe, 1982), and children (Coddington, 1972; Gersten, Langner, Eisenberg, & Orzek, 1974) may not be simply an artifact of information source. However, a cross-sectional study like this one cannot establish the direction of causality. Risk factor data from sources independent of the diagnosis, in contrast, showed little association with diagnosis (Table 7, section I). The only statistically significant difference between the ANX and the NO DIAG groups was the high proportion of the ANX children who repeated a grade. Race and socioeconomic status, however, may not have emerged as correlates of anxiety disorder because of the relatively small number of black (19%) and poor (18%) children in the sample.

The study of correlates and risk factors is the first stage in the search for etiology, and is a crucial stage in the search for "patterns of disease occurrence in human populations" (Lilienfeld and Lilienfeld, 1980, p.3), which is a major function of epidemiology. The results of this study are consistent with those summarized in Table 9 in many respects. They reinforce the evidence that anxiety disorders in children have risk factors that distinguish them from "externalizing" disorders, which are more common in boys, in children with lower socioeconomic status and lower IQ, and in children with school difficulties, stressful lives, and family psychiatric histories, whereas only the last three distinguished anxious from "normal" children. In general, our findings concur with those summarized by Werry and colleagues (1987) in their review of factors distinguishing among diagnostic groups, and between normal and diagnosed children. They too found that ANX groups contained a higher proportion of girls than other patient groups; came from relatively normal homes and had normal motor and intellectual development, but had a higher rate of grade repetitions than normal children, and more mental illness in parents. They conclude that "children with ANX seem on the whole less disturbed than children with. . . . externalizing disorders, but they resemble other patients more than they differ" (Werry et al., 1987, p. 140). It appears that the risk factors and correlates identified in this community sample are similar to those found in the mainly clinical studies reviewed by Werry et al.

5. Impaired Functioning

There is a considerable gap between different schools of thought about the significance of anxiety for impaired functioning and long-term risk of damaging consequences. The psychodynamic schools have always viewed anxiety as a construct "central to the psychoanalytic model of intrapsychic conflict and its resolution" (Michels, Frances, & Shear, 1985), with serious implications for functioning in both childhood and adulthood. The more phenomenological approach embodied in the ICD and DSM nosologies has produced data suggesting that childhood anxieties, while very common, are usually relatively benign in the sense of causing less current impairment or long-term damage than other disorders (Graham & Rutter, 1973; Rutter, 1985). For example, in their longitudinal study of children in Mannheim, West Germany, Laucht and Schmidt (1987) found that 72% of children with "neurotic and emotional disorders" at age 8 had no disorder of any sort at age 13, compared with only 9% of those with conduct disorder at age 8. In an analysis of the long-term significance of adult anxiety from the Sterling County study, Murphy, Oliver, Monson, Sobol, and Leighton (1988) found that anxiety, controlling for depression, did not predict a poor outcome, whereas depression, controlling for anxiety, did. Using data from their longitudinal study sample at age 15, McGee et al. (1989) found no association between current social functioning and the likelihood of an anxiety disorder. In our study, in contrast, there was a clear association between anxiety diagnoses and impaired functioning, but once again there was a link between informant and information. Parents judged the anxious children to be no more impaired than "normal" children in the areas of functioning measured by the CBCL, whereas teachers judged them to be significantly more impaired—as much so as the BHVR group. However, it should be noted that none of the three groups had a mean social competence score within the clinical range according to the normative data on the Teacher Report Form (Achenbach and Edelbrock, 1986). Similarly, although the clinicians who interviewed the children and parents judged the ANX group to be functioning less well than the NO DIAG group, using the CGAS, the mean score for the group was around 70, a level associated with minor or transient impairment in functioning (Shaffer et al., 1983).

If we include the measures of school functioning included in Table 7 as indicators of functional impairment, here also the anxious children appeared to be having more difficulties than the NO DIAG group. Of course, in a cross-sectional study we cannot determine whether anxious children are more likely to fail a grade, or whether failing a grade makes children anxious. But in general, we believe that the data from this study do not provide as optimistic a picture of the impact of anxiety disorders on children in the community as the literature has suggested.

Despite the limitations inherent in a community study of moderate size, the results presented here have one or two characteristics which, we believe, give them significance for the study of childhood anxiety disorders. First, they enable us to begin to examine the information about symptoms, disorders, and correlates separately for different informants, and this proves to be very illuminating. Until consensus is reached about how to use various sources of information to reach a diagnosis, we believe that the field will be best served if data are analyzed and, if necessary, presented separately. Second, there were clear differences in prevalence rates by sex, which may prove in larger samples to interact with informant; data should also wherever possible, be analyzed separately by sex. Third, comorbidity among anxiety disorders was high, varying considerably by diagnosis. Anxiety disorders also increased the likelihood of depression in boys and behavioral disorders in girls. Finally, we believe that these data underline the amount of distress and impaired functioning caused by anxiety of various kinds that is experienced by children and not being seen in a clinical setting.

REFERENCES

Achenbach, T.A., & Edelbrock, C. (1983), *Manual for the Child Behavior Checklist and Revised Child Behavior Profile*, Burlington, VT: University of Vermont Department of Psychiatry.

Achenbach, T.A., & Edelbrock, C. (1986). *Manual for the Teacher's Report Form and teacher version of the Child Behavior Profile*. Burlington, VT: University of Vermont Department of Psychiatry.

Achenbach, T.A., McConaughy, S.H., & Howell, C.T. (1987). Child/adolescent behavioral and emotional problems: implications of cross-informant correlations for situational specificity. *Psychological Bulletin*, **101**, 213–232.

Agras, S., Sylvester, D., & Oliveau, D. (1969). The epidemiology of common fears and phobias. *Comprehensive Psychiatry*, **10**, 151–156.

American Psychiatric Association (1980). *Diagnostic and statistical manual of mental disorders* (3rd ed.). Washington, DC: Author.

American Psychiatric Association (1987). *Diagnostic and statistical manual of mental disorders* (3d ed., Revised). Washington, DC: Author.

Anderson, J.C., Williams, S., McGee, R., & Silva, P.A. (1987). *DSM-III* disorders in preadolescent children. *Archives of General Psychiatry*, **44**, 69–80.

Angold, A. (1989). Structured assessments of psychopathology in children and adolescents. W.C. Thompson (Ed), *The Instruments of Psychiatric Research.* Chichester: John Wiley, 271.

Angold, A. (January 1990). *Comorbidity in child and adolescent depression: mixed disorders or multiple pathways?* Presented to the Division of Child and Adolescent Psychiatry, Columbia University.

Bird, H.R., Canino, G., Rubio-Stipec, M., Gould, M.S., Riberga, J., Sesman, M., Woodbury, M., Huertas-Goldman, S., Pagan, A., Sanchez-Lacay, A., & Moscoso, M. (1987). Estimates of the prevalence of childhood maladjustment in a community survey in Puerto Rico. *Archives of General Psychiatry,* **45,** 1120–1126.

Coddington, R.D. (1972). The significance of life events as etiological factors in the diseases of children: A study of a normal population. *Journal of Psychosomatic Research,* **16,** 205–213.

Cohen, P. (1990). Personal communication.

Costello, E.J. (1989). Developments in child psychiatric epidemiology. *Journal of the American Academy of Child and Adolescent Psychiatry,* **28,** 851–855.

Costello, E.J., Loeber, R., & Stouthamer-Loeber, M., Pervasive and situational hyperactivity–confounding effect of informant (in press) *Journal of Child Psychology and Psychiatry.*

Costello, A.J., Edelbrock, C.S., Kalas, R., Kessler, M.K. & Klaric, S.A. (1982). *Diagnostic Interview Schedule for Children.* Rockville, MD: National Institute of Mental Health.

Costello, E.J., Costello, A.J., Edelbrock, C., Burns, B.J., Dulcan, M.K., Brent, D., & Janiszewski, S. (1989). Psychiatric disorder in pediatric primary care. *Archives of General Psychiatry,* **45,** 1107–1116.

Edelbrock, C., Costello, A.J., Dulcan, M.K., Kalas, R., & Conover, N.C. (1985). Age differences in the reliability of the psychiatric interview of the child. *Child Development.* **56,** 265–275.

Eme, R.F., & Schmidt, D. (1978). The stability of children's fears. *Child Development.* **49,** 1277–1279.

Gersten, J.C., Langner, T.S., Eisenberg, J.G., & Orzeck, L. (1974). Child behavior and life events. In B.S. Dohrenwend & B.P. Dohrenwend (Eds.), *Stressful life events.* New York: Wiley.

Glidewell, J.C., Mensh, I.N., & Gilea, M. (1957). Behavior symptoms in children and degree of sickness. *American Journal of Psychiatry,* **114,** 47–53.

Goldberg, D.P. (1972). *Manual of the General Health Questionnaire.* London: National Foundation for Education.

Graham, P. & Rutter, M. (1973). Psychiatric disorder in the young adolescent: a follow-up study. *Proceedings of the Royal Society of Medicine,* **66,** 1226–1229.

Herjanic, B., & Reich, W. (1982). Development of a structured psychiatric interview for children: agreement between child and parent on individual symptoms. *Journal of Abnormal Child Psychology,* **10,** 307–324.

Hoehn-Saric, E., Maisami, M., & Wiegand, D. (1987). Measurement of anxiety in children and adolescents using semistructured interviews. *Journal of the American Academy of Child and Adolescent Psychiatry,* **26,** 541–545.

Hollingshead, A.B. (1975). *Four factor index of social status.* Unpublished paper. New Haven, CT: Yale University, Department of Sociology.

Holmes, T.H., & Masuda, M. (1974). Life change and illness susceptibility. In B.S. Dohrenwend & B.P. Dohrenwend (Eds.)., *Stressful life events.* New York: Wiley.

Kashani, J.H., Beck, N.C., Hoeper, E.W., Fallahi, C., Corcoran, C.M., McAllister, J.A., et al. (1987). Psychiatric disorders in a community sample of adolescents. *American Journal of Psychiatry,* **144,** 584–589.

Lapouse, R., & Monk, M., (1959). Fears and worries in a representative sample of children. *American Journal of Orthopsychiatry,* **29,** 803–818.

Last, C.G., Hersen, M., Kazdin, A.E., Finkelstein, R., & Strauss, C.C. (1987). Comparison of *DSM-III* separation anxiety and overanxious disorders: Demographic characteristics and patterns of comorbidity. *Journal of the American Academy of Child and Adolescent Psychiatry,* **26,** 527–531.

Laucht, M.E. & Schmidt, M.H. (1987), Psychiatric disorders at the age of 3: results and problems of a long-term study. In B. Cooper (Ed), *Psychiatric Epidemiology: Progress and Prospects.* London: Croom Helm.

Lilienfeld, A.M. & Lilienfeld, D.E. (1980). Foundations of Epidemiology. New York: Oxford University Press.

MacFarlane, J.W., Allen, L., & Honzik, M.P. (1954). *A developmental study of the behavior problems of normal children between twenty-one months and fourteen years.* Los Angeles: University of California Press.

Marks, I.M. (1986). Epidemiology of anxiety. *Social Psychiatry,* **21,** 167–171.

Mattison, R.E., & Bagnato, S.J. (1987). Empirical measurement of overanxious disorder in boys 8 to 12 years old. *Journal of the American Academy of Child and Adolescent Psychiatry,* **26,** 536–540.

McGee, R., & Williams, S. (1989, June). *Social competence in adolescence: Preliminary findings from a longitudinal study of New Zealand 15-year-olds.* Paper presented at Life History Research Society Meeting. Montreal, Canada.

Michels, R., Frances, A.J., & Shear, M.K. (1985). Psychodynamic models of anxiety. In A.H. Tuma & J. Maser (Eds). *Anxiety and the Anxiety Disorders,* New Jersey: Erlbaum.

Monroe, S.W. (1982). Life events assessment: Current practices, emerging trends. *Clinical Psychology Review,* **2,** 435–454.

Murphy, J.M., Olivier, D.C., Monson, R.R., Sobol, A.M., & Leighton, A.H. (1988). Incidence of depression and anxiety: The Stirling County study. *American Journal of Public Health,* **78,** 534–540.

Offord, D.R., Boyle, M.H., Szatmari, P., Rae-Grant, N.I., Links, P.S., Cadman, D.T., et al. (1987). Ontario Health Study: Six-month prevalence of disorder and rates of service utilization. *Archives of General Psychiatry,* **44,** 832–836.

Pilkonis, P.A., Imber, S.D., & Rubinsky, P. (1984). Influence of life events on outcome in psychotherapy. *The Journal of Nervous and Mental Disease,* **172,** 468–474.

Reich, J. (1986). The epidemiology of anxiety. *The Journal of Nervous and Mental Disease,* **174,** 129–136.

Richman, N., Stevenson, J., & Graham, P.J. (1982). *Preschool to school: A behavioral study.* London: Academic Press.

Rutter, M. (1980). The longterm effects of early experience. *Developmental Medicine and Child Neurology,* **22,** 800–815.

Rutter, M. (1985). Psychopathology and development: Links between childhood and adult life. In M. Rutter & L. Hersov (Eds.) *Child and adolescent psychiatry: Modern approaches. 2nd edition.* Oxford: Blackwell Scientific, 720–739.

Rutter, M., Tizard, J. & Whitmore, K. (1970). Health, education and behavior. London: Longman.

Shaffer, D., Gould, M.S., Brasic, J. Ambrosini, P., Fisher, P., Bird, H., & Aluwahlia, S. (1983). A children's Global Assessment Scale (CGAS). *Archives of General Psychiatry,* **40,** 1228–1231.

Sheperd, M., Opphenheim, A.N., & Mitchell, S. (1971). *Childhood behavior and mental health.* London: University of London Press.

Shrout, P.E., Skodol, A.E., & Dohrenwend, B.P. (1986). A two-stage approach for case identification and diagnosis. In J.E. Barrett & R.M. Rose (Eds), Mental disorders in the community: progress and challenge. New York: Guilford Press.

Strauss, C.C., Last, C.G., Hersen, M., & Kazdin, A. (1988). Association between anxiety and depression in children and adolescents with anxiety disorders. *Journal of Abnormal Child Psychiatry,* **16,** 57–68.

Velez, C.N., Johnson, J.G., & Cohen, P. (1989). The children in the community project: A longitudinal analysis of selected risk factors for childhood psychopathology., *Journal of the American Academy of Child and Adolescent Psychiatry,* **28,** 861–864.

Weissman, M.M. (1985). The epidemiology of anxiety disorders: Rates, risks, and familial patterns. In A.H. Tuma and J. Maser (Eds.), *Anxiety and the anxiety disorders.* New Jersey: Erlbaum, pp. 275–296.

Weissman, M..M. & Orvaschel, H. (1986). Epidemiology of anxiety disorders in children: A review. In R. Gittleman (Ed.), *Anxiety disorders of childhood.* New York: The Guilford Press.

Weissman, M.M., Leckman, J., Merikangas, K., Gammon, G., & Prusoff, B. (1984). Depression and anxiety disorders in parents and children. *Archives of General Psychiatry,* **41,** 845–852.

Werry, J.S., Reeves, J.C. & Elkind, G.S. (1987). Attention deficit, conduct, oppositional, and anxiety disorders in children: I. A review of research on differentiating characteristics. *Journal of the American Academy of Child and Adolescent Psychiatry,* **26,** 133–143.

World Health Organization. (1979). *The international classification of diseases (9th revision).* Geneva: Author.

22

Psychological Effects of Chronic Disease

Christine Eiser

University of Exeter, U.K.

Recent years have seen a tremendous growth and reconceptualization in approaches to understanding the impact of chronic disease on children and their families. The traditional deficit-centered model is slowly being replaced. The trend is towards models that take account of coping resources and individual competence. The emphasis is away from identifying psychopathology within families, and towards an understanding of how ordinary families deal with specific crises that arise. Increasingly, our models are being drawn from mainstream psychology, with the result that families and children dealing with chronic disease are not seen as deviant, but as ordinary people in exceptional circumstances. At the same time, there has been a move away from the focus on mother–child interactions. Instead, the reciprocal relationships between all family members is increasingly being acknowledged.

These trends are sadly not reflected in all current research. For this reason, this review is organized firstly in terms of the psychological effects on the child, and secondly on the family. The very complex nature of the relationship between child, parents and siblings has hardly been unravelled yet.

AFFECTS ON THE CHILD

Introduction

The weight of scientific evidence continues to point to the increased vulnerability, in terms of emotional and behavioural development, of children with a chronic disease. However, some progress has been made in determining the mag-

Reprinted with permission from *Journal of Child Psychology and Psychiatry*, 1990, Vol. 31, No. 1, 85–98. Copyright © 1990 by the Association for Child Psychology and Psychiatry.
Acknowledgment—The author is funded by the E.S.R.C., Swindon, U.K.

nitude of risk in relation to different diseases, and in identifying psychosocial and environmental variables that contribute to a child's vulnerability. Issues concerning the type of mental health problems that are most prevalent in any specific disorder, and the processes whereby disease affects development, are not well understood.

The premise on which much research is still based is that chronic disease exerts a negative impact on development at a diffuse and global level. The work is daunted by methodological difficulties. There is an emphasis placed on the child who fails to manage effectively, with the result that we know very little about the effective coping strategies that are clearly employed by large numbers of children. However, a slow shift in theoretical and empirical interest is occurring. The search for global deficits in chronically sick children continues, but increasingly researchers are also considering how some children learn appropriate coping strategies. In turn, this approach has considerable implication for new approaches to education and prevention.

The Incidence of "Maladjustment" in Chronically Sick Children

Problems of definitions. Concepts of "adjustment", "adaptation", "coping", "stress" and "competence" are used interchangeably in the literature (Rutter, 1981; Compas, 1987; Perrin, Ramsey & Sandler, 1987). The focus is, however, away from definitions of maladjustment and deviance and increasingly toward identifying individual and family coping strategies and skills (Varni & Wallander,, 1988). This approach has important implications for the development of intervention programmes (Fehrenbach & Peterson, 1989).

Methodological issues. Population-based studies are often considered preferable to clinic-based ones (Starfield, 1985), especially since they are more likely to be based on representative samples and the data are therefore widely generalizable. Despite this, most research is based on small, often specially selected clinic samples. No attention is paid to differences between clinics in terms of characteristics of their populations or approaches to care and management. Control groups are not always included, and even where they are, insufficient attention is often paid to relevant variables (Lemanek, Moore, Gresham, Williamson & Kelley, 1986). In the absence of any comprehensive theoretical framework, there is little indication of appropriate outcome measures. Psychiatric interviews and symptom reports are being replaced, for example, by assessments of behaviour (Achenbach & Edelbrook, 1983), self-concept (Piers, 1969) or depression (Kovacs, 1981; Birleson, Hudson, Buchanan & Wolff, 1987). Teacher reports of behaviour, school absence and achievement are also popular. Other measures include competence (Harter, 1981), self-esteem (Lipsitt, 1958), and locus of control (Nowicki & Strickland, 1973).

Theoretical Approaches

According to Wallander, a set of intrapersonal, interpersonal and social–ecological factors can be identified. *Intrapersonal* factors include the severity of the handicap and functional independence as well as personality factors such as temperament or coping style. *Interpersonal* factors include temperament and coping style of the mother, since there is evidence that child and maternal temperament are related (Chess & Thomas, 1986).

Finally, *social–ecological* factors include marital and family functioning, socio-economic status, family size and service utilization. The focus of the model is on the potentially reciprocal nature of these relationships. Varni and Wallander (1988) go on to suggest that the reason why families with a chronically sick child are at a greater risk for maladjustment relates to the increased number of stressful situations to which they are exposed. "Stress" is viewed "as the occurrence of problematic situations requiring a solution or some decision-making process for appropriate action" (Varni & Wallander, 1988, p. 215). A taxonomy of problematic situations for any chronic disease needs to be defined.

If stress is understood in terms of a series of problematic situations or stressors, it follows that adjustment should be determined in part by individual competence in dealing with the situations. "Competence is defined in terms of the effectiveness of the coping responses emitted when an individual is confronted with problematic situations" (Varni & Wallander, 1988, p. 215). Effective, active coping responses result in a change so that the situation is no longer problematic, while at the same time producing a maximum of additional positive consequences.

This model reflects an underlying change in professional attitudes to chronically sick children and their families, and makes specific implications about education and prevention. The task of professionals is to foster the acquisition of relevant coping skills, ultimately leading to greater independence and competence in dealing with stress. At the same time, the potential for psychosocial maladjustment and need for continuous professional involvement is reduced.

Empirical Research

Population-based work. Cadman, Boyel, Szatmari and Offord (1987) surveyed 1869 families in Ontario, Canada, including 3294 children aged between 4 and 16 years. The incidence of chronic disease was 14% , including 3.7% of children who also suffered from physical disability. (These data are broadly consistent with earlier epidemiological surveys; e.g. Hobbs & Perrin, 1985.) Children with chronic disease and physical disability were at greater than three times the risk for psychiatric disorder and at "considerable" risk for social maladjustment compared with healthy children. Those with chronic disease (but no physical disability) were less at risk:

a two-fold increase in psychiatric disorder, but little measurable increase in social maladjustment.

Clinical-based studies of single disease groups. Part of the difficulty in interpreting the results of empirical work concerned with adjustment of children with asthma can be attributed to the way in which the disease is clinically manifested. Renne and Creer (1985) have suggested that difficulties arise because of three characteristics of asthma: the disease can be intermittent, variable in severity and reversible. There remain considerable inconsistencies in the way in which objective severity of asthma is assessed (Mrazek, 1986).

Given these difficulties, it is small wonder that empirical research has failed to clarify the psychological implications of asthma. Recent work by Mrazek, Anderson and Strunk (1985) compared 26 children with asthma aged between 3 and 6 years with controls, and reported that 35% of those with asthma showed emotional disturbance (compared with none of the controls). Those with asthma were also more likely to be depressed. In contrast, Kashani, Koenig, Shepperd, Wilfley and Morris (1988) reported that 56 asthma patients (aged 7–16 years) did not differ from controls on a measure of self-concept, nor in terms of DSM-III diagnosis. Parents of those with asthma were more likely to report that their children showed psychiatric symptoms (especially in terms of overanxious or phobic behavior) than were parents of controls. No relationship was found between the incidence of psychiatric symptoms and severity of the child's asthma (as assessed by medication).

Perrin, MacLean and Perrin (1989) emphasize that there is no simple relationship between adjustment and disease severity. The authors emphasize the importance of parental perceptions of severity: adjustment was significantly worse among children rated as "moderately" affected by parents, compared with those rated as having "mild" or "severe" disease. Perrin *et al.* (1989) conclude that clinical interventions need to be available for all children with asthma, and not only for those with objectively measured severe disease.

The psychological adjustment of children with *cancer* continues to receive considerable attention. This is disproportionate in terms of the numbers of children affected by cancer compared with other diseases. However, significant improvements in prognosis, as well as concerns about the potentially damaging effects of treatment, ensure that children with cancer have a high profile in the research literature. Psychological problems, for example in learning disabilities and academic failure (Taylor, Albo, Phebus, Sachs & Bierl, 1987; Mulhern, Ochs & Fairclough, 1987; Wheeler, Keiper, Janoun & Chessells, 1988), behaviour and adjustment (Wasserman, Thompson & Wilimas, 1987) and depression (Worchel *et al.*, 1988), have all been reported. A meta-analysis including 17 studies concerned with intellectual deficits by Cousens, Waters, Said and Stevens (1988) concluded that children undergoing CNS irradiation showed substantial deficits in I.Q., and that this deficit was especially pronounced in those undergoing treatment at younger ages.

Largely because of the uncertainty surrounding the question of how radiation and chemotherapy might affect development, there have been efforts to assess psychological functioning of long-term survivors. While Malpas (1988) reported that achievements at school leaving age (in terms of examination passes) compared very favourably with those of the general population, Mulhern, Wasserman, Friedman and Fairclough (1989) identified some more subtle deficits. Long-term survivors showed a four-fold increase in school problems and somatic complaints of unknown origin over the general population. The presence of functional, but not cosmetic, impairment increased the risk of both academic and adjustment problems. Children who were older on diagnosis, were treated by cranial irradiation and lived in one-parent families were at most risk. Peckham, Meadows, Bartel and Marrero (1988) also studied long-term survivors (8–10 years following diagnosis). Although there was enormous variability in achievement outcome, children generally achieved less well in both reading and mathematics than would be expected. Peckham *et al.* (1988) consider that the pattern of deficits indicates specific learning disabilities rather than a global dysfunction. Again, deficits were greater for children who were *older* on diagnosis (in contrast to work concerned with more immediate follow-up, when it has consistently been shown that greater deficits occur for children who are *younger* on diagnosis and treatment). Studies of survivors of childhood cancer point to the increased vulnerability of the group, and suggest that greater efforts should be made to provide appropriate education and intervention throughout, and beyond, treatment.

Adjustment problems have also been reported among children with *diabetes*, especially those in poorer health and from dysfunctional families (Johnson, 1988). It has often been argued that children in "better" diabetic control show improved adjustment scores over those in "poor" control.

Recent work challenges this view. Work by Fonagny, Moran, Lindsay, Kurtz and Brown (1987) and by Close, Davies, Price and Goodyer (1986) suggests that the efforts to maintain good control may be so demanding that children become more poorly adjusted (i.e. more depressed). Parents and doctors should be careful that children are not expected to achieve unrealistic levels of glycaemic control.

The extent to which children with *juvenile rheumatoid arthritis* are affected appears dependent both on the severity of the condition and age. Billings, Moos, Miller and Gottlieb (1987) categorized 43 children as "severely" and 52 as "mildly" affected (based on objective indices such as disease activity and functional status), and compared them with matched healthy children in terms of psychosocial functioning. Parents reported more psychological and physical problems for those with severe disease. Among those with severe disease, older children experienced restricted social activities both with family and friends. Similar results were reported by Ungerer, Horgan, Chaitow and Champion (1988). Increased maladjustment and social isolation was found among older children and adolescents. Both studies point to the need for help, particularly in the early adolescent period, to enable those with arthritis to maintain and develop social relationships and activities.

A series of reports concerned with children with *sickle-cell anaemia* yield conflicting results. Lemanek *et al.* (1986) found no differences between a group with sickle-cell anaemia and controls, and attribute this finding to careful selection of the control group, especially in terms of appropriate social variables. In contrast, Hurtig and White (1986) studied 50 children aged between 8 and 16 years and found that greater maladjustment occurred among the older children. Effects were most pronounced in terms of social maladjustment, and for boys compared with girls. Similar problems in social maladjustment were reported by Morgan and Jackson (1986).

Hurtig, Koepke and Park (1989) used a number of measures of adjustment and severity, and also asked children to assess the intensity of pain associated with their disease and frequency of painful attacks. The results support earlier findings in suggesting greater maladjustment among adolescent boys than adolescent girls and younger groups. Although global (objective) measures of severity did not predict adjustment, frequency of pain experiences was inversely related to school performance. Hurtig *et al.* (1989) suggest that children who experience frequent pain should be monitored especially carefully.

Isolated reports on other disease groups have also been reported. Among survivors of *end-stage renal disease*, maladjustment (as measured by distorted body image, social immaturity and poor self-esteem) was directly related to the presence of visible impairments (Beck, Nethercut, Crittenden & Hewins, 1986). Children with chronic renal failure showed significant psychiatric maladjustment (Garralda, Jameson, Reynolds & Postlethwaite, 1988) compared with healthy controls. Although more marked difficulties were reported among those with severe disease, those who were less severely ill showed particular difficulties in school adjustment and loneliness. Children with *birth defects* (cardiac disease, cleft lip or palate, and hearing impairment) showed behaviour problems two or three times the normal rate (Heller, Rafman, Zvagulis & Pless, 1985).

Studies involving more than one disease group. Very few studies have involved comparisons of adjustments between children with different diseases. Studies of this type are based on the assumption that maladjustment is related to the specific demands of different conditions, which are perceived to be more critical than the general restrictions common to any chronic condition.

A longitudinal 5-year study by Breslau and Marshall (1985) suggests clear differences in adjustment between children with different conditions. Those with disorders involving the brain showed persistent and severe problems over the period, especially in the areas of mental retardation and social isolation. Children with cystic fibrosis showed improved adjustment over the period.

In contrast, Wallander, Varni, Babani, Banis and Wilcox (1988) argue that the emotional demands of any chronic disease are more important predictors of adjustment that the idiosyncratic demands of any particular disease. They found few differences between children suffering from diabetes, spina bifida, haemophilia, chronic obesity and cerebral palsy. The children were reported by their mothers to show more behavioral and social competence problems than would be predicted from standardized norms (Achenbach & Edelbrook, 1983). However, these data are based purely on parental reports of behaviour. Comparing the scores of children with chronic disease against standardized norms may be inadequate in terms of controlling for social class and other differences between the ill and general population.

SUMMARY

Children with chronic disease are somewhat more likely than healthy children to show maladjustment. The risk appears to increase for those with disorders involving the CNS or physical disability. Parental perceptions of severity are more predictive of a child's adjustment than physician-rated severity or estimates based on drug use. There are indications that age affects adjustment. Younger children seem more affected in terms of school tasks and achievement (Allen & Zigler, 1986; Rovet, Ehrlich & Hoppe, 1987); older children in terms of social adjustment (Ungerer *et al.*, 1988; Hurtig & White, 1986). Levels of adjustment also vary depending on the informant. Reports based on parental responses generally indicate more maladjustment than those based on teacher or physician reports, or those indicated by objective measures (Kashani *et al.*, 1988). While maternal reports of child behaviour are a useful and valid source of information, they are likely to yield as much about mother–child interaction as about the child's behaviour (Lancaster, Prior & Adler, 1989).

Undoubtedly, part of the confusion lies with the inconsistent selection of outcome measures. However, in the absence of a theoretical framework to enable predictions to be made about the kind of deficits experienced, this confusion is inevitable. More importantly, few researchers have considered the implications of adjustment for the child or family, either in terms of disease-related behaviour (e.g. compliance with treatment) or for everyday coping and achievement.

Coping Strategies in Relation to Chronic Disease

It is clear from the review so far that a sizeable majority of children with chronic disease "cope" effectively with both the disease and demands of treatment. This should not result in an underestimation of the number and variety of stressful situations with which the child must cope. Research concerned with these issues should be an integral part of intervention programmes aimed at helping children with chronic disease. Work by Band and Weisz (1988), Brown, O'Keefe, Sanders and Baker (1986), and Compas and colleagues (Compas, 1987; Compas, Malcarne & Fondacaro, 1988) gives some indication of the situations found to be stressful by healthy children and the strategies adopted. Although the work is based on theoretical models of adult copy (cf. Lazarus & Folkman, 1984), it is applicable to children, given certain caveats (Compas, 1987). This approach has been applied by Spirito and colleagues (Spirito, Stark & Tyc, 1989) to work with chronically sick groups. Tentative conclusions point to differences in coping strategies used by boys and girls, and the influence of factors such as number of hospital admissions, or age of diagnosis in determining type of strategy employed. Spirito, Stark, Williams, Stamonlis and Alexan (1988) reported that children with chronic disease referred for adjustment problems used different coping strategies from children with chronic disease and no apparent adjustment problems.

Coping with Invasive Medial Procedures

By far the most work on coping has taken place in relation to the question of how children can be helped to cope with painful medical procedures. Children can become extremely distressed by such procedures, resulting in disruptive and emotional behaviour (Jay, Elliot, Ozolins, Olson & Pruitt, 1985). Others suffer from anticipatory nausea (Ludwick-Rosenthal & Neufeld, 1988). In some cases anticipatory nausea can severely compromise compliance with treatment. Recent recognition of the degree of distress associated with medical procedures has resulted in a number of attempts at intervention, including hypnosis (Katz, Kellerman & Ellenberg, 1987), puppet therapy (Linn, Beardslee & Patenande, 1986), and cognitive coping strategies (Worchel, Copeland & Barker, 1987). All of these authors report some success in reducing children's anxiety and increasing a sense of mastery (for reviews, see Bush, 1987; McGrath & Unruh, 1987).

General Intervention Strategies

Attempts to improve adaptation by increasing children's disease-related knowledge have been partially successful (cf. Rubin *et al.* 1986), but increased knowledge alone does not predict adaptation. Knowledge may be primarily important in enabling children to become responsible for their own self-care, and some interventions have focused on improving self-care skills. Work by Johnson and colleagues (cf. Johnson, 1988) with children with diabetes, and McNabb, Wilson-Pessano & Jacobs (1986) with those with asthma, are particularly exemplary in this regard.

Other approaches have attempted to develop the social skills necessary to manage disease and treatment. For example, children are helped to understand difficulties they have in complying with treatment in different situations (diabetics may handle their diet well at home but feel embarrassed at school).; These "social skills" approaches have some success in educating well children about health issues (Eiser & Eiser, 1988), and would seem to have considerable potential with chronically sick children (Kaplan, Chadwick & Schimmel, 1985).

Summer camps, too, are becoming extremely popular, both in providing children with an opportunity to separate from parents while being well cared for, and allowing them to share experiences with peers (Drotar & Bush, 1985). Children with cancer who attended summer camp (which involved no formal cancer discussions) showed an increase in play activity 2 weeks later (but not at subsequent follow-up). Increased frequency of social activity was found immediately after camp and at follow-up. Camp experience was also related to increased interaction between family members (Smith, Gotlieb, Gurwich & Blotcky, 1987).

EFFECTS ON THE FAMILY

Introduction

Most work continues to point to the close relationship between child and family adjustment (Burr, 1985; Hauser, Jacobson, Wertlieb, Brink & Wentworth, 1985; Wertlieb, Hauser & Jacobson, 1986; Blotcky, Raczynski, Gurwich & Smith, 1985). Traditionally, research concerned with the impact of a child with chronic disease on the family has been based on the assumption that the experience is associated with marital disruption, divorce, distress, or psychopathology in both parents and children (for reviews, see Lavigne & Burns, 1981; Eiser, 1985). As a result, much is known about the incidence of maladjustment, but little about coping resources within the family. At the same time, greater impact of the disease is assumed to fall on the mother as primary caregiver, and the role of the father in facilitating either the child's adjustment, or the mother's, is neglected.

Recent work emphasizes the enormous range of coping resources displayed by families in relation to both practical and emotional difficulties. The move is toward understanding children with chronic disease and their families as normal people coping with specific stressors (Kazak, 1989). Perrin and MacLean (1988) argue that children with chronic illness are best understood as "normal children in an abnormal situation" (p. 1331).

Methodological Issues

In line with this shift in focus of research has been a change in the type of methodologies employed. There is some decrease in exclusive reliance on maternal reports of behaviour. Instead, a number of standardized assessments of family functioning are available, suitable for general use (Moos & Moos, 1981). Other measures, to assess communication and family relationships (Hauser *et al.*, 1986), and observation studies of parent–child behaviour (Dunn-Geier, McGrath, Rourke, Latter & D'Astons, 1986), have also been reported.

Empirical Research

Effects on marital adjustment. An excellent review by Sabbeth and Leventhal (1984) has done much to dispel the myth that parents of chronically ill children are more likely to divorce than others. Perrin and MacLean (1988) concluded that the incidence of divorce is not higher than among the general population. However, marital strain can result from increases in stress that are imposed on parents in bringing up a chronically sick child. Help to alleviate these specific stresses should not be seen as indicative of gross family pathology

Maternal health. Mothers and fathers differ in their perceptions of the demands and goals of treatment. Mothers are more likely than fathers to respond in a distressed manner and show depressive symptoms. However, maternal adjustment is affected as much by her perceptions of the severity of the child's condition as by any objective assessment of severity, as well as by her relationship with the father (Walker, Ford & Donald, 1986). Blotcky *et al.* (1985) present convincing evidence that the child's adjustment is affected by the responses of both parents.

Family interaction. A number of studies point to the deleterious effect of a chronically sick child on family functioning. Mothers may be described as over-protective or restrictive, and families are reported to show greater conflict, lack ability to take decisions, or may show rigid, enmeshed behaviours (Gustafsson, Kjellman Ludvigsson & Cederblad, 1987). However, such a negative view of family interaction is not inevitable (Spaulding & Morgan, 1986).

More broadly based ecological models of family interaction are called for (Dadds, Sanders, Behrens & James, 1987). These models suggest that parenting can be affected by a range of contextual factors which are independent of moment-to-moment encounters between parent and child. Parenting difficulties are not uniformly distributed throughout the day; parenting skills are more difficult to apply in some situations than others (Dadds *et al.*, 1987). Models that take account of the particular demands of chronic illness in specific situations or contexts may better predict parenting behaviour. Interventions based on ecological approaches can focus on problem situations, while preserving satisfactory aspects of family dynamics.

Variables that Mediate Family Adjustment

Social support. There is some evidence that social support networks in families with a chronically sick child are smaller, denser and qualitatively different from those of healthy families (Kazak, Reber & Carter, 1988). Families of children with PKU, for example, with large, less dense networks, reported less maternal distress than families with smaller, close-knit networks.

Work concerned with social support has gone beyond a simple linear model, where it was assumed that social support directly ameliorates stress. Cohen and Wills (1985) argue for an interactive model, in which the effects of social support become especially important under conditions of high distress. The role of social support in mediating adjustment in families of chronically sick children has not kept pace with theoretical understanding of the concept. There has been an unnecessary concentration on examining structural aspects of family networks, and less concern with more subjective indices, especially in terms of the functions that various social supports provide (Sarason, 1988).

Siblings. A number of studies point to maladjustment in siblings of chronically sick children (for reviews see Drotar & Crawford, 1985; Lobato, Faust & Spirito, 1988). The indications are that healthy siblings have lower self-concepts, can be socially isolated and resentful of parents' involvement with the sick child. Other research suggests that siblings may be involved in excessive amounts of child care and other domestic responsibilities, especially girls (Powell & Ogle, 1985; Lobato, Barbour, Hall & Miller, 1987).

The focus on much of this work has been on identifying the potentially negative aspects of illness on healthy siblings. However, there are no accurate estimates of the extent of the problem in non-referred samples; neither are there real indications of factors which determine maladjustment in siblings. Findings broadly parallel those relating to children with chronic illness themselves: namely (1) there is no one-to-one correlation between disease and adjustment; (2) maladjustment is selective and varies with age, sex and outcome measure employed; and (3) in interaction with other variables, chronic disease in the family places healthy siblings at increased risk of maladjustment (Drotar & Crawford, 1985).

More recent work has moved away from this deficit-centred perspective. Greater attention is being paid to the sibling relationship itself. Siblings derive a great deal of mutual benefit from each other. In particular, siblings socialize and educate each other, mediate parental attention and provide a peer-like context for emotion and power negotiation. Sibling relationships are among the most important precursors to peer and later adult relationships (Hartup, 1983; Lamb & Sutton-Smith, 1982). From this point of view, it is unfortunate that so much research has focused rather narrowly on atypical sibling pairs and negative aspects of sibling relationships (aggression, hostility, teasing) while ignoring the development of altruistic and empathic behaviours. Neither does this approach take into account the interdependence between sibling influence and other family factors (Brody & Stoneman, 1986; Daniels, Miller, BIllings & Moos, 1986). More direct observation studies are called for.

The extent to which healthy children are influenced by, or influence, their sick siblings remains unclear. Dunn (1988) argues that this is partly due to the fact that the chronically sick child can have a complex effect on family functioning generally, and this in itself may influence the healthy child.

EPILOGUE

There have been impressive advances made in the medical care of children with chronic disease. Despite this, they remain vulnerable in terms of physical health, and behavioural, social and emotional maladjustment. Research has led to a greater understanding of the impact of disease, of disease parameters that place children at special risk, and of coping resources that are potentially valuable. It is time that this accumulated knowledge was put to better use to provide sick children and their families with tangible help and guidance.

REFERENCES

Achenbach, T. & Edelbrook, C. (1983). *Manual for the child behavior checklist and revised child behaviour profile.* Burlington: University of Vermont.

Allen, L. & Zigler, E. (1986). Psychological adjustment of seriously ill children. *Journal of the American Academy of Child and Adolescent Psychiatry,* **25,** 708–712.

Bend, E.B. & Weisz, J.R. (1988). How to feel better when it feels bad: children's perspectives on coping with everyday stress. *Developmental Psychology,* **24,** 247–253.

Beck, A.L., Nethercut, G.E., Crittenden, M.R. & Hewins, J. (1986). Visibility of handicap, self-concept, and social maturity among young adult survivors of end-stage renal disease. *Developmental and Behavioral Pediatrics,* **7,** 93–96.

Billings, A.G., Moos, R.H., Miller, J.J. & Gottlieb, J.E. (1987). Psychosocial adaptation in juvenile rheumatic disease: a controlled evaluation. *Health Psychology,* **6,** 343–359.

Birleson, P., Hudson, I, Buchanan, D.G. & Wolff, S. (1987). Clinical evaluation of a self-rating scale for depressive disorder in childhood (depression self-rating scale). *Journal of Child Psychology and Psychiatry,* **28,** 43–60.

Blotcky, A.D., Raczynski, J.M., Gurwich, R. & Smith, K. (1985). Family influences on hopelessness among children early in the cancer experience. *Journal of Pediatric Psychology,* **10,** 479–494.

Breslau, N. & Marshall, I.A. (1985). Psychological disturbance in children with physical disabilities: continuity and change in a 5–year follow-up. *Journal of Abnormal Child Psychology,* **13,** 199–216.

Brody, G. & Stoneman, L. (1986). Contextual issues in the study of sibling socialization. In J.J. Gallagher & P.M. Vietze (Eds), *Families of handicapped persons: Research, programs and policy issues.* Baltimore: Paul H. Brookes.

Brown, J.M., O'Keeffe, J., Sanders, J.H. & Baker, B. (1986). Developmental changes in children's cognition to stressful and painful situations. *Journal of Pediatric Psychology*, **11**, 343–358.

Burr, C.K. (1985). Impact on the family of a chronically ill child. In N. Hobbs & J.M. Perrin (Eds), *Issues in the care of children with chronic illness* (pp. 24–40). San Francisco: Jossey-Bass.

Bush, P. (1987). Pain in children: a review of the literature from a developmental perspective. *Psychology and Health*, **1**, 215–236.

Cadman, D., Boyle, M., Szatmari, P. & Offord, D.R. (1987). Chronic illness, disability, and mental and social well-being: findings of the Ontario Child Health Study. *Pediatrics*, **79**, 805–812.

Chess, S. & Thomas, A. (1986). *Temperament in clinical practice*. New York: Guilford.

Close, H., Davies, A.G., Price, D.A. & Goodyer, I.M. (1986). Emotional difficulties in diabetes mellitus. *Archives of Disease in Childhood*, **61**, 337–340.

Cohen S. & Wills, T. (1985). Stress, social support and the buffering hypothesis. *Psychological Bulletin*, **98**, 310–357.

Compas, B.E. (1987). Coping with stress during childhood and adolescence. *Psychological Bulletin*, **101**, 393–403.

Compas, B.E., Malcarne, V.L. & Fondacaro, K.M. (1988). Coping with stressful events in older children and young adolescents. *Journal of Consulting and Clinical Psychology*, **56**, 405–411.

Cousens, P., Waters, B., Said, J. & Stevens, M. (1988). Cognitive effects of cranial irradiation in leukaemia: a survey and meta-analysis. *Journal of Child Psychology and Psychiatry*, **29**, 839–852.

Dadds, M.R., Sanders, M.R., Behrens, B.C. & James, J.E. (1987). Marital discord and child behavior problems: a description of family interactions during treatment. *Journal of Consulting and Clinical Psychology*, **16**, 192–203.

Daniels, D., Miller, J.J., Billings, A.G. & Moos, R.H. (1986). Psychosocial functioning of siblings of children with rheumatic disease. *Journal of Pediatrics*, **109**, 379–383.

Drotar, D. & Bush, M. (1985). Mental health issues and services. In N. Hobbs & J.M. Perrin (Eds), *Issues in the care of children with chronic illness* (pp. 827–863). San Francisco: Jossey-Bass.

Drotar, D. & Crawford, P. (1985). Psychological adaptation of siblings of chronically ill children: research and practice implications. *Developmental and Behavioral Pediatrics*, **6**, 355–362.

Dunn, J. (1988). Sibling influence on childhood development. *Journal of Child Psychology and Psychiatry*, **29**, 119–128.

Dunn-Geier, B.J., McGrath, P.J., Rourke, B.P., Latter, J. & D'Astons, J. (1986). Adolescent chronic pain: the ability to cope. *Pain*, **26**, 23–32.

Eiser, C. (1985). *The psychology of childhood illness*. New York: Springer.

Eiser, C. & Eiser, J.R. (1988). *Drug education in schools: An evaluation of the "Double Take" video package*. New York: Springer.

Fehrenbach, A.M.B. & Peterson, L. (1989). Parental problem-solving skills, stress, and dietary compliance in phenylketonuria. *Journal of Consulting and Clinical Psychology*, **57**, 237–241.

Fonagny, P., Moran, G.S., Lindsay, M.K.M., Kurtz, A.B. & Brown, R. (1987). Psychological adjustment and diabetic control. *Archives of Disease in Childhood*, **62**, 1009–1013.

Garralda, M.E., Jameson, R.A., Reynolds, J.M. & Postlethwaite, J.R. (1988). Psychiatric adjustment in children with chronic renal failure. *Journal of Child Psychology and Psychiatry*, **29**, 79–90.

Gustafsson, P.A., Kjellman, N.I.M., Ludvigsson, J. & Cederblad, M. (1987). Asthma and family interaction. *Archives of Disease in Childhood*, **62**, 258–263.

Harter, S. (1981). The perceived competence scale for children. *Child Development*. **53**, 87–97.

Hartup, W.W. (1983). Peer relations. In P.H. Mussen & E.M. Hetherington (Eds), *Handbook of child psychology* (Vol. 4), *Socialization, personality and social development* (pp. 103–196). New York: Wiley.

Hauser, S., Jacobson, A., Wertlieb, D., Brink, S. & Wentworth, S. (1985). The contribution of family environment to perceived competence and illness adjustment in diabetic and acutely ill adolescents. *Family Relations*, **34**, 99–108.

Hauser, S., Jacobson, A., Wertlieb, D., Weiss-Perry, B., Follansbee, D., Wolfsdorf, J.I., Herskowitz, R.D., Houlihan, J. & Rajapark, D.C. (1986). Children with recently diagnosed diabetes: interactions within their families. *Health Psychology*, **5**, 273–296.

Heller, A., Rafman, S., Zvagulis, I. & Pless, I.B. (1985). Birth defects and psychosocial adjustment. *American Journal of Diseases of Children*, **139**, 257–263.

Hobbs, N. & Perrrin, J.M. (eds)(1985). *Issues in the care of children with chronic illness*. San Francisco: Jossey-Bass.

Hurtig, A.L., Koepke, D. & Park, K.B. (1989). Relation between severity of chronic illness and adjustment in children and adolescents with sickle cell disease. *Journal of Pediatric Psychology*, **14**, 117–132.

Hurtig, A.L. & White, L.A. (1986). Psychosocial adjustment in children and adolescents with sickle cell disease. *Journal of Pediatric Psychology*, **11**, 411–428.

Jay, S.M., Elliot, C.H., Ozolins, M., Olson, R.A. & Pruitt, S. (1985). Behavioral management of children's distress during painful medical procedures. *Behavioral Research and Therapy*, **23**, 513–520.

Johnson, S.B. (1988). Psychological aspects of childhood diabetes. *Journal of Child Psychology and Psychiatry*, **29**, 729–739.

Kaplan, R.M., Chadwick, M.W. & Schimmel, C.E. (1985). Social learning intervention to promote metabolic control in type I diabetes mellitus: pilot experiment results. *Diabetes Care*, **8**, 152–155.

Kashani, J.H., Koenig, P., Shepperd, J.A., Wilfley, D. & Morris, D.A. (1988). Psychopathology and self-concept in asthmatic children. *Journal of Pediatric Psychology*, **13**, 509–520.

Katz, E.R., Kellerman, J. & Ellenberg, L. (1987). Hypnosis in the reduction of acute pain and distress in children with cancer. *Journal of Pediatric Psychology*, **12**, 379–394.

Kazak, A.E. (1989). Families of chronically ill children: a systems and social-ecological model of adaptation and challenge. *Journal of Consulting and Clinical Psychology*, **57**, 25–30.

Kazak, A.E., Reber, M. & Carter, A. (1988). Structural and qualitative aspects of social networks in families with young chronically ill children. *Journal of Pediatric Psychology*, **13**, 171–182.

Kovacs, M. (1981). Rating scales to assess depression in school-aged children. *Acta Paedopsychiatrica*, **46**, 305–315.

Lamb, M.E. & Sutton-Smith, D. (Eds)(1982). *Sibling relationships: Their nature and significance across the life-span*. Hillsdale, NJ: Erlbaum.

Lancaster, S., Prior, M. & Adler, R. (1989) Child behavior ratings: the influence of maternal characteristics and child temperament. *Journal of Child Psychology and Psychiatry*, **30**, 137–150.

Lavigne, J.W. & Burns, W.J. (1981). *Pediatric psychology: Introduction for pediatricians and psychologists*. New York: Grune & Stratton.

Lazarus, R.S. & Folkman, S. (1984). *Stress, appraisal and coping*. New York: Springer.

Lemanek, K.L., Moore, S.L., Gresham, F.M., Williamson, D.A. & Kelley, M.L. (1986). Psychological adjustment of children with sickle cell anemia. *Journal of Pediatric Psychology*, **11**, 397–426.

Linn, S., Berdslee, W. & Patenande, A.F. (1986). Puppet therapy with pediatric bone marrow transplant patients. *Journal of Pediatric Psychology*, **11**, 37–46.

Lipsitt, L.P. (1958). A self-concept scale for children and its relation to the children's form of manifest anxiety. *Child Development*, **29**, 463–472.

Lobato, D., Barbour, L., Hall, L.J. & Miller, C.T. (1987). Psychosocial characteristics of preschool siblings of handicapped and non-handicapped children. *Journal of Abnormal Child Psychology*, **15**, 329–338.

Lobato, D., Faust, D. & Spirito, A. (1988). Examining the effects of chronic disease and disability on children's sibling relationships. *Journal of Pediatric Psychology*, **13**, 389–408.

Ludwick-Rosenthal, R. & Neufeld, R.W.J. (1988). Stress management during noxious medical procedures: an evaluative review of outcome studies. *Psychological Bulletin*, **104**, 326–342.

Malpas, J.S. (1988). Cancer: the consequences of cure. *Clinical Radiology*, **39**, 166–172.

McGrath, P. & Unruh, A. (1987). *Pain in children and adolescents*. Amsterdam: Elsevier.

McNabb, W.L., Wilson-Pessano, S.R. & Jacobs, A.M. (1986). Critical self-management competencies for children with asthma. *Journal of Pediatric Psychology*, **11**, 103–118.

Moos, R.H. & Moos, B.S. (1981). *Family environment scale manual*. Palo Alto, CA: Consulting Psychologists Press.

Morgan, S.A. & Jackson, J. (1986). Psychological and social concomitants of sickle cell anemia. *Journal of Pediatric Psychology*, **11**, 429–440.

Mrazek, D.A. (1986). Childhood asthma: two central questions for child psychiatry. *Journal of Child Psychology and Psychiatry*, **27**, 1–5.

Mrazek, D., Anderson, I. & Strunk, R. (1985). Disturbed emotional development of severely asthmatic pre-school children. In J.E. Stevenson (Ed.), *Recent research in developmental psychopathology* (pp. 81–93). Oxford: Pergamon.

Mulhern, R.K., Ochs, J. & Fairclough, D. (1987). Intellectual and academic achievement status after CNS relapse: a retrospective study of 40 children treated for acute lymphoblastic leukemia. *Journal of Clinical Oncology*, **5**, 933–940.

Mulhern, R.K., Wasserman, A.L., Friedman, A.G. & Fairclough, D. (1989). Social competence and behavioral adjustment of children who are long-term survivors of cancer. *Pediatrics*, **83**, 18–25.

Nowicki, S. & Strickland, B.R. (1973). A locus of control scale for children. *Journal of Consulting and Clinical Psychology*, **40**, 148–154.

Peckham, V.C., Meadows, A.T., Bartel, N. & Marrero, O. (1988). Educational late effects in long-term survivors of childhood acute lymphocytic leukemia. *Pediatrics*, **81**, 127–133.

Perrin, E.C., Ramsey, B.K. & Sandler, H.M. (1987). Competent kids: children and adolescents with a chronic illness. *Child Care, Health and Development*, **13**, 13–32.

Perrin, J.M. & MacLean Jr, W.E. (1988). Children with chronic illness: the prevention of dysfunction. *Pediatric Clinics of North America*, **35**, 1325–1337.

Perrin, J.M., MacLean, W.E. & Perrin, E.C. (1989). Parental perceptions of health status and psychologic adjustment of children with asthma. *Pediatrics*, **83**, 26–30.

Piers, E.Y. (1969). *Manual for the Piers-Harris children's self-concept scale (The way I feel about myself)*. Nashville, TN: Counselor Researchings and Tests.

Powell, T.H. & Ogle, P.A. (1985). *Brothers and sisters—A special part of exceptional families*. Baltimore: Paul H. Brookes.

Renne, C.M. & Creer, T.L. (1985). Asthmatic children and their families. In *Advances in developmental and behavioral pediatrics* (Vol. 6). Greenwich, CT: JAI Press.

Rovet, J.F., Ehrlich, R.M. & Hoppe, M. (1987). Intellectual deficits associated with early onset of insulin-dependent diabetes mellitus in children. *Diabetes Care*, **10**, 510–515.

Rubin, D.H., Leventhal, J.M., Sadock, R.T., Letovsky, E., Schottland, P., Clemente, I. & McCarthy, P. (1986). Educational intervention by computer in childhood asthma: a randomized clinical trial testing the use of a new teaching intervention in childhood asthma. *Pediatrics*, **77**, 1–10.

Rutter, M. (1981). Stress, coping and development: some issues and some questions. *Journal of Child Psychology and Psychiatry*, **22**, 323–356.

Sabbeth, B.F. & Leventhal, J.M. (1984). Marital adjustment to chronic childhood illness: a critique of the literature. *Pediatrics*, **73**, 762–768.

Sarason, I.G. (1988). Social support, personality and health. In M.P. Janisse (Ed.), *Individual differences, stress and health psychology* (pp. 109–128). New York: Springer-Verlag.

Smith, K.E., Gotlieb, S., Gurwich, R.H. & Blotcky, A.D. (1987). The impact of a summer camp experience on daily activity and family interaction among children with cancer. *Journal of Pediatric Psychology*, **12**, 533–542.

Spaulding, B.R., & Morgan, S.B. (1986). Spina bifida children and their families: a population prone to family dysfunction. *Journal of Pediatric Psychology*, **11**, 359–374.

Spirito, A., Stark, L. & Tyc, V. (1989). Common coping strategies employed by children with chronic illness. *Newsletter of the Society of Pediatric Psychology*, **13**, 3–7.

Spirito, A., Stark, L.J., Williams, C., Stamonlis, D. & Alexan, D. (1988). Coping strategies utilized by referred and on referred pediatric patients and a healthy control group. Poster presented at the Society of Behavioral Medicine Annual Meeting, Boston, MA.

Starfield, B. (1985). The state of research on chronically ill children. In N. Hobbs & J.M. Perrin (Eds), *Issues in the care of children with chronic illness* (pp. 109–132). San Francisco: Jossey-Bass.

Taylor, H.G., Albo, V.C., Phebus, C.K., Sachs, B.R. & Bierl, P.G. (1987). Postirradiation treatment outcomes for children with acute lymphocytic leukemia: clarification of risks. *Journal of Pediatric Psychology*, **12**, 395–412.

Ungerer, J., Horgan, B., Chaitow, J. & Champion, G.B. (1988). Psychosocial functioning in children and young adults with juvenile arthritis. *Journal of Pediatrics*, **81**, 195–202.

Varni, J.W. & Wallander, J.L. (1988). Pediatric chronic disabilities: hemophilia and spina bifida as examples. In D. Routh (Ed.), *Handbook of pediatric psychology* (pp. 190–221). New York: Guilford Press.

Walker, L., Ford, M.B. & Donald, W.D. (1986). Stress in families with cystic fibrosis. Paper presented at the Annual Meeting of the American Psychological Association, Washington, DC.

Wallander, J.L., Varni, J.W., Babani, L., Banis, H.T. & Wilcox, K.T. (1988). Children with chronic physical disorders: maternal reports of their psychological adjustment. *Journal of Pediatric Psychology*, **13**, 197–212.

Wasserman, A.L., Thompson, E.L. & Wilimas, J.A. (1987). The psychological status of survivors of childhood/adolescent Hodgkin's disease. *Archives of Disease in Childhood*, **141**, 626–631.

Wertlieb, D., Hauser, S.T. & Jacobson, A. (1986). Adaptation to diabetes: behavior symptoms and family context. *Journal of Pediatric Psychology*, **11**, 463–480.

Wheeler, K., Keigper, A.D., Janoun, L. & CHessells, J.M. (1988). Medical cost of curing childhood acute lymphoblastic leukaemia. *British Medical Journal*, **296**, 162–166.

Worchel, F.F., Copeland, D.R., & Barker, D.G. (1987). Control-related copying strategies in pediatric oncology patients. *Journal of Pediatric Psychology*, **12**, 25–38.

Worchel, F.F., Nolan, B.F., Willson, V.L., Purser, J.S., Copeland, D. & Pfefferbaum, B. (1988). Assessment of depression in children with cancer. *Journal of Pediatric Psychology*, **13**, 101–112.

Part VI

DIAGNOSIS AND TREATMENT

What do diagnostic tests diagnose and what do treatments treat? These two questions form the common theme of the papers included in this section. Piven, Berthier, Starkstein, Nehme, Pearlson, and Folstein, performed magnetic resonance imaging (MRI) scans on 13 high-functioning, fragile-X negative, male autistic subjects who were without evidence of frank neurologic disease and 13 male nonautistic controls who were comparable in age and nonverbal IQ.

Abnormalities compatible with developmental cerebral cortical malformations were demonstrated in seven of the autistic individuals and in none of the nonautistic controls. Malformations of the kind observed, polymicrogyria (N = 5), schizencephaly, and macrogyria (N = 1), have their origins in a disturbance before the sixth month of gestation. Cortical abnormalities such as these, having been reported in association with several other conditions, are not specific to autism. However, they are consistent with the findings of numerous other studies demonstrating the presence of neurophysiologic, neurochemical, and neuroimmunologic abnormalities in autistic persons; and with a smaller but growing body of evidence suggesting that the brain abnormalities responsible for autism may have their origins during the first six months of gestation. As the authors clearly state, autism, like most behaviorally defined syndromes, is etiologically heterogeneous, and it is unlikely that the MRI lesions they have demonstrated play a direct role in its pathogenesis. Rather, in a subgroup of autistic individuals, such lesions may reflect a surface manifestation of underlying mechanisms. Consistent with this suggestion is the fact that some factors associated with cerebral cortical malformations, most particularly immunologic abnormalities and abnormalities in serotonin, also have been demonstrated to occur in autism. Clearly, the possibility of a relationship between cortical malformations and prenatal immunologic, neurochemical, and genetic abnormalities in autistic persons is intriguing and warrants further study.

Although mental retardation is averted if dietary treatment of phynylketonuria (PKU) is introduced early and controlled consistently during childhood, it is still possible that PKU may cause subtle, specific cognitive deficits that are not typically detected by traditional cognitive measure.

Welsh, Pennington, Ozonoff, Rouse, and McCage explore this hypothesis in a study of 11, early-treated PKU preschoolers (M age = 4.64) and a sample of age and IQ matched unaffected peers (N = 11) who were evaluated on a battery of measures assessing executive functions (EF), including set maintenance, planning, and organized search. In addition, a "non-executive" function task, recognition memory,

451

was administered to all subjects. Group comparisons demonstrated that the PKU children were significantly impaired on an EF composite score; but there were no group differences in recognition memory.

Although the generalizability of the finding of a specific deficit in EF is limited by the small size of the sample and awaits replication, the results call into question the use of standardized intelligence measures as the sole measure of assessing the early-treated PKU child's cognitive function. Rather, measures that focus on ability to plan and ability to flexibly shift set may be more sensitive indicators of cognitive development in children with PKU. Furthermore, the findings are important to students of normal cognitive development as well. The results provide preliminary information about the neurobiologic mechanisms underlying various cognitive functions in early childhood. Executive functions are dissociable from other cognitive skills—recognition memory and to some extent IQ. This investigation offers a model of how integration across the different research traditions of clinical neuropsychology and developmental psychology might occur.

Jacobvitz, Sroufe, Stewart, and Leffert begin their review of the treatment of attentional and hyperactivity problems in children with sympathomimetic drugs with the observation that the practice is widespread and apparently increasing. The rate of medication use has doubled every two to four years since 1971, and some have suggested that pharmacological treatment should be extended into the adolescent period and beyond. Individual clinicians who are developing treatment plans for children with ADHD and associated problems of conduct and learning will find this review invaluable. Short-term drug effects on behavior and performance are well documented, but a case for the long-term effectiveness of stimulant medication is yet to be made.

To date, follow-up studies reveal few differences in school achievement, peer relationships, or behavior problems during adolescence between medicated and unmedicated groups of children with ADHD. Moreover, questions remain concerning development of tolerance in children, ways to define subgroups of disordered children who may respond uniquely to stimulants, the efficacy of medication in combination with other treatments, and the possible long-term negative consequences of medication. Urging greater caution and a much more restricted use of stimulant treatment pending further clarification of these questions, the authors make the provocative suggestion that one of the most noteworthy negative consequences of adopting stimulants as the treatment of choice for ADHD is the paucity of research on nonorganic contributors to the disorder and on educational and psychological interventions.

The focus of the last paper in this section is the treatment not of a disorder or a syndrome, but of a symptom—aggression. Stewart, Myers, Burket, and Lyles begin their review of the pharmacotherapy of aggression in children and adolescents by noting that aggressive behavior is a heterogeneous phenomenon, occurring in a wide variety of illnesses, and that no single etiologic model seems adequate to explain its occurrence. Principles of pharmacological treatment of adults, which apply equally well to children and adolescents, include: treat the primary illness (when treating empirically, use the most benign interventions), have some quantifiable means of assessing efficacy, and institute drug trials systematically.

Consistent with these principles, the authors review available information on the psychopharmacology of aggressive behavior as it may occur in individuals with conduct disorder, ADHD, depression, bipolar affective disorder, schizophrenia, epilepsy, mental retardation, and autistic disorder. Specific consideration is given to the role of neuroleptics, antidepressants, stimulants, lithium, anticonvulsant agents such as carbamazepine, as well as beta blockers in these various conditions. Not only does the nature of the underlying disorder lend some degree of specificity to the treatment of aggressive behavior, but the place of pharmacological treatment in the overall treatment plan must be individualized. In some instances, pharmacotherapy constitutes the cornerstone of treatment, but in others pharmacotherapy may only be an adjunct to psychotherapeutic or behavioral interventions. The importance of the authors' reminder that a comprehensive plan of treatment not limited to medication must be developed for every aggressive child or adolescent cannot be overemphasized.

23

Magnetic Resonance Imaging Evidence for a Defect of Cerebral Cortical Development in Autism

Joseph Piven

Johns Hopkins University School of Medicine, Baltimore, Maryland

Marcelo L. Berthier

Institute of Neurological Research, Buenos Aires, Argentina

Sergio E. Starkstein, Eileen Nehme,

Godfrey Pearlson, and Susan Folstein

Johns Hopkins University School of Medicine, Baltimore, Maryland

Magnetic resonance imaging (MRI) scans were performed in 13 high-functioning male autistic subjects and 13 male nonautistic control subjects comparable in age and nonverbal IQ. Scans were rated for the presence of cerebral cortical malformations. Five autistic subjects had polymicrogyria, one had schizencephaly and macrogyria, and one had macrogyria. None of the control subjects had abnormalities of this type. These abnormalities result from a defect in the migration of neurons to the cerebral cortex during the first 6 months of gestation. The detection of these malformations by MRI, their pathogenesis, and the implications regarding the pathogenesis of autism are discussed.

Autism is a developmental syndrome defined by the presence of marked social deficits, specific language abnormalities, and stereotyped, repetitive behaviors[1].

Reprinted with permission from *American Journal of Psychiatry,* 1990, Vol. 147, 734–739. Copyright © 1990 by American Psychiatric Association.

Supported in part by the Interdisciplinary Committee for Nuclear Magnetic Resonance, Johns Hopkins University School of Medicine; the John Merck Fund; NIMH grant MH-39936; a grant from the University of Buenos Aires; The National Alliance for Research in Schizophrenia and Depression; and the Instituto de Investigaciones Neurologicas FLENI, Buenos Aires.

The authors thank Dr. George Thomas of the cytogenetics laboratory at the John F. Kennedy Institute for Handicapped children for his assistance with fragile X testing.

Behavioral abnormalities are typically observed before a child is 30 months of age; although they show progressive changes across different periods of development, they generally persist throughout life[2].

Like most behaviorally defined syndromes, autism is etiologically heterogeneous. A small percentage of cases appear in association with particular neurogenetic conditions (e.g., tuberous sclerosis, fragile X syndrome)[3], and autistic individuals have been shown to have a higher rate than control subjects of nonspecific risk factors for prenatal injury[4-6]. In the majority of cases, however, there are no associated neurogenetic conditions and there is no evidence of unfavorable prenatal factors. In these cases of unknown etiology, the importance of hereditary factors has been demonstrated.[3]

Although the pathogenesis of autism is unknown, overwhelming evidence suggests that a neurobiologic mechanism underlies the disorder. Numerous studies have demonstrated the presence of neurophysiologic, neurochemical, and neuroimmunologic abnormalities in autistic persons[7]. In addition, brain imaging and neuropathologic studies have described a variety of structural abnormalities in autistic subjects. Reversed cerebral asymmetries[8], enlargement of the lateral and third ventricles[9-11], and a decrease in the radiodensities of the caudates[11] have been demonstrated in CT studies. Other CT studies[12,13], however, have not found abnormalities in these structures. Magnetic resonance imaging (MRI) studies have focused on the morphometry of the posterior fossa. Courchesne et al.[14] reported a decrease in the size of the cerebellar vermis, and Gaffney et al. demonstrated enlargement of the fourth ventricle[15] and a decrease in the area of the pons of midsagittal view[16]. Finally, Gaffney and Tsai[17], in an MRI study, noted gray matter heterotopia in one autistic individual.

Autopsy studies have also reported neuronal abnormalities in autism. The most consistent finding across studies has been a decrease in number of Purkinje cells in the cerebellum[18-21]. In addition, Bauman and Kemper[18,19] reported the presence of an increased number of small, densely packed neurons in the hippocampus, amygdala, entorhinal cortex, and mamillary bodies, along with loss of granular cells of the cerebellum and neurons of the deep cerebellar nuclei. Kemper[19] and Ritvo et al.[20] independently reported finding polymicrogyria in two of the seven autistic individuals they examined for neuropathology.

Recently, one of us (M.L.B.) noted polymicrogyria on the MRI scans of two individuals with Asperger's syndrome. Individuals with this syndrome have social deficits that are qualitatively similar to but milder than those seen in autism[22]; these have been hypothesized to be etiologically related to autism[23,24].

Polymicrogyria is one of a group of malformations of the cerebral cortex, including pachygyria, schizencephaly, and heterotopia, which result from a disturbance in brain development that occurs during the first 6 months of gestation[25-29]. These malformations are thought to result from a defect in the migration of neurons to the cortical layers during the period of major cell migration[25,26,30,31].

The ability of MRI to detect developmental malformations of the cerebral cortex (as a result of its multiplanar capabilities and its high resolution, which is superior to that of CT) has recently been demonstrated[32-34]. The findings of polymicrogyria in two individuals with Asperger's syndrome on MRI and in two autistic individuals at autopsy prompted us to examine MRI scans of a series of high-functioning male autistic subjects and control subjects for the presence of developmental cortical malformations.

METHODS

Subjects

Fifteen male autistic subjects were selected from a list of 100 autistic subjects ascertained during an ongoing family study of autism being conducted at the Johns Hopkins University School of Medicine. Subjects were selected for the present study if they were 1) 18 years of age or older and 2) likely to be able to complete a 45-minute MRI scan without requiring sedation. During the course of the study, the parents of a younger family-study subject requested MRI for their child, and he was included in the sample. Three of the 16 autistic subjects were unable to complete the 45-minute MRI series, leaving 13 autistic subjects in our study group.

Parental informants for all autistic subjects were interviewed with the Autism Diagnostic Interview[35]; the subjects met both the *DMS-III-R* and the Autism Diagnostic Interview algorithm criteria for autistic disorder. The Autism Diagnostic Interview is a standardized, investigator-based interview for autism that has shown good interrater reliability and discriminant validity. Parents were also interviewed regarding the subjects' medical and neurological histories.

The autistic subjects were assessed with a structured neurodevelopmental examination which included a standard evaluation of the motor system and an examination for evidence of neurocutaneous disorders that have been reported to be associated with autism (i.e., tuberous sclerosis, neurofibromatosis)[36]. No autistic subject had a major medical condition or a neurological disorder, including seizures, by history or on examination. All autistic subjects were tested and found to be fragile X negative.

The Raven Standard Progressive Matrices[37] was administered to 10 of the autistic subjects. Two other subjects had recently been give the WAIS-R, and one had recently been given the WISC-R. The performance IQ results from these measures, along with the Raven scores, were used to evaluate the comparability of the autistic subjects and the control subjects with respect to nonverbal IQ.

The control subjects were males selected for their comparability in age and nonverbal IQ to the autistic subjects. On this basis we recruited 10 Johns Hopkins

Hospital employees, two patients attending the hospital's outpatient psychiatric clinic (one with attention deficit hyperactivity disorder and one with conduct disorder and drug abuse), and one client from a local association for retarded adults. Each control subject (or, when appropriate, an informant) was interviewed regarding his medical, neurological, and psychiatric history. Except for the two subjects we have mentioned, no control subject was known to have a neurological or medical condition or a psychiatric or developmental disorder requiring treatment.

Procedure

Before the MRI scans were done, parental informants were given a structured interview regarding the subjects' prenatal history that had been derived from two standard questionnaires about the perinatal period[4,38] and previous autism studies[4-6]. The mothers' histories during their pregnancies were reviewed to determine whether they had had 1) trauma requiring medical attention., 2) staining after the first trimester or bleeding any time during the pregnancy, 3) generalized edema, 4) severe nausea and vomiting after the first trimester, 5) systemic infection that required treatment by a physician or that lasted more than 2 days, 6) physician-prescribed medications (except iron and vitamins) taken for longer than 1 week, and 7) age greater than 34 years at the time of delivery. All seven of these clinical variables have been reported to be associated with an increased risk of autism[4-6].

After explanation of the MRI procedure, informed consent (and in the case of the one subject under 18, informed assent) was obtained from each subject and the following procedure was carried out. MRI was done with a General Electric (Signa) 1.5-tesla whole-body scanner using a standard head coil. Spin-lattice relaxation time (T_1) weighted sequences were performed in the sagittal plane (repetition time [TR] = 600 msec; echo time [TE] = 20 msec) and the coronal plane (TR = 800 msec; TE = 20 msec) with interleaved 3-mm slices. Proton weighted and spin-spin (T_2) images were performed in the axial plane (TR = 2500 msec; TE = 30/80 msec), parallel to the orbitomeatal line, with interleaved 5-mm slices.

Scans were blindly rated by consensus of two neurologists (S.E.S. and M.L.B.) who have extensive experience in rating MRI scans clinically and for research studies. Scans were rated for the presence or absence of polymicrogyria, pachygyria, heterotopia, and schizencephaly on the basis of previous published findings[31,32,39] and definitions and examples published in textbooks of neuropathology[25,26,29]. Polymicrogyria is defined as the focal or diffuse presence of an excessive number of cerebral convolutions with or without cortical thickening. Pachygyria is defined as the presence of broad, flat, and shallow gyri associated with an underlying area of increased cortical thickness ranging from involvement with one gyrus (macrogyria) to involvement of the entire cortex (agyria). Heterotopia refers to focal collections of gray matter in abnormal locations, and schizencephaly is defined as the presence of bilateral, symmetrical clefts in the cerebral cortex, with evidence of lining by gray matter, **with or without** extension into the ventricles.

Student's t test (two-tailed) was used to assess the comparability of autistic subjects and control subjects in age and nonverbal IQ. Frequency results were analyzed with chi-square tests with Yates' modification for small expected cell sizes.

RESULTS

The mean age of the autistic subjects was 27.8 years (range = 8–53 years). The mean age of the control subjects was 26.8 years (range = 11–46 years) (t = 0.53, df = 24, n.s.). The mean ±SD nonverbal IQ of the autistic group was 96.5±22.8; the mean nonverbal IQ of the control group was 100.4±18.0) (t = 0.48, df = 24, n.s.). Three autistic subjects had nonverbal IQs between 60 and 70, one had a nonverbal IQ between 70 and 90, and nine had nonverbal IQs between 90 and 130.

Developmental cortical malformations were detected in seven (53.8%) of the 13 autistic subjects and none of the control subjects $\chi^2 = 7.04$, df = 1, p = 0.008, with Yates' correction). Five autistic subjects had polymicrogyria (two in the frontal lobe, one in the parietal lobe, one in the temporal-occipital, and one in both the temporal- and parietal-occipital lobes); one had schizencephaly with bilateral parietal macrogyria; and one had a unilateral frontal macrogyria (figure 1). Three subjects had malformations localized in the left hemisphere, two had them in the right hemisphere, and two had bilateral malformations.

Autistic subjects with cortical malformations (N = 7) and without (N = 6) on MRI were compared for the presence of risk factors in their mothers' pregnancy histories. Six autistic subjects (three with and three without malformations) had mothers with pregnancy histories of one or more factors that have been shown in previous studies to be associated with autism. Theses abnormalities, all noted in either the first or second trimester, included 1) first trimester spotting and use of Bendectin (the mother of one subject with cortical malformations), 2) gastroenteritis and use of chlordiazepoxide (the mother of one subject with cortical malformations), 3) use of penicillin for influenza and use of Fiorinal (the mother of one subject without cortical malformations), 4) use of an unknown medication for prevention of miscarriage (the mother of one subject without cortical malformations), and 5) maternal age⩾35 years (mothers of one subject with and one subject without cortical malformations).

DISCUSSION

We found MRI abnormalities compatible with developmental cortical malformations in a significant number of high-functioning, strictly diagnosed autistic indi-

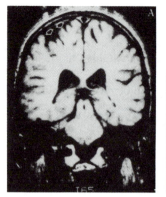
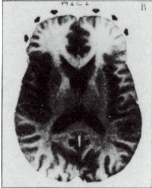
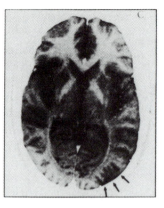

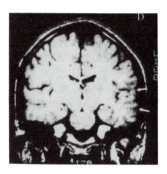
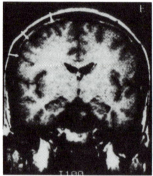
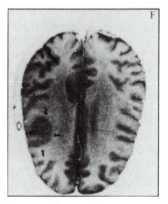

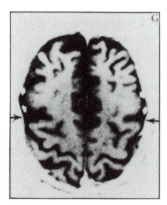

A. 19-year-old male; nonverbal IQ=116. T_1-weighted coronal image showing a right superior parietal polymicrogyria (open arrows).

B. 27-year-old male; nonverbal IQ=107. Inverted T_2-weighted axial image showing a bilateral frontopolar polymicrogyria (black arrows).

C. 35-year-old male; nonverbal IQ=67. Inverted T_2-weighted axial image showing a left parieto-occipital polymicrogyria (black arrows).

D. 22-year-old male; nonverbal IQ=95. T_1-weighted coronal image showing a left temporal polymicrogyria (white arrows). This subject also had left temporal-occipital and left-middle frontal polymicrogyria.

E. 21-year-old male; nonverbal IQ=65. T_1-weighted coronal image showing a right superior parietal polymicrogyria (white arrows).

F. 30-year-old male; nonverbal IQ≤130. Inverted T_2-weighted axial image showing a left precentral macrogyria (open arrows) and a focal region of thickened cortex (black arrows).

G. 53-year-old male; nonverbal IQ≤130. Inverted T_2-weighted axial image showing bilateral central parietal clefts (schizencephaly) (black arrows) and a wide postcentral gyrus (macrogyria) (open arrows).

Figure 1. Magnetic resonance imaging evidence of developmental cortical malformations in seven autistic subjects

viduals. There has been previous independent reports of polymicrogyria in two autistic subjects at autopsy[19,20] and heterotopia in one subject on MRI[17]. These cortical abnormalities, however, are not specific to autism and have been reported in association with several other conditions. Crome[28] reported that among 500 "severely subnormal" subjects he examined for neuropathology, 27 had brains showing polymicrogyria. Barkovich et al.[32], in a record review of 537 MRI scans of subjects in the pediatric age group, found 13 individuals with developmental cortical anomalies. All 13 individuals presented with seizures, and eight were described as having unspecified developmental delay. Finally, in a neuropathologic study of four consecutively autopsied dyslexic male patients, Galaburda et al.[40] reported developmental cortical anomalies in all four cases.

Several strengths and limitations of this study should be noted. First, with regard to selection of our study group, all subjects met criteria for autistic disorder as defined by *DSM-III-R* and by the Autism Diagnostic Interview algorithm, a detailed and standardized investigator-based instrument with established reliability and validity. The subjects were a relatively homogeneous group of high-functioning, non-fragile-X males without histories of major neurological abnormalities (including seizures) or medical abnormalities. Although the homogeneity of our subjects may be helpful in our search for a common neuroanatomical abnormality, it also limits the generalizability of our findings. Additionally, the small size of our study group limited the conclusions we can draw from our results. Control subjects for this study were selected on the basis of their comparability to the autistic subjects in age, nonverbal IQ, and sex. While comparability on these parameters was a strength of the study, the comparability of the autistic and control subjects on IQ may have been limited by our use of nonverbal IQ scores only. Finally, with regard to the design of the study, our assessment of the presence or absence of cortical malformations on MRI would have been strengthened if ratings had been made by two independent raters with high interrater agreement.

Our findings of a high rate of cortical malformations in individuals with autism has a number of implications with respect to the pathogenesis of this disorder. These findings support an accumulating body of evidence that brain abnormalities responsible for the disorder have their origin during the first 6 months of gestation. Courchesne[41], in his MRI study of autism, hypothesized that the neocerebellar hypoplasia which he observed was a result of abnormal granular call and/or Purkinje cell migration in the cerebellum that occurred between the third and fifth months prenatally. Bauman and Kemper[18] concluded from their neuropathologic case studies of autism that their findings were consistent with a lesion occurring early in development, perhaps before 30 weeks' gestation. Kemper[19] also postulated that an abnormality of cerebellar granular cells, observed in one subject, suggested early damage to glial cells and an arrest of granular cell migration. Our finding of cerebral cortical malformations is consistent with the timing of a disturbance in brain development that these other studies have hypothesized to occur. In addition, in each of these studies, abnormal neuronal migration was implicated in the disturbance.

In our study, cortical malformations were not confined to any particular lobe and were detected at the same rate in both hemispheres. The failure of these lesions to coincide topographically suggests that it is unlikely that they have a direct role in the pathogenesis of autism but, rather, that in a subgroup of autistic individuals, they are linked to the underlying mechanism in the disorder. This hypothesis is supported by experimental studies demonstrating that early acquired lesions may have effects on reorganizations and connectivity of the cortical architecture at distances remote from the site of the original lesions[42].

Both extrinsic and intrinsic factors, including fetal anoxia[43], maternal cytomegalovirus infection[44], and single gene defects[45], have been implicated in the pathogenesis of cerebral cortical malformations. Rakic[30], in addition, has hypothesized that cell-cell interactions resulting from viral infection, cell-mediated immune reactions, or defects in the recognition of specific proteins essential for cell movement may be responsible for abnormal neuronal migration. Immunologic abnormalities have been demonstrated in autism[46,47], as have abnormalities in serotonin[48], a neurotransmitter that has been implicated in the regulation of neurogenesis[49]. These studies suggest that the relationship between cortical malformations and prenatal immunologic, neurochemical, and genetic abnormalities in autistic subjects warrants further exploration.

Our findings raise several questions regarding the validity of MRI in detecting cerebral cortical malformations. The advantage of MRI over CT in detecting these abnormalities has been established[32-34]. Barkovich et al.[32], in reviewing the use of MRI in diagnosing migration abnormalities, suggested that these anomalies are readily detectable with MRI if at least two planes with both T_1 and T_2 weighted images and a 5-mm slice thickness are used. In our study, all subjects were imaged in three planes. Cortical malformations were detected in some cases in only the axial plane, in others in only the coronal plane, and in some in all three planes. This finding was seen as support for the efficacy of MRI in diagnosing these disorders.

Barkovich et al.[32] also emphasized that "recognition depends on awareness of the characteristic appearance of the entities" (p. 1017). However, although the capability of MRI to detect cortical malformations has been established, the sensitivity and specificity of MRI in diagnosing these disorders have received only limited attention in studies with clinical-pathological correlations and will require further investigation[32].

In summary, abnormalities compatible with developmental cerebral cortical malformations were demonstrated by MRI in seven of 13 high-functioning autistic individuals. These malformations have their origins in a disturbance before the sixth month of gestation. The small size and skewed IQ distribution of our study group do not allow us to make definitive inferences from the results of this study. However, the significance of our results and their agreement with the results of other studies suggest that future studies should be conducted on larger groups to replicate these findings and to investigate the presence of clinical and biological correlates.

REFERENCES

1. Rutter M, Schopler E: Autism and pervasive developmental disorders: concepts and diagnostic issues, in Diagnosis and Assessment in Autism. Edited by Schopler E, Mesibov GB. New York, Plenum, 1988

2. Paul R: Natural history, in Handbook of Autism and Pervasive Developmental Disorders. Edited by Cohen, DJ, Donnellan AM. New York, John Wiley & Sons, 1987

3. Folstein SE, Rutter ML: Autism: familial aggregation and genetic implications. J. Autism Dev Disord 1988; 18:3–29.

4. Gillberg C, Gillberg IC: Infantile autism: a total population study of reduced optimality in the pre-, peri-, and neonatal period. J Autism Dev Disord 1983; 13:153–166

5. Deykin EY, MacMahon B: Pregnancy, delivery, and neonatal complications among autistic children. Am J Dis Child 1980; 134:860–864

6. Finegan J, Quarrington B: Pre-, peri-, and neonatal factors and infantile autism. J Child Psychol Psychiatry 1979; 20:119–128

7. DeMyer MK, Hingtgen JN, Jackson RK: Autism: a decade of research. Schizophr Bull 1981; 3:388–451

8. Hier DE, LeMay M, Rosenberg PB: Autism and unfavorable left-right asymmetries of the brain. J Autism Dev Disord 1979; 9:153–159

9. Damassio H, Maurer RGG, Damasio AR, et al: Computerized tomorgraphic scan findings in patients with autistic behaviour. Arch Neurol 1980; 37:504–510

10. Campbell M, Rosenbloom S, Perry R, et al: Computerized axial tomography in young autistic children. Am J Psychiatry 1982; 1399:510–512

11. Jacobson R, Le Couteur A, Howlin P, et al: Selective subcortical abnormalities in autism. Psychol Med 1988; 18:39–48

12. Creasey H, Rumsey JM, Schwartz M, et al: Brain morphometry in autistic men as measured by volumetric computed tomography. Arch Neurol 1986; 43:669–672

13. Rumsey JM, Creasey H, Stepanek JS, et al: Hemispheric asymmetries, fourth ventricular size, and cerebellar morphology in autism. J Autism Dev Disord 1988; 18:127–137

14. Courchesne E. Yeung-Courchesne R, Press GA, et al: Hypoplasia of cerebellar vermal lobules VI and VII in autism. N Engl J Med 1988; 318:1349–1354

15. Gaffney GR, Kuperman S, Tsai LY, et al: Midsagittal magnetic resonance imaging of autism. Br J Psychiatry 1987; 151:831–833

16. Gaffney GR, Kuperman, S, Tsai LY, et al: Morphological evidence for brainstem involvement in infantile autism. Biol Psychiatry 1988; 24:578–586

17. Gaffney GR, Tsai LY: Magnetic resonance imaging of high level autism. J Autism Dev Disord 1987; 17:433–438

18. Bauman ML, Kemper T: Histoanatomic observations of the brain in early infantile autism. Neurology 1985; 35:866–874

19. Kemper TL: Neuroanatomic studies of dyslexia and autism, in Disorders of the Developing Nervous System: Changing Views on Their Origins, Diagnosis, and Treatments. Edited by Swann JW, Messer A. New York, Alan R Liss, 1988

20. Ritvo ER, Freeman BJ, Scheibel AB, et al: Lower Purkinje cell counts in the cerebella of four autistic subjects: initial findings of the UCLA-NSAC autopsy research report. Am J Psychiatry 1986; 143:862–866

21. Williams RS, Hauser SL, Purpura DP, et al: Autism and mental retardation: neuropathologic studies performed in four retarded persons with autistic behavior. Arch Neurol 1980; 37:749–753

22. Wing L: Asperger's syndrome: a clinical account. Psychol Med 1981; 11:115–129

23. Van Krevelen DA: Early infantile autism and autistic psychopathy. J Autism Child Schizo 1971; 1:82–86

24. Piven J, Gayle J, Chase G, et al: A family history study of neuropsychiatric disorders in the adult siblings of autistic individuals. J Am Acad Child Adolesc Psychiatry (in press)

25. Friede RL (ed): Developmental Neuropathology. Vienna, Springer, 1975

26. Larroche JC: Malformations of the nervous system, in Greenfield's Neuropathology, 4th ed. Edited by Adams JH, Corsellis JAN, Duchen LW. New York, John Wiley & Sons, 1984

27. Yakovlev PI, Wadsworth RC: Schizencephalies: a study of the congenital clefters in the cerebral mantle, I: clefts with hydrocephalus and lips separated. J Neuropathol Exp Neurol 1946; 5:169–207

28. Crome L: Pachygyria. J Pathology and Bacteriology 1956; 71:335–352

29. Ludwin SD, Malamud N: Pathology of congenital anomalies of the brain, in Radiology of the Skull and Brain, vol 3: Anatomy and Pathology. Edited by Newton TH, Potts DG. St Louis, CV Mosby, 1977

30. Rakic P: Neuronal migration and contact guidance in the primate telencephalon. Postgrad Med J 1978; 54:25–40

31. Dvorak K, Feit J: Migration of neuroblasts through partial necrosis of the cerebral cortex in newborn rats—contribution to the problems of morphological development and developmental period of cerebral microgyria: histological and autoradiographical study. Acta Neuropathol (Berl) 1977; 38:203–212

32. Barkovich AJ, Chuang SH, Norman D: MR of neuronal migration anomalies. AJNR 1987; 8:1009–1017

33. Kuzniecki R, Berkovic S, Andermann F, et al: Focal cortical myoclonus and rolandic cortical dysplasis: clarification by magnetic resonance imaging. Ann Neurol 1988; 23:317–325

34. Marchal G, Andermann F, Tampieri D, et al: Generalized cortical dysplasia manifested by diffusely thick cerebral cortex. Arch Neurol 1989;; 46:430–434

35. Rutter M, Le Couteur A, Lord C, et al: Diagnosis and subclassification of autism: con-

cepts and instrument development in Diagnosis and Assessment in Autism. Edited by Schopler E, Mesibov GB. New York, Plenum, 1988

36. Gillberg C: Annotation: the neurobiology of infantile autism. J Child Psychol Psychiatry 1988; 29:257–266

37. Raven JC (ed): Guide to the Standard Progressive Matrices. London, HR Lewis, 1960

38. Sameroff AJ: The etiology of cognitive competence: a systems perspective, in Infants at Risk: Assessment of Cognitive Functioning. Edited by Kearsley K, Segel I. New York, John Wiley & Sons, 1979

39. Barkovich, AJ, Normal D: MR imaging of schizencephaly. AJNR 1988; 9:297–302

40. Galaburda AM, Sherman GF, Rosen GD, et al: Developmental dyslexia: four consecutive patients with cortical anomalies. Ann Neurol 1985; 18:222–233

41. Courchesne E: Cerebellar changes in autism, in Disorders of the Developing Nervous System: Changing Views on Their Origins, Diagnoses, and Treatments. Edited by Swann JW, Messer A. New York, Alan R Liss, 1988

42. Goldman-Rakic PS, Rakic P: Prenatal removal of the frontal association cortex in the fetal rhesus monkey: anatomical and functional consequences in postnatal life. Brain Res 1978; 152:451–485

43. Hallervorden J: Ueber eine Kohlenoxydvergiftung im Fotalleben mit Entwicklungsstoorung der Hirnrinde. Allgemeine Zeitschrift fur Psychiatrie 1949; 124:289–298

44. Diezel P: Mikrogyrie infolge cerebrater speicheldrusenvirusinfektion im Rahmen einer generalisierten Cytomegalie bei einem Saugling Zugleich ein Beitrag zur Theorie der Windungbildung. Virchows Archiv fur Pathologie und Anatomie 1954; 325:109

45. Dobyns WB, Stratton RF, Greenberg F: Syndromes with lissencephaly, I: Miller-Dieker and Norman-Roberts syndromes and isolated lissencephaly. Am J Med Genet 1984; 18:509–526

46. Warren RP, Foster A, Margaretten NC: Reduced natural killer cell activity in autism. J Am Acad Child Adolesc Psychiatry 1987; 3:333–335

47. Todd RD, Ciaranello RD: Demonstration of inter- and intraspecies differences in serotonin binding sites by antibodies from an autistic child. Proc Natl Acad Sci USA 1985; 82:612–616

48. McBride PA, Anderson GM, Hertzig ME, et al: Serotonergic responsivity in young male adults with autistic disorder. Arch Gen Psychiatry 1989; 46:213–221

49. Lauder JM, Krebs H: Serotonin as a differentiation signal in early neurogenesis. Dev Neurosci 1978; 1:15–30

24

Neuropsychology of Early-treated Phenylketonuria: Specific Executive Function Deficits

Marilyn C. Welsh

Fordham University, New York

Bruce F. Pennington and Sally Ozonoff

University of Denver

Bobbye Rouse

University of Texas Medical Branch

Edward R.B. McCabe

Baylor College of Medicine, Waco, Texas

This study explored the hypothesis that children with early-treated phenylketonuria (PKU) are selectively impaired on executive function measures, even when still on diet. The rationale for this hypothesis is that even mild elevations in phenylalanine (Phe) can lead to lower central levels of biogenic amines, including dopamine (DA). We hypothesize that this mild DA depletion causes subtle prefrontal dysfunction, which in turn affects executive functions such as set maintenance, plan-

Reprinted with permission from *Child Development*, 1990, Vol. 61, 1697–1713. Copyright © 1990 by The Society for Research in Child Development, Inc.

This research was supported by the following grants to the first author: NIMH Postdoctoral Fellowship (MH 15442–07), March of Dimes project grant (12–85), and seed money from the Developmental Psychobiology Research Group Endowment Fund of the University of Colorado School of Medicine (141). The second author was supported by the following grants: NIMH RSDA (MH 00419) and project grants from NIMH (MH 38820), NICHD (HD 19423), and March of Dimes (12–135). We gratefully acknowledge the participation of the patients and families of the PKU clinics at the University of Colorado Health Sciences Center and the University of Texas Medical Branch. We also thank the staff of these clinics for their help in recruiting participants, Warren Tryon, for his guidance in statistical analysis, and Suzanne Miller for help in manuscript preparation. The helpful comments of anonymous reviewers on earlier drafts of this manuscript are also acknowledged. Portions of this research were presented at the fifteenth annual meeting of the International Neuropsychological Society, February 1987, Washington, DC.

ning, and organized search. 11 preschool early-treated PKU children (M age = 4.64) and a sample of age- and IQ-matched unaffected peers (n = 11) were evaluated on a battery of executive function (EF) measures. In addition, a "non-executive function" task recognition memory, was administered to all subjects. Group comparisons demonstrated that PKU children were significantly impaired on an executive function composite score; there were no group differences, however, in recognition memory. These results supported the hypothesized specific deficit in executive function. Furthermore, within the PKU group the executive function composite score was significantly negatively correlated with concurrent phenylalanine levels, even after controlling for the correlation between IQ and executive function skills. This second finding provides support for the proposed biochemical mechanism underlying the specific cognitive deficits.

Studies of clinical populations can make a unique contribution to our understanding of normal cognitive development because such studies can reveal dissociations among cognitive mechanisms that may not be readily apparent in normally developing populations. Conversely, basic research in normal cognitive development provides theories and methods needed to analyze cognitive processes in clinical populations. In our research, we are particularly interested in specific cognitive processes that are relatively IQ-independent and contribute to clinically significant individual differences. In the present investigation, we use methods from the study of normal cognitive effects of the biochemical variations produced by a natural experiment, early-treated phenylketonuria (PKU). The hypothesis tested here is that PKU causes specific cognitive effects in the domain of executive function that may be due to mild dopamine depletion in the prefrontal cortex.

PKU is a well-known genetic cause of mental retardation, affecting one in 10,000 to 20,000 live births (Benson & Fensom, 1985). The disorder is the consequence of mutations in the gene that codes for the enzyme phenylalanine hydroxylase (DiLella, Marvit, Lidsky, Guttler, & Woo, 1986; Woo, DiLella, Marvit, & Ledley, 1986; Woo, Lidsky, Guttler, Chandra, & Robson, 1983). This enzyme is essential for hydroxylation of dietary phenylalanine (Phe) to tyrosine in the liver (Choo, Cotton, Jennings, & Danks, 1979; Guttler & Lou, 1986). Given normal dietary intake of the amino acid Phe, severe mental handicap results (Primrose, 1983). Today, newborn screening programs identify individuals with PKU (Guthrie & Susi, 1963; Levy, 1973; Veale, 1980) so that a diet low in Phe may be initiated early in development. If this treatment is begun early and controlled consistently during childhood, mental retardation is averted (Bickel, Gerrard, & Hickmans, 1954; Hudson, Mordaunt, & Leahy, 1970; Williamson, Koch, Azen, & Chang, 1981).

Even with early treatment, it is possible that PKU may cause subtle, specific cognitive deficits that are not typically detected by traditional cognitive measures. This possibility has only rarely been considered or studied. Recently, a prefrontal dysfunction hypothesis of early-treated PKU has been suggested by several investigators (Chamove & Molinaro, 1978; Pennington, van Doorninck, McCabe, & McCabe, 1985; Spreen, Tupper, Risser, Tuokko, & Edgell, 1984). However, this hypothesis has not been systematically specified or tested. In what follows, we delineate this prefrontal dysfunction hypothesis and describe the methodology used in the current study to test parts of it.

The prefrontal dysfunction hypotheses proposes that PKU has a relatively specific effect on neurochemistry. Individuals with PKU cannot convert phenylalanine to tyrosine (McKean, 1972); this contributes to low tyrosine levels in the brain, as does the fact that high Phe levels interfere with brain transport of tyrosine from other sources (Curtius, Baerlocher, & Vollmin, 1972; Curtius, Vollmin, & Baerlocher, 1972). Since the conversion of tyrosine to L-dopa is the rate-limiting step in the synthesis of dopamine and norepinephrine (Cooper, Bloom, & Roth, 1982), elevations in Phe lead to catecholamine depletion through reduction of tyrosine. Thus, central levels of dopamine and norepinephrine are expected to be depressed in individuals with PKU. Reduced levels have been found in untreated PKU individuals (Butler, O'Flynn, Seifert, & Howell, 1981; Pratt, 1980; Sandler, 1982). More evidence for the relation between Phe and brain chemistry comes from experimental "Phe loading" studies. When Phe levels of early-treated PKU subjects are manipulated, correlated reductions in dopamine precursors and metabolites are found (Krause et al., 1985; Lou, Guttler, Lykelund, Bruhn, & Niederwieser, 1985), as well as concomitant changes in electrophysiological measures (Krause, Epstein, Averbrook,, Dembure, & Elsas, 1986). Lowered serotonin levels have also been found and appear to be caused by the inhibiting effects of high Phe levels on the uptake of serotonin precursors (Butler et al., 1981).

The prefrontal dysfunction hypothesis proposes that the main effects on cognition in PKU are caused specifically by dopamine depletion. Norepinephrine and serotonin projections in the neocortex are diffusely distributed and appear to make less specific contributions to cognition than the dopaminergic projections to the neocortex, which are found primarily in the frontal lobes (Divac, Bjorklund, Lindvall, & Passingham, 1978; Porrino & Goldman-Rakic, 1982). The depletion of dopamine is hypothesized to impair prefrontal functioning and result in deficits in executive function. Studies in nonhuman primates support this notion, demonstrating that depletion of prefrontal dopamine impairs performance on the delayed response task, a classic behavioral test of prefrontal function in these species (Arnsten & Goldman-Rakic, 1985; Brozoski, Brown, Rosvold, & Goldman, 1979).

The concept of executive function has been offered as a potential behavioral marker of prefrontal functioning in developing humans and nonhuman primates (Luria, 1966; Shallice, 1982; Stuss & Benson, 1984). Welsh and Pennington (1988) discuss how this overarching term may be applicable to the study of prefrontal functioning in developing children. Executive function is defined as the ability to maintain an appropriate problem solving set for attainment of a future goal. Appropriate set maintenance allows for strategic planning, impulse control, organized search, and flexibility of thought and action. Frontal damage in human adults has been found to impair anticipation, planning, goal establishment, self-monitoring, and flexibility (Fuster, 1980, 1985; Luria, 1973; Stuss & Benson, 1984, 1987). Furthermore, patients with conditions associated with dopamine deficiency (e.g., Parkinson's disease, attention deficit disorder) also display impairment in executive function skills (Douglas, 1983; Taylor, Saint-Cyr, & Lang, 1986; Weinberger, Berman, & Chase, 1987).

The behavioral and cognitive sequelae of PKU in untreated, late-treated, and early-treated individuals provide support for the hypothesis that executive functions are differentially affected in PKU. In addition to severe mental retardation, untreated PKU individuals manifest a range of behavioral impairments, including hyperactivity, attention and perceptual-motor problems, aggressiveness, negative mood, and motor disturbance (MacLeod, Munro, Ledingham & Farquhar, 1983; Paine, 1957; Primrose, 1983). Motor deficits can be similar to those observed in Parkinson's disease, a dopamine-deficient disorder in adults (Kolb & Whishaw, 1985). Cognitive and behavioral deficits seen in late treatment (i.e., after infancy) are similar but less extreme (Margolin et al., 1978; McKean, 1971). Thus, the specific cognitive impairments of untreated and late-treated PKU individuals appear more related to putative executive function processes, such as problem solving, attention, and perceptual-motor functioning, than to non-executive function processes, such as language and memory.

Studies of cognitive functioning in early-treated individuals have also been done. Most published follow-up studies investigating the consequences of early-initiated dietary treatment have focused on IQ scores of school-aged children. A synthesis of reports from the large Collaborative Study (Koch, Azen, Friedman, & Williamson, 1984; Williamson, Dobson, & Koch, 1977) and from smaller, independent projects (Berry, O'Grady, Perlmutter, & Bofinger, 1979; Fuller & Shulman, 1987; Netley, Hanley, & Rudner, 1984; O'Grady, Berry, & Sutherland, 1971), makes it clear that the IQ scores of early-treated PKU children are typically in the normal range, although they are often significantly lower than those of unaffected siblings or parents. Recent findings from the Collaborative Study suggest that extending dietary treatment until age 8 results in IQ levels more similar to those of family members (Holtzman, Kronmal, van Doorninck, Azen, & Koch, 1986).

Although intelligence tests can be helpful in identifying some general depression in neuropsychological functioning, they are relatively inadequate in detecting *specific* cognitive deficits. This is particularly true for impairments due to prefrontal dysfunction (Pollack, 1950; Teuber, 1959; Warrington, James, & Maciejewski,

1986; Weinstein & Teuber, 1957). Recently, research on early-treated individuals has turned to exploring specific cognitive functions that are not readily evaluated by traditional IQ tests. The few relevant studies differ in the measures used, but some preliminary generalizations seem warranted. While language, perception, memory, and motor functions appear to be normal, the studies document impairments in several domains, including attention (Cabalska et al., 1977; Crowie, 1971; Griffen, Clarke, & d'Entremont, 1980), perceptual-motor functioning (Brunner, Jordan, & Berry, 1983; Cabalska et al., 1977; Koff, Boyle, & Pueschel, 1977; Pennington et al., 1985; Seashore, Friedman & Norelly, 1979), planning and organizational skills (Crowie, 1971; Koff et al., 1977), flexible application of strategies (Pennington et al., 1985), and concept formation (Brunner et al., 1983; Pennington et al., 1985).

We have summarized several studies of untreated, late-treated, and early-treated PKU individuals. While none of the investigations was specifically designed to test the executive function hypothesis, results are generally consistent with it.

Two studies (Krause et al., 1985; Lou et al., 1985) that *have* examined the relation between Phe and executive function demonstrated both the hypothesized inverse relation between Phe and dopamine and concomitant deficits in executive function. Using a Phe-loading technique to induce a dopamine-deficient condition in an early-treated PKU individual, impaired attention was demonstrated. Deficits in sustained attention can be conceptualized as reflecting prefrontal dysfunction, since sustained attention is a by-product of the executive functions of set maintenance and goal-directed activity. While these studies demonstrated immediate cognitive effects of manipulated biochemical levels, a range of executive functions was not examined, nor were results related to prefrontal dysfunction.

A second area of PKU research that has been relatively neglected is the cognitive development of very young early-treated PKU children. The few studies that have investigated cognitive functioning in PKU infants and toddlers have demonstrated normal linguistic functioning (Melnick, Kimberlee, Michals, & Matalon, 1981) and developmental status (Fuller & Shulman, 1971), given early and appropriate treatment. Similarly, IQ scores were normal in early-treated PKU preschoolers when dietary treatment was initiated during the first month of life (Dobson, Williamson, Azen, & Koch, 1977; Williamson et al., 1981). However, as discussed above, average intelligence does not rule out specific cognitive deficits. Missing from this research are investigations of underlying cognitive processes more directly related to the skills impaired in older early-treated PKU children. Specifically, no studies have yet been done investigating the quality of executive function in infants or preschoolers with PKU.

A final issue that deserves attention in the PKU literature concerns when abnormal Phe levels have their greatest effect on cognition. For example, the issue of whether current, lifetime, or infant Phe level is the best predictor of cognitive function remains unresolved. There is some evidence that cognitive deficits are correlated with Phe level in the blood at the time of testing (Brunner et al., 1983; Koch et al., 1984; Krause et al., 1985); such cognitive deficits may be transient and reversible (Krause et al., 1985). Data also suggest that lifetime dietary compliance (as indexed by an average measure of Phe over the lifespan) contributes to cognitive performance, particularly IQ (Koch et al., 1984; Waisbren, Mahon, Schnell, & Levy, 1987). The relations of current, infant, and lifetime Phe levels to cognitive functioning are further explored in the current research.

In the present study, four tasks were selected from a larger Executive Function Battery that has been used recently with normally functioning subjects spanning a wide age range (Welsh, Pennington, & Groisser, in press). Three of these tasks, Visual Search, Verbal Fluency, and Motor Planning, were found to load on the same principal component; this factor seemed to reflect "speeded, organized responding." The developmental courses for these tasks ranged from adult-level performance achieved by age 6 (Visual Search) to adult-level skill emerging sometime after age 12 (Motor Planning, Verbal Fluency). The fourth executive function measure, Tower of Hanoi, loaded on a separate "planning" factor; optimal performance on this task was reached by age 6 years. Thus, the tasks used in the present study represented at least two domains of executive functions and ranged in difficulty level. Moreover, the normative study (Welsh et al., in press) found little association between performance on these tasks and sex or IQ-measured intelligence.

These executive function measures and a memory task assumed to be relatively free of executive function demands were administered to a group of early-treated PKU children and to an age- and IQ-matched group of unaffected controls. The objective of this design was to test two hypothesis: (1) that specific executive function deficits are present in young, early-treated PKU children still on diet, and (2) that these impairments are associated with higher concurrent Phe levels, and possibly with higher lifetime and infant Phe levels as well. A more direct index of dopaminergic functioning, such as metabolite level, could not be measured in these subjects. Therefore, the neurochemical aspect of the prefrontal hypothesis was tested only indirectly by examining the relation between Phe level and executive function performance.

METHOD

Subjects

The early-treated PKU group was comprised of nine female and two male Caucasian children (M age $=$ 4.64 years). All had IQ scores in the normal range and none attended special education programs. All subjects had been continuously maintained on a low-Phe diet since the first 2–4 weeks of life (M $=$ 22.7 days, range = 14–28 days). Subjects were recruited by personnel from two regional PKU clinics. Families expressing interest in the study were sent consent forms and subsequently contacted by the principal investigator. Eleven of the 17 families contacted agreed and were able to participate (65%).

Only children with IQ scores in the normal range (above 80) were included in the sample. Table 1 provides the IQ scores and the following three Phe levels for each PKU subject: (1) the Phe level concurrent with testing, (2) the mean lifetime Phe level, from diet initiation and stabilization through the testing day, and (3) the highest Phe level during infancy, prior to dietary restriction. The first two Phe levels indicate there was dietary compliance in the group as a whole, while all three levels also indicate individual differences. Infant Phe level was unavailable for one PKU subject.

The control group consisted of 11 unaffected Caucasian children, seven females and four males (*M* age = 4.99 years); they were recruited from two metropolitan preschools and from the University of Denver subject pool. An important aspect of the study design was to group-match the control children with the PKU children in IQ. Therefore, teachers at the two schools were asked to suggest children who appeared to be "average" in cognitive ability. From this subset, children with informed parental consent were randomly selected. The control group was matched with the early-treated PKU group on IQ, chronological age, and ethnicity; there was no substantial or significant difference in sex distribution across the two groups.

Children with sensory, intellectual, or emotional handicaps were excluded from both the PKU and control groups. Hollingshead's Social Index (1975) was calculated for each PKU subject and for 10 of the 11 control subjects (demographic information

TABLE 1
IQ and Phe Levels of the Early-treated PKU Sample

Subject	Sex	Age (Years)	FSIQ	CPhe	MPhe	IPhe
1	F	4.25	114	13.0	9.2	44.5
2	F	5.75	120	8.4	9.9	45.3
3	F	4.08	116	10.6	7.9	36.1
4	F	5.17	82	9.9	10.5	31.9
5	F	4.50	101	9.9	11.4	51.1
6	F	4.83	115	4.9	10.3	31.9
7	F	4.50	94	17.9	14.0	50.1
8	M	4.67	112	9.5	7.3	20.0
9	M	4.42	93	7.5	8.3	[a]
10	F	4.33	119	10.8	7.4	19.1
11	F	4.50	86	1.1	9.5	43.0

NOTE.—CPhe = concurrent Phe level, MPhe = mean lifetime Phe level, IPhe = infant Phe level. Intelligence test given was the WPPSI, except in the cases of subjects 7 and 8, who were administered the Gesell Developmental Assessment.
[a] Infant Phe level not available for subject 9.

was unavailable for one control child). The mean Hollingshead scores were 41.59 and 52.40 for the PKU and control groups, respectively. The lower SES for the PKU sample is possibly due to the fact that these subjects came from both urban and rural environments, whereas the control children were all from an urban environment. As will be seen below, this SES difference was not a significant confound.

MEASURES

Both groups were administered four executive function tasks and a discriminant recognition memory task. To obtain a general intelligence quotient, the early-treated PKU group was administered either the Wechsler Preschool and Primary Intelligence Scale (WPPSI; $n = 9$) or the Gesell Preschool Developmental Schedule ($n = 2$). The Gesell was given to these two subjects due to pragmatic constraints within the clinic from which both children were recruited. All subjects in the control group were given the WPPSI.

Executive Function Measures

Visual search. This organized search task was adapted from one used by Teuber, Battersby, and Bender (1955) with brain-injured adults; it has been shown to be differentially sensitive to frontal lesions (Teuber, Battersby, & Bender 1955). On each trial, subjects were shown an 8 ½ × 11-inch sheet of white paper, upon which 40 black-and-white drawings of common objects (e.g., food, animals, clothing, shapes) were printed. A target object was circled at the top of the page; eight occurrences of the target were scattered among 32 distractors in the page below. Eight trials were given within the test; the same pool of figures was used for targets and background stimuli across the eight trials. This method provided an opportunity for perseveration across trials; for example, some subjects continued to point out occurrences of objects which had been targets on previous trials but were no longer correct on the current trial.

On each trial, the picture array was placed on the table in front of the child within easy viewing and pointing distance. Subjects were instructed to find all the figures that "looked the same" as the circled target at the top of the page; they were told to do so as quickly as possible. Once the subject pointed to a figure, it was crossed out by the experimenter. The subject was timed from presentation of the stimulus until he or she said "done." One practice trial was administered before the eight test trials.

Two variables, reaction time and number of correct responses, were calculated for each of the eight trials; the variable "correct responses" was defined as the number of correct figures selected in a trial, minus the number of false alarms, or nontargets, chosen. An "inefficiency score" was calculated for each trial by dividing reaction time by correct responses. Inefficiency scores for the eight test trials were then averaged to obtain an overall inefficiency score for the test; higher scores reflected greater inefficiency. The second dependent measure of the Visual Search task was a perseveration index, defined as the percentage of errors that were perseverative. It was calculated by dividing the number of false alarms that had been targets on previous items by the total number of errors across trials. Nonperseverative errors were not analyzed in this study.

Verbal fluency. This task measured systematic search of the semantic network. Deficits on phonemic verbal fluency tasks have been found in frontal-damaged adults (Milner, 1964). Since Milner's (1964) task is inappropriate for young nonreading subjects, a semantic fluency task was substituted, adapted from the McCarthy Scales of Children's Abilities (McCarthy, 1972). Subjects were required to produce as many different members of the requested semantic category as possible in 40 sec; they were explicitly told that modifications of a previously given response (e.g., dog, small dog) would not be given credit. The procedure was demonstrated and practiced using the semantic category "colors." The four test categories were "food," "clothing," "animals," and "things to ride." The demand to shift set, at both the category and the word level, provided opportunities to observe perseveration.

Again, the two dependent variables involved efficiency and perseveration. Efficiency was defined as the number of correct, unique words generated within the time limit, summed across the four categories. Two types of perseveration were scored: (1) incorrect responses that represented members of previous categories, and (2) repetitions (e.g., dog, cat, dog), and modifications (e.g., dog, mommy dog) of appropriate words within a category. The perseveration index was calculated by dividing perseverative errors of both types by total responses (correct and incorrect). Nonperseverative incorrect responses were not analyzed.

Motor planning task. This finger-sequencing task was taken from the Luria-Nebraska Neuropsychological Battery for Adults (Golden, 1981). Subjects were instructed to touch each of their four fingers to their thumb (in the order ring finger to "pinky") without missing a finger or striking any finger twice. After one or two practice trials, children were asked to perform the sequences as quickly as possible, first using the right hand, then with the left hand. The dependent measure, efficiency, was defined as the number of completed, correct motor sequences performed in 10 sec, averaged across both hands.

Tower of Hanoi. This disk-transfer task has been used to study the planning capacities of normal and retarded children and adults (Borys, Spitz, & Dorans, 1982; Simon, 1975). The Tower of Hanoi evaluates the ability to plan and execute a sequence of moves that transform an initial configuration of disks into a goal state that duplicates the experimenter's disk configuration. A factor-analytic study of executive function measures (Welsh et al., in press) found that this task loads most highly on a "planning" factor when used with children. Efficient performance also requires the ability to inhibit irrelevant responses. Performance on the Tower of Hanoi is not significantly correlated with IQ (Welsh et al., in press). A deficit in this type of planning behavior has been demonstrated in frontal-damaged adults (Shallice, 1982) and in individuals with Parkinson's disease (Saint-Cyr, Taylor, & Lang, 1988).

Identical apparatuses were set up in front of the subject and the experimenter. Each apparatus consisted of a wooden base (5¼ × 19 inches) with three vertical pegs inserted in it, spaced 3½ inches apart; three disks of different sizes and colors rested on the pegs. The plastic pegs and disks were obtained from Fisher-Price Rock-a-Stack toys.

Subjects were given an age-appropriate explanation of the task objectives and rules. To reduce the abstractness of the task demands, a cover story concerning a family of monkeys (disks) jumping around trees (pegs) was used (Klahr & Robinson, 1981).

The peg apparatuses were set up in front of both the subject and the experimenter. The experimenter's disks were arranged on the experimenter's right-hand peg to form a tower, with the largest disk on the bottom and the smallest disk on the top. This disk arrangement represented the goal state that the subject was trying to achieve on all problems. Disks were moved in compliance with three rules: (1) a larger disk could not be placed on a smaller disk, (2) only one disk could be moved at a time, and (3) the disks had to be on a peg or in the subject's hand at all times. All subjects exhibited their understanding of these rules by demonstrating legal and illegal moves before continuing to the practice problems. Subjects were required to solve two practice problems. Individual moves were recorded by the experimenter, creating an exact record of the moves generated by each subject on each trial.

Six problems varying in initial disk configuration and difficulty were administered; the easiest problem required only two moves to solve, while the most difficult could be completed in seven moves. All subjects began the test with the two-move problem. Subjects had to complete the problem in the fewest number of moves possible, with no rule violations, twice in succession; they were given six trials to achieve this criterion for each problem. Testing continued until the subject was unable to complete a problem within the six trials allowed.

The scoring system for the Tower of Hanoi was developed by Borys et al. (1982). If a problem was solved in the first two trials, a score of 6 was given. Point total decreased with the number of trials required to solution; for example, solution on trials 2 and 3 received a score of 5, solution on trials 3 and 4 received a score of 4, and so on. This procedure resulted in scores ranging from 0 to 6 (excepting a score of 1) for each problem. The dependent variable was a "planning efficiency" score that was obtained by summing the scores received on the six problems of the test; this total score ranged from 0 to 36 (excepting a total score of 1).

Discriminant Task

Continuous picture recognition task This recognition memory test was developed by Brown and Scott (1971); rather than measuring deliberate monitoring strategies that may be frontally mediated, the task was designed to tap a relatively non-strategic, automatic recognition memory function (Brown & DeLoache, 1978).

The test was constructed as described by Brown and Scott (1971). It consisted of 100 pictures of cartoon characters familiar to preschool children (e.g., Smurfs) mounted on 8 × 8-inch pieces of black cardboard. Forty-four of the pictures were repeated once in the stack of cards, after lags of either 0 (immediate repetition), 5, 10, 25, or 50 pictures; the remaining 12 cards were filler items.

Subjects were first administered a practice session with a smaller deck of 10 cards; four of these pictures were repeated once within the deck. Children were instructed to say "yes" if they remembered seeing the picture earlier in the stack of 10 cards and "no" if they did not remember seeing the picture. During practice, it was clarified that a "yes" response should not be given if they had seen the picture on TV or in their own books, but should be reserved only for pictures appearing earlier in the stack. All of the children demonstrated understanding of the procedure, as evidenced by good performance on the practice trials. That is, all subjects correctly identified at least eight of the 10 practice pictures as having appeared earlier or having not appeared earlier in the deck. Following the practice session, the 100 test trials were administered. The directions were the same as for the practice trials.

Responses were scored as hits ("yes" to an item previously seen, "no" to a new item), false alarms ("yes" to a new item), or misses ("no" to an item previously seen). The dependent measure was the total number of hits; the maximum score possible was 100.

Procedure

All children were tested on the five experimental measures during a 45-min session that included several breaks. The following test order was constant across all subjects: Visual Search (VS), Tower of Hanoi (TOH), Verbal Fluency (VF), Motor Planning (MP), and Picture Recognition (PR). Early-treated PKU children were administered the IQ assessment either later on the day of testing ($n = 7$) or no more than 6 months prior to testing ($n = 4$). Control children were administered the WPPSI either on the day of testing ($n = 9$) or no more than 4 months prior to testing ($n = 2$). In addition, the concurrent Phe level of each PKU subject was obtained by drawing ½ cc of blood from the finger on the day of testing.

RESULTS

Two questions were addressed in the current study: (1) Do PKU preschoolers exhibit specific impairments in the domain of executive function (EF) when compared with unaffected age-mates? and (2) What are the specific contribution of concurrent, mean, and infant Phe levels to EF performance in PKU preschoolers on diet? Moreover, does Phe level continue to predict EF after controlling for the contribution of general intelligence?

GROUP DIFFERENCES

To reduce the number of statistical comparisons, and EF composite score was derived by converting raw scores on the EF measures to Z scores, using the grand mean and standard deviation of the EF measures. After converting them to Z scores, the six EP variables (Motor Planning, Verbal Fluency Efficiency, Verbal Fluency Perseveration, Tower of Hanoi, Visual Search Inefficiency, and Visual Search Perseveration) were averaged to obtain the EF composite score. This composite was the primary variable used to examine the two questions posed by this study.

Quantitative differences. Sex, age, IQ, and test performance data for the groups are presented in Table 2. Since the two groups were matched on age and FSIQ, they did not differ significantly on these variables; there were also no significant

TABLE 2
Group Differences on Age, IQ, SES, and Performance Measures

| | PKU | | CONTROL | | |
MEASURE	M	SD	M	SD	GROUP DIFFERENCE
Age (years)	4.64	.47	4.99	.36	N.S.
FSIQ	104.73	13.94	108.00	9.74	N.S.
VIQ	106.80	10.80	106.30	15.70	N.S.
PIQ	107.00	7.80	100.00	10.10	N.S.
SES	41.59	11.53	52.40	9.29	$p < .03$
Picture Recognition	94.09	6.35	94.72	4.36	N.S.
Executive function composite	−.56	.90	.46	.37	$p < .004$
Motor Planning	1.91	.86	2.64	.98	$p < .08$
Verbal Fluency (VF) efficiency	14.09	4.57	20.82	3.71	$p < .001$
VF perseveration[a,b]	19.09	14.50	10.55	5.47	$p < .08$
Tower of Hanoi	7.46	7.74	18.82	6.37	$p < .001$
Visual Search (VS)[b] inefficiency	7.36	5.31	3.88	1.58	$p < .05$
VS perseveration[a,b]	34.00	36.73	20.09	32.00	N.S.

NOTE.—$N = 11$ in each group for all the analyses, with the exception of the test of SES group differences. In this one analysis, $N = 10$ in the control group.
[a] Percent of the baseline response that is perseverative.
[b] Higher score reflects poorer performance.

group differences on Verbal or Performance IQ. The two groups did differ significantly on SES, however.

The dependent variable of primary interest was the EF composite score. As can be seen, the PKU group's score on the EF compositive was 1 SD lower than that of the control group; this difference is significant, $t(13.26) = -3.50$, $p<.004$, separate variance estimate. In contrast, there were no group differences on the discriminant measure, Picture Recognition.

Performance on the individual EF variables is also presented in Table 2. Independent t tests revealed three measures on which the groups differed significantly, with the early-treated PKU group performing more poorly in each case: (1) Verbal Fluency efficiency $t(20) = 3.79$, $p<.001$; (2) Tower of Hanoi, $t(20) = 3.76$, $p<.001$; and (3) Visual Search inefficiency, $t(20) = 2.09$, $p<.05$. In addition, there were trends toward early-treated PKU children being less efficient in Motor Planning, $t(20) = 1.85$, $p <.08$, and more perseverative in Verbal Fluency, $t(20) = 1.83$, $p<.08$.

Given that there was a significant difference between the two groups in SES, $t(19) = 2.35$, $p<.03$, an ANCOVA controlling for SES was also conducted. The results reported above were retained, with the exception of those for Verbal Fluency perseveration, $F(1,18) = .96$, $p <.34$, and Visual Search inefficiency, $F(1,18) = 2.31$, $p<.15$. Most importantly, both the significant group difference on the EF composite, $F(1,18) = 6.47$, $p<.02$, and the lack of difference on Picture Recognition, $F(1,18) = 0$, $p<.97$, were maintained.

In view of the relatively small sample sizes, it was important to evaluate whether the group differences reflected very poor performance of only one or two PKU children. For those measures in which significant or marginally significant group differences were found, the following percentages of the PKU group scored below the control group mean: EF Composite (73%, 8/11), Motor Planning (82%, 9/11), Verbal Fluency efficiency (91%, 10/11), Verbal Fluency perseveration (64%, 7/11), Tower of Hanoi (82%, 9/11), and Visual Search inefficiency (91%, 10/11). In addition, nonparametric Sign Tests were conducted to evaluate the significance of the number of differences across age-matched pairs of PKU and control subjects. Sign tests were significant for the EF composite ($p<.03$), Verbal Fluency efficiency ($p<.006$), Tower of Hanoi ($p<.03$), and Visual Search inefficiency ($p<.03$); they were marginally significant for Motor Planning ($p<.09$) and Verbal Fluency perseveration ($p<.11$).

Thus, despite the small sample sizes utilized in this study, very clear and consistent differences in executive functions were found in the PKU children relative to controls of similar age, IQ, and sex.

Qualitative differences. To provide a clearer picture of the performance differences between the groups, we analyzed qualitative aspects of performance on the Tower of Hanoi, a task that is amenable to such an analysis and that revealed large group differences. The three-move problems as chosen for analysis because it was of intermediate difficulty and required employment of a relatively counterintuitive strategy (rings first had to be moved away from the goal state before being moved back toward it). The three-move problem was easy enough to be attempted by a majority (73%) of the PKU subjects; three PKU subjects were unable to reach criterion on the simpler two-move problem and testing was discontinued before administering the three-move problem.

We first asked if PKU subjects committed more rule violations than controls, which would suggest that, despite adequate performance on the practice trials, they had understood the rules less well than controls. However, there were no group differences in the frequency of rule violations. After eliminating this possibility, we next analyzed the efficiency of the two groups in solving the three-move problem. First, more controls (11/11) attempted the three-move problem than PKU subjects (8/11). Also, more controls (11/11 or 100%) solved the problem correctly twice in a row than did PKU children (3/8 or 38%), $\chi^2(1, N = 19) = 7.04, p<.01$. An additional two PKU children solved the three-move problem correctly once but not twice in a row; still, however, the proportion of the PKU group solving the problem at least once (5/8 or 63%) was significantly lower than controls (11/11 or 100%), $\chi^2(1, N = 19) = 4.71, p<.05$. Moreover, more than half (6/11 or 55%) of the PKU group failed the three-move problem, while none of the controls did. In fact, all but one of the controls also solved problems of four moves or more.

So it is not simply that the PKU children were less efficient at solving these problems. Rather, it appeared that they had difficulty planning moves in advance, as indicated by the commission of what we call "the typical first move error." This error occurs when a ring is moved directly toward the goal, when the correct move requires that the subjects first move the ring (counterintuitively) away from the goal. In fact, this strategy of moving the ring directly to the goal peg had been correct on the previous two-move problem. Seven of eight PKU subjects (88%) committed the typical first move error, while only two of 11 controls (18%) did so $\chi^2(1, N = 19) = 8.93, p<.01$. Thus, it appears that PKU subjects were "captured" (Shallice, 1982) by the previously established response set and had difficulty engaging in the internal planning necessary to avoid this error. In other words, PKU children tended to perseverate on previously correct problem-solving strategies more than control subjects; this is consistent with their higher rates of perseveration on the Visual Search and Verbal Fluency tasks as well.

CONTRIBUTIONS OF PHE LEVEL TO EXECUTIVE FUNCTIONS

Given that executive function impairments were observed in the PKU group, it was important next to evaluate the contribution of Phe levels and other variables to executive function performance. As seen in Table 3, the EF composite was sig-

TABLE 3
Correlations Among Measures and Between Measures and Phe Levels

Task	FSIQ (N = 22)	PR (N = 22)	CPhe (N = 11)	MPhe (N = 11)	IPhe (N = 10)
FSIQ	...	.30	.02	-.42	-.30
Picture Recognition	.30	...	.14	.39	.49
Partial r	...	...	.09	.69**	.71**
EF composite	.61***	.18	-.54*	-.62*	-.37
Partial r	...	-.01	-.88****	-.51	-.24

NOTE.—Performance measures are correlated with concurrent Phe (CPhe), mean Phe (MPhe), and infant Phe (IPhe). Concurrent Phe reflects Phe level on the day either the IQ test or the experimental measures were administered. The values in the partial r rows are the partial correlations controlling for FSIQ.

* $p < .05$.
** $p < .01$.
*** $p < .001$.
**** $p < .0001$.

nificantly correlated ($p<.001$) with FSIQ, but not with Picture Recognition. Picture Recognition was also not correlated significantly with FSIQ. This pattern of correlations supports the role of Picture Recognition as a discriminant measure. Because of the significant positive correlation between FSIQ and the EF composite, we controlled for FSIQ when examining the relation between Phe levels and EF.

To test our hypothesis regarding Phe level and executive function deficits, we analyzed the relative contributions of the three Phe levels to variability in the EF composite within the PKU group. First, we examined the intercorrelations among the three measures of Phe level. Concurrent Phe level was correlated with neither means Phe $r(9) = .38$, $p<.12$, nor infant Phe, $r(8) = .17$, $p<.32$, levels; however, infant and mean Phe level were significantly correlated with each other, $r(8) = .73$, $p<.01$. Despite this significant association, we felt that infant and mean Phe level provided conceptually distinct information. Therefore, the three Phe levels were kept separate in the analysis of the univariate and partial correlations presented in Table 3.

We found significant associations between the EF composite score and both concurrent, $r(9) = -.54$ $p<.05$, and mean lifetime, $r(9) = -.62$, $p<.05$, Phe levels. When FSIQ was partialed out, the correlation with mean lifetime Phe was only slightly reduced, $r(8) = -.51$, $p<.07$, while the correlation with concurrent Phe increased, $r(8) = -.88$, $p<.0001$. Thus, EF deficits within the PKU group were associated with high Phe levels; these results support our hypothesis regarding the biochemical mechanism underlying EF deficits in PKU. The results also indicate that EF deficits are most strongly related to concurrent Phe levels and hence to potentially reversible neurochemical perturbations.

In contrast, none of the Phe levels was significantly correlated with recognition memory, although these null results may be the result of low statistical power. If reliable, this result once again validates Picture Recognition as a discriminant measure.

The relation between Phe levels and Picture Recognition was also examined. When FSIQ was partialed out, a surprising positive correlation between both mean and infant Phe levels and Picture Recognition emerged, $r(9) = .69$, $p<.02$, and $r(8) = .71$, $p<.02$, respectively. Possible interpretations of this result are considered below. Correlations between individual EF measures and IQ, Picture Recognition and Phe levels can be found in the Appendix.

DISCUSSION

In this early-treated PKU group, we found specific deficits in executive function relative to age- and IQ-matched controls. Moreover, within the PKU group, executive function performance was significantly correlated with concurrent and mean lifetime Phe levels. Thus, the present results provide preliminary support for the prefrontal dysfunction hypothesis of PKU outlined in the introduction. Since executive function performance was related to both concurrent and mean lifetime Phe levels, it appears that the biochemical anomaly of PKU has both transient and long-lasting effects on executive functions. In this discussion, we first consider interpretive issues, then implications for research and clinical work with PKU, and finally broader implications for research in cognitive development.

Interpretive issues. Several interpretive issues will be considered in this section, including the relation of the present results to previous studies, neuropsychological interpretation of results, possible confounds in the present study, and interpretation of the pattern of correlations among Phe levels, EF, recognition memory, and IQ. In view of the small sample sizes in this study, however, it is important that we consider the present results exploratory and await results of future replication studies.

The present results are consistent with those of previous studies (Krause et al., 1985; Lou et al., 1985; Pennington et al., 1985) finding EF deficits in early-treated PKU individuals. Moreover a recent French study of children with PKU (Sonneville, Schmidt, & Michel, 1989) found deficits in sustained attention and visual search that were correlated with concurrent Phe levels.

Regarding neuropsychological interpretation, the overall pattern of cognitive impairment found in this study parallels that found in frontal-damaged adults (Luria, 1973; Milner, 1964; Shallice, 1982; Stuss & Benson, 1984). However it is an empirical question whether perseverative behavior and impairments in planning and organized search indicate prefrontal dysfunction in *children*. Also, there is not yet independent neurological validation that these executive function tasks are selectively sensitive to prefrontal functioning in preschool children. Thus, our assumption that these executive function tasks are indeed prefrontal measures in this age range must be considered tentative. Second, we do not know if the PKU subjects had *specific* deficits in executive functions. To truly assess specificity, a more comprehensive test battery must be used, one that includes additional measures of nonexecutive function abilities, such as language and memory. Such a study is currently being conducted in our laboratory to explore whether previously undetected nonexecutive function impairments are present in early-treated PKU children.

A possible confound in the present study is the SES difference between the two groups. However, group differences in EF skills were generally maintained when SES was covaried out. Moreover, the significant correlation between EF performance and concurrent Phe level within the PKU group was maintained after covarying out SES, $r(8) = .57$, $p < .04$. Since concurrent Phe levels of the two groups differed, it is a likely explanation for the group difference in EF. Nonetheless, future studies should match on SES, as well as on IQ and sex.

A second potential confound is ascertainment bias. It is possible that PKU children with more cognitive problems were included in the study. Then our results might not accurately represent the prevalence of EF problems in the general population of children with PKU. At the extreme ascertainment bias could provide an artifactual basis for group differences. Ascertainment bias was a problem in an earlier study by Pennington et al. (1985), which found perseverative behavior on the Wisconsin Card Sorting Test in an older PKU sample referred to a clinic for learning and/or behavior problems. Such ascertainment bias did not exist in the current study, however; the preschool-age subjects were not selected because they had experienced problems. Since the results of the two studies were generally convergent, ascertainment bias also appears to be an unlikely explanation of earlier results (Pennington et al., 1985). Taken together, the two studies indicate EF problems in both preschool and school-age PKU children. An intriguing question to explore longitudinally is whether early-treated PKU preschoolers with elevated Phe levels and executive function deficits are more likely to exhibit learning and behavior difficulties later in life.

Another interpretive issue concerns the different relations found among Phe levels and EF, IQ, and recognition memory. In this study, all PKU subjects had IQ scores in the normal range; neither infant, mean, nor concurrent Phe level was significantly correlated with intelligence. The lack of correlation between both infant and concurrent Phe levels and IQ is not surprising, since IQ measures skills and knowledge accumulated across the lifespan and thus should be relatively insensitive to transient neurochemical states. Given this logic, however, we might expect a significant correlation between mean lifetime Phe and IQ. Although that correlation only approached significance in the current small sample, it was larger than the correlations between IQ and the two other Phe level measures. In contrast, concurrent Phe level was more strongly associated with performance on the EF composite, suggesting that these measures are more sensitive than IQ to concurrent neurochemical perturbations.

One quite unexpected result concerns the emergence of *positive* correlations between Picture Recognition and both mean lifetime and infant Phe levels. The memory task was selected as a discriminant measure, and the nonsignificant correlations between Picture Recognition and the majority of executive function tasks support this selection. Thus, a nonsignificant correlation between Picture Recognition and Phe level was predicted; indeed, this was true of concurrent Phe. However, the partial correlation analysis demonstrated that high mean and infant Phe levels were associated with *better* scores on the memory task. It appears that partialing out the weak, negative correlation between Phe and IQ strengthened the previously nonsignificant positive correlations between these two Phe levels and recognition memory. These results may reflect the spurious effects that can emerge when sample size is small and power is limited. Consequently, this result must await replication on a larger sample of children and further testing with a broad range of memory measures. If it is a reliable result, one possible explanation is compensatory development of cognitive skills that lie outside the range of the primary deficit. A similar process is thought to underlie the "splinter skills" observed in other developmental disabled populations. At the very least, this result suggests that recognition memory operates differently from executive functions, which were adversely affected by high Phe level.

Implications for PKU. These results have several implications for research and clinical work with PKU individuals. First, these findings are important because they call into question the use of standardized intelligence measures as the sole, or primary, method of assessing the early-treated PKU child's cognitive functioning (Woolfe, 1979). They suggest that EF measures, which require planning and ability to flexibly shift set, may be more sensitive indicators of cognitive development in children with PKU. The perseverative behavior exhibited by these children may be analogous to the perseveration seen on the Wisconsin Card Sorting Test (WCST) in a sample of older early-treated PKU children (Pennington et al., 1985). The WCST is the most widely accepted neuropsychological measure of prefrontal function in adults, but is not appropriate for use with preschoolers.

In the present study, the early-treated PKU children were poor planners on the Tower of Hanoi and were less likely to flexibly modify unsuccessful strategies from trial to trial. For example, the majority of the PKU sample (73%) could not solve problems beyond the two-move level, while the vast majority of the control children (91%) could solve problems of four moves or more. Failure on the three-move problem, described above, has implications for the "depth of search" (Borys et al., 1982) or "look-ahead" skills of these children. That is, the three-move problem demanded that subjects plan one move *in advance of action* to successfully solve the problem. All of the control children could engage in this internal planning, but only three of 11 PKU children could. In addition, the unsuccessful PKU children (all of whom were older than 4) committed a first-move error that is characteristic of developmental normal 3-year-olds (Welsh, in press); this error seems to reflect difficulty inhibiting prepotent, but incorrect, moves directly toward the goal. Thus, it appears that PKU preschoolers have difficulty guiding and inhibiting behavioral responses in accordance with covert or internal plans. In future research, it will be important to evaluate how early in development such problems are manifest in children with PKU. Detecting deficits in infancy may aid clinical management of and cognitive intervention with these children.

Since EF deficits are most strongly correlated with concurrent Phe level, it is possible that EF impairment is reversible. An important clinical implication of the current research is that dietary compliance or direct biochemical intervention might improve EF performance in these children.

Finally, it is important to note that there was variability in EF performance within the PKU group; thus, EF problems are not an inevitable consequence of the disorder. Variation in performance among PKU children suggests that the disorder may be an ideal one in which to study risk and protective mechanisms in the development of EF impairment.

Implications for cognitive development research. The present data are relevant to research on cognitive development, both in other clinical groups and in normal children. For example, we expect analogous patterns of performance in other clinical groups suspected of executive dysfunction; conversely, we expect normal performance in clinical groups not suspected of such problems. Preliminary data from our laboratory support this dissociation. We have found that children from 5 to 9 years of age, referred for attentional deficits, exhibit selective impairments on the Tower of Hanoi, Verbal Fluency, and Visual Search tasks when compared with an age- and IQ-matched clinical control group referred for speech and language difficulties (Welsh, Wall, & Towle, 1989).

The current study also has several implications for research on normal cognitive development. First, it provides another way of thinking about domains of cognition of particular interest to developmentalists, namely, metacognition and future-oriented behavior. Much of what is studied in these areas can be classified as executive functions, as we have defined them in this article.

Second, to the extent that this identification is correct, the present study also has implications for the disociability of metacognition and future-oriented behavior from other cognitive domains. The results of the present study provide evidence that executive functions are dissociable from one other cognitive skill, recognition memory, and, to a certain extent, from IQ (since separate variance in executive function was accounted for by Phe, apart from IQ). Therefore the present study provides preliminary information about the neurobiological mechanisms underlying executive and other cognitive functions in early childhood. For example, the strong relation found between concurrent Phe level and executive function suggests that EF is particularly influenced by the individual's current neurochemical state, while neither recognition memory nor IQ appear to be so state-dependent.

Third, this research has implications for theories of intelligence and how it develops. In the history of psychology, there is a long tradition of distinguishing cognitive tasks that require novel problem solving from those that rely more heavily on memory. Wertheimer's (1945) distinction between productive (insightful) and reproductive (memory based) thinking, Hebbs's distinction between A and B type intelligence, Horn's (1985) distinction between fluid and crystallized intelligence, and Sternberg's (1982) distinction between routine and nonroutine problem solving all come to mind. Thus, it is important to investigate whether executive functions are the same as or similar to what psychometricians call fluid intelligence. In any case, the present results show that clinical data provide important constraints for validating theories of intelligence, as well as demonstrating how integration across the different research traditions of clinical neuropsychology and developmental psychology might occur.

APPENDIX

TABLE A1
Correlations Between Individuals EF Measures and IQ, Recognition Memory, and Phe Levels

Task	FSIQ ($N = 22$)	PR ($N = 22$)	CPhe ($N = 11$)	MPhe ($N = 11$)	IPhe ($N = 10$)
Motor	.34	.39*	−.13(−.21)	.01(.21)	.32(.51)
Verbal Fluency (VF)	.59**	.24	.19(.15)	−.38(−.07)	−.22(.05)
VF perseveration[a]	−.48**	−.04	.52*(.82**)	.70**(.60*)	.53*(.46)
Tower of Hanoi	.17	−.15	−.46(−.49)	−.06(−.01)	−.46(−.44)
Visual Search (VS)[a]	−.48**	−.06	.63*(.81**)	.68**(.59*)	.28(.16)
VS perseveration[a]	−.61**	−.03	.47(.65*)	.56*(.43)	.43(.34)

NOTE.—Performance measures are correlated with concurrent Phe (CPhe), mean Phe (MPhe), and infant Phe (IPhe). Concurrent Phe reflects Phe level on the day either the IQ test or the experimental measures were administered. In light of the small sample sizes in the EF-Phe correlations, nonparametric Spearman rank-order correlations were tested and confirmed five of the six significant associations. Values in parentheses are partial correlations controlling for FSIQ. Since the IQ scores of two PKU subjects were obtained from a different test than the majority of the sample, the partial correlation analysis was repeated with a reduced sample ($n = 9$), all of whom had been given the same IQ test (WPPSI). This small sample size reduces the statistical power of such an analysis and increases the risk of Type I error. Nevertheless, of five significant correlations in the original analysis above, the three correlations with concurrent Phe level were maintained in the same direction and at an acceptable level of significance in this subsequent analysis. Finally, all the analyses in the table above were repeated separating the data of the PKU and control groups; all the significant effects were maintained.
[a] Higher score reflects poorer performance.
* $p < .05$.
** $p < .01$.

REFERENCES

Arnsten, A.F.T., & Goldman-Rakic, P.S. (1985). Alpha-adrenergic mechanisms in prefrontal cortex associated with cognitive decline in aged nonhuman primates. *Science*, **230**, 1273–1276.

Benson, P.F., & Fensom, A.H. (1985). *Genetic biochemical disorders.* Oxford: Oxford University Press.

Berry, H.K., O'Grady, D.J., Perlmutter, L.J., & Bofinger, M.K. (1979). Intellectual development and academic achievement of children treated early for phenylketonuria. *Developmental Medicine and Child Neurology*, **21**, 311–320.

Bickel, H., Gerrard, J., & Hickmans, E.M. (1954). The influence of phenylalanine intake on the chemistry and behavior of a phenylketonuric child. *Acta Paediatrica*, **43**, 64–77.

Borys, S.V., Spitz, H.H., & Dorans, B.A. (1982). Tower of Hanoi performance of retarded young adults and nonretarded children as function of solution length and goal state. *Journal of Experimental Child Psychology*, **33**, 87–110.

Brown, A.L., & DeLoache, J.S. (1978). Skills, plans, and self-regulation. In R.S. Siegler (Ed.), *Children's thinking? What develops?* (pp. 3–35). Hillsdale, NJ: Erlbaum.

Brown, A.L., & Scott, S.S. (1971). Recognition memory for pictures in preschool children. *Journal of Experimental Child Psychology*, **11**, 401–412.

Brozoski, T., Brown, R.M., Rosvold, H.E., & Goldman, P.S. (1979). Cognitive deficit caused by regional depletion of dopamine in prefrontal cortex of rhesus monkey. *Science*, **205**, 929–932.

Brunner, R.L., Jordan, M.K., & Berry, H.K. (1983). Early-treated PKU: Neuropsychologic consequences. *Journal of Pediatrics*, **102**, 831–835.

Butler, I.J., O'Flynn, M.E., Seifert, W.E., & Howell, R.R. (1981). Neurotransmitter defects and treatment of disorders of hyperphenylalaninemia. *Journal of Pediatrics*, **98**(5), 729–733.

Cabalska, B., Durzynska, N., Borzymonwska, J., Zorska, K., Kaslacz-Folga, A., & Bozkowa, K. (1977). Termination of dietary treatment in phenylketonuria. *European Journal of Pediatrics*, **126**, 253–262.

Chamove, A.S., & Molinaro, T.J. (1978). Monkey retarded learning analysis. *Journal of Mental Deficiency Research*, **22**, 223.

Choo, K.H., Cotton, R.G.H., Jennings, I.G., & Danks, D.M. (1979). Observations indicating the nature of the mutation in phenylketonuria. *Journal of Inherited Metabolic Disease*, **2**, 79–84.

Cooper, J.R., Bloom, F.E., & Roth, R.H. (1982).*The biochemical basis of neuropharmacology* (4th ed.). New York: Oxford University Press.

Crowis, V.A. (1971). Neurological and psychiatric aspects of phenylketonuria. In H. Bickell, F. Hudson, & L. Woolf (Eds.), *Phenylketonuria and some other inborn errors of amino acid metabolism* (pp. 29–39). Stuttgart: Verlag.

Curtius, H.C., Baerlocher, K., & Vollmin, J.A. (1972). Pathogenesis of Phenylketonuria: Inhibition of dopa and catecholamine synthesis in patients with phenylketonuria. *Clinica Chemica Acta*, **42**, 235–239.

Curtius, H.C., Vollmin, J.A., & Baerlocher, K. (1972). The use of deuterated phenylalanine for the elucidation of the pheynlalanine-tyrosine metabolism. *Clinica Chemica Acta*, **37**, 277–285.

DiLella, A.G., Marvit, J., Lidsky, A.S., Guttler, F., & Woo, S.L.C. (1986). Tight linkage between a splicing mutation and a specific DNA haplotype in phenylketonuria. *Nature*, **322**, 799–803.

Divac, I., Bjorklund, A., Lindvall, O., & Passingham, R. (1978). Converging projections from the mediodorsal thalamic nucleus and mesencephalic dopaminergic neurons to the neocortex in three species. *Journal of Comparative Neurology*, **180**, 59–72.

Dobson, J.C., Williamson, M.L., Azen, C., & Koch, R. (1977). Intellectual assessment of 111 four-year-old children with phenylketonuria. *Pediatrics*, **60**, 822–827.

Douglas, V.I. (1983). Attention and cognitive problems. In M. Rutter (Ed.), *Developmental neuropsychiatry*, (pp. 280–329). New York: Guilford.

Fuller, R. & Shulman, J. (1971). Treated phenylketonuria: Intelligence and blood phenylalanine levels. *American Journal of Mental Deficiency*, **75**, 539–545.

Fuster, J.M. (1980). *The prefrontal cortex*. New York: Raven.

Fuster, J.M. (1985). The prefrontal cortex, mediator of cross-temporal contingencies. *Human Neurobiology,* **4,** 169–179.

Golden, C.J. (1981). A standardized version of Luria's neuropsychological tests. In S. Filskov & T.J. Boll (Eds.), *Handbook of Clinical Neuropsychology* (pp. 608–642). New York: Wiley-Interscience.

Griffin, F.D., Clarke, J.T.R. & d'Entremont, D.M. (1980). Effect of dietary phenylalanine restriction on visual attention span in mentally retarded subjects with phenylketonuria. *Journal Canadien des Sciences Neurologiques,* **128,** 127–131.

Guthrie, R.E., & Susi, A. (1963). A simple phenylalanine method for detecting phenylketonuria in large populations of newborn infants. *Pediatrics,* **32,** 338–343.

Guttler, F., & Lou, H. (1986). Dietary problems of phenylketonuria: Effect on CNS transmitters and their possible role in behavior and neuropsychological function. *Journal of Inherited Metabolic Disease,* **9**(Suppl. 2), 169–177.

Hollingshead, A.B. (1976). *Four-Factor Index of Social Status.* New Haven, CT: Yale University Press.

Holtzman, N.A., Kronmal, R.A., van Doornick, W., Azen, C., & Koch, R. (1986). Effect of age at loss of dietary control on intellectual performance and behavior of children with phenylketonuria. *New England Journal of Medicine,* **34,** 593–598.

Koff, E., Boyle, P., & Pueschel, S.M. (1977). Perceptual-motor functioning in children with phenylketonuria. *American Journal of Disorders of Children,* **313,** 1084–1087.

Kolb, B., & Whishaw, I.Q. (1985). *Fundamentals of human neuropsychology* (2nd ed.). New York: Freeman.

Krause, W.L., Epstein, C., Averbrook, A., Dembure, P., & Elsas, L. (1986). Phenylalanine alters the mean power frequency of electroencephalograms and plasma L-dopa in treated patients with phenylketonuria. *Pediatric Research,* **220,** 1112–1116.

Krause, W.L., Halminski, M., McDonald, L., Dembure, P., Salvo, R., Freides, D., & Elsas, L.J. (1985). Biochemical and neuropsychological effects of elevated plasma phenylalanine in patients with treated phenylketonuria: A model for the study of phenylalanine and brain function in man. *Journal of Clinical Investigation,* **75,** 40–48.

Levy, H.L. (1973). Genetic screening. *Advance in Human Genetics,* **4,** 1–104.

Lou, H.C., Guttler, G., Lykelund, C., Bruhn, P., & Niederwieser, A. (1985). Decreased vigilance and neurotransmitter synthesis after discontinuation of dietary treatment of phenylketonuria in adolescents. *European Journal of Pediatrics,* **144,** 17–20.

Luria, A.R. (1966). *Higher cortical functions in man.* London: Tavistock.

Luria, A.R. (1973). *The working brain.* New York: Basic.

MacLeod, M.D., Munro, J.F., Ledingham, J.G. & Farquhar, J.W. (1983). Management of extra pyramidal manifestations of phenylketonuria with L-dopa. *Archives of Diseases of Childhood,* **58,** 457–466.

Margolin, D., Pohl, R.E., Stewart, R.M., Touchette, P.E., Townsend, N.M., & Kolodny, E.H. (1978). Effects of diet and behavior therapy on social and motor behavior of retarded phenylketonuric adults: An experimental analysis. *Pediatric Research,* **12,** 179–187.

McCarthy, D.A. (1972). *Manual for the McCarthy Scales for Children's Abilities.* New York: Psychological Corp.

McKean, C.M. (1971). Effect of totally synthetic low phenylalanine diet on adolescent phenylketonuric patients. *Archives of Diseases in Childhood, 46,* 606–615.

McKean, C.M. (1972). The effects of high phenylalanine concentrations on serotonin and catecholamine metabolism in the human brain. *Brain Research, 47,* 469–476.

Melnick, C.K., Kimberlee, M.A., Michals, K., & Matalon, K. (1981). Linguistic development of children with phenylketonuria and normal intelligence. *Journal of Pediatrics, 98,* 269–272.

Milner, B. (1964). Some effects of frontal lobectomy in man. In J.M. Warren & K. Akert (Eds.), *The frontal granular cortex and behavior* (pp. 313–334). New York: McGraw-Hill.

Netley, C., Hanley, W.B., & Rudner, H.L. (1984). Phenylketonuria and its variants: Observations on intellectual functioning. *Canadian Medical Association Journal, 131,* 751–755.

O'Grady, D.J., Berry, H.K., & Sutherland, B.S. (1971). Cognitive development in early-treated phenylketonuria. *American Journal of Mental Association Journal, 131,* 751–755.

Paine, R.S. (1957). The variability in manifestations of untreated patients with phenylketonuria (phenylpyruvic aciduria). *Pediatrics, 20,* 290–302.

Pennington, B.F., van Doorninck, W.J., McCabe, L.L., & McCabe, E.R.B. (1985). Neurological deficits in early-treated phenylketonurics. *American Journal of Mental Deficiency, 89,* 467–474.

Pollack, M. (1960). Effects of brain tumor on perception of hidden figures, sorting behavior and problem solving performances. *Dissertation Abstracts, 20,* 3405–3406.

Porrino, L.J., & Goldman-Rakic, P.S. (1982). Brain stem innervation of prefrontal and anterior cingulate cortex in the rhesus monkey revealed by retrograde transport of HRP. *Journal of Comparative Neurology, 205,* 63–76.

Pratt, O.E. (1980). A new approach to the treatment of phenylketonuria. *Journal of Mental Deficiency Research, 24,* 203–217.

Primrose, D.A. (1983). Phenylketonuria with normal intelligence. *Journal of Mental Deficiency Research, 27,* 239–246.

Saint-Cyr, J.A., Taylor, A.E., & Lang, A.E. (1988). Procedural learning and neostriatal dysfunction in man. *Brain, 111,* 941–959.

Sandler, M. (1982). Inborn errors and disturbances of central neurotransmission (with special reference to phenylketonuria). *Journal of Inherited Metabolic Disease, 5* (Suppl.2) 65–70.

Seashore, M., Friedman, E., & Norelly, R. (1979). Loss of intellectual function in children with PKU. *American Journal of Human Genetics, 31,* 62A.

Shallice, T. (1982). Specific impairments of planning. *Philosophical Transactions of the Royal Society of London Bulletin, 298,* 199–209.

Simon, H.A. (1975). The functional equivalence of problem solving skills. *Cognitive Psychology, 7,* 268–288.

Sonneville, L.M.J. De, Schmidt, E., & Michel, U. (1989). Information processing in early-treated PKU. *Journal of Clinical and Experimental Neuropsychology,* **11,** 362.

Spreen, O., Tupper, D., Risser, A., Tuokko, H., & Edgell, D. (1984). *Human developmental neuropsychology.* New York: Oxford University Press.

Sternberg, R.J. (1982). A componential approach to intellectual development. In R.J. Sternbrg (Ed.), *Advances in the psychology of human intelligence* (Vol. **1,** pp. 413–463). Hillsdale, NJ: Erlbaum.

Stuss, D.T., & Benson, F. (1984). Neuropsychological studies of the frontal lobes. *Psychological Bulletin,* **95,** 3–28.

Stuss, D.T., & Benson, F. (1987). The frontal lobes and control of cognition and memory. In E. Perceman (Ed.), *The frontal lobes revisited* (pp. 141–158). New York: IRBN.

Taylor, A.E., Saint-Cyr, J.A. & Lang, A.E. (1986). Frontal lobe dysfunction in Parkinson's disease: The cortical focus on neostriatal outflow. *Brain,* **109,** 845–883.

Teuber, H.L., Battersby, W.S., & Bender, M.B. (1955). Changes in visual searching performance following cerebral lesions. *American Journal of Physiology,* **159,** 592.

Veale, A.M.O. (1980). Screening for phenylketonuria. In H. Bickel, R. Guthrie, & G. H. Jammerson (Eds.), *Neonatal screening for inborn errors of metabolism* (pp. 7–18). Berlin: Springer.

Waisbren, S.E., Mahon, B.E., Schnell, R.R., & Levy, H.L. (1987). Predictors of intelligence quotient and intelligence quotient change in persons treated for phenylketonuria early in life. *Pediatrics,* **79,** 351–355.

Warrington, E.K., James, M., & Maciejewski, C. (1986). The WAIS as a lateralizing and localizing diagnostic instrument: A study of 656 patients with unilateral lesions. *Neuropsychologia,* **24,** 223–239.

Weinberger, D.R., Berman, K.F., & Chase, T.N. (1987). Prefrontal CBF during specific cognitive activation: Studies of Huntington's and Parkinson's diseases. *Journal of Clinical and Experimental Neuropsychology,* **9,** 47.

Weinstein, S., & Teubr, H.L. (1957). Effects of penetrating brain injury on intelligence test scores. *Science,* **125,** 1036–1037.

Welsh, M.C.(in press). Rule-guided behavior and self-monitoring on the Tower of Hanoi disk-transfer task. *Cognitive Development.*

Welsh, M.C., & Pennington, B.F. (1988). Assessing frontal lobe function in children: Views from developmental psychology. *Developmental Neuropsychology,* **4,** 199–230.

Welsh, M.C., Pennington, B.F., & Groisser, D.B. (in press). A normative-developmental study of executive function: A window on prefrontal function in children. *Developmental Neuropsychology.*

Welsh, M.C., Wall, B.M., & Towle, P.O. (1989, April). *Executive function in children with attention deficit: Implications for a prefrontal hypothesis.* Paper presented at the biennial meeting of the Society for Research in Child Development, Kansas City, MO.

Wertheimer, M. (1945). *Productive thinking.* New York: Harper & Row.

Williamson, M.L., Dobson, J.C., & Koch, R. (1977). Collaborative study of children trated for phenylketonuria: Study design. *Pediatrics,* **60,** 815–821.

Williamson, M.L., Koch, R., Azen, C., & Chang, C. (1981). Correlates of intelligence test results in treated phenylketonuric children. *Pediatrics*, **68**, 161–167.

Woo, S.L.C., DiLella, A.G., Marvit, J., Ledley, F.D. (1986). Molecular basis of phenylketonuria and potential somatic gene therapy. *Cold Spring Harbor Symposia on Quantitative Biology*, **51**, 395–401.

Woo, S.L.C., Lidsky, A.S., Guttler, F., Chandra, T., & Robson, K.J.H. (1983). Cloned human phenylalanine hydroxylase gene allows prenatal diagnosis and carrier detection of classical phenylketonuria. *Nature*, **306**, 151–155.

Woolfe, L.I. (1979). Late onset phenylalanine intoxication. *Journal of Inherited Metabolic Disease*, **2**, 19–20.

25

Treatment of Attentional and Hyperactivity Problems in Children with Sympathomimetic Drugs: A Comprehensive Review

Deborah Jacobvitz
University of Texas, Austin

L. Alan Sroufe
University of Minnesota

Mark Stewart
University of Iowa

Nancy Leffert
University of Minnesota

Issues concerning sympathomimetic drug treatment of children with attentional problems and hyperactivity are considered in light of cumulative and current research. These issues concern the atypical or "paradoxical" drug response of such children, predictability of drug response from neurological or biochemical assessments, and, especially, long-term outcome or effectiveness of sympathomimetic medication. Short-term drug effects on behavior and performance are well documented. However, follow-up studies that exist presently suggest little long-term impact of sympathomimetic drugs on school achievement, peer relationships, or behavior problems in adolescence. Questions remain concerning development of tolerance in children, ways to define subgroups of disordered children who may respond uniquely to stimulants, the effi-

Reprinted with permission from *Journal of the American Academy of Child and Adolescent Psychiatry,* 1990, vol. 29, No. 5, 677–688. copyright © 1990 by The American Academy of Child and Adolescent Psychiatry.

The writing of this paper was supported in part by the National Institute of Mental Health (MH-40864-04) *cacy of medication in combination with other treatments, and possible long-term negative consequences of medication.*

The practice of treating children with stimulant drugs (primarily methylphenidate) is widespread and apparently increasing. For example, a recent survey in Baltimore County revealed that by 1987 5.96% of all public elementary school students (approximately 10% of all males) were receiving stimulant medication (Safer and Krager, 1988). The rate of medication has doubled every 2 to 4 years since 1971. This study also showed the rate currently to be increasing disproportionately in females and in secondary school populations, two very recent trends. Proposals have been made to extend treatment deliberately into the adolescent period and beyond (Wender, 1987). In light of the continued use of stimulant medication with hundreds of thousands of children, it seems prudent to review the current status of research concerning the effected of stimulants on children. Data now exist on issues for which there was no information 10 or 15 years ago (Sroufe and Stewart, 1973), and numerous studies exist on issues where once there was only scant information. It is time for a comprehensive review.

Major questions that have persisted over time are the following:

1. Are the effects of stimulant medications with hyperactive children (now called children with attention deficit/hyperactivity disorder) (ADHD) atypical or "paradoxical"; that is, do stimulants affect these children uniquely? Until recently, there were no direct data on this question, though numerous studies with normal adults have suggested that the responses of hyperactive children were quite usual (Sroufe and Stewart, 1973).

2. Is there a relationship between specifiable neurological or biochemical abnormality and ADHD, and is drug response predictable from such markers? This literature has been plagued by inconsistency.

3. Do the demonstrable short-term effects of stimulant medications persist? Is enhanced attention still in evidence after several months of treatment? Are there long-term gains in school achievement and social behavior? Is there carry-over of positive effects following termination of treatment? Are there long-term negative consequences of prolonged stimulant medication? There were virtually no data on these questions 15 years ago. This issue is critical.

A related question of current interest concerns differential diagnosis, especially the problem of distinguishing ADHD from learning disabilities and conduct disorders. This issue also will be addressed.

Before examining current data on these questions, the authors will begin by briefly reviewing the overwhelming evidence for the short-term impact of stimulants on attention and behavior. These dramatic, incontrovertible effects underlie the widespread use of stimulant medication. After all, there is pressing need to address the problems of children with attentional and activity problems.

SHORT-TERM EFFECTS

Over the past 25 years, there have been hundreds of controlled studies demonstrating the short-term efficacy of stimulant drugs. These studies have been reviewed frequently, (Sroufe, 1975; Kline et al., 1980; Barkley, 1981; Ross and Ross, 1982; Solanto, 1984) and will be summarized only briefly.

Ratings by parents and professionals reveal improved behavior and performance following stimulant drug treatment. Task irrelevant activity, such as fidgetiness, finger tapping, and fine motor movement, declines, classroom disturbance lessens, and attention is enhanced, all in comparison to placebo treated control groups.

Significant drug-placebo differences also have been reported on an array of prolonged, routinized laboratory tasks. Especially after many trials on repetitive reaction time tasks, medicated hyperactive children show shorter response latency and improved performance (Rapport et al., 1982). Errors of omission and errors of commission decline on vigilance tasks and performance improves on perceptual search tasks, including matching familiar figures and maze tracing. Stimulant drugs also facilitate performance on certain subscales of standard intelligence tests.

Researchers now are examining stimulant drug effects on children in settings other than laboratory situations. Researchers observing the effects of stimulants on classroom behavior find improvements on arithmetic and graphing tasks and enhanced attention (Whalen et al., 1978). There are also reductions in gross and minor motor movements, noncompliance, interferences, and overall hyperactivity (Abikoff and Gittelman, 1985a). Taken together, these short-term effects of stimulants for ADHD children are impressive.

Though stimulants improve the ability to sustain attention, there is little evidence that stimulants enhance retention, retrieval and re-learning of material, or the control of anger. In numerous studies, hyperactive children, following stimulant treatment, failed to show improvement in achievement (Gittelman-Klein and Klein, 1976; Rie et al., 1976a,b). Based on Cunningham and Barkley's (1978) review of 17 such studies using 55 independent measures of academic achievement, Barkley (1981) concluded that "these drugs have almost no effect on scholastic achievement (p. 197).

There are various explanations for poor outcomes with achievement in the face of positive short-term outcomes on behavior. Douglas et al. (1986) suggest that methodological and conceptual weaknesses may have led to these conclusions. For example, most academic achievement tests do not contain enough items at appropriate levels of complexity to detect short-term changes, and few investigators have carefully matched forms of tests for repeated testing.

Alternatively, Sprague and Sleator (1977) offer an explanation based on differential dose response curves, with the dose of stimulants used to effect targeted behavior difficulties so high that they inhibit the child's ability to learn. This matter is unresolved. More recent studies (Douglas et al., 1986, 1988) suggest that even low doses (e.g., 0.15 to 0.3 mg/kg) lead to behavioral improvement. However, in contrast to behavioral changes that show improvements up to 0.6 mg/kg or even 1.0 mg/kg, there does appear to be a leveling off, if not a decline, in effectiveness on cognitive performance (arithmetic tasks, paired associate learning) at moderate dosages (e.g., 0.6 mg/kg). Dosages higher than 0.6 mg/kg may be ill-advised if the goal is improved cognitive task performance.

Over the past decade, stimulant drug effects on hyperactive children's relationships with mothers and teachers also have been examined. Drug treatment appears to increase child compliance and decrease maternal (Humphries et al., 1978; Tallmadge and Barkley, 1983; Barkley et al., 1985; Barkley, 1989) and teacher control (Whalen et al., 1980, 1981), though, generally, such differences appear only during structured tasks and not free play (Barkley, 1989). Although these studies used sequential analysis, it remains unclear whether the child's compliance elicits or is a consequence of less controlling behavior. Still, changes in adult behavior are important short-term outcomes.

ATYPICAL DRUG RESPONSE

A positive stimulant response by ADHD children has been used as evidence of central neurophysiological disturbance (Shaywitz et al., 1978). One assumption of this model is that reductions in task irrelevant activity in structured classroom settings and improved performance on repetitive tasks following medication distinguish those who suffer from ADHD from other children and adults (Wender, 1971).

The accumulated literature clearly refutes the notion of an atypical stimulant response of ADHD children. First, substantial work with adult military personnel showed that stimulants enhanced concentration and performance, especially in repetitive, routinized situations (Weiss and Laties, 1962; Laties and Weiss, 1967). Second, those few studies of stimulant drug effects using a normal comparison group or clinically referred non-ADHD children show that the response of these groups to stimulants is similar to that of ADHD children. For example Rapoport et al. (1978) conducted a double-blind study administering 0.5 mg/kg body weight of amphetamines to ADHD children, normal children, and normal adults. Despite differences in age and clinical status, all groups responded to amphetamines with reduced activity level and enhanced vigilance and memory performance in a laboratory task situation. Peloquin and Klorman (1986), working with normal children and adults, found methylphenidate to enhance several aspects of psychomotor performance, such as reaction time and vigilance. Werry and Aman (1984) report enhanced reaction time and vigilance following administrations of methylphenidate to ADHD children as well as enuretic non-ADHD controls.

In addition, stimulant effects on ADHD children themselves are not genuinely paradoxical. The children are not "slowed down." While researchers report reductions in activity during tasks performance or in structured classroom situations, these are in part an indirect consequence of enhanced attention and concentration, the effects stimulants have on all populations. Activity level may not be reduced in truly "free field" situations (e.g., on the playground), although the literature is inconsistent here (Ellis et al., 1974; Solanto, 1984; Cunningham et al., 1985). Finally, the increases in heart rate and blood pressure routinely reported argue against a subduing effect.

ATTENTION DEFICIT HYPERACTIVITY DISORDER AND ORGANIC DYSFUNCTION

Although not logically necessitated, an organic basis for ADHD has often served as a rationale for prescribing stimulant drugs. Despite the plethora of research findings over the past 2 decades, the underlying deficits in hyperactivity remain poorly understood, leading to dozens of labels attached to these children (minimal brain dysfunction, hyperkinetic impulse disorder, etc.).

Brain Injury

ADHD was initially traced to brain injury resulting from traumatic events such as illness, injury, and prenatal and perinatal problems (Still, 1902; Ebaugh, 1923). Research, however, has shown that neurological abnormalities have been present in only a small proportion of ADHD children (Werry, 1968; Nichols and Chen, 1981); that pregnancy and delivery complications have contributed little to the prediction of hyperactivity in school children (Nichols and Chen, 1981; Taylor, 1986; Jacobvitz, 1988, unpublished dissertation); and that brain damaged children commonly have shown no overactivity (Rutter et al., 1970). The lack of evidence concerning brain dysfunction in hyperactivity could stem from failure to locate specific sites of the dysfunction; one candidate being the frontal lobe (Lou et al., 1984; Zametkin and Rapoport, 1987; Hamdan-Allen et al., submitted for publication).

ADHD, Arousal, and Biochemical and Neurological Dysfunction

Many researchers now postulate that ADHD children rather than having any specific brain lesion, are underaroused or overaroused in autonomic and central nervous system functioning. The underarousal model (e.g., Zentall and Zentall, 1983) assumes that all organisms have a biologically determined optimal level of stimulation, and behavioral activity serves as a homeostatic regulator. Stimulant drugs have been prescribed for children with ADHD symptoms in order to increase their level of cortical arousal, thereby reducing their need to seek external stimulation. In the overarousal model, one version being a noradrenergic hypothesis, it is assumed that the effects of stimulants are paradoxical, perhaps through competition with norepinephrine at postsynaptic receptor sites (Kornetsky, 1970).

While there is abundant evidence that stimulants affect neurotransmitter functioning, there is little evidence for the underarousal theories of ADHD or overarousal theories that preceded them. Dozens of studies have examined psychophysiological indices of arousal in hyperactive children. Studies comparing heart rate, indices of skin conductance, cortical evoked potentials, and electroencephalograms of ADHD children and normal controls have been inconsistent, usually showing no significant differences. (An alternative possibility to over- or underarousal per se is that ADHD children may suffer from difficulties modulating and regulating arousal to meet situational demands [Douglas and Peters, 1979]. This is a plausible idea. The physiological mechanism underlying such difficulties, however, awaits elaboration).

More promising is research on brain neurophysiological mechanisms that may underlie ADHD. Research has focused on the hypothesis that stimulants affect catecholamines, their metabolism, or their action on receptor sites and that it may be possible to understand the exact nature of this disorder through an understanding of stimulant drug action (Zametkin and Rapport, 1987).

A major area of research has centered on differences between children with ADHD and controls on peripheral measures on CNS neurotransmitter functioning from blood and urine assays. Differences obtained from such studies have been rather uniformly disappointing (Bhagauan et al., 1975; Mikkelson et al., 1981; Shekim et al., 1982, and others). However, such peripheral measures are indirect, imperfect indicators of brain functioning.

Another active area of research has been concerned with the effect of various drugs on neurotransmitter functioning and correlated behavior change in ADHD. Drugs that would specifically interfere with or enhance functioning of particular neurotransmitters have been examined as well as drugs which, like stimulants, affect a broad range of catecholamines (e.g., monoamine oxidase inhibitors). This very complex literature has been summarized by Zametkin and Rapoport (1987) in the following way: (1) specific agents, such as dopamine against (L-dopa) or antagonist (haloperidol etc.) have not yielded impressive results in terms of behavior change; (2) more broadly acting drugs, such as methylphenidate and dextroamphetamine, do have demonstrable affects on catecholamine metabolism and behavior; (3) such changes have been shown in some studies to be correlated; that is, non-behavioral responders do not show change in the catecholamine metabolite (e.g., 3-methoxy-4-hydroxyphenylethyleneglycol [MHPG] under examination while responders do (Shekim et al., 1979; Yu-cun and Yu-feng, 1984), though not always (Brown et al., 1981).

Without proper controls, such research cannot demonstrate that any metabolite/behavioral correlations are unique to ADHD children. Nor can it demonstrate the biogenetic origins of ADHD; that is, whether any anomalous reaction of ADHD children is inherent or is the product of experience with arousal modulation problems over time. There is little information available on the prevalence of biochemical or other organic signs in the general child population and on the rates that such signs are associated with ADHD. Also, while organic deviations may produce ADHD symptoms, it is also possible that ADHD symptoms produce biological abnormalities (Connors, 1977). Experiential factors have been found to produce change in PT (plasma testosterone) hormones in male rhesus monkeys. For example, when low-ranking males were given the opportunity to sexually dominate several females, their PT hormones rose sharply, and when they later returned to a cage with high-ranking males, their PT levels decreased again (Rose et al., 1972). Similarly, levels of neurotransmitters linked with depression have been shown to increase in young monkeys following separation from the mothers (McKinney, 1977). The direction of causality between biochemical factors and behavior does not move in one direction only. Much more research, including longitudinal studies, will be needed to sort out cause-effect relationships.

Still, the authors agree with Zametkin and Rapoport that research on neurotransmitters and recent work with brain imaging has a potential for helping to identify subgroups of ADHD children, perhaps ultimately identifying a subset or subsets of children for whom medication has unique advantages. This important goal remains elusive at present.

PREDICTORS OF DRUG RESPONSE

In response to stimulant medication, the symptoms of at least 25% of the ADHD children either remain unchanged or become worse (Barkley, 1976; Safer and Krager, 1984). Dozens of studies have been conducted to isolate predictors of drug response among ADHD children (Sroufe 1975; Solanto, 1984). Symptom severity, EEG abnormalities, soft signs, ratings of inattention, activity, and tests of memory all have failed to consistently distinguish responders and nonresponders. In fact, Rie et al. (1976b) found that hyperactive children with organic impairments actually responded more poorly to stimulants. The few studies demonstrating organic predictors have either not been replicated or show contradictory results. For example, responders, compared with nonresponders, have shown greater visual and auditory average evoked responses (Satterfield et al., 1972; Buchsbaum and Wender, 1973) but also smaller responses (Prichep et al., 1976). Skin conductance responses can be interpreted as showing underarousal (Satterfield et al., 1972) or overarousal (Zahn et al., 1975). Heart rates of responders have been reported to be slower (Porges et al., 1975) and faster (Barkley and Jackson, 1978). Variations in predrug catecholamine metabolites (e.g., MHPG) do not distinguish stimulant responders and nonresponders, though they do distinguish ADHD children from normal controls (Shekim et al., 1979; Yu-cun and Yu-Feng, 1984).

The difficulty in establishing predictors of drug response may be due to a number of factors. There are serious methodological difficulties, including wide variations in drug response measurements across studies, the confounding of pharmacological effects with who will take the drug, and the lack of reliable methods for determining the psychological and physiological effects of different doses for different children. Nevertheless, it remains the case that there is no biochemical aberration or other market that has been established as specific to ADHD children or which can guide the decision to medicate. This remains an important area for additional research.

LONG-TERM OUTCOME OF DRUG TREATMENT

Researchers and clinicians agree that ADHD is not a passing phase (Weiss and Hechtman, 1986). Rather, problems of these children undergo developmental transformation. Hyperactivity per se is not the critical feature beyond middle childhood. However, some ADHD symptoms, such as impulsiveness and inattentiveness, persist into adolescence and adulthood with associated academic failure (Lambert, 1988; Mannuzza et al., 1988), low self-esteem, and poor peer relations during adolescence (Hoy et al., 1978), although a substantial minority are functioning normally in adulthood, perhaps especially in the work arena (Weiss and Hechtman, 1986). In adolescence, delinquency and antisocial behavior are also reported (Feldman et al., 1979; Satterfield et al., 1982; Weiss, 1983), presumably a continuation of the conduct disorder that is so often associated with ADHD.

Critical questions regarding long-term effects of stimulants drugs can be divided into two areas: (1) do children habituate to the drug, losing beneficial effects; and (2) does mediating ADHD children predict overall long-range behavioral improvement?

Whether children develop a tolerance to stimulant drugs is still not resolved. Although side effects usually disappear after a few weeks, particularly if the dosage is monitored and adjusted, it is still logically possible that positive effects persist. For logistical reasons, however, studies following ADHD children who are taking stimulants, with some notable exceptions, have generally not lasted more than a few weeks or months, so the persistence of positive effects often is not fully investigated. The observation of deteriorating performance on removal from stimulants is not conclusive, because deterioration in performance would be expected if tolerance had developed (a disruptive effect) *or* if the drug were still being effective. To resolve this question, patients would need to be tested regularly (e.g., weekly) for several months.

Most critical is the overall long-term effectiveness of stimulants in treating ADHD children. Developmental psychologists agree that the crucial challenges adolescents face are successful adjustment to school, formation of close friendships, a relative absence of substance abuse, and other problems such as antisocial behavior. The long-term efficacy of stimulant drug treatment will first be evaluated with respect to these criteria.

Academic Performance

Researchers have reported immediate improvement in performance on arithmetic (Whalen et al., 1980; Rapport et al., 1982; Pelham et al. 1985); and spelling (Stephens et al., 1984). Such changes occur too quickly to reflect an actual increase in math and reading achievement and are best interpreted as improved ability to function in the test setting. Here, the authors examine data concerning actual change in achievement scores over time.

To date, there is no evidence that stimulants enhance academic performance. In the 5-year follow-up conducted by Weiss et al. (1975), there were no differences between treated and untreated hyperactive children in the number of grades failed. In addition, lower performance during adolescence on achievement tests such as the Wide-Range Achievement Test, (WRAT) (Riddle and Rapoport, 1976), the spelling subtest on the Stanford Achievement Test (SAT), and the word knowledge subtest on the Metropolitan Achievement Test (MAT)(Hoy et al., 1978) reveal persistent problems in retaining and mastering new materials. Other studies also show that treated ADHD children do not significantly differ from untreated children on achievement tests such as the WRAT (Riddle and Rapoport, 1976; Blouin et al., 1978; Charles and Schain, 1981) and Peabody Individual Achievement Test (PIAT)(Charles and Schain, 1981). These results held up whether stimulant drug treatment lasted 2 years (Riddle and Rapoport, 1976) or 4 years, (Charles and Schain, 1981) and even when positive and poor drug responders were compared (Blouin et al., 1978).

Only one study has examined the scholastic performance of ADHD children followed into young adulthood (16 to 24 years old). Hechtman et al. (1984) compared 20 hyperactive children receiving methylphenidate, 20 untreated hyperactive children, and 20 normal controls. Without regard to medication, hyperactive children attended fewer junior colleges and universities and in high school failed more grades and dropped out more frequently due to poor marks than did normal controls. (Such differences suggest that these measures have adequate reliability and validity.) Medicated hyperactive children, however, did not significantly differ from untreated hyperactive children on any of these variables. Though more studies of school performance are needed, at present there is no evidence that learning, as assessed by school work and achievement tests, is enhanced by stimulant drug treatment. Rather than using global measures of academic performance, such as college enrollment, studies that address particular abilities such as writing or mathematical computation skills might reveal specific stimulant drug effects, but this is yet to be established in long-term outcome studies.

These negative results have been subject to a number of critiques (Douglas et al., 1986; Pelham, 1986). Pelham (1986), for example, raises questions about the "sensitivity of achievement tests, individual differences, drug dosage, compliance, and time-course effects" (p. 267). In addition, the presence of learning disabilities or gaps in knowledge before drug treatment may influence the results. These are leads for additional research.

Peer Relations

Peer relationship problems of ADHD children have been well documented (King and Young, 1982; Johnston et al., 1985; Carlson et al., 1987). In comparison with normal children, ADHD children more often engage in controlling and dominating behaviors (Cunningham et al., 1985) and negative, aggressive interactions with peers (Pelham and Bender, 1982; Clark et al., 1988). They are more likely to be targets for others' aggression (Klein and Young, 1979) and receive lower sociometric nominations by their peers (Pelham and Bender, 1982), compared with controls. Recent work suggests that ADHD children communicate less effectively with peers, failing to modulate their social communications as task demands shifted (Landau and Milich, 1988) and engaging in fewer reciprocal verbal exchanges, compared with non-ADHD dyads (Clark et al., 1988). Grenell et al. (1987) report that ADHD children's peer difficulties are apparent during actual peer interactions as well as on assessments of their social knowledge. Researchers have linked poor peer relations during middle childhood with an increased risk for later adjustment difficulties in general (Kohlberg et al., 1972) and specifically, with delinquency and academic problems in adolescence (Kupersmidt, 1983) and psychiatric problems in adulthood (Cowen et al., 1973). Difficulties with peers is clearly a critical concern.

Studies of the immediate effects of stimulant medication show few significant positive effects and a high incidence of negative effects. Pelham and Bender (1982) failed to find declines in negative nonverbal behavior in either direct observations or the sociometric rankings of ADHD children by their peers. This could be because methylphenidate leads to decreased social interactions and adversely affects mood (Schleifer et al., 1975), with medicated children rated as less happy and pleased with themselves and more dysphoric (Whalen et al., 1979). Such negative findings may be the result of high drug dosages sometimes used. Cunningham et al. (1985)

compared the interactions of children at different dosage levels. At the lowest dose (0.15 mg/kg), but not at higher doses commonly used, they reported a significant decline in controlling and dominating behaviors of ADHD children and a reciprocal decrease in controlling responses by normal peers. Significant differences, however, were found only in a highly structured, simulated school setting. Consistent with previous work (Pelham and Bender, 1982), peer interactions of ADHD children following drug administration did not significantly change in free play and cooperative tasks settings where most peer interactions take place. The decline in controlling responses in structured classroom situations reported by Cunningham et al. may be related to the significant increase in the percent of time spent on-task at both dosage levels. Additionally, there was no change in popularity following medication at any dosage. Studies of longer duration are needed to determine if stimulant drug treatment helps break the chain of negative interactions allowing ADHD children to develop better social skills and form lasting friendships. At present, no studies have examined the effects of drug treatment during the school years on children's formation of friendships during adolescence. There is critical need for additional research here.

Antisocial Behavior

Antisocial behavior and delinquency during adolescence are more likely among children previously diagnosed as ADHD. Hyperactive children were more likely to have been arrested for a serious offense (Satterfield et al., 1982), appeared in court more often (Mendelson et al., 1971), had more frequent difficulties with police, and had more frequent detentions in the principal's office (Hoy et al., 1978). Depending on diagnosis (minimal brain dysfunction verses ADHD) and seriousness of the offense (difficulties with police versus third time arrest), prevalence estimates of antisocial behavior range from 10% (Feldman et al., 1979) to 25% (Mendelson et al., 1971; Weiss, 1983) to 45% (Satterfield et al., 1982) during the early high school years. To some degree, the link between ADHD and later delinquent behavior may be due to the comorbidity of attention and aggressive behavioral/conduct disorder symptoms (August and Stewart, 1983).

Neither Blouin et al. (1978) nor Weiss et al. (1975) found significant differences in delinquency during adolescence between hyperactive children treated and not treated with drugs. In a 10-year follow-up of 110 ADHD boys and 88 controls. Satterfield et al. (1982) found significantly more delinquency (placement in juvenile halls and probation camps) among hyperactive children compared with controls even though most of the ADHD children were treated with stimulant drugs for at least 25 months. (A later study where evidence is presented for the efficacy of medication plus psychological treatment is discussed below.) If delinquency during adolescence is due to aggression rather than ADHD, it is not surprising that stimulant drug effects targeted at reducing the core symptoms of ADHD do not diminish antisocial behavior. Many physicians currently argue against prescribing stimulant medication for conduct disorders (Cantwell, 1987; Garfinkel, 1987).

Overview of Long-Term Studies of Stimulant Treatment

Comprehensive studies of long lasting effects of stimulants have been conducted on five different samples of ADHD children, each carried out by a different group of researchers (Weiss et al., 1975; Riddle and Rapoport, 1976; Blouin et al., 1978; Charles and Schain, 1981; Satterfield et al., 1982). These studies focused primarily on academic performance (Weiss et al., 1975; Riddle and Rapoport, 1976; Blouin et al., 1978; Charles and Schain, 1981) or antisocial behavior (Mendelson et al., 1971; Blouin et al., 1978; Satterfield et al., 1982), and, on the whole, show little support for the efficacy of drug treatment.

Hechtman, Weiss and colleagues (e.g., Weiss and Hechtman, 1986) reported some positive effects on questionnaire measures of self-esteem in young adults. Results were not fully consistent (with some differences favoring the nonmedication group), were noted within many statistical tests, and were not supported by more objective measures. Nonetheless, the subjects' feelings are important, and this is a lead for additional research.

A variety of explanations are possible for the failure to find lasting improvement on academic tasks or a reduction in delinquent behavior among ADHD children following treatment with stimulant drugs. Increasing attention has been given to the overlap among children with symptoms of both ADHD and conduct disorder (Schachar et al., 1981; Taylor, 1986; Hindshaw, 1987; Rutter and Tuma, 1988). Since antisocial behavior during childhood predicts similar behavior during adolescence and adulthood (Robins, 1978), some researchers argue that antisocial behavior during adolescence may be more related to childhood aggression and conduct disorder than to ADHD symptoms. After separating children with antisocial behavior from those manifesting core ADHD symptoms (inattention, impulsivity, and overactivity), Loney et al., (1981) found that aggressiveness, not ADHD symptoms, predicted antisocial behavior. Gittelman et al. (1983) prospectively followed 107 males originally diagnosed as hyperactive (between 6 and 12 years old) into young adulthood. They found that the greatest risk factor for developing antisocial behavior was the maintenance of ADHD symptoms even after separating out ADHD children who were also diagnosed with conduct disorder during childhood. Overlapping symptoms of impulsivity and aggression (but not necessarily conduct disorder) in children diagnosed ADHD may account for the high incidence of antisocial behavior during adolescence. Additional research is needed in this area.

Another explanation for finding relatively few enduring drug effects is that none of the studies were experimental, with children randomly assigned to drug and no drug conditions. It is possible that children placed on medication had more severe problems than nonmedicated children. Also, in such studies, there are concerns about drug compliance. The disappointing long-term drug effects reported may stem from children's inconsistent drug intake or discontinuation of stimulant drugs entirely. While some researchers have checked whether children were taking stimulant drugs by contacting schools weekly. (Satterfield et al., 1987), others did not examine such factors (Weiss et al., 1975; Blouin et al., 1978) or report how many children discontinued medication (Charles and Schain, 1981).

Charles and Schain (1981) explored the relationship between length of treatment on stimulants and ADHD children's performance on achievement tests as a 4-year follow-up. Children were separated into five groups on the basis of length of treatment—0 to 6 months to 2 years, 2 to 3 years, 3 to 4 years, and children still on medication. Although there were significant differences between some of the groups on their academic achievement test scores at the 4-year follow-up, ADHD children in all groups were functioning well below the norms for children their age. Additionally, children still on stimulants were not different from children who had discontinued medication.

Subject attrition in studies of long-term drug effects may also influence the findings reported. Subjects who dropped out of the study may be those who improved on the drug and discontinued drug usage leaving those who were functioning more poorly. In Riddle and Rapoport's (1976) 2-year follow-up, only 5% of the subjects dropped out, but in the other four outcome studies discussed above (Weiss et al., 1975; Blouin et al., 1978; Charles and Schain, 1981; Satterfield et al., 1982), attrition ranged from about 30% to 50%. Sometimes attrition stemmed primarily from difficulties in locating subjects rather than in subjects declining participation (Charles and Schain, 1981). In other cases, subjects were deliberately excluded to make comparison groups more homogeneous (Weiss et al., 1975) or to tighten standards for inclusion of subjects (Satterfield et al., 1982). Although most of the researchers found no significant differences on relevant measures such as IQ, socioeconomic status (SES), symptom severity, age, and parent education between subjects who dropped out of the study and those who remained (Weiss et al., 1975; Charles and Schain, 1981; Satterfield et al., 1982), one study did not examine differences between the two groups (Blouin et al., 1978).

Finally, failure to include relevant control groups limits interpretation of the research findings. In some cases, ADHD children were not initially matched on relevant variables such as IQ which could have influenced achievement test scores at the 2-year follow-up (Riddle and Rapoport, 1976); while other studies did not include an untreated ADHD group (Riddle and Rapoport, 1976), a nonclinical "normal" comparison group (Weiss et al., 1975; Blouin et al., 1978; Charles and Schain, 1981; Satterfield et al., 1987), or a non-ADHD clinical control group (Weiss et al.,

1975; Riddle and Rapoport, 1976; Charles and Schain, 1981; Satterfield et al., 1987).

Satterfield and his colleagues (1987) compared ADHD children who received drug treatment and brief counseling (the Drug Treatment Only (DTO) group) with ADHD children who underwent both drug treatment and intensive psychological treatment (the Multiple Method Treatment (MMT) group). The MMT group showed significantly less delinquency than the DTO group. This does suggest that medication should be used within a broader treatment approach. However, it cannot be taken as evidence for the effectiveness of medication. There was no psychological treatment alone group. Thus, it is unclear whether finding reductions in delinquency over a 2- to 3-year period among ADHD boys in the MMT group, compared with the DTO group, was due to the combination of drugs and psychological intervention or to the psychological intervention alone.

To date, evidence of long-term benefits following stimulant drug treatment is inconclusive. The available data base remains limited, and additional studies exploring long-term stimulant effects are clearly needed.

Multimodal Treatment

Multimodal treatment programs have increased dramatically during the 1970s and 1980s. Using medication alone has been increasingly challenged. Specifically, concerns have been raised over the prolonged use of medication (Ross and Ross, 1982); lack of evidence for altering the eventual outcome for ADHD children; the heterogeneity of children diagnosed ADHD; the limited evidence for effects on important aspects of cognitive ability, such as learning, problem solving, and reasoning (Abikoff and Gittelman, 1985); reluctance of parents to give children psychoactive drugs; and the dislike many ADHD children have of taking medications (Firestone, 1982). Given the limitations of solely treating ADHD children with psychoactive drugs, the relative benefits of alternative interventions alone and in combination with stimulant drugs will be examined.

Cognitive-behavioral training (CBT) has been one of the most frequently researched adjuncts or alternatives to medication (Abikoff and Gittelman, 1985; Pelham and Murphy, 1986). CBT has been found effective primarily for brief durations, in circumscribed contexts, and with nonclinical samples of children experiencing difficulties with self-control (Kendall and Braswell, 1984). While some short-term benefits on ADHD children's capacity for self-control have been reported (Hindshaw et al., 1984b), lasting effects on ADHD children have been disappointing (Abikoff and Gittelman, 1985; Brown et al., 1986). Even when using multiple materials, trainers, and settings and encouraging teachers and parents to continue the treatment at home and at school, CBT has shown limited generalization for ADHD children (Cohen et al., 1981; Brown et al., 1985; Abikoff, 1987).

Whether ADHD children benefit more from stimulants by themselves or in combination with CBT remains inconclusive. Some researchers report little additional benefit of combining treatments (Abikoff and Gittelman, 1985; Brown et al., 1986). Others, such as Hindshaw and his colleagues, were able to increase ADHD children's capacity to cope with anger (Hindshaw et al., 1984a) and to accurately self-monitor their own behavior (Hindshaw et al., 1984b) using a combination of pharmacotherapy and cognitive-behavioral methods. Pelham and Murphy (1986) argue that available multimodal studies are filled with methodological limitations, such as, among others, failure to provide uniform treatment across conditions, small sample sizes, and inadequate outcome measures, that may obscure combination treatment effects. To date, few studies have investigated the long-term effects of combined treatments.

Other approaches are currently being developed including educational training and psychotherapy with the child and family. Recent work by Satterfield and his colleagues lends evidence for the beneficial effects of psychotherapy for each ADHD child or each child and family as part of a comprehensive treatment plan (Satterfield et al., 1982). In light of the poor prognosis for children diagnosed ADHD and the limitations of current treatment programs, there is a pressing need for more effective treatment programs. More work which considers individual needs and then examines the effectiveness of various treatment combinations is required.

NEGATIVE CONSEQUENCES OF STIMULANT MEDICATION

Potential negative consequences of the widespread use of the stimulant medication are both indirect and direct. Perhaps one of the most noteworthy consequences of adopting stimulants are the treatment of choice for ADHD is the paucity of research on nonorganic contributors to this disorder. Likewise, relatively little research has been done on educational or psychological interventions, although this may be changing (see above). When organic dysfunction in the child is viewed as the problem, and medication as the solution, motivation to deal more comprehensively with these children may be compromised. This is an addition to possible physical side effects.

Most of the physical side effects of stimulant drugs commonly reported, including appetite loss, insomnia, weight loss, headaches, irritability, and sudden mood changes are transient, disappearing after a short while, and are reversible either with dosage reduction or drug withdrawal (see Klein et al., 1980, for a detailed review of side effects).

Growth suppression, the most widely researched side effect, was first described by Sager et al. in 1972. Decrements in height were estimated to be as much as 3 cm per year for children given dosages of methylphenidate exceeding 20 mg for at least 3 years (Safer and Allen, 1973; Mattes and Gittelman, 1979) and after only

1 and 2 years (Greenhill et al., 1981). Others report that height rebounds toward normal after the first year of treatment (Gross, 1976). The most extensive investigation of growth effects to date is that of Rachel Gittelman-Klein and colleagues. In one report (Gittelman-Klein et al., 1988), a growth rebound effect during summer vacations from medication was demonstrated. After one such summer, weight was higher for the group removed from medication; after 2 summers, height, but not weight, showed a rebound effect. (See also Safer et al., 1975, for other evidence of growth rebound following termination of stimulant treatment). In a second paper, Gittelman-Klein and Mannuzza (1988) report that adult height of treated children did not differ from a nontreated, non-ADHD normal control group. While not an experimental study, groups were matched on key variables of SES and race, and age differences at outcome were controlled statistically. These data attest to the possibility that height rebounds following termination of stimulant treatment. However, the average duration of treatment for these subjects was 2.24 years, and almost all were under age 13 when treatment was terminated. Consequences of longer treatment, and treatment through the adolescent growth spurt, remain to be investigated.

Researchers have sought to understand the mechanism underlying the documented growth suppression during stimulant drug treatment. An important lead has been discovered here. Research reveals that methylphenidate stimulates daytime release of growth hormone, disrupting the usual nocturnal release (Greenhill et al., 1977; Jensen and Garfinkel, 1988). This finding is troublesome since disturbances in the normal cycle of release of growth hormone may not only influence height velocity but may also have an impact on other critical aspects of physical development such as sexual maturation. This would be of special concern if stimulant treatment is increased for adolescents. For some children, especially those treated over time, the growth hormone suppression disappears. This finding, of course, raises questions as to whether tolerance develops.

In recent years, much has been written concerning a possible link between stimulant treatment and either onset or exacerbation of tics, especially in children having or predisposed to having Tourette syndrome. Such a connection was implied by early case studies (Denckla et al., 1976; Golden, 1977). As recently as 1982, a report in the *Journal of the American Medical Association*, based on careful monitoring of 15 cases (Lowe, 1982), concluded that the presence of tics, or Tourette syndrome, or a family history of such problems contraindicates using stimulant medications. Others, however, have interpreted these data differently (Shapiro and Shapiro, 1981; Comings and Comings, 1987), arguing that the association between tics and stimulants, if any, is quite small, may be an effect of excessive dosage, and may even be artifactual. In a large scale study, Comings and Comings (1987) report that symptoms of ADHD often precede the onset of Tourette syndrome, usually by more than 2 years. Additionally, they report that this gap is unaffected by stimulant medication. Their conclusion is that the onset of Tourette symptoms occurs independently of stimulant treatment and they, in fact, argue that stimulants may be useful in combination with haloperidol. At present, this issue is not fully resolved. It should be noted that none of these studies has been experimental, with random assignment and proper controls. Moreover, contrary to their claim, the Comings and Comings study was not prospective, but, rather, relied on questionnaire reports concerning the onset of hyperactivity and Tourette symptoms. The authors would agree with Cohen (Cohen , Leckman & Shaywitz, 1984) that at this time, stimulants should be used cautiously with ADHD children who have a close relative with TS, and should be terminated with the onset of tics in children who were previously tic free"(p. 13).

Also of concern regarding side effects of stimulation medication is the lack of information about possible health consequences in adult life. Given the recent advocacy of extending treatment into the adolescent years, children may now be on such medication for 8 to 10 years or more. Only a handful of children treated extensively with stimulant have reached middle age. It will be important to begin conducting such follow-up research. The foci of an investigation might be vascular, cardiac, or kidney function.

FUTURE DIRECTIONS FOR RESEARCH

Some researchers suggest that the lack of long-term effectiveness of these treatments is due to the heterogeneity of the disorder, in terms of definition and etiology. There are several ways to decrease the heterogeneity among children who are being investigated. One is to apply strict criteria; that is, to be faithful to the letter of the *DSM-III-R* when diagnosing children. Another is to insist that children's symptoms are "pervasive" versus "situational" (Taylor, 1988). Last, reliability and validity would be improved by using a batter of diagnostic instruments and administering these tests more than once, with at least a month between examinations.

When studying children with ADHD, reading disability and conduct disorder should be targets as well, since they were the most obvious correlates of ADHD (August et al., 1983). Conduct disorder has been associated with ADHD along a continuum, from no "acting out" to a full blown aggressive conduct disorder. In a large scale epidemiologic study (August and Garfinkel, 1989), two types of children with attention deficits and hyperactivity were found, the first marked by behavior problems, and the second by reading disability. A third group had both the behavioral and cognitive problems. This analysis may provide clues as to which subtypes of ADHD will benefit the most from stimulant drugs or other treatments.

Longitudinal studies of children before they develop the disorder are needed to identify various etiological influences. At present, only one study has followed children from birth through age 8 and examined both early caregiving and biological variables (Jacobvitz and Sroufe, 1987; Jacobvitz, 1988, unpublished dissertation). In this study, three assessments of the early child-caregiver relationship (parental intrusiveness at 6 months and overstimulation at 24 and 42 months) were examined. The 42 biological variables assessed included temperament measures (e.g., activity level, distractability, impulsivity, sociability), physical anomalies, prematurity, delivery complications, and indicators of early neurological dysfunction (e.g., newborn reflexes). Two of the three caregiving measures, intrusiveness at 6 months and overstimulation at 42 months, and one of the 42 biological measures (a 7- and 10-day composite of motor immaturity during the newborn period) significantly distinguished 27 children, later showing ADHD symptoms, from 27 normal controls during kindergarten and the early school years (Jacobvitz and Sroufe, 1987; Jacobvitz, 1988; unpublished dissertation). This study suggests that experiential factors should not be overlooked in searching for the etiology of ADHD and that there may be multiple pathways to this disorder. Much more work is needed along these lines.

Jensen and Garfinkel (1988) and Taylor (1988), among others, emphasize the need to identify biological markers of ADHD and to confirm their validity through replication. Establishing prevalence rates of such markers and their unique presence in ADHD children is an important goal. Screening children whose difficulties stem from exogenous experiences could aid in distinguishing children with organic problems and help identify any subset of children who are indeed true responders to stimulant drugs.

CONCLUSIONS

The regulation of attention and activity are often problematic in childhood, and such anomalies can give rise to painful conflicts for children, families, and teachers. And while the manifest form of the misbehavior changes with age, children with such problems often suffer for years, if not for a lifetime. The motivation of professionals to deal swiftly and efficiently with such problems is therefore reasonable. This motivation and the often clear, dramatic, short-term impact of stimulant medication make it understandable how the widespread practice of stimulant medication came into being.

However, the paucity of data showing continued or lasting impact of stimulant medication for these children is disconcerting. A case for the long-term effectiveness of stimulant medication simply cannot be made at this time. This is especially troubling because some of the very aspects of functioning and development we would most hope to impact—school achievement, relationships with peers, and the behavior problems common to adolescence—have been the central focus in the outcome studies that have been done. ADHD children often continue to have problems in adolescence and having been treated with stimulant medication in childhood has had little demonstrable effect. Nor is there evidence that stimulant medication continues to benefit children after several months, though here the situation is mostly a lack of pertinent evidence rather than negative findings.

There are several possible explanations for the absence of demonstrable long-term benefits of stimulant drug medication. First, children with attentional and behavioral problems likely are a very heterogeneous group. If only a subset of these children, especially if that subset is small, have a specific biochemical abnormality, drug treatment effects would be obscured. Second, drug treatment alone may represent inadequate treatment for most children, even those having an organic contribution to their problems. (Thus, studies using medication in combination with other treatments, such as that by Satterfield et al. (1987) are of great importance.) Finally, children, like adults, may commonly develop tolerance for stimulant medication so that drug effects in time disappear. Existing evidence does not allow firm conclusions concerning the relative importance of each of these factors.

At present, the decision to prescribe stimulant medication remains an individual clinical decision. Current research would not seem to justify sustained treatment with medication alone, widespread drug trials as a diagnostic procedure, or unrestrained use of stimulant medication. The Baltimore County study (Safer and Krager, 1988) revealed that 6% of public school children were being treated with stimulant medication. While rates certainly vary locally, this figure is striking. The estimated prevalence of ADHD is 3% (American Psychiatric Association, 1987), and only a yet to be defined subset of these children are appropriate targets of stimulant medication. The authors would urge greater caution and a much more restricted use of stimulant treatment pending more research on long-term effects, both concerning positive and negative consequences, and an increased ability to identify the subset of children having a specific biochemical abnormality.

REFERENCES

Abikoff, H. (1987), An evaluation of cognitive behavior therapy for hyperactive children. In: *Advances in Clinical Child Psychology*, Vol. 10, eds. B.B. Lahey & A.E. Kazdin, New York: Plenum, pp. 171–216.

————Gittelman, R. (1985a), The normalizing effects of methylphenidate on the classroom behavior of ADHD children. *J. Abnorm. Child Psychol.*, 13:33–44.

——————(1985b), Hyperactive children treated with stimulants: is cognitive trailing a useful adjunct? *Arch. Gen. Psychiatry*, 42:953–961.

American Psychiatric Association, Committee on Nomenclature and Statistics. (1987), *Diagnostic and Statistical Manual of Mental Disorders, (3rd ed.–Revised)*. Washington, DC: American Psychiatric Association.

August, G.J. & Garfinkel, B.D. (1989), Behavioral and cognitive subtypes of ADHD. *J. Am. Acad. Child Adolesc. Psychiatry*, 28:739–748.

————Stewart, M.A. & Holmes, C.S. (1983), A four-year follow-up of hyperactive boys with and without conduct disorder. *Br. J. Psychiatry*, 143:192–198.

Barkley, R.A. (1976), Predicting the response of hyperkinetic children to stimulant drugs: a review. *J. Abnorm. Child Psychol.* 4:327–348.

————(1981), *Hyperactive Children: A Handbook for Diagnosis and Treatment.* New York: Guilford Press.

————(1989), Hyperactive girls and boys: stimulant drug affects on mother-child interaction. *J. Child Psychol. Psychiatry*, 30:379–390.

————Jackson, T. (1978), Hyperkinesis, autonomic nervous system activity and stimulant drug effects. *J. Child Psychol. Psychiatry*, 18:347–358.

————Karlsson, J., Pollard, S. & Murphy, J. (1985), Developmental changes in the mother-child interactions of hyperactive boys: effects of two dose levels of Ritalin. *J. Child Psychol. Psychiatry*, 26:705–715.

Bhagauan, H.N., Coleman, M. & Coursina, D.B. (1975), The effect of pyridoxine hydrochloride on blood serotonin and pyridoxal phosphate contents in hyperactive children. *Pediatrics*, 55:437–441.

Blouin, A.G., Bornstein, R.A. & Trites, R.L. (1978), Teenage alcohol use among hyperactive and nonhyperactive children: a five-year follow-up study. *J. Pediatr. Psychol.*, 3:188–194.

Brown, G.L., Ebert, M.H., Hunt, R.D. & Rapoport, J.L. (1981), Urinary 3-methoxy-4-hydroxyphenylglycol and homovanillic acid response to d-amphetamine in hyperactive children. *Biological Psychiatry*, 16:779–787.

Brown, R.T., Borden, K.A., Wynne, M.E., Schleser, R. & Clingermann, S.R. (1986), Methylphenidate and cognitive therapy with ADD children: a methodological reconsideration. *J. Abnorm. Child Psychol.*, 14:481–497.

————Wynne, M.E. & Medenis, R. (1985), Methylphenidate and cognitive therapy: a comparison of treatment approaches with hyperactive boys. *J. Abnorm. Child Psychol.*, 13:69–87.

Buchsbaum, M. & Wender, P. (1973), Average evoked responses in normal and minimally brain dysfunctioned children treated with amphetamine: a preliminary report. *Arch. Gen. Psychiatry*, 29:764–770.

Cantwell, D. (1987, June). *Developmental and Longitudinal Aspects of Attention Deficit Disorders.* Workshop at the Conference on Attention Deficit Hyperactivity in Children and Adolescents: Assessment and Intervention, Minneapolis, Minnesota.

Carlson, C.L., Lahey, B.B., Frame, C.L., Walker, J. & Hynd, G.W. (1987), Sociometric status of clinic-referred children with attention deficit disorders with and without hyperactivity. *J. Abnorm. Child Psychol.*, 15:537–547.

Charles, L. & Schain, R. (1981), A four-year follow-up study of the effects of methylphenidate on the behavior an academic achievement of hyperactive children. *J. Abnorm. Child Psychol.*, 9:495–505.

Clark, M.L., Cheyne, J.A., Cunningham, C.E. & Siegel, L.S. (1988), Dyadic peer interaction and task orientation in attention-deficit-disordered children. *J. Abnorm. Child Psychol.*, 16:1–15.

Cohen, D., Leckman, J. & Shaywitz, B. (1984), The clinical guide to child psychiatry. In: *The Tourette Syndrome and Other Tics*, eds. Shatler, A. Eberhard & L. Greenhill, New York: Free Press, pp. 3–28.

Cohen, N.J., Sullivan, J., Minde, K., Novak, C. & Helwig, C. (1981). Evaluations of the relative effectiveness of methylphenidate and cognitive behavior modification in the treatment of kindergarten-aged hyperactive children. *J. Abnorm. Child. Psychol.*, 9:43–54.

Comings, D.E. & Comings, B.G. (1987), A controlled study of tourette syndrome. I. Attention-deficit disorder, learning disorders and school problems. *Am. J. Hum. Genet.*, 41:701–741.

Conners, C.K. (1977), Discussion of Rapoport's chapter. In: *Depression in Childhood*, eds. J. Schulterbrandt & A. Raskin. New York: Raven Press, pp. 101–104.

Cowen, E.L., Pederson, A., Babijian, H., Izzo, L. & Trost, M.A. (1973), Long-term follow-up of early detected vulnerable children. *J. Consult. Clin. Psychol.*, 41:438–446.

Cunningham, C.E., & Barkley, R.A. (1978), The role of academic failure in hyperactive behavior. *Journal of Learning Disabilities*, 11:15–21.

———Siegel, L.S. & Offord, D.R. (1985), A developmental dose-response analysis of the effects of methylphenidate on the peer interactions of attention deficit disordered boys. *J. Child Psychol. Psychiat.*, 26:955–971.

Denckla, M.B., Bemporad, J.R. & Mackay, M.C. (1976), Tics following methylphenidate administration. *JAMA*, 235:1349–1351.

Barr, R.G., O'Neill, M.E., & Britton, B.G. (1986), Short term effects of methylphenidate on the cognitive learning and academic performance of children with attention deficit disorder in the laboratory and the classroom. *J. Child Psychol. Psychiat.* 27:191–211.

———Amin, K., O'Neill, M.E. & Britton, B.G. (1988). Dosage effects and individual responsivity to methylphenidate in attention deficit disorder. *J Child Psychol. Psychiat.*, 29:453–475.

Ebaugh, F.G. (1923), Neuropsychiatric sequelae of acute epidemic encephalitis in children. *Am. J. Dis. Child.*, 25:89–97.

Ellis, M.J., Witt, P.A., Reynolds, R. & Sprague, R.L. (1974), Methylphenidate and the activity of hyperactives in the informal setting. *Child Dev.*, 45:217–220.

Feldman, S., Denhoff, E. & Denhoff. (1979), The attention disorders and related syndromes. Outcome in adolescence and young adult life. In: *Minimal Brain Dysfunction: A Developmental Approach*: eds L. Starr & E. Denhoff. New York: Mason, pp. 133–148.

Firestone, P., Peters, S., Rivier, M. & Knights, R.M. (1978), Minor physical anomalies in hyperactive, retarded and normal children and their families. *J. Child Psychol. Psychiat.*, 19:155–160.

Garfinkel, B. (1987, June), *Treatment strategies for Ad-HD*. Paper presented at the conference on Attention-Deficit Hyperactivity Disorders in Children and Adolescents. Minneapolis.

Gittelman Klein, R. & Klein, D.F. (1976), Methylphenidate effects in learning disabilities. Psychometric changes. *Arch. Gen. Psychiatry*, 33:655–664.

———Mannuzza, S. (1988), Hyperactive boys almost grown up. III. Methylphenidate effects on ultimate height. *Arch. Gen. Psychiatry*, 45:1131–1134.

————Landa, B., Mattes, J.A. & Klein, D.F. (1988), Methylphenidate and growth in hyperactive children: a controlled withdrawal study. *Arch. Gen. Psychiatry*, 45:1127–1130.

Golden, G.S. (1977), The effect of central nervous system stimulants on Tourette syndrome. *Ann. Neurol.* 2:69–70.

Greenhill, L., Puig-Antich, K. & Sassin, J. (1977), Hormone and growth response in hyperkinetic children on stimulant medication. *Psychopharmacol Bull.*, 12:33–34.

————Puig-Antich, J., Chambers, W., Rubinstein, B., Halpern, F. & Sachar, E.J. (1981), Growth hormone, prolactin, and growth responses in hyperkinetic males treated with D-amphetamine. *J. Am. Acad. Child Psychiatry*, 20:84–103.

Grenell, M.M., Glass, C.R. & Katz, K.S. (1987), Hyperactive children and peer interaction: knowledge and performance of social skills. *J. Abnorm. Child Psychol.*, 15:1–13.

Gross, M.D. (1976), Dextroamphetamine, desipramine, growth, hyperkinetic syndrome, imipramine, methylphenidate. *Pediatrics.* 58:423–431.

Hechtman, L., Weiss, G., Perlman, T. & Amsel, R. (1984), Hyperactives as young adults: initial predictors of adult outcome. *J. Am. Acad. Child Adolesc Psychiatry*, 23:250–260.

Hindshaw, S.P. (1987), On the distinction between attentional deficits/hyperactivity and conduct problems/aggression in child psychopathology. *Psychol. Bull.*, 101:443–463.

————Henker, B. & Whalen, C.K. (1984a). Cognitive-behavioral and pharmacological interventions for hyperactive boys: comparative and combined effects. *J. Consult. Clin. Psychol.*, 52:739–749.

————————(1984b), Self-control in hyperactive boys in anger-inducing situations: effect of cognitive-behavioral training and methylphenidate. *J. Abnorm. Child Psychol.*, 12:55–77.

Hoy, E., Weiss, G., Minde, K. & Cohen, N. (1978), The hyperactive child at adolescence: emotional, social, and cognitive functioning. *J. Abnorm. Child Psychol.*, 6:311–324.

Humphries, T., Kinsbourne, M. & Swanson, J.M. (1978), Stimulant effects on cooperation and social interaction between hyperactive children and their mothers. *J. Child Psychol. Psychiat.*, 19:13–22.

Jacobvitz, D. & Sroufe, L.A. (1987), The early caregiver-child relationship and Attention Deficit Disorder with Hyperactivity in kindergarten: a prospective study, *Child Dev.*, 58:1488–1495.

Jensen, J.B. & Garfinkel, B.D. (1988), Neuroendocrine aspects of attention deficit Hyperactivity disorder. *Endocrinol. Metab. Clin. NorthAm.*, 17:111–127.

Johnston, C., Pelham, W.E. & Murphy, H.A. (1985), Peer relationships in ADHD and normal children: a developmental analysis of peer and teacher ratings. *J. Abnorm. Child Psychol.*, 13:89–100.

Kendall, P.C. & Braswell, L. (1984), *Cognitive-behavioral Therapy for Impulsive Children.* New York: Guilford Press.

King, L.A. & Young, R.D. (1982), Attentional deficits with and without hyperactivity: teacher and peer perceptions. *J. Abnorm. Child Psychol.*, 10:483–495.

Klein, A.R. & Young, R.D. (1979), Hyperactive boys in their classroom: assessment of teachers and peer perceptions, interactions, and classroom behavior. *J. Abnorm. Child Psychol.*, 7:425–442.

Klein, D.F., Gittelman, R., Quitkin, A. & Rifkin, A. (1980), Side effects of antipsychotic drugs and their treatment. In: *A Diagnosis and Treatment of Psychiatric Disorder: Adults and Children, (2nd ed).* eds. D.F. Klein, R. Gittelman, A. Quitkin & A. Rifkin. Baltimore: William & Wilkins, pp. 174–214.

Kohlber, L. LaCrosse, J. & Ricks, D. (1972), The predictability of adult mental health from childhood behavior. In: *Manual of Child Psychopathology,* ed. B.B. Wolman. New York: McGraw-Hill, pp. 1217–1284.

Kornetsky, C. (1970), Psychoactive drugs in the immature organism. *Psycho-pharmacologia,* 17:105–136.

Kupersmidt, J.B. (1983, April), Predicting delinquency and academic problems from childhood peer status. *Strategies for identifying children at social risk: longitudinal correlates and consequences.* Symposium presented at the biennial meeting of the Society for Research in Child Development, Detroit.

Lambert, N.M. (1988), Adolescent outcomes for hyperactive children: perspectives on general and specific patterns of childhood risk for adolescent educational, social and mental health problems. *Am. J. Psychol.,* 43:786–799.

Landau, S. & Milich, R. (1988), Social communication patterns of attention-deficit-disordered boys. *J. Abnorm. Child Psychol.,* 16:69–81.

Laties, V.G. & Weiss, B. (1967), Performance enhancement by the amphetamines: a new appraisal. In: *Neuropharmacology,* eds. H. Brill, J.O. Cole, P. Deniker, H. Hopkins, & P.D. Bradley, Amsterdam: Excerpta Medica Foundation, pp. 800–808.

Loney, J., Kramer, J. & Milich, R. (1981), The hyperactive child grows up: predictors of symptoms, delinquency, and achievement at follow-up. In: *Psychosocial Aspects of Drug Treatment for Hyperactivity,* eds. K. Gadow & J. Loney. Boulder, CO: Westview Press, pp. 381–415.

Lou, H.C., Henricksen, & Bruhn, P. (1984), Focal cerebral hypoperfusion in children with dysphasia and/or attention deficit disorder. *Arch. Neurol.* 41:825–829.

Lowe, T.L., Cohen, D.J., Detlor, J., Kaeonenitzer, M.W. & Shaywitz, B.A. (1981), Stimulant medications precipitate Tourette's syndrome. *JAMA,* 247:1729–1731.

Mannuzza, S., Gittleman-Klein, R., Bonagura, N., Horowitz-Konig, P. & Shenker, R. (1988), Hyperactive boys almost grown up. *Arch. Gen. Psychiatry,* 45:13–18.

Mattes, J. & Gittelman, R. (1979), Drug linked to growth problem in children. *Psychiatric News,* 14:17.

McKinney, W. (1977), Animal behavioral/biological models relevant to depression and affective disorders in humans. In: *Depression in Childhood,* eds. J. Schulterbrandt & A. Raskin. New York: Raven Press, pp. 10–122.

Mendelson, J.H. Johnson, N.E. & Stewart, M.A. (1971), Hyperactive children as teenagers: a follow-up study. *J. Nerv. Ment. Dis.,* 153:273–279.

Mikkelson, E., Lake, C.R., Brown, G.L., Ziegler, M.G. & Ebert, M.H. (1981), The hyperactive child syndrome: peripheral sympathetic nervous system function and the effect of d-amphetamine. *Psychiatry Res.,* 4:157–169.

Nichols, P.L. & Chen, T.C. (1981), *Minimal Brain Dysfunction: A Prospective Study,* Hillsdale, NJ: Erlbaum.

Pelham, W. (1986), The effects of psychostimulant drugs on learning and academic achievement in children with attention-deficit disorders and learning disabilities. In: *Psychological and Educational Perspectives on Learning Disabilities*, eds. J. Torgesen & B. Wong. New York: Academic Press, pp. 259–295.

——————Caddell, J., Booth, S., & Moore, S. (1985), Methylphenidate and children with attention deficit disorder. Dose effects on classroom academic and social behavior. *Arch. Gen. Psychiatry*, 42:948–952.

——Bender, M.E., (1982), Peer relationships in hyperactive children: description and treatment. In: *Advances in Learning and Behavioral Disabilities, Vol. 1*, eds. K. Gadow & I. Bailer. Greenwich, CT: JAI Press, Inc., pp. 365–436.

——Murphy, H.A. (1986), Behavioral and pharmacological treatment of hyperactivity and attention deficit disorders. In: *Pharmacological and Behavioral Treatment: An Integrative Approach*. eds. M. Hersen & S.E. Breuning. New York: Wiley, pp. 108–147.

Peloguin, L.J. & Klorman, R. (1986), Effects of methylphenidate on normal children's mood, event-related potentials and performance in memory, scanning & vigilance. *J. Abnorm. Psychol.*, 95:88–98.

Porges, S.W., Walter, G.F., Korb, R.J. & Sprague, R.L. (1975), The influence of methylphenidate on heart rate and behavioral measures of attention in hyperactive children. *Child Dev.*, 46:727–733.

Prichep, L., Sutton, S. & Hakerem, G. (1976), Evoked potentials in hyperkinetic and normal under certainty and uncertainty. *Psychophysiology*, 13:419–428.

Rapport, M.D., Murphy, H.A. & Bailey, J.S. (1982), Ritalin vs. response cost in the control of hyperactive children: a within-subject comparison. *J. Appl. Behav. Anal.*, 15:205–216.

Rapoport, J.L., Buchsbaum, M., Zahn, T.P., Weingartner, H., Ludlow, G. & Mikkelsen, E. (1978), Dextroamphetamine: cognitive and behavioral effects in normal prepurtal boys. *Science*, 199:560–562.

Riddle, K.D. & Rapoport, J.L. (1976), A 2-year follow-up of 72 hyperactive boys. *J. Nerv. Ment. Dis.*, 162:126–134.

Rie, H.E., Rie, E.D., Stewart, M. & Ambuel, J.P. (1976a), Effects of methylphenidate on underachieving children. *J. Consult, Clin. Psychol.* 44:250–260.

——————————(1976b), Effects of Ritalin on underachieving children: a replication. *J. Orthopsychiatry*, 46:313–322.

Robins, L.N. (1978), Sturdy childhood predictors of adult outcomes: replications from longitudinal studies. *Psychol. Med.* 8:611–622.

Rose, R.M., Gordon, T.P. Bernstein, I.S. (1972), Plasma testosterone in the male rhesus: influences of sexual and social stimuli. *Science*, 178:643–645.

Ross, D. & Ross, S. (1982), *Hyperactivity*. New York: Wiley.

Rutter, M. & Tuma, A.H. (1988), Diagnosis and classification: Some outstanding issues. In: *Assessment and Diagnosis in Child Psychopathology*, eds. M. Rutter, A.H. Tuma & I.S. Lanor. New York: Guilford Press, pp. 3–17.

——Graham, P. & Yule, W. (1970), A neuropsychiatric study in childhood. In: *Clinics in Developmental Medicine, Nos. 35–36*. London: Spastics International Medical Publications/Heinemann Medical Books.

Safer, D.J., & Allen, R.P. (1973), Factors influencing the suppressant effects of two stimulant drugs on the growth of hyperactive children. *Pediatrics*, 51:660–667.

———Krager, J.M. (1984), Trends in medication therapy for hyperactivity: national and international perspectives. *Adv. Learn. Behav. Dis.*, 3:125–149.

—————(1988). A survey of medication treatment for hyperactive/inattentive students. *JAMA*, 260:2256–2258.

————Barr, E. (1972), Depression of growth inn hyperactive children on stimulant drugs, *N. Engl. J. Med.*, 287:217–220.

—————(1975), Growth rebound after termination of stimulant drugs. *J. Pediatr.*, 86:113–116.

Satterfield, J. Cantwell, D., Lesser, L. & Posodin, R. (1972), Physiological studies of the hyperkinetic child:I. *Am. J. Psychiatry*, 128:1418–1424.

———Hoppe, C.M. & Schell, A.M. (1982), A prospective study of delinquency in 110 adolescent boys with attention deficit disorder and 88 normal adolescent boys. *Am. J. Psychiatry*, 139:797–798.

———Satterfield, B.T. & Schell, A.M. (1987), Therapeutic interventions to prevent delinquency in hyperactive boys. *J. Am. Acad. Child Adolesc. Psychiatry*, 26:56–64.

Schachar, R., Rutter, M & Smith, A. (1981), Situationally and pervasively hyperactive children. *J. Child Psychol. Psychiatry*, 22:375–392.

Schleifer, M., Weiss, G., Cohen, N., Elman, M., Crejic, H. & Kruger, E. (1975), Hyperactivity in preschoolers and the effect of methylphenidate. *Am. J. Orthopsychiatry*, 45:33–50.

Shapiro, A.K. & Shapiro, E. (1981), Do stimulants provide, cause or exacerbate tics and Tourette Syndrome? *Compr. Psychiatry.* 22:265–273.

Shaywitz, S.E., Cohen, D.J. & Shawitz, S.E. (1978), The biochemical basis of minimal brain dysfunction. *Am. J. Dis. Child.*, 92:179–187.

Shekim, W.O., Davis, L.G., Bylund, D.B., Brunngraber, E., Fikes, L., & Lanham, J. (1982), Platelet MASO in children with attention deficit disorder and hyperactivity. A pilot study. *Am. J. Psychiatry*, 139:936–938.

———Dekirmenjian, H. & Chapel, J.L. (1979), Urinary MHPG excretion in minimal brain dysfunction and its modification by d-amphetamine. *Am. J. Psychiatry*, 136:667–671.

Solanto, M.V. (1984), Neuropharmacological basis of stimulant drug action in deficit disorder with hyperactivity: a review and synthesis. *Psychol. Bull.*, 95:387–409.

Sprague, R.L. & Sleator, E.K. (1977), Methylphenidate in hyperkinetic children: differences in dose effects on learning and social behavior. *Science*, 198: 1274–1276.

Sroufe, L.A. (1975), Drug treatment of children with behavior problems. In: *Review of Child Development Research, Vol. 4*, In: F. Horowitz. Chicago: University of Chicago Press, pp. 347–407.

———Stewart, M.A. (1973), Treating problem children with stimulant drugs. *N. Engl. J. Med.*, 289:407–413.

Stephens, R., Pelham, W.E. & Skinner, R. (1984), The state-dependent and main effects of pemoline and methylphenidate on paired-associate learning and spelling in hyperactive children. *J. Consult. Clin. Psychol.*, 52:104–113.

Still, G.F. (1902), The Coulstonian Lectures on some abnormal physical conditions in children. *Lancet*, 1:1008–1012, 1077–1082, 1163–1168.

Tallmadge, J. & Barkley, R.A. (1983). The interactions of hyperactive and normal boys with their fathers and mothers. *J. Abnorm. Child Psychol.*, 11:565–580.

Taylor, E.A. (1988), Attention deficit and conduct disorder syndromes. In: *Assessment and Diagnosis in Child Psychopathology.* eds. M. Rutter, A.H. Tuma, & I.S. Lann. New York: Guilford Press, pp. 377–407.

———(1986), Childhood hyperactivity. *Br. J. Psychiatry*, 149:562–573.

Weiss, G. (1983), Long term outcome of hyperkinetic syndrome: empirical findings, conceptual problems and practical implications. In: *Developmental Neuropsychiatry*, ed. M. Rutter, New York, Guilford Press, pp. 422–436.

———Laties, V.G. (1962), Enhancement of human performance by caffeine and the amphetamines, *Pharmacol. Rev.*, 14:1–36.

———Hechtman, L.T. (1986), *Hyperactive children grown up*. New York: Guilford.

———Kruger, E., Danielson, V. & Elman, M. (1975), Effects of long-term treatment of hyperactive children with methylphenidate. *Can. Med. Assoc. J.*, 112:159–165.

Wender, P.H. (1971), *Minimal Brain Dysfunction in Children*. New York, Wiley-Interscience.

———(1987), *The hyperactive child, adolescent, and adult: attention deficit disorder through the lifespan*. New York: Oxford University Press.

Werry, J.S. (1968). Studies on the hyperactive child, IV. An empirical analysis of the minimal brain dysfunction syndrome. *Arch. Gen. Psychiatry*, 19:9–16.

———Aman, M. (1984), Methylphenidate in hyperactive and enuretic children. In B. Shospin, & L. Greenhill (Eds.): *The psychobiology of childhood: Profile of current issues* (pp. 183–195). Jamaica, NY: Spectrum.

Whalen, C.K. & Henker, B. (1980) The social ecology of psychostimulant treatment: a model for conceptual and empirical analysis. In C.K. Whalen & B. Henker (Eds.), *Hyperactive children: The social ecology of identification and treatment* (pp. 3–51). New York: Academic Press.

———Alkus, S.R., Adams, D. & Stapp, J. (1978), Behavior observations of hyperactive children and methylphenidate (Ritalin) effects in systematically structured classroom environments: now you see them, now you don't. *J. Pediatr. Psychol.* 3:177–184.

———Fink, D. & Dotemoto, S. (1979), A social ecology of hyperactive boys: medication effects in structured classroom environments. *J. Appl. Behav. Anal.*, 12:65–82.

———McAuliffe, S. & Vaux, A. (1979), Peer interaction in a structured communication tasks. Comparison of normal and hyperactive boys and methylphenidate (Ritalin) and placebo effects. *Child Dev.*, 50:338–401.

———Dotemoto, S. (1980), Methylphenidate and hyperactivity: effects on teachers' behaviors. *Science*, 208:1280–1282.

———(1981), Teacher response to the methylphenidate (Ritalin) versus placebo status of hyperactive boys in the classroom. *Child Dev.* 52:1005–1014.

Yu-cum, S. & Yu-feng, W. (1984). Urinary 3-methoxy-4-hydroxy-phenylglycol sulfate excretion in seventy-three school children with minimal brain dysfunction syndrome. *Biol. Psychiatry*, 19:861–870.

Zahn, T.P., Abate, F., Little, B. & Wender, P. (1975), Minimal brain dysfunction, stimulant drugs, and autonomic nervous system activity. *Arch. Gen. Psychiatry*, 32:381–387.

Zametkin, A.J. & Rapoport, J.L. (1987), Neurobiology of attention deficit disorder with hyperactivity: where have we come in 50 years? *J. Am. Acad. Chil Adolesc. Psychiatry*, 26:676–686.

Zentall, S.S. & Zentall, T.R. (1983), Optimal stimulation: a model of disordered activity and performance in normal and deviant children. *Psychol. Bull.*, 94:446–471.

26

A Review of the Pharmacotherapy of Aggression in Children and Adolescents

Jonathan T. Stewart, Wade C. Myers, Roger C. Burket, and W. Bradford Lyles

University of Florida College of Medicine, Gainesville

Aggressive behavior in children and adolescents is a heterogeneous phenomenon occurring in a wide variety of illnesses. No single etiologic model seems adequate to explain this phenomenon. In many cases, pharmacotherapy may prove to be a useful adjunct to treatment. Potentially useful medications are described in reference to psychiatric diagnosis. Pharmacological treatment can be helpful in the management of the aggressive youth when judiciously applied in the context of a comprehensive treatment plan.

Aggressive behaviors are frequently seen by clinicians who work with children and adolescents. There have been numerous attempts to develop unified theories of the pathogenesis of aggression, based on psychodynamic, neurochemical, or evolutionary data. These efforts have been reviewed extensively by Miczek (1987) and will not be discussed here. Thus far, no theory has been successful in explaining all human aggression or even the majority of human aggression. This does not seem surprising, as it is clinically obvious that aggression is a heterogeneous phenomenon, occurring in the context of numerous seemingly unrelated illnesses. Naturally, then, the treatment of aggression will be equally heterogeneous, in spite of implications to the contrary in the psychiatric literature. Accordingly, the authors have chosen to describe the pharmacologic treatment of aggression in children and adolescents as a function of diagnosis, a self-evident but surprisingly often overlooked principle.

Reprinted with permission from *Journal of the American Academy of Child and Adolescent Psychiatry*, 1990, Vol. 29, No. 2, 269–277. Copyright © 1990 by the American Academy of Child and Adolescent Psychiatry.

The authors wish to thank Ms. Eliese M. Coleman for her assistance in the preparation of this manuscript.

The vast majority of controlled studies, and even case reports, concerning the treatment of aggression have involved adult patients. On occasion this adult literature has been cited to fill significant voids in the child and adolescent literature. It should be remembered, however, that these citations may not always be applicable to adolescents and quite frequently will not be applicable to children.

This paper will specifically review physical aggression directed toward other people. It is not clear whether the treatment strategies suggested are effective for severe verbal aggression or threats, or for physical aggression directed toward animals or inanimate objects. This judgment is left to the clinician, as there is very little in the literature that addresses these distinctions. Aggression directed towards the self, including suicide, self-mutilation, and head-banging, constitutes an entirely different set of problems and will not be addressed in this review.

Eichelman (1988) described four important principles for the pharmacologic treatment of aggressive adults: treat the primary illness, use the most benign interventions when treating empirically, have some quantifiable means of assessing efficacy, and institute drug trials systematically. These principles are perhaps even more important with children and adolescents than with adults.

Finally, and perhaps most importantly, it must be remembered that there is virtually no situation in which an aggressive child or adolescent should be treated only pharmacologically. In some instances, pharmacotherapy constitutes the cornerstone of treatment, whereas in other cases, pharmacotherapy may act only as an adjunct to more definitive therapies such as psychotherapeutic or behavioral interventions. Although this paper will deal exclusively with pharmacologic issues, a comprehensive plan of treatment, not limited to medications, must be developed for virtually every aggressive child or adolescent.

CONDUCT DISORDER

Aggression in child and adolescent psychiatric disorders is most commonly thought to occur with the diagnosis of conduct disorder. *DSM-III-R* lists 13 criteria to be used for the diagnosis of conduct disorder, 10 of which specifically probe for symptoms of aggression. The prevalence of conduct disorder in children and adolescents is estimated to be 9% for males and 2% for females according to *DSM-III-R*, although actual rates tend to vary widely according to the method of measurement used and the type of population studied (Quay, 1987).

Pharmacologic treatment of aggression in the conduct disordered youth must be part of a comprehensive plan that also includes psychosocial and behavioral interventions. There is no research currently available to justify the use of pharmacologic agents alone in treating the violent youth (O'Donnell, 1985).

Anticonvulsants were among the first drugs studied to treat aggression in children and adolescents. Phenytoin is the only anticonvulsant to have been studied adequately for the management of aggression in youthful populations; double-blind, placebo-controlled studies by Lefkowitz (1969), Looker and Conners (1970), and Conners et al. (1971) failed to show positive results. Controlled trials to determine the efficacy of carbamazepine specifically in conduct disorder are lacking, although there are positive reports in undiagnosed aggressive children (Kuhn-Gebhart, 1976; Remschmidt, 1976).

Psychostimulants were also used in early studies for the treatment of aggressive children and adolescents. Several investigators reported positive results with the use of amphetamine sulfate in treating aggressive youths, although these studies were open, uncontrolled trials with poorly defined populations (Bradley, 1937; Bender and Cottington, 1942). Continued support for the use of amphetamines in delinquent populations was found in double-blind, placebo-controlled studies by Eisenberg et al. (1963), Conners et al. (1971), and Maletzky (1974). However, these studies are characterized by ambiguous results, as well as lack of information concerning methodology and results, clinical significance, and/or clear diagnostic criteria (Rifkin et al., 1986). Furthermore, the increased probability of antisocial behavior or conduct disorder in children with attention deficit disorder (Hechtman, 1985; Weiss, 1985) creates additional complexity in interpreting these studies.

The existence of major depression as a diagnostic entity in children and adolescents has been well accepted. Antisocial behavior as a form of "masked depression" in children has been described by Cytryn and McKnew (1972); Carlson and Cantwell (1980) reported a similar association between depression and conduct disorder in children and adolescents. In a study of 60 children and adolescents referred for depression, 18% were found to have concomitant affective disorder and conduct disorder (Marriage et al., 1986). Additionally, Geller et al. (1985) found that in both pre- and postpubertal subjects antisocial behaviors began after the onset of depressive features. Puig-Antich et al. (1978) found that in a group of prepubertal boys with concomitant major depression and conduct disorder, the depressive symptoms preceded the conduct disorder symptoms in four of the five cases. Puig-Antich et al. (1982) reported on another group of children with diagnoses of both major depression and conduct disorder; 11 of these 13 children had remission of conduct disorder symptoms following antidepressant response to a tricyclic. Thus, the use of antidepressants in juveniles with conduct disorder and accompanying depressive symptoms seems to be a reasonable treatment approach. The efficacy of antidepressants for the treatment of "pure" conduct disorder awaits further investigation.

Studies addressing the use of neuroleptics for aggression in children and adolescents generally yield positive findings. In double-blind studies, Cunningham et al. (1968) reported the effectiveness of haloperidol for aggressive, destructive children; Alderton and Hoddinott (1964) reported the effectiveness of thioridazine for aggressive, hyperactive children; and Campbell et al. (1982) found both haloperidol and chlorpromazine useful in the treatment of aggression in children. These afore-mentioned studies, however, refer to the treatment of aggressive children who may or may not have met criteria for conduct disorder. More recent double-blind studies have addressed the use of neuroleptics for aggression, specifically in conduct disorder, and the efficacy of haloperidol has been demonstrated (Werry and Aman, 1975; Campbell et al., 1984).

Several open studies support the use of lithium for children with such charac-teristics as unmanageability, aggressiveness, and impulsivity (Lena, 1979; Siassi, 1982). A controlled study by Sheard et al. (1976) also found lithium to be effective for aggression in a population of incarcerated males whose ages ranged from 16 to 24 years, some of whom might have met criteria for conduct disorder. In another open study, Delong and Aldershot (1987) reported limited success (15% response rate) in the use of lithium for children with conduct disorder. Finally, the use of lithium for aggression in children with conduct disorder was found to be superior to placebo—and as effective as haloperidol—in a double-blind study by Campbell et al. (1984).

Beta blockers have recently assumed an important role in the treatment of mental disorders, including aggressive behavior. In this regard, they have proved especially useful in aggressive patients with a variety of organic mental disorders. An open study by Kuperman and Stewart (1987) reported the use of propranolol to decrease aggressive outbursts in four of seven youthful subjects diagnosed with under-socialized aggressive conduct disorder. However, one of the responders had addi-tional diagnoses of attention deficit disorder and mental retardation.

Benzodiazepines are rarely if ever used in the treatment of aggressive conduct disorder. The adult literature is inconclusive regarding the use of benzodiazepines for aggression (Azcarate, 1975; Rogers and Waters, 1985). Brown and Sleator (1979) reported worsening of aggression in prisoners treated with diazepam or oxazepam. There does, however, appear to be a valid subgroup of delinquent youths who are "overinhibited" or "anxious" (Cavior and Schmidt, 1978). Whether antianxiety agents might be useful for this type of aggressive child remains to be investigated. The risk of these drugs being abused by the patient with conduct disorder is another important consideration.

In summary, there is great need for continued controlled studies to further define the pharmacologic treatment of aggression in children and adolescents with conduct disorder. Haloperidol and lithium have been shown to be useful in this population. Stimulants may have a role in treating aggressive conduct disorder with accom-panying signs of attention deficit disorder (i.e., impulsivity, hyperactivity). Antidepressants appear to be helpful in some conduct disorders with accompanying depressive symptomatology. Beta blockers and carbamazepine show some promise, but further controlled studies in rigorously defined populations are necessary. The efficacy of benzodiazepines in this population is unclear, and the risks of using these agents may outweigh the benefits in most patients.

ATTENTION DEFICIT HYPERACTIVITY DISORDER

Attention-deficit hyperactivity disorder (ADHD) is the current term for a chronic, heterogenous disorder characterized by developmentally inappropriate degrees of inattention, impulsiveness, and hyperactivity. Although aggression is not one of the *DSM-III-R* criteria for diagnosis, it is commonly observed in children and adolescents with ADHD (Cantwell, 1977; Loney et al., 1978; Prinz et al., 1981). The presence, meaning, and implications of aggression in ADHD was recently reviewed by Hinshaw (1987), who found considerable overlap in the behavioral dimensions of hyperactivity/attention deficits and aggression/conduct problems.

Psychostimulants (i.e., methylphenidate, dextroamphetamine, and pemoline) remain the cornerstone of pharmacologic treatment for ADHD, and their efficacy has been well established in over 100 double-blind studies (Gittelman-Klein and Klein, 1987). In addition to beneficial motor and cognitive effects, aggressive behavior is markedly improved with stimulants, as noted specifically in double-blind studies of decreased classroom disruption (Barkley, 1979; Whalen et al., 1979; 1981). Additionally, three well-designed double-blind studies (Arnold et al., 1978; Amery et al., 1984; Klorman et al., 1988) have demonstrated the efficacy of psychostimulants in controlling aggressive behavior in children with ADHD. Other studies have not relied on rigorous diagnosis: a placebo-controlled study found dextroamphetamine to be effective in reducing aggression in 28 juveniles with antisocial behavior (Maletzky, 1974); the aggressive youngsters most likely to respond had a history of "hyperactive behavior." Interestingly, Allen et al., (1975) concluded that the anti-aggressive effects of dextroamphetamine are independent of the activity-reducing effects in aggressive hyperactive children. Finally, it appears that the maximum benefits in behavioral control with methylphenidate occur at a higher dose than the cognitive effects (Sprague and Sleator, 1977; Porges and Smith, 1980). Cognitive performance may in fact be impaired at drug levels at which behavior is improved (Sprague and Sleator, 1977; Kupietz et al., 1982).

Tricyclic antidepressants have been demonstrated to be as effective or slightly less so than the stimulants in treatment of ADHD in numerous double-blind studies (Winsberg et al., 1972; Gittelman-Klein, 1974; Rapoport et al., 1974; Waizer et al., 1974; Yepes et al., 1977). The specific anti-aggressive effects of antidepressants in ADHD have generally not been addressed in these studies, although Winsburg et al. (1972) did find a preferential response to imipramine over methylphenidate in a group of hyperkinetic and aggressive children. Tricyclics may also prove useful in the presence of coexisting depression (Pliszka, 1987) or enuresis, or in children who prove refractory to or intolerant of stimulants.

The use of neuroleptics as an alternative treatment for ADHD is increasingly controversial, primarily due to the adverse side-effect profile of these agents. Moreover, aggression has not been specifically addressed in studies of neuroleptics in ADHD. Lithium has also occasionally been reported as useful in ADHD. One open study (Siassi, 1982) demonstrated a specific anti-aggressive effect of lithium in a heterogeneous group of aggressive children; 25% met diagnostic criteria for ADHD.

In summary, psychostimulants remain the mainstay of treatment in the aggressive child or adolescent with ADHD; their efficacy in this population is well-documented. The utility of tricyclics and lithium is far less clear, and further research is needed.

DEPRESSION

There is a developing consensus among clinicians and researchers that *DSM-III-R* criteria are generally valid for diagnosing depressive disorders in children and adolescents (Cytryn and McKnew, 1987; Mitchell et al., 1988). Children may frequently have somatic complaints, irritability, temper tantrums, and aggressive behaviors in addition to other adult depressive features.

As described above, there are complex links between depression and assaultiveness in children (Puig-Antich, 1982; Geller et al., 1985; Marriage et al., 1986). Although the exact relationship between depression and aggressive behaviors remains uncertain, it would appear that the potential for aggression is present in a significant minority of depressed children and adolescents. Thus, there is considerable evidence that the clinician should carefully evaluate aggressive children and adolescents for the presence of endogenous depression (Curry et al., 1988).

The use of tricyclic antidepressants in this age group has increased over the past decade; however, their efficacy is not as well established as in adult depression. There are a significant number of open trials generally suggesting the usefulness of imipramine, amitriptyline, desipramine, or nortriptyline in at least some depressed children, although aggression is not specifically addressed (Weller and Weller, 1984). However, as yet double-blind studies have not demonstrated superiority of these medications over placebo in children or adolescents; this may be related to inadequate dosages used, however (Puig-Antich et al., 1987).

In summary then, it would appear that despite much promise and anecdotal clinical experience, conclusive proof of the usefulness of tricyclics in this age group and especially of their usefulness for aggression in "pure" depressive illness remains elusive. There are no well-controlled studies of the use of Monoamine Oxidase (MAO) inhibitors in children and adolescents.

BIPOLAR AFFECTIVE DISORDER

Although *DSM-III-R* criteria for bipolar affective disorder are applicable to children, various authors have reported that psychotic symptoms and aggression are more prominent than in adults (McGlashan, 1988; Varanka et al., 1988). Adolescents with mania are sometimes difficult to distinguish from those with schizophrenia because of their florid psychotic presentation and atypical mood expressions, while those with hypomania can be confused with conduct disorders because of hostility, rebelliousness, or substance abuse (Carlson, 1985). Furthermore, bipolar disorder may not initially be recognized in the depressed child or adolescent: in one prospective study of 60 adolescents hospitalized for major depression, 20% developed mania in a 3- to 4-year follow-up period (Strober and Carlson, 1982).

Several recent studies (Delong and Aldershot, 1987; Varanka et al., 1988) have demonstrated the efficacy of lithium in bipolar children and adolescents. While no studies address aggression specifically, a trial of lithium along with other treatment modalities is reasonable in children and adolescents who present with bipolar features, especially if there is a family history of bipolar disorder or lithium responsiveness.

Finally, while the utility of carbamazepine in treating bipolar adults is well-established, there have been several reports of increased aggression in children and adolescents treated with this agent (Pleak et al., 1988; Myers and Carrera, 1989). Clearly, this phenomenon requires further investigation.

SCHIZOPHRENIA

Schizophrenia is one of the most severe clinical conditions encountered in child psychiatry. Aggressive behaviors is likely to be a frequent and distressing problem in children with schizophrenia: Inamdar et al. (1982) reported that two-thirds of the 51 adolescent schizophrenics he studied had histories of serious assaultive behavior against others.

Very few studies of treatment of children with *DSM-III-R* schizophrenia exist, and no controlled trials of psychotropic medication in specifically aggressive schizophrenic children have been reported to date. There is only one double-blind, placebo-controlled study of the use of neuroleptics in 75 schizophrenic adolescents; both loxapine and haloperidol were superior to placebo in alleviating schizophrenic symptomatology (Pool et al., 1976). A single-blind study by Realmuto et al. (1984) found thiothixene and thioridazine to be effective in controlling schizophrenic symptoms, but only half of the subjects were responders. Aggressive symptoms were not addressed directly in these studies. The risks of extrapyramidal side effects including tardive dyskinesia, and behavioral toxicity, including depression, irritability, temper tantrums and enuresis (Campbell, 1985), must be weighed against potential benefits when using neuroleptics in this population.

Although its use in adult schizophrenics has been increasingly studied of late, there have been no specific studies of the utility of lithium in childhood schizophrenia. However, Campbell et al. (1972) reported limited success with the use of lithium for symptoms of explosiveness, aggressiveness, hyperactivity, and psychotic speech in a group of ten severely disturbed children, six having the diagnosis of childhood schizophrenia.

In summary, although their utility in childhood and adolescent schizophrenia is not well established, the neuroleptics probably remain the pharmacologic treatment of choice in the aggressive schizophrenic child or adolescent, although they have not been studied specifically for aggression, and many children may not respond. Surprisingly, lithium has not been studied in this population.

ORGANIC MENTAL DISORDERS

Although less common than in adults, organic mental disorders are not rare in children and adolescents. Perhaps the most common etiology in this population is traumatic brain injury, either by mechanical trauma or anoxia. Other common etiologies include various metabolic derangements and degenerative illnesses. All of these illnesses can have quite diverse psychiatric presentations, from which aggression may arise for a variety of reasons. The clinician must, therefore, be alert to evidence of a specific phenomenologic syndrome in the aggressive, organically impaired child, since definitive therapy may be possible. For example, a child with an irritable depression and aggression secondary to metachromatic leukodystrophy might be treatment initially with antidepressant agents rather that with other agents such as neuroleptics or beta-blockers. Empirical approaches, as described below, should be employed only when no specific treatable syndrome can be identified.

Numerous authors (Maletzky and Klotter, 1974; Elliot, 1987; Eichelman, 1988) have described the so-called "episodic dyscontrol syndrome" in both children and adults, characterized by intermittent, uncontrollable fits of rage, typically precipitated by frustration. Elliot (1987) has maintained that an organic etiology may be implicated in the majority of such patients. Episodic dyscontrol is not however, a single diagnostic entity with uniform treatment and should be thought of as a purely descriptive term.

In terms of empirical treatment for aggression in the organically impaired child or adolescent, neuroleptics are probably the most commonly used agents. However, aside from aggression related to overt psychotic symptoms, there is little evidence to suggest a specific anti-aggressive effect to these agents. In practice, relatively high doses are generally necessary for treatment of aggression, and this anti-aggressive effect generally seems to be only a function of sedation (Miczek, 1987; Yudofsky et al., 1987). The use of these agents is further complicated by numerous risks. For example, children and adolescents are at high risk for development of tardive dyskinesia (Campbell et al., 1983), and neuroleptic agents may decrease the seizure threshold in epileptic patients (James, 1986). Finally, behavioral toxicity, as mentioned above, may be problematic. Therefore, neuroleptics should be considered only as a last resort in the empirical treatment of aggression in this population. If these agents are used, high potency agents seem to be best tolerated by children (Campbell, 1985), and the smallest effective dosages should be prescribed.

One double-blind study (Greendyke et al., 1986) and several case series (Elliot, 1977; Yudofsky et al., 1981; Greendyke et al., 1984) have demonstrated the safety and efficacy of the beta-adrenergic blocker propranolol in the empirical treatment of aggression or "episodic dyscontrol" in adults with a variety of organic mental disorders. These agents are frequently described as effective in patients for whom neuroleptic therapy has failed. Schreier (1979) first reported the utility of propranolol for children in an aggressive 12-year old with a history of encephalitis. Williams et al. (1982) and Kuperman and Stewart (1987) have since published studies of propranolol for aggression in organically impaired children and adolescents, and these studies reported success rates of 60 to 80%. The side effects noted were comparable to those noted in adults, including hypotension, bronchospasm, and depression.

Several authors have suggested an anti-aggressive effect of lithium in a variety of organic mental disorders, again primarily in adults (Williams and Goldstein, 1979; Yudofsky et al., (1987), although there have been no well-designed studies to date. It should be remembered that lithium may exacerbate some seizure disorders (Jus et al., 1973). Schiff et al. (1982), in fact, have reported increased aggression in an adult with temporal lobe epilepsy who was treated with lithium.

Benzodiazepines are occasionally considered in the treatment of these patients, although it is well documented that these agents may occasionally disinhibit organically impaired adults, increasing aggressive behavior (Salzman, 1988). Although not systematically studied in aggressive children and adolescents, the possibility of a paradoxical increase in aggression must be borne in mind should the clinician consider these agents.

In summary, both propranolol and lithium appear to show promise in the empirical treatment of the aggressive organically impaired child. Anticonvulsants, such as carbamazepine, have not been specifically studies in this population. Neuroleptics may be effective, but their efficacy may be merely a function of sedation, and their use is complicated by numerous side effects.

EPILEPSY

There has been a controversy about the exact relationship, if any, between aggression and seizures for many years, and this controversy shows few signs of resolution. In the course of any discussion of this subject, it must be remembered that epileptic patients have seizures due to underlying organic brain disease which may, in and of itself, be associated with aggression. To further complicate matters, such psychodynamically significant factors as severe physical abuse or serious injury may contribute to longstanding personality difficulties as well as to the development of a seizure disorder. Conversely, patients with personality difficulties may be at increased risk for head injury as a result of risk-taking behavior. Finally, the presence of an active seizure disorder may be, in and of itself, a significant psychodynamic stressor that may contribute to the development of aggressive behavior in children.

The question of whether a seizure may be accompanied by violent or criminal behavior has been of great concern for many years. The consensus of the literature is that ictal aggression is quite rare (Delgado-Escueta et al., 1981; Devinsky and Bear, 1984). When ictal aggression does occur, it almost invariably consists merely of non-directed swinging and/or fearful defensiveness (Delgado-Escueta et al., 1981; Devinsky and Bear, 1984; Treiman, 1986) and is hardly ever problematic if by-standers stay farther than at arm's reach from the seizing patient. Delgado-Escueta et al. (1981) reported seven patients with more sustained or directed ictal aggression, but all of these patients had a history of severe non-ictal aggression, as well as co-existing severe organic mental disorders. The treatment of ictal aggression consists of confirmation that it is indeed ictal, followed by treatment of the underlying seizure disorder.

The most common form of aggression in epileptic patients is post-ictal aggression. This consists simply of defensive aggression in reaction to post-ictal confusion, and clears rapidly. No treatment is necessary (Devinsky and Bear, 1984; Treiman, 1986).

The greatest controversy in this field concerns the nature and prevalence of inter-ictal aggression. Several authors have indicated a higher incidence of seizure disorders or EEG abnormalities in incarcerated adolescents (Lewis et al., 1982) and adults (Williams, 1969; Treiman, 1986), as well as in patients with a history of aggression (Eichelman, 1988), but this has also been demonstrated in prisoners with a history of non-violent crime and even socieconomically matched non-offenders (Treiman, 1986), suggesting the importance of coexistent organic and psychodynamic factors as mentioned above.

If the existence of pure inter-ictal aggression in the absence of underlying organic or functional psychopathology is not clear, then treatment of these patients is even less clear. Many studies have assumed the existence of this pure inter-ictal aggression, but these studies have looked collectively at epileptics, patients with non-specific EEG abnormalities, and even patients with symptoms of "episodic dyscontrol" but no EEG data (Reynolds, 1983). Traditionally, the anti-aggressive effects of anticonvulsant agents have been most studied in this population. Maletzky and Klotter (1974) initially reported that phenytoin was effective for "episodic dyscontrol" but no EEG data was reported. This has not been replicated since. The most recent reports concern the use of carbamazepine, although results have been mixed. The empirical use of carbamazepine in aggressive adolescents and adults with seizure foci, especially temporal lobe seizure foci, has shown promise (Yudofsky et al., 1987; Eichelman, 1988; Yathen and McHale, 1988), although it has not been systematically studied. Other authors (Bear and Fedio, 1977; Devinsky and Bear, 1984) have found carbamazepine to be effective in the treatment of inter-ictal aggression.

In summary, although not specifically studied in aggressive epileptic children and adolescents, carbamazepine may be a reasonable option in such patients with inter-ictal aggression when no other specific organic or functional psychopathology is evident, especially if a temporal lobe seizure focus is present. Carbamazepine has the additional advantage of potentially controlling both seizures and aggression in such patients. It is probably the treatment of choice in well-documented ictal aggression as well. Its use in non-epileptic children with normal EEGs or non-specific EEG abnormalities is far more dubious, and the risks of blood dyscrasias and a paradoxical increase in aggression, although low, must be kept in mind. Lithium and neuroleptics should be used with caution in epileptics, as they may decrease the seizure threshold.

MENTAL RETARDATION

The mentally retarded probably represent the most overmedicated and under-diagnosed segment of society. At least 40 to 50% of institutionalized mentally retarded patients and 25 to 35% of those in the community are treated chronically with psychotropic medications, mostly neuroleptics, and these figures are virtually the same for those under eighteen years of age (Intagliata and Rinck, 1985). In marked contrast, only 3% to 5% of these patients receive psychotropic medications for specific diagnoses; the vast majority are treated for "aggression," "overactive behavior," or simply "mental retardation" (Hill et al., 1985).

Mental retardation, per se, does not lead to aggression. However, mentally retarded patients are not immune to functional psychiatric illnesses which may lead to aggression. In fact, functional psychiatric illnesses are two to six times as common among the mentally retarded as in the general population (Matson, 1985) and generally respond to appropriate treatment. However, diagnosis becomes increasingly difficult as IQ decreases and the patient becomes less verbal. For example, bipolar illness may be manifested only by periods of hyperactivity and aggression alternating with periods of apathy and anorexia. Additionally, diagnostic issues become less important in severely and profoundly retarded patients (Gualtieri and Keppel, 1985), and treatment issues merge with those of the organic mental disorders.

In spite of extensive diagnostic efforts, frequently no specific treatable etiology for aggression will be found in a retarded child or adolescent. In these instances, empirical pharmacologic treatment may be pursued. The best studied and most commonly used agents for treatment of aggressive mentally retarded patients are the neuroleptics, with the majority of studies employing thioridazine. Although there are numerous reports of the efficacy of neuroleptics in aggression at low doses (Lipman, 1986), the prevalence of tardive dyskinesia in mentally retarded children and adolescents receiving neuroleptics is as high as 34% (Gualtieri et al., 1986), and exacerbation of seizure disorders and behavioral toxicity may be problematic. Additionally, several reports (Lipman, 1986) have noted impairment of cognitive function and work performance in mentally retarded patients treated with thioridazine. In light of this, neuroleptics should be used with caution in the treatment of aggression in the mentally retarded child or adolescent unless there is strong evidence suggestive of schizophrenia or another treatable psychosis, or in the rare case of intractable aggression unresponsive to all other behavioral and pharmacologic interventions.

Perhaps the most promising anti-aggressive agent studied in recent years for the mentally retarded patient is lithium. Three double-blind (Worrall et al., 1975; Tyrer et al., 1984; Craft et al., 1987) and numerous open (Dostal and Zvolsky, 1970; Goetzl et al., 1977; Dale, 1980; Sovner and Hurley, 1981) studies have demonstrated its safety and efficacy in the empirical treatment of aggression in this population. Although mostly used with adult patients, there are several reports of its utility in mentally retarded children and adolescents (Dostal and Zvolsky, 1970; Dale, 1980). The strongest predictors of response to lithium seem to be hyperactive behavior and emotional liability (Dostal and Zvolsky, 1970; Goetzl et al., 1977; Sovner and Hurley, 1981; Tyrer et al., 1984). It should be remembered, however, that lithium may exacerbate seizure disorders and enuresis (Dostal and Zvolsky, 1970). The clinician must also remember to closely monitor non-verbal patients for objective signs of lithium toxicity.

Beta-adrenergic blockers have also been studied in aggressive mentally retarded patients. Propranolol has been most studied in adults (Yudofsky et al., 1981; Ratey et al., 1986) as well as children and adolescents (Kuperman and Stewart, 1987). One must be especially diligent in monitoring the non-verbal patient for evidence of depression when using these agents.

Carbamazepine was shown to be effective in a group of 12 hyperactive, aggressive mentally retarded adults, independent of any history of seizures or EEG abnormality, in one double-blind study (Reid et al., 1981), and also in one mentally retarded adolescent (Rapport et al., 1983). There have been no other studies to date. Benzodiazepines have not been extensively studied in this population, although the same cautions about disinhibition that apply to organically impaired patients probably apply to the mentally retarded child or adolescent as well. Finally, although aggression has not been specifically addressed, Gadow (1985) has noted a good response to psychostimulants in mentally retarded children with evidence of coexistent ADHD, especially in those with relatively higher IQs.

In summary, the first step in managing an aggressive mentally retarded child or adolescent is accurate diagnosis. Failing identification of a definitively treatable condition, lithium, and neuroleptics are probably the most reasonable options for empirical treatment, although there are significant problems with the latter. Beta-blockers and carbamazepine seem to be promising agents, and clearly more studies are needed with these. Psychostimulants may be effective in selected patients with coexistent ADHD.

AUTISM

The pharmacologic treatment of autistic children and adolescents has been for the most part rather disappointing. Behavior modification is considered the treatment of choice for aggressive behavior in this population (Rutter, 1985), although pharmacotherapy may in some instances be a useful adjunct to treatment in refractory patients. It should be noted that 75% of autistic children are also mentally retarded, and that often a specific organic etiology for the autistic syndrome can be found (DeMyer, 1987). Thus, previously described treatment options may be appropriate for these patients as well.

Of all agents studied, low-dose neuroleptics remain the best studied agents in treating the hyperactive, agitated, and aggressive autistic child. Haloperidol is the best studied agent, and has been noted to decrease hyperactivity, agitation, and stereotypy (Campbell et al., 1978; Anderson et al., 1984; Joshi et al., 1988), as well as overt aggression (Joshi et al., 1988), in numerous well-designed studies. Dosages for children have been relatively low, and side effects have reportedly been limited to occasional dystonias and sedation at higher dosages (Campbell et al., 1978; Anderson et al., 1984; Joshi et al., 1988). These studies have not commented on the incidence of tardive dyskinesia or behavioral toxicity on this population, although there is no reason to believe that autistic children are immune to such effects. Most importantly, the use of haloperidol at these low dosages does not seem to impair cognitive function; in fact, one double-blind study has indicated an actual increase in language acquisition (Anderson et al., 1984). Neuroleptics seem most effective in hyperactive children; behavioral problems in hypoactive autistic children seem to be exacerbated by neuroleptics (Anderson et al., 1984).

Quite surprisingly, there have been virtually no studies on the use of lithium in aggressive autistic children. Kerbeshian et al. (1987) reported on two autistic children whose aggression responded dramatically to the use of lithium carbonate at serum levels greater than 1.0 mEq/L. Although the authors felt that there was evidence of an atypical bipolar illness in both children, one is reminded of the nonspecific antiaggressive effects of lithium in mentally retarded and organically impaired children. This is clearly an area for future controlled studies.

Although previously considered contraindicated in autistic children, several open studies have demonstrated the utility of psychostimulants in autistic children with coexistent hyperactivity and aggression (Geller et al., 1981; Birmaher et al., 1988). Previously reported increases in stereotypy have not been noted in these studies.

There has been a great deal of interest in the use of fenfluramine in autistic patients since initial reports suggested an increase in social interaction and intelligence with this drug (Ritvo et al., 1983; Stubbs et al., 1986). Although there is some evidence that fenfluramine may decrease hyperactivity and stereotypy somewhat (Stubbs et al., 1986), there is also evidence of increased irritability. Stubbs et al. (1986), in studying eight autistic children, noted increased irritability in five and overt aggression in two. More recently, a study by Campbell et al. (1988) of 28 autistic children failed to demonstrate the superiority of fenfluramine over placebo in their treatment.

In summary, low-dose haloperidol remains the best studied drug for treatment of aggression in autistic children, especially when accompanied by an overall hyperactive picture, although the incidence of adverse effects such as tardive dyskinesia has not been adequately addressed to date. Lithium has not been systematically studied. Psychostimulants may be helpful in patients with evidence of coexistent ADHD, although this population needs to be more clearly defined. Fenfluramine should be used with caution in children with autism, and its efficacy remains uncertain.

CONCLUDING REMARKS

The aggressive child or adolescent constitutes one of the most distressing and urgent referrals in child psychiatry. The consequences of aggressive behavior can be devastating to the child's family, his friends, his school, society at large, and especially to the child himself. The clinician who is well versed in the pharmacologic treatment of these disorders, and especially in the limitations of pharmacotherapy, will find the treatment of these patients especially rewarding.

REFERENCES

Alderton, H. R., & Hoddinott, B. A. (1964), A controlled study of the use of thioridazine in the treatment of hyperactive and aggressive children in a children's psychiatric hospital. *Canadian Psychiatric Association Journal*, 9:239–247.

Allen, R. P., Safer, D. & Covi, L. (1975), Effects of psychostimulants on aggression. *J. Nerv. Ment. Dis.*, 160:138–145.

Amery, B., Minichiello, M. D., & Brown, G. L. (1984), Aggression in hyperactive boys: response to d-amphetamine. *J. Am. Acad. Child Psychiatry*, 23:291–294.

Anderson, L. T., Campbell, M., Grega, D. M. et al. (1984), Haloperidol in the treatment of infantile autism: effects of learning and behavioral symptoms. *Am. J. Psychiatry*, 141:1195–1202.

Arnold, L. E., Christopher, J., Huestis, R. et al. (1978), Methylphenidate vs dextroamphetamine vs caffeine in minimal brain dysfunction. *Arch. Gen. Psychiatry*, 35:463–473.

Azcarate, C. L. (1975), Minor tranquilizers in the treatment of aggression. *J. Nerv. Ment. Dis.*, 160:100–107.

Barkley, R. A. (1979), Using stimulant drugs in the classroom. *School Psychology Review*, 8:412–425.

Bear, D. M. & Fedio, P. (1977), Quantitative analysis of inter-ictal behavior in temporal lobe epilepsy. *Arch. Neurol.*, 34:454–467.

Bender, L. & Cottington, F. (1942), The use of amphetamine sulfate in child psychiatry. *Am J. Psychiatry*, 99:116–121.

Birmaher, B., Quintana, H. & Greenhill, L. L. (1988), Methylphenidate treatment of hyperactive autistic children. *J. Am. Acad. Child Adolesc. Psychiatry*, 27:248–251.

Bradley, C.(1937), The behavior of children receiving benzedrine. *Am. J. Psychiatry*, 94:577–584.

Brown, R. T. & Sleator, E. K. (1979), Methylphenidate in hyperkinetic children: differences in dose effects on impulsive behavior. *Pediatrics*, 64:408–411.

Campbell, M., (1985), On the use of neuroleptics in children and adolescents. *Psychiatric Annals*, 15:101, 105–107.

Campbell, M., Fish, B., Korein, J. et al. (1972), Lithium and chlorpromazine: a controlled cross-over study of hyperactive severely disturbed young children. *Journal of Autism and Childhood Schizophrenia*, 2:234–263.

Campbell, M., Anderson, L. T., Meier, M. et al. (1978), A comparison of haloperidol and behavior therapy and their interaction in autistic children. *J. Am. Acad. Child Psychiatry*, 17:640–655.

Campbell, M., Cohen, I. L. & Small, A. M. (1982), Drugs in aggressive behavior. *Am. J. Child Psychiatry*, 21:107–117.

Campbell, M., Grega, D. M., Green, W. H., et al. (1983), Neuroleptic-induced dyskinesis in children. *Clin. Neuropharmacol.*, 6:207–222.

Campbell, M., Small, A. M., Green, W. H. et al. (1984), A comparison of haloperidol and lithium in hospitalized aggressive conduct disordered children. *Arch. Gen. Psychiatry*, 41:650–656.

Campbell, M., Adams, P., Small, A. M. et al. (1988), Efficacy and safety of fenfluramine in autistic children. *J. Am. Acad. Child Adolesc. Psychiatry*, 27:434–439.

Cantwell, D. (1977), Hyperkinetic syndrome. In: *Child Psychiatry: Modern Approaches*, ed. M. Rutter & L. Harsov. Oxford, England: Blackwell, pp. 524–555.

Carlson, G. A. (1985), Bipolar disorder in adolescence. *Psychiatric Annals*, 15: 375–386.

Carlson, G. & Cantwell, D. (1980), unmasking masked depression. *Am. J. Psychiatry*, 137:445–449.

Cavior, H. E. & Schmidt, A. A. (1978), Test of the effectiveness of a differential treatment strategy at the Robert F. Kennedy Center. *Criminal Justice and Behavior*, 5:131–139.

Conners, C. K., Kramer, R., Rothschild, G. H. et al. (1971), Treatment of young delinquent boys with diphenylhydantoin sodium and methylphenidate. *Arch. Gen. Psychiatry*, 24:156–160.

Craft, M., Ismail, I. A., Krishnamurti, D. et al. (1987), Lithium in the treatment of aggression in mentally handicapped patients. *Br. J. Psychiatry*, 150:685–689.

Cunningham, M. A., Pillai, V. & Blachford-Rogers, W. J. (1968), Haloperidol in the treatment of children with severe behavior disorders, *Br. J. Psychiatry*, 114:845–854.

Curry, J., Pelissier, B., Woodford, D., et al. (1988). Violent or assaultive youth: dimensional and categorical comparisons with mental health samples. *J. Am. Acad. Child Adolesc. Psychiatry*, 27:226–232.

Cytryn, L. & McKnew, D. (1972), Proposed classification of childhood depression. *Am. J. Psychiatry*, 129:148–155.

——————(1987), Treatment of childhood depression. In: *Basic Handbook of Child Psychiatry (Vol. V)*, ed. in chief J. Noshpitz. New York: Basic Books, pp. 439–443.

Dale, P. G. (1980), Lithium therapy in aggressive mentally subnormal patients. *Br. J. Psychiatry*, 137:469–474.

Delgado-Escueta, A. V., Mattson, R. H., King, L. et al. (1981), The nature of aggression during epileptic seizures. *N. Engl. J. Med.*, 305:711–716.

DeLong, G. R. & Aldershot, A. L. (1987), Long-term experience with lithium treatment in childhood: correlation with clinical diagnosis. *J. Am. Acad. Child Adolesc. Psychiatry*, 26:389–394.

DeMyer, M. K. (1987). Treatment of psychotic children. In: *Basic Handbook of Child Psychiatry (Vol. V)*, ed. in chief J. D. Noshpitz. New York: Basic Books, pp. 502–511.

Devinsky, O., & Bear, D. (1984), Varieties of aggressive behavior in temporal lobe epilepsy. *Am. J. Psychiatry*, 141:651–656.

Dostal, T. & Zvolsky, P. (1970), Anti-aggressive effect of lithium salts in severe mentally retarded adolescents. *International Pharmacopsychiatry*, 5:203–207.

Eichelman, B. (1988), Toward a rational pharmacotherapy for aggressive and violent behavior. *Hosp. Community Psychiatry*, 39:31–39.

Eisenberg, L., Lachman, R., Molling, P. et al. (1963). A psychopharmacologic experiment in a training setting for delinquent boys: methods, problems, findings. *Am. J. Orthopsychiatry*, 33:431–447.

Elliot, F. A. (1977), Propranolol for the control of belligerent behavior following acute brain damage. *Ann. Neurol.*, 1:489–491.

————1987, Neuroanatomy and neurology of aggression. *Psychiatric Annals*, 17:385–389.

Gadow, K. D. (1985), Prevalence and efficacy of stimulant drug use with mentally retarded children and youth. *Psychopharmacol. Bull.*, 21:291–303.

Geller, B., Guttmacher, L. B. & Bleeg, M. (1981), Coexistence of childhood onset pervasive development disorder and attention deficit disorder with hyperactivity. *Am. J. Psychiatry*, 138:388–389.

Geller, B., Chestnut, E., Miller, D. et al. (1985), Preliminary data on DSM-III associated features of major depressive disorder in children and adolescents. *Am. J. Psychiatry*, 142:643–644.

Gittelman-Klein, R. (1974), Pilot clinical trial of imipramine in hyperkinetic children. In: *Clinical Use of Stimulant Drugs in Children*, ed. C. K. Conners, Amsterdam: Excerpta Medica, pp. 192–201.

Gittelman-Klein, R. & Klein, D. F. (1987), Pharmacotherapy of childhood hyperactivity: an update. In: *Psychopharmacology: The Third Generation of Progress*, ed. H. Y. Meltzer. New York: Raven Press, pp. 215–1221.

Goetzl, Grunberg, F. & Berkowitz, B. (1977), Lithium carbonate in the management of hyperactive aggressive behavior of the mentally retarded. *Compr. Psychiatry*, 18:599–606.

Greendyke, R. M., Schuster, D. B. & Wooton, J. A. (1984), Propranolol in the treatment of assaultive patients with organic brain disease. *J. Clin. Psychopharmacol.*, 4:282–285.

Greendyke, R. M., Kantner, D. R., Schuster, D. B. et al. (1986), Propranolol treatment of assaultive patients with organic brain disease: a double-blind crossover, placebo-controlled study. *J. Nerv. Ment. Dis.*, 174:290–294.

Gualtieri, C. T. & Keppel, J. M. (1985), Psychopharmacology in the mentally retarded and a few related issues. *Psychopharmacol. Bull.*, 21:304–309.

Gualtieri, G. T., Schroeder, S. R., Hicks, R. E. et al. (1986), Tardive dyskinesia in young mentally retarded individuals. *Arch. Gen. Psychiatry*, 43:335–340.

Hechtman, L. (1985), Adolescent outcome of hyperactive children treated with stimulants in childhood: a review. *Psychopharmacol. Bull.*, 21:178–191.

Hill, B. K., Barlow, E. A. & Bruininks, R. H. (1985), A national study of prescribed drugs in institutions and community residential facilities for mentally retarded people. *Psychopharmacol. Bull.*, 21:279–284.

Hinshaw, S. P. (1987), On the distinction between attentional deficits/hyperactivity and conduct problems/aggression in child psychopathology. *Psychopharmacol. Bull.*, 101:443–463.

Inamdar, S. C., Lewis, D. O., Siomopoulis, G. et al. (1982), Violent and suicidal behavior in psychotic adolescents. *Am. J. Psychiatry*, 139:932–935.

Intagliata, J. & Rinck, C. (1985), Psychoactive drug use in public and community residential facilities for mentally retarded persons. *Psychopharmacol. Bull.*, 21:268–278.

James, D. H. (1986), Neuroleptics and epilepsy in mentally handicapped patients. *J. Ment. Defic. Res.*, 30:185–189.

Joshi, P. T., Capozzoli, J. A. & Coyle, J. T. (1988), Low-dose neuroleptic therapy for children with childhood-onset pervasive development disorder. *Am. J. Psychiatry*, 145:335–338.

Jus, A., Villeneuve, A., Gautier, J. et al. (1973), Some remarks on the influence of lithium carbonate on patients with temporal lobe epilepsy. *Int. J. Clin. Pharmacol. Ther. Toxicol.*, 7:67–74.

Kerbeshian, J., Burd, L. & Fisher, W. (1987), Lithium carbonate in the treatment of two patients with infantile autism and atypical bipolar symptomatology. *J. Clin. Psychopharmacol.*, 7:401–405.

Klorman, R., Brumaghim, J. T., Salzman, L. F. et al. (1988), Effects of methylphenidate on attention-deficit hyperactivity disorders with and without aggressive/noncompliant features. *J. Abnorm. Psychol.* 97:413–422.

Kuhn-Gebhart, V. (1976), Behavioral disorders in non-epileptic children and their treatment with carbamazepine. In: *Epileptic Seizure-Behavior-Pain, International Symposium at St. Moritz*, ed. W. Birkmayer. Baltimore: University Park Press, pp. 264–276.

Kuperman, S. & Stewart, M. A. (1987), Use of propranolol to decrease aggressive outbursts in younger patients. *Psychosomatics*, 28:315–319.

Kupietz, S. S., Winsberg, B. G. & Sverd, I. (1982), Learning ability and methyphenidate (Ritalin) plasma concentration in hyperactive children: a preliminary investigation. *J. Am. Acad. Child Psychiatry*, 21:27–30.

Lefkowitz, M. M. (1969), Effects of diphenylhydantoin on disruptive behavior: study of male delinquents. *Arch. Gen. Psychiatry*, 20:63–651.

Lena, B. (1979), Lithium therapy in hyperaggressive behavior in adolescence. In: *Psychopharmacology of Aggression*, ed. M. Sandler. New York: Raven Press, pp. 197–203.

Lewis, D. O., Pincus, J. H., Shanok, S. S., et al. (1982), Psychomotor epilepsy and violence in a group of incarcerated adolescent boys. *Am. J. Psychiatry*, 139:882–887.

Lipman, R. A. (1986), Overview of research in psychopharmacological treatment of the mentally ill/mentally retarded. *Psychopharmacol. Bull.*, 22:1046–1054.

Loney, J., Langhorne, J. E. & Paternite, C. E. (1978), An empirical basis for subgrouping the hyperkinetic/minimal brain dysfunction syndrome. *J. Abnorm. Psychol.*, 87:431–441.

Looker, A. & Conners, C. K. (1970), Diphenylhydantoin in children with severe temper tantrums. *Arch. Gen. Psychiatry*, 23:80–89.

Maletzky, B. M., (1974), D-amphetamine and delinquency: hyperkinesis persisting? *Diseases of the Nervous System*, 35:543–547.

Maletzky, B. M. & Klotter, J. (1974), Episodic dyscontrol: a controlled replication. *Disease of the Nervous System*, 35:175–179.

Marriage, K., Fine, S., Moretti, M. et al. (1986), Relationship between depression and conduct disorder in children and adolescents. *J. Am. Acad. Child Adolesc. Psychiatry*, 25:687–691.

Matson, J. L. (1985), Emotional problems in the mentally retarded: the need for assessment and treatment. *Psychopharmacol. Bull.*, 21:258–261.

McGlashan, T. (1988), Adolescent versus adult onset of mania. *Am. J. Psychiatry*, 145:221–223.

Miczek, K. A. (1987), The psychopharmacology of aggression. In: *Handbook of*

Psychopharmacology, Vol. 19, ed. L. L. Iversen, S. D. Iversen & S. H. Snyder. New York: Plenum Press, pp. 183–328.

Mitchell, J., McCauley, E., Burke, P. et al. (1988), Phenomenology of depression in children and adolescent. *J. Am. Acad. Child Adolesc. Psychiatry*, 27:12–20.

Myers, W. C. & Carrera, F. (1989), Carbamazepine-induced mania with hypersexuality in a 9-year old boy. *Am. J. Psychiatry*, 146:400.

O'Donnell, D. J. (1985), Conduct disorders. In: *Diagnosis and Psychopharmacology of Childhood and Adolescent Disorders*, ed. J. M. Weiner. New York: Basic Books, pp. 249–287.

Pleak, R. R., Birmaher, B., Gavrilescu, A. et al. (1988), Mania and neuropsychiatric excitation following carbamazepine. *J. Am. Acad. Child Adolesc. Psychiatry*, 27:500–503.

Pliszka, S. R. (1987), Tricyclic antidepressants in the treatment of children with attention deficit disorder. *J. Am. Acad. Child Adolesc. Psychiatry*, 26:127–132.

Pool, D., Bloom, W., Mielke, D. H. et al. (1976), A controlled evaluation loxitane in seventy-five adolescent schizophrenic patients. *Current Therapeutic Research Clinical and Experimental*, 19:99–104.

Porges, S. W. & Smith, K. M. (1980), Defining hyperactivity: psychophysiological and behavioral strategies. In: *Hyperactive Children*, ed. C. K. Whalen & B. Henker. New York: Academic Press, pp. 75–104.

Prinz, R. J., Conner, P. A. & Wilson, C. C. (1981), Hyperactive and aggressive behaviors in childhood: intertwined dimensions. *J. Abnorm. Child Psychol.*, 9:191–202.

Puig-Antich, J. (1982), Major depression and conduct disorder in prepuberty. *J. Am. Acad. Child Psychiatry*, 21:118–128.

Puig-Antich, J., Blau, S., Marx, N. et al. (1978), Prepubertal major depressive disorder. *J. Am. Acad. Child Psychiatry*, 17:695–707.

Puig-Antich, J., Perel, J., Lupatkin, W. et al. (1987), Imipramine in prepubertal major depressive disorders. *Arch. Gen. Psychiatry*, 44:81–89.

Quay, H. C. (1987), Patterns of delinquent behavior: In: *Handbook of Juvenile Delinquency*, ed. H. C. Quay. New York: Wiley, pp. 118–138.

Rapport, J. L., Quinn, P. O., Bradbard, G. et al. (1974), Imipramine and methylphenidate treatments of hyperactive boys. *Arch. Gen. Psychiatry*, 30:789–793.

Rapport, M. D., Sonis, W. A., Fialkov, M. J. et al. (1983), Carbamazepine and behavior therapy for aggressive behavior. *Behav. Modif.*, 7:255–265.

Ratey, J. J., Mikkelsen, E.J., Smith, G. B. et al. (1986), Beta-blockers in the severely and profoundly mentally retarded. *J. Clin. Psychopharmacol.*, 6:103–107.

Realmuto, G. M., Erickson, W. D., Yellin, A. M. et al. (1984), Clinical comparison of thiothixene and thioridazine in schizophrenic adolescents. *Am. J. Psychiatry*, 141:440–442.

Reid, A. H., Naylor, G. J. & Kay, D. S. (1981), A double-blind, placebo-controlled, cross-over trial of carbamazepine in overactive, severely mentally handicapped patients. *Psycol. Med.*, 11:109–113.

Remschmidt, H. (1976), The psychotropic effect of carbamazepine in non-epileptic patients with particular reference to problems posed by clinical studies. In: *Epileptic Seizure-*

Behavior-Pain, International Symposium at St. Moritz, ed. W. Birkmayer. Baltimore: University Park Press, pp. 253–258.

Reynolds, E. H. (1983), Interictal behavior in temporal lobe epilepsy, Br. Med. J., 286:918–919.

Rifkin, A., Wortman, R., Reardon, G., et al. (1986), Psychotropic medication in adolescents: a review. *J. Clin. Psychiatry*, 47:400–408.

Ritvo, E. R., Freeman, B. J., Geller, E. et al. (1983), Effects of fenfluramine on 14 outpatients with the syndrome of autism. *J. Am. Acad. Child Psychiatry*, 22:549–558.

Rogers, R. J. & Waters, A. N. (1985), Benzodiazepines and their antagonists: a pharmacothological analysis with particular reference to effects on "aggression." *Neurosci. Biobehav. Rev.*, 9:21–35.

Rutter, M. (1985), Infantile autism and other pervasive developmental disorders. In: *Child and Adolescent Psychiatry: Modern Approaches (2nd Ed.)*, ed. M. Rutter & L. Hersov. St. Louis: Blackwell Scientific Publications, pp. 545–566.

Salzman, C. (1988), Treatment of agitation, anxiety, and depression dementia. *Psychopharmacol. Bull.*, 24:39–42.

Schiff, H. B., Sabin, T. D., Geller, A. et al. (1982), Lithium in aggressive behavior. *Am. J. Psychiatry*, 139:1346–1348.

Schreier, H. A. (1979), Use of propranolol in treatment of post-encephalitic psychosis. *Am. J. Psychiatry*, 136:840–841.

Sheard, M. H., Marini, J. L. & Bridges, C. I. (1976), The effect of lithium on impulsive aggression (or aggressive behavior) in man. *Am. J. Psychiatry*, 133:1409–1413.

Siassi, I. (1982), Lithium treatment of impulsive behavior in children. *J. Clin. Psychiatry*, 43:482–484.

Sovner, R. & Hurley, A. (1981), The management of chronic behavior disorders in mentally retarded adults with lithium carbonate. *J. Nerv. Ment. Dis.*, 169:191–195.

Sprague, R. L., & Sleator, E. K. (1977), Methylphenidate in hyperkinetic children: differences in dose effects on learning and social behavior. *Science*, 198:1274–1276.

Strober, M. & Carlson, G. (1982), Bipolar illness in adolescents with major depression. *Arch. Gen. Psychiatry*, 39:549–555.

Stubbs, E. G., Budden, S. S., Jackson, R. H. et al. (1986), Effects of fenfluramine on eight outpatients with the syndrome of autism. *Dev. Med. Child Neurol.*, 28:229–235.

Treiman, D. M. (1986), Epilepsy and violence: medical and legal issues. *Epilepsia*, 27(Suppl. 2):S77–S104.

Tyrer, S. P., Walsh, A., Edwards, D. E. et al. (1984), Factors associated with a good response to lithium in aggressive mentally handicapped subjects. *Prog. Neuropsychopharmacol. Biol. Psychiatry*, 8:751–755.

Varanka, T., Weller, R., Weller, E. et al. (1988), Lithium treatment of manic episodes with psychotic features in prepubertal children. *Am. J. Psychiatry*, 145:1557–1559.

Waizer, J., Hoffman, S., Polizos, P. et al. (1974), Outpatient treatment of hyperactive school children with imipramine. *Am. J. Psychiatry*, 131:587–591.

Weiss, G. (1985), Follow-up studies on outcome of hyperactive children. *Psychopharmacol. Bull.*, 21:169–177.

Weller, R. & Weller, E. (1984), Use of tricyclic antidepressants in prepubertal depressed children. In: *Current Perspectives on Major Depression Disorders in Children*, ed. E. Weller & R. Weller. Washington, DC: American Psychiatric Press, pp. 50–63.

Werry, J. S. & Aman, M. G. (1975), Methylphenidate and haloperidol in children. *Arch. Gen. Psychiatry*, 32:790–795.

Whalen, C. K., Henker, B. E., Finck, D. et al. (1979), A social ecology of hyperactive boys: medication effects in structured classroom environments. *J. Appl. Behav. Annal.*, 12:65–81.

——————————(1981), Medication effects in the classroom: three naturalistic indicators. *J. Abnorm. Child Psychol.* 9:419–433.

Williams, D. (1969), Neural factors related to habitual aggression: consideration of differences between those habitual aggressive and others who have committed crimes of violence. *Brain*, 92:503–520.

Williams, D. T., Mehl, R., Yudofsky, S., et al. (1982), The effect of propranolol on uncontrolled rage outbursts in children and adolescents with organic brain dysfunction. *J. Am. Acad. Child Psychiatry*, 21:129–135.

Williams, K. H. & Goldstein, G. (1979), Cognitive and affective responses to lithium in patients with organic brain syndrome. *Am. J. Psychiatry*, 136:800–803.

Winsberg, B. G., Bialer, A., Kupietz, S. et al. (1972), Effects of imipramine and dextroamphetamine on behavior of neuropsychiatrically impaired children. *Am. J. Psychiatry*, 128:1425–1431.

Worrall, E. P., Moody, J. P. & Naylor, G. J. (1975), Lithium in nonmanic-depressives, antiaggressive effect and red blood cell lithium values *Br. J. Psychiatry*, 126:464–468.

Yatham, L. N. & McHale, P. A. (1988), Carbamazepine in the treatment of aggression: a case report and a review of the literature. *Acta. Psychiatr. Scand.*, 78:188–190.

Yepes, L., Balka, E., Winsberg, B. et al. (1977), Amitriptyline and methylphenidate treatment of behaviorally disordered children. *J. Child Psychol. Psychiatry*, 18:39–52.

Yudofsky, S., Williams, D. & Gorman, J. (1981), Propranolol in the treatment of rage and violent behavior in patients with chronic brain syndromes. *Am. J. Psychiatry*, 138:218–220.

——————Silver, J. M. & Schneider, S. E. (1987), Pharmacologic treatment of aggression. *Psychiatric Annals*, 17:397–406.

Part VII

PSYCHOSOCIAL ISSUES

The issues addressed in this section are of importance not only to those charged with the care and treatment of children and adolescents, but also to those whose responsibilities include the formulation of public policy. In the first paper, Shedler and Block add a longitudinal perspective to our understanding of the causes and correlates of drug use among adolescents. The findings of this carefully conducted investigation of the relation between psychological characteristics and drug use in 101 subjects who were studied from preschool to late adolescence raise serious questions about current approaches to drug prevention.

On the basis of drug use information collected from 18-year-olds, subjects were divided into nonoverlapping groups of frequent drug users, experimenters, and abstainers. Q-sort descriptions of personality characteristics of both abstainers and frequent users differed significantly (albeit in different ways) from the psychologically healthier group of adolescents who had used marijuana experimentally. Adolescents who used drugs frequently were alienated interpersonally, showed poor impulse control, and manifested emotional distress, whereas those who by age 18 had never experimented with any drug were relatively anxious, emotionally constricted, and lacking in social skills. Moreover, psychological differences between the groups were evident during childhood. When compared with experimenters, frequent users were judged to be relatively insecure, unable to form healthy relationships, and emotionally distressed as children, whereas abstainers were judged to be relatively anxious, inhibited, and morose as children. Additionally, both frequent users and abstainers were judged to have received poorer maternal parenting than experimenters, as assessed by direct observations of mother-child interactions when the subjects were five years old. In comparison with the mothers of experimenters, both the mothers of frequent users and the mothers of abstainers were perceived to be cold, critical, pressuring, and unresponsive to their children's needs.

In a thoughtful discussion examining the implications of the findings for theory and social policy, the authors underscore the importance of distinguishing between experimentation and abuse, noting that patterns of drug use in adolescence are not adequately explained in terms of peer influence, but rather, they have developmental antecedents. The widely held assumption that abstinence is categorical evidence of psychological health, is persuasively questioned, as is the effectiveness of drug prevention programs aimed at discouraging experimentation. Serious consideration needs to be given to the alternative proposal that society's limited resources be invested in interventions focusing on the personality syndrome underlying problem drug use.

New Zealand's freedom from nuclear weaponry has been legislatively guaranteed since the mid-eighties. Oliver, utilizing data derived from interviews and question-naires, has assessed the impact of this "experiment in public policy" on New Zealand youth. Responses indicate that in comparison with lower efficacy percep-tions of young people in other countries New Zealanders between the ages of nine and 18 years strongly believe that ordinary adults and even very small nations are able to effectively influence the process of nuclear weapons reduction and war pre-vention. However, with the exception of those who were close to adults active in the "nuclear free" movement, this sense of efficacy does not generalize to a personal level for most young people. Oliver's conclusion that direct exposure to effective adult models is required if young people are to acquire a belief in their own ability to help shape the future, to gain a sense of social responsibility in general, is of impor-tance to all concerned with the development of a responsible citizenry.

The study by Lee, Brooks-Gunn, Schnur, and Liaw examines the sustained effects of Project Head Start for disadvantaged black children into kindergarten and first grade. Children who participated in generic Head Start programs in two American cities in 1969–1970 were compared with those who had no preschool experience or those who attended other preschool programs. Why is there yet another study of the effectiveness of Head Start? As the authors underscore, this study has advantages over other Head Start impact studies. Both preprogram back-ground and cognitive differences were controlled in a covariance analysis design, using dependent measures in the cognitive, verbal, and social domains. The findings are consistent with those of earlier reports, indicating that strong effects favoring Head Start, relative to both comparison groups at the end of the preschool year have been attenuated, but not completely dissipated by the end of the first grade. The importance of this report lies in the finely reasoned section on implications in which the authors highlight Zigler's assertion, "We simply cannot inoculate children in 1 year against the ravages of a life of deprivation" (*Annual Progress*, 1988, p. 171).

As concerns about the effectiveness of American education are increasingly the focus of public debate, the findings of this study provide solid scientific evidence in support of the assertion that this nation cannot salve its conscience only through the provision of preschool experience.

In the final paper in this section, Hersov surveys the history of adoption, noting changing trends in adoption practices. Until fairly recently, adoption was considered primarily a service for childless couples to provide them with a child of their own to cement the marriage and meet the adults' emotional needs. Currently, however, adoption is increasingly seen as a form of child care, one of several ways of bringing up children whose parents are unable or unwilling to look after them. As a conse-quence, criteria for placement have shifted—any child in need can be considered for adoption regardless of color, family history, state of health or handicap, and level of intelligence. Transracial adoptions have increased in number, as have adoptions of older children. Increasingly, single persons of both sexes have sought to become adoptive parents. Hersov observes that the outcome for adopted children is generally good, although they are overrepresented in clinical populations. As older children with histories of severe deprivation, neglect, abuse, and institutionalization are placed, this trend is likely to continue, thereby increasing the risk of adoption disruption.

Hersov's summary of developmental studies of "telling," are of particular value to professionals advising parents regarding the timing and content of adoptive status. Sensitivity to the developmental course of a child's capacity to comprehend and integrate knowledge regarding his or her adoptive status may well forestall some of the problems of behavior and relationships that commonly arise in adoptive families during late childhood and early adolescence.

27

Adolescent Drug Use and Psychological Health: A Longitudinal Inquiry

Jonathan Shedler and Jack Block

University of California, Berkeley

The relation between psychological characteristics and drug use was investigated in subjects studied longitudinally, from preschool through age 18. Adolescents who had engaged in some drug experimentation (primarily with marijuana) were the best-adjusted in the sample. Adolescents who used drugs frequently were maladjusted, showing a distinct personality syndrome marked by interpersonal alienation, poor impulse control, and manifest emotional distress. Adolescents who, by age 18, had never experimented with any drug were relatively anxious, emotionally constricted, and lacking in social skills.

Psychological differences between frequent drug users, experimenters, and abstainers could be traced to the earliest years of childhood and related to the quality of parenting received. The findings indicate that (a) problem drug use is a symptom, not a cause, of personal and social maladjustment, and (b) the meaning of drug use can be understood only in the context of an individual's personality structure and developmental history. It is suggested that current efforts at drug prevention are misguided to the extent that they focus on symptoms, rather than on the psychological syndrome underlying drug abuse.

Drug abuse among young people is one of the greatest challenges of our time. Almost daily, we are besieged by media reports of drug-related tragedy,

Reprinted with permission from *American Psychologist*, 1990, Vol. 45, No. 5, 612–630. Copyright © 1990 by the American Psychological Association, Inc.

The study was supported by National Institute of Mental Health Grant MH 16080 to Jack and Jeanne H. Block.

Correspondence concerning this article should be addressed to Jonathan Shedler or Jack Block, Department of Psychology, University of California, Berkeley, CA 94720.

of shootings in our schools, gang warfare, and overdose-related deaths. Many see the drug problem as epidemic (Robins, 1984). As an increasing share of society's resources is diverted toward coping with the drug problem and its consequences, the need for sound, scientific information on the factors contributing to drug use is urgent.

Considerable research has already been directed toward studying the causes and correlates of drug use, and important recognitions have developed (for reviews, see Bush & Iannotti, 1985; Cox, 1985; Hawkins, Lishner, & Catalano, 1985; Jessor, 1979; Jones & Battjes, 1985; Kandel, 1980). Nevertheless, many studies to date have been interpretively constrained by various research-design or empirical limitations.

Large-scale epidemiological studies (e.g., Jessor, Chase, & Donovan, 1980; Johnston, O'Malley, & Bachman, 1984, 1986; National Institute on Drug Abuse [NIDA], 1986) have provided much-needed information about the prevalence and patterns of drug use, about the demographics of drug users, and about certain psychosocial characteristics of drug users. In general, however, these studies have been unable to provide the kind of in-depth, psychologically rich, clinically oriented information needed to inform intervention efforts. And by their very nature, cross-sectional studies and panel studies of relatively brief duration can offer only limited or confounded understandings of the antecedents of drug use.

Recognizing the crucial importance of prospective inquiry into the psychological antecedents of drug use, a number of longitudinal studies of adolescent development have been undertaken and have deepened our understanding of the interplay of psychosocial forces during adolescence (e.g., Brook, Gordon, & Whiteman, 1985; Brook, Whiteman, Gordon, & Cohen, 1986; Jessor & Jessor, 1977, 1978; Smith & Fogg, 1978; see Kandel, 1978, for a review). In general, however, these studies have also been interpretively constrained because they have studied adolescents already well along in years (subjects have rarely been younger than age 13) and because they have tended to track these adolescents for no more than three or four years, from junior high school into high school or from high school into college. Also, these studies have tended to depend, perhaps too heavily, on self-administered, mailed, or impersonally offered questionnaires.

To date, only two *truly* long-term investigations into the childhood antecedents of drug use have appeared. The Woodlawn study of Kellam and his associates (Kellam, Branch, Agrawal, & Ensminger, 1975; Kellam, Brown, Rubin, & Ensminger, 1983) traced the development of a group of poor, Black, urban children beginning at ages 6 to 7. In the Woodlawn study, Kellam et al. found that psychological characteristics assessed at ages 6 to 7 foretold drug use at ages 16 to 17, a decade later. The longitudinal study initiated by Jeanne and Jack Block (see J. H. Block & J. Block, 1980) followed a group of San Francisco Bay area children from nursery school on and found numerous, theoretically coherent relations between psychological characteristics assessed in nursery school and subsequent drug use in early adolescence, at age 14 (Block, Block & Keyes, 1988). These studies converge in demonstrating the existence of important psychological antecedents of drug use, antecedents dating to the earliest years of childhood. Conjointly, they suggest that early psychological factors may be central to an understanding of drug use, and they highlight the need for prospective research.

The present study further reports on the Block and Block sample, studied again in late adolescence when the subjects had reached age 18. This later age represents a different developmental era, one in which the implications of drug use and nonuse can well take on psychological significance different from the significance of drug use and nonuse in early adolescence. The findings we report span 13 years, from preschool through age 18. By virtue of their prospective nature, these data allow inferences about the antecedents of drug use that cannot be made from retrospective, cross-sectional, or short-term panel studies.

Beyond the length of time spanned by the present investigation, the study differs from previous studies in two important ways. In most empirical studies, psychological descriptions are limited to a small number of variables that are selected by researchers on a priori grounds. In the present study, psychological descriptions are, for all practical purposes, comprehensive and open-ended. They are based on extensive evaluations of participants by panels of psychologists, and they encompass the full range of constructs subsumed by the California Adult Q-sort (CAQ; Block, 1961/1978) and the California Child Q-sort (CCQ; J. Block & J. H. Block, 1980)—personality assessment instruments specifically designed to allow clinicians to provide in-depth, comprehensive psychological descriptions. The intention was to gather information psychologically rich enough to speak to clinical concerns and to inform intervention efforts.

The study also differs from previous studies in its approach to data analysis. Previous investigators have tended to assume (and test for) linear relations between level of drug use and measures of psychosocial disturbance. In effect, such an approach assumes that occasional experimentation with drugs is psychologically problematic, if not quite as problematic as regular use, and that complete avoidance of drugs is psychologically optimal.

However, the majority of young adults in the United States, nearly two thirds, have experimented with marijuana at one time or another (Johnston et al., 1986; Johnston, Bachman, & O'Malley, 1981a, 1981b; Miller et al., 1983; NIDA, 1986), and the vast majority of these young people do not subsequently become drug *abusers*. Little is known about the relative psychosocial adjustment of adolescents who have experimented with drugs on an occasional basis and of adolescents who have avoided drugs entirely. Indeed, a number of researchers have suggested that occasional drug use among adolescents may be best understood as a manifestation of *developmentally appropriate* experimentation. Newcomb and Bentler (1988), for example, have observed that

> one defining feature of adolescence is a quest for or establishment of independence and autonomous identity and functioning. This may involve experimentation with a wide range of behaviors, attitudes, and activities before choosing a direction and way of life to call one's own. This process of testing attitudes and behavior may include drug use. In fact, experimental use of various drugs, both licit and illicit, *may be considered a normative behavior among United States teenagers in terms of prevalence, and from a developmental task perspective.* (p. 214, emphasis added)

These empirical and developmental considerations suggest that the relations between psychological variables and level of drug use may not be linear at all. To the extent that drug experimentation may represent normative behavior during the prolonged adolescent period, as individuals seek a sense of self and possibility, it may be wrong to pathologize adolescents who experiment with drugs by assuming that they fall between nonusers and drug abusers on a continuum of psychosocial adjustment. To evaluate this conceptual possibility in the present study, we identify and contrast discrete groups of nonusers, experimenters, and frequent drug users. Additionally, we employ quadratic regression methods to formally test for curvilinear relations, when the data indicate that such relations may exist. These approaches permit the emergence of findings not discernible through conventional correlational methods with their assumption of linearity.

METHOD

Subjects

Subjects were 101 18-year-olds, 49 boys and 52 girls, from an initial sample of 130 participating in a longitudinal study of ego and cognitive development. The subjects were initially recruited into the study at age 3, while attending either a university-run nursery school or a parent-cooperative nursery school in the San Francisco Bay area. They were assessed on wide-ranging batteries of psychological measures at ages 3, 4, 5, 7, 11, 14, and 18 (see J. H. Block & J. Block, 1980, for an extended description of the study). Because so few subjects were lost over the years, there can be little influence of differential attrition.

The subjects live primarily in urban settings and are heterogeneous with respect to social class and parent education. About two thirds are White, one fourth are Black, and one twelfth are Asian. Not all subjects are used in all analyses to be reported, as will be discussed.

Measuring Drug Use

Information about drug use was collected at age 18 during individual interviews with the subjects. Skilled clinicians conducted these interviews, which ranged over a variety of topics including schoolwork, peer relations, family dynamics, personal interests, dating experiences, and so on. Total interview time was typically four hours per subject, and all interviews were videotaped.

The subjects were asked whether they "smoked pot or used it in another form." Their responses were coded from the interview videotapes as follows: (0) never used marijuana; (1) used once or twice; (2) used a few times; (3) used once a month; (4) used once a week; (5) used two or three times a week; and (6) used daily. The subjects were also given a list of other substances and were asked to check which (if any) they had used at least once on a "recreational" basis. The list included inhalants (e.g., glue, nitrous oxide), cocaine, hallucinogens, barbiturates, amphetamines, tranquilizers, heroin, and an open-ended category for "other" drugs not specifically listed.

Although self-report data on drug use are always subject to underreporting, the findings of a number of investigations indicate that such data have high validity (e.g., Block et al., 1988; Haberman, Josephson, Zanes, & Elinson, 1972; Jessor & Jessor, 1977; Perry, Killen, & Slinkard, 1980; Single, Kandel, & Johnston, 1975). Additionally, there is every reason to believe that the subjects in this investigation answered our questions honestly. The interviewers were skilled in gaining rapport and in eliciting information without inducing discomfort. Moreover, the subjects had been involved in the longitudinal study from earliest childhood; they not only had been assured that their individual responses would be held in confidence, but they knew from years of prior experience that this promise had been honored.

Measuring Personality

Age 18 assessment. At age 18, the personality characteristics of each subject were described by four psychologists, using the standard vocabulary of the California Adult Q-sort (Block, 1961/1978). The CAQ is a personality assessment instrument that allows psychologists to provide comprehensive personality descriptions in a conceptually systematic, quantifiable, and readily comparable form. The CAQ consists of 100 personality-descriptive statements, each printed on a separate index card. The psychologist sorts these statements into a fixed nine-step distribution, according to their evaluated salience via-á-vis the person being described. Thus, the CAQ yields a score of 1 through 9 for each of 100 personality-descriptive statements; higher scores indicate that a statement is relatively characteristic of a person, and lower scores indicate that it is relatively uncharacteristic. The validity and usefulness of Q-sort personality descriptions has been demonstrated frequently (see, e.g., Bem & Funder, 1978; Block, 1961/1978; Block, 1971; Gjerde, Block, & Block, 1988; Mischel, Shoda, & Peake, 1988).[1]

The psychologists based their CAQ descriptions of each subject on observations made while administering a variety of experimental procedures designed to tap various aspects of psychological functioning. These psychologists were *not* the interviewers who gathered information about drug use; they had no knowledge of subjects' drug use or of any other information elicited during the interviews. Each of the four psychologists who provided CAQ-based personality descriptions saw the subjects in a different assessment context, so that four entirely independent Q-sort descriptions were available per subject. The scores assigned to each Q-sort item were then averaged across the four psychologists, to yield a final, composite Q-sort for each subject. These composite Q-sorts thus represent the consensual judgment of four independent assessors. The reliabilities of the composite Q-sorts differed somewhat from subject to subject, and were of the order of .70 and .90.

Childhood assessments. At ages 7 and 11, the personality characteristics of the subjects were described in a similar manner, each time by entirely different sets of psychologists, using the standard vocabulary of the California Child Q-sort (CCQ). The CCQ is an age-appropriate modification of the California Adult Q-sort, and consists of statements describing the personality, cognitive, and social characteristics of children (see J. Block & J. H. Block, 1980; J. H. Block and J. Block, 1980). At age 7, the standard 100-item CCQ was used; at age 11, an abridged 63-item version was used. Three psychologists observed the children at age 11, while administering a variety of age-appropriate experimental procedures. The scores assigned to the CCQ items were averaged across the psychologists to produce a composite Q-sort for age 7 and a composite Q-sort for age 11. Again, the reliabilities of the composite Q-sorts were of the order of .70 to .90.

Measuring the Quality of Parenting

When the subjects were five years old they participated in a joint assessment session with their mothers and in a separate joint assessment session with their fathers. The purpose of the joint sessions was to allow observations of parent–child interactions under standard conditions.

---

[1]The specific personality-descriptive statements that make up the California Adult Q-Sort are the result of a lengthy selection process, aimed at developing an item set of sufficient richness to allow a comprehensive description of an individual's psychological functioning. Experienced clinicians employed an initial set of descriptive statements to describe a variety of individuals, including psychiatric cases, they knew well. In the process, important item omissions were revealed, ambiguities of wording noted, and redundancies recognized. Needed items were then added, ambiguities clarified, and redundancies eliminated. This process iterated through a number of cycles until the item set was deemed sufficiently comprehensive to do justice to the clinical psychologists' formulations. A detailed description of the development of the California Adult Q-Sort is found in Block (1961/1978).

During each joint assessment session, the children were given a variety of age-appropriate tasks to perform, such as assembling objects from wooden blocks, arranging plastic pieces according to shape and color, solving mazes, and so on. The parents were instructed to respond to their child's eventual difficulties with the tasks and to provide whatever help they felt was needed. The tasks were designed to be of interest to parent and child, to be appropriately challenging to the child, and to be readily understandable to all parents. The order of the sessions and the order of the tasks within sessions were counterbalanced. The joint assessment procedure has been described in more detail elsewhere (Block & Block, 1971; Gjerde, 1988).

Parent and child were left alone to work on the tasks while a trained observer watched the interaction through a one-way mirror. Additionally, the sessions were video-taped. After the session, the observer described the parent's manner of interacting with the child using a 49-item Parent-Child Interaction Q-sort (PCIQ) specially developed for this purpose (Block & Block, 1971). A second observer provided an additional Q-sort description after watching the session on videotape. The two Q-sorts describing the mother–child interaction were composited, as were the two Q-sorts describing the father–child interaction.

RESULTS

Rates of Drug Use

The primary purpose of this study was to investigate the relations between drug use and psychological characteristics. However, it is first useful to consider the rate of drug use in the sample in absolute terms.

Of the 101 subjects for whom information about drug use was available, 68% had tried marijuana (four years earlier, 51% of the subjects had used marijuana; see Keyes & Block, 1984). Thirty-nine percent of the subjects reported using marijuana once a month or more, and 21% reported using it weekly or more than weekly. These figures are comparable to figures obtained in nationwide probability samples of adolescents and young adults (Johnston et al., 1986; Johnston, Bachman & O'Malley, 1981a, 1981b; Miller et al., 1983; NIDA, 1986).

Approximately 37% of the subjects reported trying cocaine, and 25% reported trying hallucinogens. Approximately 10% of the subjects reported trying amphetamines, barbiturates, tranquilizers, or inhalants. Only one subject reported that she had used heroin.

Creation of Comparison Groups

Based on the drug use information collected at age 18, the subjects were divided into three nonoverlapping groups, as follows.

Abstainers were defined as subjects who had never tried marijuana or any other drug. This group contained 29 subjects, 14 boys and 15 girls.[2]

Experimenters were defined as subjects who had used marijuana "once or twice," "a few times," or "once a month," and who had tried *no more* than one drug other than marijuana. This group contained 36 subjects, 16 boys and 20 girls. The mean number of other drugs tried by the subjects in this group was 0.31 (i.e., 11 of the 36 subjects had tried one drug other than marijuana).

Frequent users were defined as subjects who reported using marijuana frequently, that is, once a week or more, and who had tried *at least* one drug other than marijuana. This group contained 20 subjects, 11 boys and 9 girls. The mean number of other drugs tried by the subjects in this group was 2.70.[3]

Sixteen subjects "fell between the cracks" of the classification scheme, and did not meet the definitional criteria for any of the groups. In general, these were subjects who were excluded from the abstainer and experimenter groups because of their use of drugs other than marijuana.

The basis for the groupings derives from conceptual considerations, as well as from some recognitions derived from prior evaluation of the subjects in early adolescence (Block et al., 1988). Obviously, a degree of arbitrariness is unavoidable in any such classification scheme; however, the results to be reported are robust with respect to the various group definitions. That is, we considered both broader and narrower definitions for the various groups (e.g., excluding from the group of experimenters subjects who had tried any drug other than marijuana, or including subjects who had tried as many as two other drugs). As long as the sample was divided into three groups that could be broadly construed in terms of nonusers, experimenters, and regular users, the pattern of results we report emerged reliably.

The groups were first compared on the control variables of socioeconomic status, as assessed by both the Duncan (1961) and Warner, Meeker, and Eells (1949) indexes and IQ, as measured by the Wechsler Preschool and Primary Scale of Intelligence (WPPSI) at age 4, the Wechsler Intelligence Scale for Children (WISC) at age 11, and the Wechsler Adult Intelligence Scale (WAIS) at age 18. No associations approaching significance were observed; consequently, these variables cannot be readily invoked to explain subsequent findings.

---

[2]Although it would have been preferable to analyze the sexes separately in order to either investigate sex differences or to cross-validate the relations observed, the resulting small group sizes would have inordinately weakened the power of statistical tests. Because there is an appreciable similarity of the sexes with respect to the psychological correlates of drug use (e.g., Block et al., 1988; Jessor & Jessor, 1978; Newcomb & Bentler, 1988; Stein, Newcomb, & Bentler, 1986), the decision to merge the sexes seemed warranted.

[3]The most frequently mentioned drugs were cocaine, hallucinogens, and amphetamines, which had been used by 81%, 65%, and 43% of the frequent users, respectively.

PERSONALITY CONCOMITANTS OF DRUG USE

The major findings from the age 18 personality assessment are presented in Table 1, which lists mean scores for the CAQ items differentiating between frequent drug users, experimenters, and abstainers.

Findings are presented using the experimenters as a reference group, and the personality characteristics associated with the other groups are elucidated through comparison with them. The experimenters are used as a frame of reference for two reasons: (a) they constitute the largest group and reflect the pattern of drug use most typical for this sample and most typical for adolescents in the nation as a whole; (b) the group of experimenters lies between the other groups on the continuum of frequency of drug use; therefore, its use as a reference group facilitates the discernment of possible curvilinear relations between drug use and personality measures. As will be seen, this second consideration takes on considerable importance.

Personality Characteristics of Frequent Users

The frequent users were compared with the experimenters on each of the 100 Q-sort items, by means of separate *t*-tests. The number of statistically significant differences between the groups is striking and far exceeds the number to be expected by chance. Fully 51 of the 100 Q-sort items revealed differences at the .05 significance level (hypothesis tests are two-tailed unless otherwise noted).[4]

The following set of Q-sort items, all of which discriminate beyond the .05 level, serve to characterize the frequent users. The items are grouped according to general conceptual similarity. Inspection of Table 1 will reveal additional items that supplement this summary characterization.

Relative to experimenters, frequent users are described as not dependable or responsible, not productive or able to get things done, guileful and deceitful, opportunistic, unpredictable and changeable in attitudes and behavior, unable to delay gratification, rebellious and nonconforming, prone to push and stretch limits, self-indulgent, not ethically consistent, not having high aspiration, and prone to express hostile feelings directly.

Relative to experimenters, frequent users are also described as critical, ungiving, not sympathetic or considerate, not liked and accepted by others, not having warmth

Continued on p. 557

---

[4]The number of statistically significant findings and the theoretical coherence of these findings leaves little doubt that the observed differences between groups are both reliable and robust. The reader is cautioned, however, not to overemphasize the statistical "significance" or lack of significance of any single statistical test. The use of the .05 level as a threshold for determining significance is always arbitrary. Moreover, given the sheer number of *t*-tests computed, there may be instances of both Type I and Type II errors.

TABLE 1
Mean Scores for Age 18 California Adult Q-sort (CAQ) Items

CAQ item	Group Abstainers	Experimenters	Frequent users
1. Is critical, skeptical, not easily impressed.	4.9	4.6	5.6***
2. Is a genuinely dependable and responsible person.	7.7	7.5	5.9***
5. Behaves in a giving way with others.	6.4	6.5	5.5***
6. Is fastidious.	5.3**	4.9	4.2**
7. Favors conservative values in a variety of areas.	5.6**	5.0	3.6***
13. Thin-skinned; sensitive to anything that can be construed as criticism.	4.2	4.0	4.7**
17. Behaves in a sympathetic or considerate manner.	7.2	7.3	6.2***
18. Initiates humor.	5.3*	5.7	5.3
19. Seeks reassurance from others.	5.0	4.9	4.3*
21. Arouses nurturant feelings in others.	5.1*	5.4	4.7***
22. Feels a lack of personal meaning in life.	2.6	2.7	3.8***
23. Extrapunitive; tends to transfer or project blame.	3.7*	3.4	4.0**
24. Prides self on being "objective," rational.	6.2***	5.5	5.1
25. Overcontrols needs and impulses; delays gratification unnecessarily.	4.8***	3.9	3.3**
26. Is productive; gets things done.	7.1**	6.7	5.6***
27. Shows condescending behavior to others.	2.5	2.2	3.0***
28. Tends to arouse liking and acceptance in people.	7.0***	7.6	6.2***
29. Is turned to for advice and reassurance	5.0	5.0	4.3***
30. Gives up and withdraws in face of frustration, adversity.	3.6	4.0	4.7*
31. Regards self as physically attractive.	5.4**	5.8	5.4
34. Overreactive to minor frustrations; irritable.	3.5	3.4	4.4***
35. Has warmth, capacity for close relationships.	7.2	7.5	6.7***
36. Is subtly negativistic; tends to undermine, sabotage.	2.9	2.5	4.0***

37.	Is guileful and deceitful, manipulative, opportunistic.	1.7	1.6	2.4***
38.	Has hostility toward others.	3.5	3.3	4.4***
39.	Thinks and associates to ideas in unusual ways.	4.2	4.3	5.0**
41.	Is moralistic.	4.6***	4.2	3.9
42.	Delays or avoids action.	3.4*	3.8	4.1
43.	Is facially and/or gesturally expressive.	5.2***	5.9	5.5
45.	Has a brittle ego-defense system; maladaptive under stress.	3.0	2.9	3.6**
48.	Keeps people at a distance; avoids close interpersonal relationships.	3.7**	3.0	3.9**
49.	Is basically distrustful of people in general.	3.4	3.1	4.2***
50.	Is unpredictable and changeable in behavior, attitudes.	3.7**	4.0	4.9***
51.	Genuinely values intellectual and cognitive matters.	7.0*	6.5	6.0
53.	Undercontrols needs and impulses; unable to delay gratification.	2.9***	3.7	4.4***
54.	Emphasizes being with others; gregarious.	5.6**	6.2	5.3***
55.	Is self-defeating.	3.2	3.0	4.1***
56.	Responds to humor.	6.8*	7.2	6.8
58.	Enjoys sensuous experiences (touch, taste, smell, physical contact).	5.3***	5.7	6.0**
62.	Tends to be rebellious and nonconforming.	3.5	3.8	5.8***
63.	Judges self and others in conventional terms (e.g., "popularity").	5.4	5.2	4.4***
65.	Characteristically pushes and tries to stretch limits.	3.6	3.7	5.2***
67.	Is self-indulgent.	4.1	4.2	4.9***
68.	Is basically anxious.	4.3**	3.8	4.3
69.	Is sensitive to anything that can be construed as a demand.	4.7	4.4	5.1**
70.	Behaves in an ethically consistent manner.	6.8	6.5	6.0**
71.	Has high aspiration level for self.	7.0	6.4	5.4***

Continued

TABLE 1
Continued

CAQ item	Group		
	Abstainers	Experimenters	Frequent users
72. Concerned with own adequacy as a person.	5.4	5.0	6.0***
73. Tends to perceive many different contexts in sexual terms.	3.9***	4.3	4.7*
74. Subjectively unaware of self-concern, satisfied with self.	5.1	5.5	4.9*
75. Has clear-cut, internally consistent personality.	6.7	6.6	5.9***
76. Tends to project own feelings and motivations onto others.	4.5	4.5	4.9**
77. Appears straightforward, forthright, candid with others.	7.1***	7.6	6.0***
78. Feels cheated and victimized by life; self-pitying.	2.2	2.1	3.0***
80. Interested in members of the opposite sex.	6.1***	6.6	6.6
81. Is physically attractive; good-looking.	5.9***	6.6	6.1*
82. Has fluctuating moods.	4.8	4.9	5.5***
84. Is cheerful.	6.9*	7.6	5.7***
86. Handles anxiety and conflict by denial, repression.	4.5	4.2	4.7*
88. Is personally charming.	5.9**	6.5	5.5***
92. Has social poise and presence; is socially at-ease.	6.3**	6.9	5.6***
93. Is sex-typed (masculine/feminine).	6.8	7.0	6.4**
94. Expresses hostile feelings directly.	3.8	3.9	4.3**
96. Values own independence and autonomy.	7.0	7.1	7.8***

* Differs from experimenters, $p < .10$. ** Differs from experimenters, $p < .05$. *** Differs from experimenters, $p < .01$.

or the capacity for close relationships, having hostility toward others, prone to avoid close relationships, distrustful of people, not gregarious, not personally charming, and not socially at ease.

Finally, frequent users are described as relatively overreactive to minor frustrations, likely to think and associate to ideas in unusual ways, having brittle ego-defense systems, self-defeating, concerned about the adequacy of their bodily functioning, concerned about their adequacy as persons, prone to project their feelings and motives onto others, feeling cheated and victimized by life, and having fluctuating moods.

Consistent with the CAQ descriptions suggesting alienation and poor impulse control, the frequent users attain significantly lower high school grade point averages than the experimenters, 2.3 versus 3.0 ($p < .01$).

When the Q-sort descriptions are considered as a set, the picture of the frequent user that emerges is one of a troubled adolescent, an adolescent who is interpersonally alienated, emotionally withdrawn, and manifestly unhappy, and who expresses his or her maladjustment through undercontrolled, overtly antisocial behavior.

Personality Characteristics of Abstainers

The abstainers were compared with the experimenters on each of the 100 Q-sort items, by means of separate *t*-tests. Once again, the number of statistically significant CAQ items well exceeds chance, with 19 of the 100 CAQ items showing differences between the groups at the .05 level.

The following Q-sort items, all significant beyond the .05 level, serve to characterize the abstainers.

Relative to experimenters, abstainers are described as fastidious, conservative, proud of being "objective" and rational, overcontrolled and prone to delay gratification unnecessarily, not liked or accepted by people, moralistic, unexpressive, prone to avoid close interpersonal relationships, predictable in attitudes and behavior, not gregarious, not able to enjoy sensuous experiences, basically anxious, not straightforward and forthright with others, not physically attractive, not personally charming, and not socially at ease.

The abstainers and the experimenters achieve identical high school Grade Point Averages, 3.0 in both cases.

When the Q-sort items are considered as a set, the picture of the abstainer that emerges is of a relatively tense, overcontrolled, emotionally constricted individual who is somewhat socially isolated and lacking in interpersonal skills.

PERSONALITY ANTECEDENTS OF DRUG USE

An unusual feature of the present study is that psychological descriptions of subjects are available from early childhood on. Moreover, the psychological descriptions obtained at different ages are wholly independent of one another. We wish to emphasize this independence: The psychologists who saw the subjects at different ages were different people, they saw the subjects under different conditions, they saw the subjects only at the age at which they served as assessors, and they had no contact with one another. Because of the safeguards taken to ensure the independence of the data, relations between psychological characteristics observed at age 18 and psychological characteristics observed in early childhood must be attributed to continuities in psychological development over time (and not to artifacts of the research design).

On the basis of the CAQ descriptions obtained at age 18, a priori directional hypotheses were generated for virtually all at the age 11 and age 7 California Child Q-Sort items. Specifically, it was hypothesized that abstainers would show signs of impulse overcontrol, and frequent users would show signs of impulse undercontrol, relative to experimenters; and that abstainers and frequent users would both show signs of interpersonal alienation and psychological distress, relative to experimenters.[5] In view of the existence of directional hypotheses and the independence of the data collected at different ages, one-tailed statistical tests were employed in evaluating the childhood CCQ data. Table 2 lists the mean scores for the age 11 CCQ items discriminating between the groups (recall that an abridged 63-item Q-sort was used at the age 11 assessment, so fewer significant relationships can be expected), and Table 3 lists the mean scores for the age 7 CCQ items discriminating between groups.[6]

The Childhood Personality of Frequent Users

The frequent users were compared with the experimenters on each of the CCQ items by means of separate *t*-tests. At age 11, frequent users were described (in comparison to experimenters) as visibly deviant from their peers, emotionally labile, inattentive and unable to concentrate, not involved in what they do, stubborn (preceding items significant at the .05 level), unhelpful and uncooperative, pushing and

Continued on p. 563

---

[5]These hypotheses are based on conceptual considerations as well as on results of factor analytic examination of the age 18 CAQ data. See the section entitled Underlying Personality Factors: Linear and Curvilinear Relationships.

[6]The use of one-tailed tests may seen insufficiently conservative to some. However, the thrust of the findings would be the same regardless of whether one- or two-tailed statistical tests were employed. Moreover, there is an inherent trade-off between the level of Type I and Type II errors. Given an exploratory study involving difficult-to-obtain data, it seems scientifically strategic to lessen the likelihood of Type II errors, rather than to overprotect against Type I errors (cf. Block, 1960).

TABLE 2
Mean Scores for Age 11 California Child Q-sort (CCQ) Items

CCQ item	Group		
	Abstainers	Experimenters	Frequent users
1. Prefers nonverbal methods of communication.	4.6	4.5	5.1*
3. Is warm and responsive.	5.3**	6.2	5.2**
6. Is helpful and cooperative.	7.0	7.2	6.5**
8. Tends to keep thoughts, feelings, or products to self.	5.6*	4.7	5.3
13. Characteristically pushes and tries to stretch limits.	3.0*	3.6	4.2
14. Is eager to please.	6.0	6.1	5.3**
21. Tries to be the center of attention.	3.1**	3.8	3.9
23. Is fearful and anxious.	4.5***	3.3	4.0
25. Uses and responds to reason.	7.3**	6.6	6.5
26. Is physically active.	5.2**	5.9	5.7
27. Is visibly deviant from peers in physical appearance.	3.3	3.0	3.7**
28. Is vital, energetic, lively.	4.9**	5.9	5.2
30. Tends to arouse liking and acceptance in adults.	6.1	6.5	5.9*
34. Is restless and fidgety.	3.7***	4.6	5.1
35. Is inhibited and constricted.	5.1**	3.9	4.4
37. Likes to compete; tests and compares self with others.	4.1**	4.5	4.6
39. Becomes rigidly repetitive or immobilized under stress.	4.2*	3.5	4.2*
40. Is curious, eager to learn, open to new experiences.	5.4***	6.4	5.7*
41. Is persistent in activities; does not give up easily.	5.9	5.6	5.1*
42. Is an interesting, arresting child.	5.1**	5.8	5.1*
45. Tends to withdraw and disengage when under stress.	5.0*	4.2	5.2**
47. Has high standards of performance for self.	6.1	5.9	5.1**
52. Is physically cautious.	5.1***	4.0	4.5
54. Has rapid shifts in mood; is emotionally labile.	3.5	3.4	4.2**
59. Is neat and orderly in dress and behavior.	6.5***	5.5	5.2
60. Becomes anxious in unpredictable environment.	4.9**	4.0	4.8*
62. Is obedient and compliant.	6.5*	5.8	5.6

63.	Has a rapid personal tempo; reacts and moves quickly.	4.2**	5.0	4.6
64.	Is calm and relaxed, easy-going.	5.0*	5.6	5.2
66.	Is attentive and able to concentrate.	7.0	6.6	5.9*
67.	Is planful; thinks ahead.	6.9**	6.1	5.9
71.	Looks to adults for help and direction.	5.6*	5.0	4.6
73.	Responds to humor.	4.9**	5.7	5.7
74.	Becomes strongly involved in what she or he does.	5.8	6.2	5.2**
75.	Is cheerful (low placement implies unhappiness).	5.4**	6.3	5.6
79.	Tends to be suspicious and distrustful of others.	3.8**	2.9	3.8*
82.	Is self-assertive.	4.4**	5.3	5.2
84.	Is a talkative child.	4.6*	5.4	4.6*
85.	Is aggressive (physically or verbally).	2.9*	3.4	3.8
88.	Is self-reliant, confident; trusts own judgment.	5.4*	5.9	5.8
90.	Is stubborn.	4.3	4.0	4.8**
94.	Tends to be sulky or whiny.	3.7	3.1	4.0**
95.	Overreacts to minor frustrations; is easily irritated.	3.5	3.1	3.9**
98.	Is shy and reserved; makes social contacts slowly.	5.6**	4.3	5.0
99.	Is reflective; deliberates before speaking or acting.	6.7*	6.0	6.1

* Differs from experimenters, $p < .10$. **Differs from experimenters, $p < .05$. ***Differs from experimenters, $p < .01$.

TABLE 3
Mean Scores for Age 7 California Child Q-sort (CCQ) Items

CCQ item	Abstainers	Experimenters	Frequent users
		Group	
1. Prefers nonverbal methods of communication.	4.6*	4.4	4.7**
3. Is warm and responsive.	5.6	5.7	5.5*
4. Gets along well with other children.	6.1	5.8	5.3**
5. Is admired and sought out by other children.	5.1	5.2	4.8*
7. Seeks physical contact with others (touching, hugging, etc.).	4.9	4.9	4.6*
8. Tends to keep thoughts, feelings, or products to self.	5.0*	4.7	5.1*
14. Is eager to please.	5.6*	5.4	5.3
15. Shows concern for moral issues (fairness, reciprocity).	5.4	5.5	5.1*
16. Tends to be pleased with his/her accomplishments.	5.6*	5.8	5.6*
20. Tries to take advantage of others.	4.1**	3.8	4.0
23. Is fearful and anxious.	4.5	4.3	4.5*
26. Is physically active.	5.4*	5.6	5.5
28. Is vital, energetic, lively.	5.6	5.7	5.3**
32. Tends to give, lend, and share.	5.7*	5.4	5.2
34. Is restless and fidgety.	4.5*	4.8	4.8
35. Is inhibited and constricted.	4.6**	4.3	4.6
38. Has unusual thought processes.	4.6***	5.2	5.2
39. Becomes rigidly repetitive or immobilized under stress.	4.2*	4.0	4.3*
40. Is curious, eager to learn, open to new experiences.	5.5	5.6	5.4*
43. Can recoup or recover after stressful experience.	5.3	5.2	5.0*
44. When in conflict with others, yields and gives in.	4.7	4.5	4.9**
45. Tends to withdraw and disengage when under stress.	4.6	4.5	4.8*

50. Has bodily symptoms as a function of stress.	4.2	4.2	4.9***
53. Tends to be indecisive and vacillating.	4.3	4.3	4.6**
55. Is afraid of being deprived.	4.4	4.2	4.5*
59. Is neat and orderly in dress and behavior.	5.7***	5.2	5.2
62. Is obedient and compliant.	5.6*	5.3	5.4
67. Is planful; thinks ahead.	5.1**	5.4	5.1**
69. Is verbally fluent; can express ideas well.	5.2***	5.7	5.5*
72. Has a readiness to feel guilty; puts blame on self.	4.1**	4.5	4.4
76. Can be trusted; is dependable.	6.1	6.1	5.7*
77. Appears to feel unworthy; thinks of self as "bad."	4.0	4.0	4.5**
81. Can admit to own negative feelings.	5.1	5.0	4.5***
83. Seeks to be independent and autonomous.	5.1**	5.4	5.2
84. Is a talkative child.	5.1	5.3	5.0*
86. Likes to be by him/herself, enjoys solitary activities.	4.8	4.6	5.1**
87. Tends to imitate characteristics of those admired.	4.8	4.9	4.5**
88. Is self-reliant, confident; trusts own judgment.	5.4	5.5	5.3*
89. Is competent, skillful.	5.6*	5.9	5.7
91. Is inappropriate in emotive behavior.	4.1	4.4	4.8**
92. Is physically attractive, good-looking.	5.9***	5.5	5.7
96. Is creative in perception, work, thought, or play.	5.3*	5.5	5.3
97. Has an active fantasy life.	4.9	4.9	5.3*
100. Is easily victimized or scapegoated by other children.	4.1	4.1	4.6**

* Differs from experimenters, p < .10. ** Differs from experimenters, p < .05. *** Differs from experimenters, p < .01.

stretching limits, not eager to please, immobilized under stress, not curious and open to new experience, likely to give up easily, likely to withdraw under stress, not having high performance standards, suspicious and distrustful, and overreactive to minor frustrations (preceding items significant at the .10 level).

At age 7, the frequent users were described as not getting along well with other children, not showing concern for moral issues (e.g., reciprocity, fairness), having bodily symptoms from stress, tending to be indecisive and vacillating, not planful or likely to think ahead, not trustworthy or dependable, not able to admit to negative feelings, not self-reliant or confident (preceding items significant at the .05 level), preferring nonverbal methods of communication, not developing genuine and close relationships, not proud of their accomplishments, not vital or energetic or lively, not curious and open to new experience, not able to recoup after stress, afraid of being deprived, appearing to feel unworthy and "bad," not likely to identify with admired adults, inappropriate in emotive behavior, and easily victimized and scape-goated by other children (preceding items significant in the .10 level).

In short, the frequent users appear to be relatively maladjusted as children. As early as age 7, the picture that emerges is of a child unable to form good relation-ships, who is insecure, and who shows numerous signs of emotional distress. These data indicate that the relative social and psychological maladjustment of the fre-quent users predates adolescence, and predates initiation of drug use.

The Childhood Personality of Abstainers

The abstainers were compared with the experimenters on each of the CCQ items. At age 11, the abstainers were described as relatively fearful and anxious, using and responding to reason, not physically active, not vital or energetic or lively, inhibited and constricted, not liking to compete, not curious and open to new expe-riences, not interesting or arresting, physically cautious, neat and orderly (implies fussiness), anxious in unpredictable environments, not having a rapid personal tempo, looking to adults for help and direction, not responsive to humor, not self-assertive, not self-reliant or confident, shy and reserved (preceding items significant at the .05 level), cold and unresponsive, immobilized under stress, obedient and compliant, not calm or relaxed, planful and likely to think ahead, not cheerful, not talkative, and not aggressive (preceding items significant at the .10 level).

At age 7, the abstainers were described as relatively eager to please, inhibited and constricted, conventional in thought, neat and orderly, planful and likely to think ahead, not verbally expressive, not seeking to be independent and autonomous (preceding items significant at the .05 level), not proud of their accomplishments, not physically active, immobilized under stress, obedient and compliant, not self-assertive, not competent and skillful, and not creative (preceding items significant at the .10 level).

These descriptions present a picture of a child who is relatively overcontrolled, timid, fearful, and morose. While the characterizations of these children as "anxious," "inhibited," and "immobilized under stress" are telling, more telling, perhaps, may be the descriptions of what these children are not; relative to the reference group of experimenters, they are not warm and responsive, not curious and open to new experience, not active, not vital, and not cheerful.

QUALITY OF PARENTING

Table 4 lists the mean scores for the PCIQ items that discriminate between the mothers of frequent users, experimenters, and abstainers. These data reflect direct observations of mother–child interactions when the subjects were five years of age. Hypothesis tests are two-tailed.

Quality of Parenting: Frequent Users

Compared with the mothers of the experimenters, the mothers of the frequent users are described as hostile, not spontaneous with their children, not responsive or sensitive to their children's needs, critical of their children and rejecting of their ideas and suggestions, not supportive and encouraging of their children, tending to dramatize their teaching, making the test situation grim and distasteful rather than fun, pressuring their children to work at the tasks, underprotective of their children, overly interested in and concerned with their children's performance, conducting the session in such a way that their children do not enjoy it (preceding items significant at the .05 level), appearing to lack pride in and be ashamed of their children, seeming to be confused about what is expected of them in the test situation, conducting the session in unusual or atypical ways, not giving their children praise, and not having a clear and coherent teaching style (preceding items significant at the .10 level).

In brief, the mothers of the frequent users are perceived as relatively cold, unresponsive, and underprotective. They appear to give their children little encouragement, while, conjointly, they are pressuring and overly interested in their children's "performance." The apparent net effect of this double-bind is that they turn a potentially enjoyable interaction into a grim and unpleasant one.

Few items discriminated between the fathers of frequent users and the fathers of experimenters.

Quality of Parenting: Abstainers

Compared with the mothers of the experimenters, the mothers of the abstainers were described as hostile, not responsive or sensitive to their children's needs, critical of their children and rejecting of their ideas and suggestions, frustrated by an

TABLE 4
Mean Scores for Parent–Child Interaction Q-sort (PCIQ) Items Describing Mothers

PCIQ item	Group		
	Abstainers	Experimenters	Frequent users
1. Is hostile.	1.8**	1.2	1.7**
3. Adult becomes involved in the situation.	4.9	4.8	5.5*
5. Is spontaneous with child.	4.4*	5.1	3.9**
7. Is responsive to child's needs from moment to moment.	4.5**	5.4	4.5*
17. Is critical; rejects child's ideas and suggestions.	3.8***	2.6	3.6**
20. Frustrated by inability to find teaching strategies.	3.4**	2.3	2.9
22. Conducts the session in unusual or atypical ways.	2.5*	1.7	2.0
23. Seems confused about what is expected in the situation.	2.1*	1.3	1.7
25. Values child's originality.	3.3*	4.3	3.7
26. Seems easy and relaxed in situation.	3.9	4.5	3.5*
28. Is supportive and encouraging of child in situation.	5.3**	6.0	5.3**
33. Makes the situation fun (versus grim or distasteful).	4.9	5.4	4.4***
34. Has clear and coherent teaching style.	4.9*	5.8	5.3
35. Pressures the child to work at tasks.	4.1	3.2	4.6***
37. Uses physical means to communicate with child.	4.9*	4.1	4.6
38. Is protective of child.	3.8	4.4	3.6**
39. Is overly invested in the child's performance.	4.4**	3.5	4.3*
40. Is impatient with child.	3.1*	2.1	2.7
44. Child appears to enjoy the situation.	5.4*	6.1	5.0***

* Differs from experimenters, $p < .10$. ** Differs from experimenters, $p < .05$. *** Differs from experimenters, $p < .01$.

inability to find adequate strategies for teaching their children, not valuing their children's originality, not supportive and encouraging of their children, overly interested in, and concerned with, their children's performance, impatient with their children (preceding items significant at the .05 level), appearing to lack pride in and be ashamed of their children, seeming to be confused about what is expected of them in the test situation, conducting the session in unusual or atypical ways, not giving their children praise, not having a clear and coherent teaching style, pressuring their children to work at the tasks, and conducting the session in such a way that their children do not enjoy it (preceding items significant at the .10 level).

Like the mothers of the frequent users, these mothers are perceived as relatively cold and unresponsive. They give their children little encouragement, while, conjointly, they are pressuring and overly interested in their children's performance. Again, the apparent net effect is that they make the interaction grim and unenjoyable.

A variety of PCIQ items discriminated between fathers of abstainers and fathers of experimenters (these items are listed here and are not presented in a separate table). Compared with the fathers of the experimenters, the fathers of the abstainers were described as relatively attentive to the cognitive elements in the test situation, not responsive or sensitive to their children's needs, not allowing open disagreement between parent and child, maintaining tight control of the session, critical of their children and rejecting of their ideas and suggestions, appearing to lack pride in and be ashamed of their children, not encouraging their children to proceed independently, not valuing their children's originality, using physical means (e.g., body language and facial expression) to communicate with their children, overly interested in, and concerned with, their children's performance, impatient with their children, conducting the session in such a way that the children do not enjoy it, not deriving pleasure from being with their children, intruding physically into their children's activities (preceding items significant at the .05 level), setting too fast a pace for their children, seeming confused about what is expected in the situation, not easy and relaxed, and pressuring their children to work at the tasks (preceding items significant at the .10 level).

The picture that emerges is of an authoritarian and domineering father who squelches spontaneity and creativity and who demands that things be done *his* way. He does not appear to enjoy being with his child, and he ensures that his child does not enjoy being with him.

UNDERLYING PERSONALITY FACTORS:
LINEAR AND CURVILINEAR RELATIONS

Up to this point, we have taken a *person-centered* approach in presenting our findings. That is, we focused on discrete groups of subjects (e.g., frequent users) and attempted to provide comprehensive and psychologically rich characterizations of these subjects. Such a person-centered approach is congruent with the orientation of clinical practitioners and facilitates the often difficult task of translating empirical findings into usable clinical insights.

The more common analytical approach is nomothetic or *variable-centered*. Such an approach emphasizes *variables* rather than persons. In the context of the present study, drug use is treated as a continuum, and the research inquiries become: "What are the major personality variables associated with drug use?" and "What is the *form* of the relations between these variables and drug use?"

Person-centered and variable-centered approaches can inform and complement one another, each illuminating different facets of the problem at hand. The variable-centered analyses that follow examine concomitant relations only (i.e., relations between drug use and personality characteristics, both assessed at age 18).

Major Personality Dimensions

Impressionistic content analysis of the age 18 Q-sort items that discriminate between frequent users, experimenters, and abstainers suggests that these items cluster around three broad themes, having to do with (a) interpersonal relations, (b) subjectively experienced emotional distress, and (c) impulse regulation. To formally evaluate the importance of these themes, the Q-sort items listed in Table 1 were subjected to factor analysis (principle factors method). This factor analysis yielded three conceptually interpretable factors after varimax rotation, which together accounted for 64% of the variance in the Q-sort descriptions. The items that best mark the factors are listed in Table 5. It can be seen from this table that the factors correspond to the three themes identified here.

Factor 1, which we have labeled *Quality of Interpersonal Relations*, reflects warm interpersonal relations versus interpersonal alienation and distrust. Factor 2, labeled *subjective distress*, reflects self-devaluation and emotional distress versus a sense of personal well-being. Factor 3, labeled *Ego-Control* (J. H. Block & J. Block, 1980), reflects impulse under-control and impetuousness, versus impulse over-control and conformity.

For each of the three factors, factor scales were constructed by averaging the relevant CAQ items, after reversing the coding of items that were negative indicators of factors. The alpha reliabilities were .96, .94, and .89 for the Quality of Interpersonal Relations, Subjective Distress, and Ego-Control factors, respectively.[7]

---

[7]These alpha coefficients are somewhat inflated because they were calculated from the same sample used to generate the factors.

TABLE 5
Factors Relevant to an Understanding of Drug Use

CAQ item	Loading
Factor 1: Quality of Interpersonal Relations	
35. Has warmth; capacity for close relationships.	.89
5. Behaves in a giving way with others.	.88
17. Behaves in a sympathetic or considerate manner.	.84
21. Arouses nurturant feelings in others.	.77
28. Tends to arouse liking and acceptance in people.	.76
77. Appears straightforward, forthright, candid with others.	.65
37. Is guileful and deceitful, manipulative, opportunistic.	−.64
38. Has hostility towards others.	−.67
49. Is basically distrustful.	−.71
36. Is subtly negativistic; tends to undermine, sabotage.	−.73
1. Is critical, skeptical, not easily impressed.	−.74
27. Shows condescending behavior to others.	−.85
Factor 2: Subjective Distress	
72. Concerned with own adequacy as a person.	.85
22. Feels a lack of personal meaning in life.	.83
45. Has a brittle ego-defense system; maladaptive under stress.	.79
78. Feels cheated and victimized by life; self-pitying.	.75
55. Is self-defeating.	.72
68. Is basically anxious.	.70
30. Gives up and withdraws in face of frustration, adversity.	.63
88. Is personally charming.	−.62
29. Is turned to for advice and reassurance.	−.69
92. Has social poise and presence; is socially at ease.	−.72
74. Subjectively unaware of self-concern, satisfied with self.	−.74
Factor 3: Ego Control	
53. Undercontrols needs and impulses; unable to delay gratification.	.84
67. Is self-indulgent.	.54
65. Characteristically pushes and tries to stretch limits.	.55
50. Unpredictable and changeable behavior, attitudes.	.51
26. Is productive; gets things done.	−.66
2. Is a genuinely dependable and responsible person.	−.67
25. Over-controls needs and impulses; delays gratification unnecessarily.	−.67

Monotonic and Nonmonotonic Relations

Examination of the Q-sort findings presented in Table 1 reveals a mixture of monotonic and nonmonotonic relations between personality characteristics and level of drug use. Specifically, scores for certain CAQ items appear to increase (or decrease) monotonically as a function of drug use, whereas scores for other CAQ items appear to manifest somewhat "U"- (or inverted "U") shaped relations with drug use. The item "Undercontrols needs and impulses; unable to delay gratification (CAQ item 53) illustrates a monotonic relation, with frequent users receiving higher scores than experimenters, who in turn receive higher scores than abstainers. In contrast, the item "Keeps people at a distance; avoids close interpersonal relationships" (CAQ item 48) illustrates a U-shaped relationship, with abstainers and frequent users both receiving higher scores than experimenters.

The pattern of monotonic and nonmonotonic relations appears to be orderly. Specifically, it appears that (a) items reflecting the Quality of Interpersonal Relations factor show somewhat U- (or inverted U) shaped relations with level of drug use, such that experimenters are judged to have healthier interpersonal relationships than either abstainers or frequent users; (b) items reflecting the Subjective Distress factor manifest somewhat U- (or inverted U) shaped relationship with level of drug use, such that experimenters are judged to have a greater sense of emotional well-being than either abstainers or frequent users; and (c) items reflecting the Ego-Control factor are related monotonically to level of drug use, such that abstainers are judged to be relatively overcontrolled with respect to impulse expression and frequent users are judged to be relatively undercontrolled. Finally, the U-shaped relations described here do not appear to be symmetric: Although both abstainers and frequent users are evaluated relatively unfavorably in terms of the Quality of Interpersonal Relations and Subjective Distress factors, it also appears that frequent users are evaluated less favorably by far.

To test these observations formally, three separate hierarchical multiple regressions were performed, in which level of marijuana use served as a predictor of the Quality of Interpersonal Relations. Subjective Distress, and Ego-Control scales, respectively.[8] Each regression equation included both a linear and a quadratic term. The regressions were "hierarchical" in the sense that the linear term entered the regression equation first, followed by the quadratic term, which provided a test of curvilinearity. The regression analyses are based on the full sample of 101 subjects for whom drug use and personality data were available; the previous distinctions between abstainers, experimenters, and frequent users were ignored.

---

[8]Marijuana use is an ordinal variable (0 = never tried marijuana, 6 = daily marijuana use; see Method section). Level of marijuana use is used as the predictor variable in these regression analyses because it carries the most fine-grained information regarding drug involvement and because it is the primary variable upon which classification as abstainer, experimenter, or frequent user was based.

Table 6 presents the results of the three regression analyses. Both linear and quadratic terms contributed significantly in the regression equation to predict Quality of Interpersonal Relations, and in the regression equation to predict Subjective Distress (i.e., the quadratic terms explained significant incremental variance, over and above the variance explained by the linear terms). The significant contributions of the quadratic terms indicate that these personality factors manifest, at least to some extent, U- or inverted U-shaped relations with level of drug use. The quadratic term did not significantly contribute to the regression equation to predict Ego-Control, indicating that the relation between drug use and Ego-Control is essentially linear. Ego-Control is quite strongly related to drug use ($R = .52$, $p < .0001$), a finding similar to that obtained when the subjects were 14 years of age (see Block et al., 1988). Quality of Interpersonal Relations and Subjective Distress are also significantly related, but less strongly ($R = .33$, $p < .005$, and $R = .29$, $p < .05$, respectively).

Figure 1 graphically illustrates the best-fit regression lines to predict Quality of Interpersonal Relations, Subjective Distress, and Ego-Control. It can be seen that both Quality of Interpersonal Relations and Subjective Distress show somewhat U- (or inverted U) shaped relations with level of drug use (i.e., moderate experimentation with marijuana is associated with more positive interpersonal relationships, and greater subjective well-being, than either no marijuana use or heavy use). These U-shaped relations are clearly asymmetric, with heavy marijuana use associated with much greater intrapersonal and interpersonal disturbance than abstention. It can also be seen from Figure 1 that the relation between drug use and Ego-Control is linear: the more impulsivity, the greater the level of drug use.

GENERAL DISCUSSION

Summary of Major Findings

On the basis of the drug use information collected at age 18, subjects were divided into nonoverlapping groups made up of frequent drug users, experimenters, and abstainers. At age 18, frequent users were observed to be alienated, deficient in impulse control, and manifestly distressed, compared with experimenters. At age 18, abstainers were observed to be anxious, emotionally constricted, and lacking in social skills, compared with experimenters.

Differences between the groups were evident during childhood as well, at the age 7 and age 11 assessments. Consistent with the age 18 findings, frequent users were judged to be relatively insecure, unable to form healthy relationships, and emotionally distressed as children, compared with experimenters. Also consistent with the age 18 findings, abstainers were judged to be relatively anxious, inhibited, and morose as children, compared with experimenters.

TABLE 6

Hierarchical Regressions of Three Personality Factors on Level of Marijuana Use

Personality factor	R	R^2	F	df	Increment in R^2	F^a
Quality of Interpersonal Relations						
Marijuana use: linear term	.22	.05	5.18*	1, 98		
linear term + quadratic term	.33	.11	5.92***	2, 97	.06	6.36**
Subjective Distress						
Marijuana use: linear term	.21	.04	4.55*	1, 98		
linear term + quadratic term	.29	.09	4.58*	2, 97	.04	4.6*
Ego Control						
Marijuana use: linear term	.52	.27	36.67***	1, 98		
linear term + quadratic term	.52	.27	18.25***	2, 97	.00	.15 ns

[a] F value associated with increment in R^2.
* $p < .05$. **$p < .01$. ***$p < .005$.

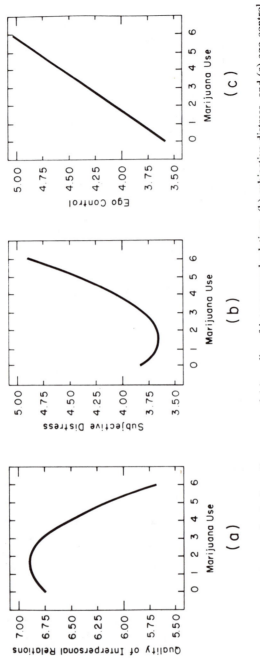

Figure 1. Relations between level of marijuana use and (a) quality of interpersonal relations, (b) subjective distress, and (c) ego control

Additionally, both frequent users and abstainers were judged to have received poorer maternal parenting than experimenters, as assessed by direct observations of mother–child interactions when the subjects were five years old. Compared with the mothers of experimenters, both the mothers of frequent users and the mothers of abstainers were perceived to be cold, critical, pressuring, and unresponsive to their children's needs.

There were no noteworthy findings involving the fathers of frequent users. However, fathers of abstainers were seen (in comparison with the fathers of experimenters) as relatively unresponsive to their children's needs and as authoritarian, autocratic, and domineering.

At age 18, the underlying personality factors relevant to an understanding of drug use appear to be Quality of Interpersonal Relations, Subjective Distress, and Ego-Control. When level of marijuana use is treated as a continuous variable, both the Quality of Interpersonal Relations and the Subjective Distress factors show somewhat U-shaped relationships with level of marijuana use. Ego-Control appears to be linearly related to level of marijuana use, with heavy users showing the poorest impulse control.

On the Relation Between Drug Use and Psychological Health

When the psychological findings are considered as a set, it is difficult to escape the inference that experimenters are the psychologically healthiest subjects, healthier than either abstainers or frequent users. Psychological health is meant here in a global and nonspecific sense, consistent with ordinary conversational usage, and consistent also with empirical recognitions by mental health researchers that a general psychological health/psychological distress factor underlies diverse clinical syndromes (e.g., Dohrenwend, Shrout, Egri, & Mendelsohn, 1980; Tanaka & Huba, 1984; Watson & Clark, 1984). The inference that there is an inverted U-shaped relation between level of drug use and psychological adjustment is supported by the patterns of Q-sort items characterizing abstainers, experimenters, and frequent users, and also by the U- (and inverted U) shaped relations observed between level of marijuana use and the two personality factors. Quality of Interpersonal Relations and Subjective Distress.

The finding that frequent users are relatively maladjusted has been obtained by many other investigators. The finding that abstainers also show some signs of relative maladjustment (albeit of a very different kind) is, perhaps, unusual. In order to understand this latter finding, we suggest it is important to consider both the *meaning* of drug use within adolescent peer culture, as well as the psychology of adolescent development.

First, it is necessary to recognize that in contemporary American culture, there is wide prevalence and apparent acceptability of marijuana use in late adolescence.

The majority of the 18-year-olds in our sample—approximately two thirds—had tried marijuana at one time or another. Such a high usage rate is consistent with the findings from national probability samples (Johnston et al., 1986; Johnston, Bachman, & O'Malley, 1981a, 1981b; Miller et al., 1983; NIDA, 1986). Thus, some experimentation with marijuana cannot be considered *deviant* behavior for high school seniors in this culture at this time. In a statistical sense it is *not* trying marijuana that has become deviant.

Second, the extended period of adolescence is a time of transition, a time when young people face the developmental task of differentiating themselves from parents and family and forging independent identities. Experimenting with values and beliefs, exploring new roles and identities, and testing limits and personal boundaries are normative behaviors during adolescence, and they serve important developmental ends (cf. Erikson, 1968; Havinghurst, 1972).

Given these factors—the ubiquity and apparent acceptability of marijuana in the peer culture and the developmental appropriateness of experimentation and limit-testing during adolescence—it is not surprising that by age 18, psychologically healthy, sociable, and reasonably inquisitive individuals would have been tempted to try marijuana. We would not expect these essentially normal and certainly normative adolescents to *abuse* the drug (and it is crucial to distinguish between experimentation and abuse) because they would have little need for drugs as an outlet for emotional distress or as a means of compensating for lack of meaningful human relationships—but we should not be surprised if they try it. Indeed, not to do so may reflect a degree of inhibition and social isolation in an 18-year-old.[9]

Although no prior study has focused explicitly on the psychology of adolescent abstainers, there is some empirical precedent for the present finding that abstainers are not the most well-adjusted of adolescents. Hogan, Mankin, Conway, and Fox (1970), using a self-report personality inventory, compared marijuana users with nonusers in a college population and found that users "are more socially skilled, have a broader range of interests, are more adventuresome, and more concerned with the feelings of others" (p. 63). Nonusers were characterized as "too deferential to external authority, narrow in their interests, and overcontrolled" (p. 61). These findings, based on entirely different methodology, are strikingly similar to our own. In a similar vein, Bentler (1987) reported a small but reliable association between marijuana use and the development of a *positive* self-concept.

We do not suggest that the inverted U-shaped relation between level of drug use and psychological health expresses a fundamental psychological "principle" or

---

[9]In a previous report on the psychological correlates of drug use in early adolescence (at age 14), the relations observed between drug use and psychological factors were essentially monotonic, with drug users characterized by undercontrol and alienation (Block et al., 1988). The curvilinear relations observed in the present study were not fully discernible then, perhaps because issues of experimentation and identity formation had not yet become paramount.

"law." Rather, we view this finding as a function of historical and social circumstances—specifically, of the current prevalence of drug use in this culture, conjoined with the developmentally appropriate propensity of adolescents to explore and experiment. Gergen's (1973) arguments regarding "social psychology as history" may be applicable here.

The U-shaped relations between psychological health and drug use are reminiscent of U-shaped relations between psychological health and alcohol use noted in an earlier generation of subjects. Thus, Jones (1968, 1971) found that moderate drinkers were psychologically healthier than either problem drinkers or abstainers. Moreover, the undercontrolled, alienated personality attributes of problem drinkers and the overcontrolled, diffident personality attributes of alcohol abstainers were quite similar to the personality attributes that characterize frequent drug users and drug abstainers in the present study. Given the prevalence and apparent acceptability of marijuana use among adolescents today, it would seem that marijuana use has taken on psychological and sociological meanings for young people that, in earlier generations, were associated with alcohol use.

Toward an Understanding of Frequent Drug Users

If drug use among experimenters reflects normative adolescent exploration and inquisitiveness, it reflects something quite different in the group we have labeled frequent users. Frequent users differ profoundly from the comparison group of experimenters, and indications of their social and psychological maladjustment are pervasive.

At age 18, the frequent users appear unable to invest in, or derive pleasure from, meaningful personal relationships. Indeed, they seem fortified against the possibility of such relationships through their hostility, distrust, and emotional withdrawal. Neither do they appear to be capable of investing in school and work, or of channeling their energies toward meaningful future goals. They are, then, alienated from the "love and work" that lend a sense of satisfaction and meaning to life. Consistent with this, they appear to *feel* troubled and inadequate. It is easy to see how these characteristics could create a vicious cycle: Feeling troubled and inadequate, these adolescents withdraw from work and relationships, and alienated from work and relationships, they feel all the more troubled and inadequate.

Such a pattern of alienation can be expected to go hand in hand with an impaired ability to control and regulate impulses. When there is little investment in either work or relationships, that is, when there is little connection with those things that give life a sense of stability and purpose, then the impulses of the moment become paramount. The impulses are not adequately transformed or mediated by a broader system of values and goals because such a system is lacking.

Shapiro (1965) has written eloquently on this point:

The normal person "tolerates" frustration or postpones the satisfaction of his whim at least in part because he is also interested in other things; his heart is set on goals and interests that are independent of the immediate frustration or extend beyond the whim and supercede it in subjective significance. This is not simply a matter of intellectual choice. Rather, the existence of these general goals and interests automatically provides a perspective, a set of dimensions in which a passing whim or an immediate frustration is experienced. In the absence of such goals and interests, the immediately present frustration or the promised satisfaction must, accordingly, gain in subjective significance, and under these conditions forbearance or tolerance is unthinkable. (pp. 145–146)

Drugs would have a special appeal to the alienated and impulsive individuals we are discussing. The temporary effects of various drugs "numb out" feelings of isolation and inadequacy; they offer transient gratification to individuals who lack deeper and more meaningful gratifications (i.e., through relationships and work); and given the poor ability of these individuals to regulate impulse, the urge toward drug use would meet with little inner resistance and would be little modified by a broader value system.

The traits that characterize the frequent users can be seen, then, to form a theoretically coherent syndrome, characterized by the psychological triad of *alienation, impulsivity,* and *subjective distress.* The data indicate that the roots of this syndrome predate adolescence and predate initiation of drug use.

As early as age 7, the frequent users show signs of the alienation, undercontrol, and emotional distress that will characterize them at age 18. Relative to experimenters, they are described as not getting along well with other children, as not developing genuine and close relationships, as not showing concern for moral issues, as not trustworthy or dependable, as having bodily symptoms from stress, as afraid of being deprived, as appearing to feel unworthy, as inappropriate in emotive behavior, and so on (see Table 2). The data clearly indicate, then, that *the relative maladjustment of the frequent users precedes the initiation of drug use.*

This relative maladjustment perhaps may be traced, at least in part, to the maternal parenting that the frequent users received, as assessed by direct observations of mother–child interactions when the subjects were five years of age. Relative to the mothers of experimenters, the mothers of frequent users were perceived as hostile, critical and rejecting, and not sensitive or responsive to their children's needs. Moreover, they seemed to place their children in a double-bind: Although they gave their children little support and encouragement, they were simultaneously pressuring and overly concerned with their children's "performance."[10]

---

[10]These findings do not necessarily imply that the emotional difficulties of frequent drug users can

Toward an Understanding of Abstainers

Adolescents who have never experimented with marijuana or any other drug have not been the subject of research attention, if only because their behavior does not pose an obvious, confronting societal problem and because it has been presumed categorically that *not* using drugs goes hand in hand with psychological health. However, our data suggest that, relative to experimenters, abstainers in late adolescence are somewhat maladjusted. Unlike the patent, blatant maladjustment of frequent drug users, however, the psychological inadequacies of abstainers are largely a private matter, limiting of life as it is led, and do not attract societal attention. The constriction, uneasiness with affect, and interpersonal deficiencies of abstainers are recognizable more by way of *omission* than commission.

By omission, we refer to personal potentialities that seem to remain unfulfilled, specifically, potentialities for emotional gratifications, friendship, and human warmth and closeness. It is the relative capacity (or rather, *incapacity*) to experience these positive qualities of life that distinguishes abstainers from experimenters. Relative to experimenters, the abstainers are described at age 18 as overcontrolled and prone to delay gratification unnecessarily, not able to enjoy sensuous experiences, prone to avoid close interpersonal relationships, not gregarious, not liked and accepted by people, and so on. Thus, their avoidance of drugs seems less the result of "moral fiber" or successful drug education than the result of relative alienation from their peers and a characterological overcontrol of needs and impulses.

It seems likely that the relative overcontrol and emotional constriction of the abstainers serves the psychological purpose of containing or masking feelings of vulnerability. There is some evidence for this hypothesis in the age 18 personality descriptions of our subjects, for the abstainers are described at this age as relatively anxious. However, the strongest support for this hypothesis comes from the childhood data, when the relative maladjustment of these subjects is most manifest. At age 11, for example, prior to initiation of drug use, the abstainers are described (relative to experimenters) as fearful and anxious, inhibited and constricted, immobilized under stress, anxious in unpredictable environments, not curious and open to new experience, not vital or energetic or lively, not confident, not responsive to humor, and not cheerful. These traits would appear to reflect a susceptibility

---

be blamed on poor mothering. Such a view may in part be correct, but it may also be too simplistic. As proponents of family therapy remind us (e.g., Haley, 1976; Hoffman, 1981; Minuchin, 1974), it is difficult to speak of simple causation when discussing a family system. If a mother is not sufficiently responsive to her child's needs, it may be because an emotionally impoverished marital relationship does not leave her with the emotional resources needed to invest in her child. In such a case, causation could just as easily be said to lie with the father as with the mother. The point here is that, given a pattern of reciprocal and circular causation within a dysfunctional family system, a "causal" relationship might be found nearly anywhere a researcher happened to look.

to anxiety and, perhaps, a consequent avoidance of circumstances or behaviors perceived as risky.

The hypothesis that emotional constriction serves the purpose of "containing" feelings of vulnerability is reinforced further by observations of mother–child interactions when the children were age five: The mothers of the abstainers were perceived (relative to the mothers of the experimenters) as unresponsive, cold, critical, and rejecting. Such parenting clearly has negative implications for psychological resiliency and well-being. It is interesting that the descriptions of the mothers of abstainers are strikingly similar to the descriptions of the mothers of the frequent users. These results at least raise the possibility that the behavior of the abstainers and the behavior of the frequent users, manifestly so different, represent alternative reactions to an underlying psychological vulnerability.

The question of why abstainers and frequent users traveled such different developmental pathways remains an open one. Character formation is a matter of complex temperamental and developmental vicissitudes, and such questions have no straightforward answer. Our findings suggest the speculation that the fathers of the abstainers played a telling role in their character development. They acted toward their children in ways that would seem to increase anxiety, but their stern, authoritarian, and autocratic manner may have also provided a model for dealing with that anxiety. It is conceivable that the children internalized their fathers' attitudes, adopting an attitude toward their own impulses that paralleled their fathers' attitudes toward them.

Implications for Theory and Social Policy

Taken as a whole, the present data indicate that drug use and drug abstinence have theoretically coherent antecedents and must be understood within the context of an individual's total psychology. Because experimenters and frequent users are, psychologically, very different kinds of people, the meaning of drug use in these two groups is very different. In the case of experimenters, drug use appears to reflect age-appropriate and developmentally understandable experimentation. In the case of frequent users, drug use appears to be a manifestation of a more general pattern of maladjustment, a pattern that appears to predate adolescence and predate initiation of drug use. Undoubtedly, drug use exacerbates this earlier established pattern but, of course, the logic of a longitudinal research design precludes invocation of drug use as causing this personality syndrome.

Current theories (e.g., Akers, Krohn, Lanze-Kaduce, & Radosevich, 1979; Jessor & Jessor, 1977, 1978; Kaplan, Martin, & Robins, 1982) tend to emphasize the role of peers in influencing drug use. The importance of peers in providing an encouraging surround for *experimentation* cannot be denied, but "peer-centered" or "environmental" explanations of *problem* drug use seem inadequate, given the present longitudinal findings (cf. Margulies, Kessler, & Kandel, 1977).

The discovery of psychological antecedents predating drug use (see also Block et al., 1988; Kellam et al., 1975; Kellam et al., 1983; Kellam, Ensminger, & Simon, 1980) can to some extent be integrated with explanations of drug use that emphasize environmental factors, once it is recognized that individuals, from early childhood, actively construct and seek out environments that, given their essential personality, motivational, and intellectual characteristics, they find particularly harmonious and vivifying (see, e.g., Scarr & McCartney, 1983). Rather than being passive recipients of "environmental" influences, by the time of adolescence, individuals are already appreciably formed psychologically and are actively evoking, actively seeking, and actively forging the circumstances that will suit them and that will then, in an adventitious way, "impinge" on them.

The recognition that *problem* drug use (and, for that matter, abstinence) has developmental antecedents, that it is a part of a broad and theoretically coherent psychological syndrome, and that it is not adequately explained in terms of peer influence has important implications for social policy.

Current social policy seems to follow from the assumption that peer influence leads to experimentation, which in turn leads to abuse. Thus, efforts at drug education are aimed at discouraging experimentation by emphasizing the need to "just say no" to peer influence. But adolescent experimentation in and of itself does not appear to be personally or societally destructive (see also Kandel, Davies, Karus, & Yamaguchi, 1986, and Newcomb & Bentler, 1988), and peer influence does not appear to be an adequate explanation for *problem* drug use. Moreover, given the developmental tasks of the prolonged adolescent period, efforts aimed at eliminating adolescent experimentation are likely to be costly and to meet with limited success.

Current efforts at drug "education" seem flawed on two counts. First, they are alarmist, pathologizing normative adolescent experimentation and limit-testing, and perhaps frightening parents and educators unnecessarily. Second, and of far greater concern, they *trivialize* the factors underlying drug *abuse*, implicitly denying their depth and pervasiveness. For so long as problem drug use is construed primarily in terms of "lack of education," so long is attention diverted from its disturbing psychological underpinnings: the psychological triad of alienation, impulsivity, and distress. Paradoxically, then, the "just say no" approach may be concerned with a "problem" that, from a developmental viewpoint, need not be seen as alarming (adolescent experimentation), and it may be dismayingly oblivious to a serious problem that is extremely alarming (the ubiquity of the psychological syndrome that appears to underlie *problem* drug use).

The concept of drug "education" may have its current popular appeal in part because the link between the problem (drugs) and the attempted solution (drug education) is self-evident and thus reassures concerned parents, educators, and policymakers that "something is being done." But educational approaches to drug prevention have had limited success (Tobler, 1986), and society's limited resources might be better invested in interventions focusing on the personality syndrome underlying problem drug use.

Given current understandings of personality development, it would seem that the psychological triad of alienation, impulsivity, and distress would be better addressed through efforts aimed at encouraging sensitive and empathic parenting, at building childhood self-esteem, at fostering sound interpersonal relationships, and at promoting involvement and commitment to meaningful goals. Such interventions may not have the popular appeal of programs that appear to tackle the drug problem "directly," but may have greater individual and societal payoff in the end.

Forfending Misinterpretation

The finding that experimenters are the psychologically healthiest adolescents, and the observation that some drug experimentation in and of itself, does not seem to be psychologically destructive, may sit badly with some. In particular, it may sit badly with drug counselors who "know" from clinical experience that there is no level of drug use that is safe, that it is dangerous to suggest otherwise, and that the most effective intervention is one aiming at total abstinence. To avoid any misunderstanding, we wish to make clear that there is no contradiction between this therapeutic perspective and the findings we have reported. On the contrary, we are in agreement with the therapeutic perspective.

The present data indicate that in a nonselected late-adolescent sample, occasional experimentation with marijuana is not personally or societally destructive. This view is supported by longitudinal studies of the consequences of drug use (as well as by the present study of the antecedents and concomitants of drug use; see, e.g., Kandel et al., 1986; Newcomb & Bentler, 1988), and by the fact that the majority of adolescents in the United States have experimented with marijuana but have not subsequently become drug abusers. The apparent contradiction between clinical wisdom, on the one hand, and the present findings, on the other, is resolved when it is recognized that individuals who present themselves for drug treatment are *not* representative of the general population of adolescents, but instead constitute a special, highly selected subpopulation. The psychological meaning of drug use is very different for this fractional group existing within the larger population of adolescents. For them, experimentation with drugs is highly destructive because drugs easily become part of a broader pathological syndrome. For adolescents more generally, some drug experimentation apparently does not have psychologically catastrophic implications.

In closing, one final clarification is in order. In presenting research on a topic as emotionally charged as drug use, there is always the danger that findings may be misinterpreted or misrepresented. Specifically, we are concerned that some segments of the popular media may misrepresent our findings as indicating that drug use might somehow improve an adolescent's psychological health. Although the incorrectness of such an interpretation should be obvious to anyone who has actually read this article, our concerns about media misrepresentation requires us to state categorically that our findings do *not* support such a view, nor should anything we have said remotely encourage such an interpretation.

REFERENCES

Akers, R. L., Krohn, M. D., Lanze-Kaduce, L., & Radosevich, M. (1979). Social learning and deviant behavior: A specific test of a general theory. *American Sociological Review, 44*, 636–655.

Bem, D. J., Funder, D. C. (1978). Predicting more of the people more of the time: Assessing the personality of situations. *Psychological Review, 85*, 485–501.

Bentler, P. M. (1987). Drug use and personality in adolescence and young adulthood: Structural models with nonnormal variables. *Child Development, 58*, 65–79.

Block, J. (1960). On the number of significant findings to be expected by chance. *Psychometrika, 25*, 369–380.

Block, J. (1971). *Lives through time.* Berkeley, CA: Bancroft.

Block, J. (1978). *The Q-sort method in personality assessment and psychiatric research.* Palo Alto, CA: Consulting Psychologists Press (Original work published 1961).

Block, J., & Block, J. H. (1980). *The California Child Q-set.* Palo Alto, CA: Consulting Psychologists Press.

Block, J., Block, J. H., & Keyes, S. (1988). Longitudinally foretelling drug usage in adolescence: Early childhood personality and environmental precursors. *Child Development, 59*, 336–355.

Block, J. H., & Block, J. (1971). *Manual for the Parent-Child Interaction Procedure.* Berkeley: University of California, Department of Psychology. CA.

Block, J. H., & Block, J. (1980). The role of ego-control and ego-resiliency in the organization of behavior. In W. A. Collins (Ed.), *Minnesota symposia on child psychology* (Vol. 13, pp. 39–101). Hillsdale, NJ: Erlbaum.

Brook, J. S., Gordon, A. S., & Whiteman, M. (1985). Stability of personality during adolescence and its relationship to stage of drug use. *Genetic, Social, and General Psychology Monographs, 111*, 317–330.

Brook, J. S., Whiteman, M., Gordon, A. S., & Cohen, P. (1986). Dynamics of childhood and adolescent personality traits and adolescent drug use. *Developmental Psychology, 22*, 403–414.

Bush, P. J., & Iannotti, R. (1965). The development of children's health orientations and behaviors: Lessons for substance use prevention. In C. L. Jones & R. J. Battjes (Eds.), *Etiology of drug abuse: Implications for prevention* (Research Monograph No. 56, pp. 45–74). Rockville, MD: National Institute on Drug Abuse.

Cox, W. M. (1985). Personality correlates of substance abuse. In M. Galizio & S. A. Maisto (Eds.), *Determinants of substance abuse: Biological, psychological, and environmental factors* (pp. 209–246). New York: Plenum.

Dohrenwend, B. S., Shrout, P. E., Egri, G., & Mendelsohn, F. S. (1980). Nonspecific psychological distress and other dimensions of psychopathology. *Archives of General Psychiatry, 37*, 1229–1236.

Duncan, O. (1961). A socioeconomic index for all occupations. In A. J. Reiss, Jr. (Ed.), *Occupation and social status* (pp. 109–138). New York: Free Press.

Erikson, E. H. (1968). *Identity: Youth and crisis.* New York: Norton.

Gergen, K. J. (1973). Social psychology as history. *Journal of Personality and Social Psychology, 36*, 309–320.

Gjerde, P. F. (1988). Parental concordance on child-rearing and the interactive emphases of parents: Gender differentiated relationships during the preschool years. *Developmental Psychology, 24*, 700–706.

Gjerde, P. F., Block, J., & Block, J. H. (1988). Depressive symptomatology and personality during late adolescence: Gender differences in the externalization-internalization of symptom expression. *Journal of Abnormal Psychology, 97*, 475–486.

Haberman, P. W., Josephson, E., Zanes, A., & Elinson, J. (1972). High school drug behavior: A methodological report on pilot studies. In S. Einstein & S. Allen (Eds.), *Proceedings of the First International Conference on Student Drug Surveys* (pp. 103–121). Farmingdale, NY: Baywood.

Haley, J. (1976). *Problem-solving therapy.* New York: Harper & Row.

Havinghurst, R. J. (1972). *Developmental tasks and education (3rd ed.).* New York: McKay.

Hawkins, J. D., Lishner, D. M., & Catalano, R. F. (1985). Childhood predictors and the prevention of adolescent substance abuse. In C. L. Jones & R. J. Battjes (Eds.), *Etiology of drug abuse: Implications for prevention* (Research Monograph No. 56, pp. 75–125). Rockville, MD: National Institute on Drug Abuse.

Hoffman, L. (1981). *Foundations of family therapy: A conceptual framework for systems change.* New York: Basic Books.

Hogan, R., Mankin, D., Conway, J., & Fox, S. (1970). Personality correlates of undergraduate marijuana use. *Journal of Consulting and Clinical Psychology, 35*, 58–63.

Jessor, R. (1979). Marijuana: A review of recent psychosocial research. In R. L. Dupont, A. Goldstein, & J. O'Donnell (Eds.), *Handbook on drug abuse* (pp. 337–355). Washington, DC: Government Printing Office.

Jessor, R., Chase, J. A., & Donovan, J. E. (1980). Psychosocial correlates of marijuana use and problem drinking in a national sample of adolescents. *American Journal of Public Health, 70*, 604–613.

Jessor, R., & Jessor, S. L. (1977). *Problem behavior and psychological development: A longitudinal study of youth.* New York: Academic Press.

Jessor, R., & Jessor, S. L. (1978). Theory testing in longitudinal research on marijuana use.

In D. B. Kandel (Ed.), *Longitudinal research on drug use: Empirical findings and methodological issues* (pp. 41–71). Washington, DC: Hemisphere.

Johnston, L. D., Bachman, J. G., & O'Malley, P. M. (1981a). *Highlights from student drug use in America 1975–1981*. Rockville, MD: National Institute on Drug Abuse.

Johnston, L. D., Bachman, J. G., & O'Malley, P. M. (1981b). *Student drug use in America 1975–1981*. Rockville, MD: National Institute on Drug Abuse.

Johnston, L. D., O'Malley, P. M., & Bachman, J. G. (1984). *Drugs and American high school students, 1975–1983* (National Institute of Drug Abuse, DHHS Publication No. ADM 84–1317). Washington, DC: Government Printing Office.

Johnston, L. D., O'Malley, P. M., & Bachman, J. G. (1986). *Drug use among American high school students, college students, and other young adults: National trends through 1985*. Rockville, MD: National Institute on Drug Abuse.

Jones, C. L., & Battjes, R. J. (Eds.). (1985). *Etiology of drug abuse: Implications for prevention*. (Research Monograph No. 56; DHHS Publication No. ADM 85-1335). Rockville, MD: National Institute of Drug Abuse.

Jones, M. C. (1968). Personality correlates and antecedents of drinking patterns in adult males. *Journal of Consulting and Clinical Psychology, 31*, 1–12.

Jones, M. C. (1971). Personality antecedents and correlates of drinking patterns in women. *Journal of Consulting and Clinical Psychology, 36*, 61–69.

Kandel, D. B. (1978). Convergences in prospective longitudinal surveys of drug use in normal populations. In D. Kandel (Ed.), *Longitudinal research on drug use: Empirical findings and methodological issues* (pp. 3–38). Washington, DC: Hemisphere.

Kandel, D. B. (1980). Drug and drinking behavior among youth. *Annual Review of Sociology, 6*, 235–285.

Kandel, D. B., Davies, M., Karus, D., & Yamaguchi, K. (1986). The consequences in young adulthood of adolescent drug involvement. *Archives of General Psychiatry, 43*, 746–754.

Kaplan, H. B., Martin, S. S., & Robbins, C. (1982). Application of a general theory of deviant behavior: Self-derogation and adolescent drug use. *Journal of Health and Social Behavior, 23*, 274–294.

Kellam, S. G., Branch, J. D., Agrawal, K. C., & Ensminger, M. E. (1975). *Mental health and going to school: The Woodlawn program of assessment, early intervention, and evaluation*. Chicago: University of Chicago Press.

Kellam, S. G., Brown, C. H., Rubin, B. R., & Ensminger, M. E. (1983). Paths leading to teenage psychiatric symptoms and substance use: Developmental epidemiological studies in Woodlawn. In S. B. Guze, F. J. Earls, & J. E. Barrett (Eds.), *Childhood psychopathology and development* (pp. 17–47). New York: Raven.

Kellam, S. G., Ensminger, M. E., & Simon, M. B. (1980). Mental health in first grade and teenage drug, alcohol, and cigarette use. *Drug and Alcohol Dependence, 5*, 273–304.

Keyes, S., & Block, J. (1984). Prevalence and patterns of substance abuse among early adolescents. *Journal of Youth and Adolescence, 13*, 1–14.

Margulies, R. Z., Kessler, R. C., & Kandel, D. B. (1977). A longitudinal study of onset of drinking among high school students. *Journal of Studies of Alcohol, 38*, 897–912.

Miller, J. D., Cisin, I. H., Gardner-Keaton, H., Harrel, A. V., Wirtz, P. W., Abelson, H. I., & Fishburne, P. M. (1983). *National survey on drug abuse: Main findings 1982.* Rockville, MD: National Institute on Drug Abuse.

Minuchin, S. (1974). *Families and family therapy.* Cambridge, MA: Harvard University Press.

Mischel, W., Shoda, Y., & Peake, P. K. (1988). The nature of adolescent competencies predicted by preschool delay of gratification. *Journal of Personality and Social Psychology, 54,* 687–696.

National Institute on Drug Abuse. (1986). *Capsules: Overview of the 1985 household survey on drug abuse.* Rockville, MD: Author.

Newcomb, M., & Bentler, P. (1988). *Consequences of adolescent drug use: Impact on the lives of young adults.* Newbury Park, CA: Sage.

Perry, C. L., Killen, J., & Slinkard, L. A. (1980). Peer teaching and smoking prevention among junior high school students. *Adolescence, 15,* 277–281.

Robins, L. N. (1984). The natural history of adolescent drug use. *American Journal of Public Health, 74,* 656–657.

Scarr, S., & McCartney, K. (1983). How people make their own environments: A theory of genotype (arrow) environmental effects. *Child Development, 54,* 424–435.

Shapiro, D. (1965). *Neurotic styles.* New York: Basic Books.

Single, E., Kandel, D., & Johnson, B. D. (1975). The reliability and validity of drug use responses in a large scale longitudinal survey. *Journal of Drug Issues, 5,* 426–443.

Smith, G. M. & Fogg, C. P. (1978). Psychological predictors of early use, late use, and nonuse of marijuana among teenage students. In D. B. Kandel (Ed.), *Longitudinal research on drug use* (pp. 101–113). New York: Wiley.

Stein, J. A., Newcomb, M. D., & Bentler, P. M. (1986). The relationship of gender, social conformity, and substance use: A longitudinal study. *Bulletin of the Society of Psychologists in Addictive Behaviors, 5,* 125–138.

Tanaka, J. S., & Huba, G. J. (1984). Confirmatory hierarchical factor analysis of psychological distress measures. *Journal of Personality and Social Psychology, 46,* 621–635.

Tobler, N. S. (1986). Meta-analysis of 143 adolescent drug prevention programs: Quantitative outcome results of program participants compared to a control or comparison group. *Journal of Drug Issues, 16,* 537–568.

Warner, W. L., Meeker, M., & Eells, K. (1949). *Social class in America.* Chicago: Science Research Associates.

Watson, D. W., & Clark, L. A. (1984). Negative affectivity: The disposition to experience aversive emotional states. *Psychological Bulletin, 96,* 465–490.

28

Nuclear Freedom and Students' Sense of Efficacy About Prevention of Nuclear War

Pam Oliver

University of Auckland

Questionnaire and interview responses of young New Zealanders, living in a nuclear-free zone, reveal general concerns about nuclear war but relatively little personal, subjective worry. Their sense of citizen and national efficacy is stronger than that reported by youngsters in other countries, but is not reflected in feelings of self-efficacy. Responses are compared to those reported in North American and European research, and the importance of adult role models in facilitating children's belief in the efficacy of antinuclear activities is highlighted.

Anecdotal reports early in the past decade from doctors, teachers, psychologists, and others working with children and teenagers indicated that young people in New Zealand were concerned about the arms race and the threat of nuclear war, and suggested that for some young people such concerns could be having harmful effects on their general development and their optimism about the future (*"Threat of the Bomb," 1984*). This suggestion was consistent with several studies in the United States and Europe which had concluded that substantial numbers of young people, especially adolescents, were fearful about the possibility of a nuclear war, and that, for some, this could be affecting their willingness and ability to plan for the future or to invest effort in personal relationships and achievements (*Beardslee & Mack, 1982; Escalona, 1982*). Some authors even suggested that the perceived threat of nuclear war could be damaging the development of young people generally, and effectively removing their sense of efficacy by making them feel helpless in the

Reprinted with permission from *American Journal of Orthopsychiatry*, 1990, Vol. 60, No. 4, 611–621. Copyright © 1990 by the American Orthopsychiatric Association, Inc.

Research was supported in part by the New Zealand Social Science Research Fund, with assistance from International Physicians for the Prevention of Nuclear War. The author is in the Department of Management Studies and Labour Relations, University of Auckland, New Zealand.

face of a seemingly irreversible and immutable path toward nuclear destruction of the world (*Beardslee & Mack; Tizard, 1986*).

More recent research and analyses, both in the United States and elsewhere (*Griffin & Prior, 1990; Hamilton, van Mouwerik, Oetting, Beauvais, & Keilin, 1987; Oliver, 1989a*), have indicated that, while young people are certainly concerned about the possibility of a nuclear war, they do not worry about it as actively as the earlier studies appeared to suggest. The earlier conclusions that substantial proportions of young people were actively worried about the nuclear threat may have been based on the failure of researchers to distinguish between a more passive concern and active worrying (*Oliver, 1989a*), and on their narrow interpretation of children's concern or anxiety as a negative and disempowering reaction (*Hamilton et al., 1987; Ingleby, 1986*). Studies which do not focus primarily on nuclear issues have found that concern about nuclear threat does not appear to interfere unduly with young people's optimism about the future in general (*Bachman, 1983*). There is also evidence from recent research that concern and even fear often are associated with a *greater* sense of efficacy or resourcefulness in relation to preventing nuclear war, rather than causing feelings of helplessness and hopelessness (*Boehnke, Macpherson, Meador, & Petri, 1988; Griffin & Prior, 1990; Sommers, Goldberg, Levinson, Ross, & LaCombe, 1984*), depending on how the fear is dealt with and whether it is used constructively. Moreover, one New Zealand study (*Barnhart-Thompson & Stacey, 1987*) which did not ask specifically about anxiety or concern found that the primary emotional response of young people to nuclear war and other nuclear issues was not fear, but anger, and a recent study in Australia (*McMurray & Prior, 1987*) demonstrated that self-reported rates of concern about nuclear issues can vary enormously within individual respondents, depending on question phraseology and response format. This potential bias has also been noted by other researchers (*Deutsch, 1984; Schuman, Ludwig, & Krosnick, 1986*).

Thus, while it is clear that many, or even most, young people in the western world are concerned about nuclear weapons, it is not at all certain that such concern causes them actually to worry to any great degree, nor that it leaves them feeling powerless to avert a nuclear war. It may even be that the recognition of one's own anxiety or fear, and an understanding that these are realistic and natural emotional responses to nuclear threat, are prerequisite stimuli to becoming involved in social action (*Boehnke et al., 1988*), which in turn can act as a protection against helplessness and despair. The vital factor in determining whether the outcome of fear and concern is helplessness or a stronger sense of efficacy may well be whether young people have effective models (*Bandura, 1977; Fernando & Oliver, 1988; Zeitlin, 1984*), that is, some clear demonstration from the actions of salient others that there is something positive *and* effective that they can do to turn the nuclear arms race around. It is well recognized that fear-arousal per se is not a sufficient stimulus to induce either personal or citizen action in response to even an urgent problem

(*Braithwaite & Law, 1977; Fiske, 1987; McMurray & Prior, 1987*); this is especially so when people do not believe they have the problem-solving skills necessary for the specific task, as is inevitably more likely with children.

Currently, some researchers in both hemispheres are beginning to focus on the role of parents and other adults as models both for social action and for antinuclear attitudes (*Falconer, 1988; Hesse, Goodman, Mack, & Beardslee, 1987*). However it is possible also that the modeling of social action can come from the activities of other children, or of an entire nation, for example when a cohesive stand is seen to be taken by a whole population, as in the case of New Zealand's antinuclear stance. This action occurred at both political and social levels, and culminated in legislation guaranteeing New Zealand nuclear freedom, which in turn resulted in aggressive political action against New Zealand by the United States. These various events, which took place over a period of approximately five years (from 1983 to 1988), took on the nature of a popular groundswell which included widespread citizen action in the early 1980s in declaring nuclear-free zones throughout the country, and assertive lobbies to have the Labour Party, then in opposition, adopt nuclear freedom as its political platform. Large contingents of school students also were involved very actively in the establishment of nuclear-free zones both in their schools and in wider local body areas (*"School Nuclear Free," 1983; "College Declared," 1983*), and in other peace activities through groups such as Schools Against the Bomb and School Children Against Nuclear Arms. (The membership of these groups appears to have atrophied substantially since, however.) Antinuclear issues remain quite salient, partly because of continuing pressure on New Zealand from the United States in relation to conflict over the ANZUS defense pact between the two nations, and partly because they constitute popular press.

The effect of these events on the nuclear attitudes of New Zealanders, including the nation's young people, has been illustrated in many ways, both anecdotal and empirical. Clements (*1989*) has described how New Zealand's nuclear-free status has become firmly incorporated into the national identity, that of both adults and children. Studies in the mid-1980s have shown that New Zealand youth are, almost without exception, strongly opposed to nuclear weapons, that they place little or no credence in the principle of deterrence and generally believe that the use of nuclear weapons would never be justifiable (*Barnhart-Thompson & Stacey, 1987; McSweeney, 1985; Patten, 1987; Shallcrass & Gavriel, 1983; Sides, 1987*). They also appear to have a robust belief in citizen and national efficacy in relation to nuclear issues, with often large majorities (50%–90%) believing that citizens in general or New Zealand as a nation can do a lot to help prevent a nuclear war from happening. These findings appear to compare favorably with the few northern hemisphere studies which have asked young people specifically about their sense of their own and other people's efficacy in relation to nuclear war prevention. Questionnaire surveys in Canada, Italy, and Finland have revealed that the majority of adolescents in those countries believe that neither they personally nor citizens in general could have any significant influence on the nuclear arms race (*Ponzo, 1986; Solantaus, Rimpela, Taipale, & Rahkonen, 1984; Sommers et al., 1984*), and that they feel discouraged and helpless because of this perception. Even amongst young Finnish adults aged 17–18, less than half of those asked believed that an ordinary individual could do anything to prevent war or that citizen activities such as peace marches had any impact on disarmament (*Wahlstrom, 1984*). Moreover, the studies showed a clear tendency for young people to believe that adults are not particularly concerned about nuclear weapons or trying to oppose their proliferation (*Tizard, 1985*).

It is interesting, then, to speculate on whether clearly effective modeling of antinuclear attitudes and behavior at a citizen and national level, such as has been demonstrated in New Zealand, is sufficient to provide young people with a sense of self-efficacy. While it is apparent that young New Zealanders have a strong sense of efficacy at the group level, for example believing that politicians, whole nations, or citizen groups are able to take concerted social action, there is no evidence that this will necessarily translate into a sense of personal efficacy. The collective work on self-efficacy (*Bandura, 1984, 1986*) suggests that one's own personal experiences of mastery may be essential to developing a sense that one is personally able to have some effect on control in a particular context, and that neither vicarious experience nor mastery in other areas will necessarily be a sufficient basis for developing self-efficacy in relation to a novel challenge (*Bandura, 1984*).

The present study sought, inter alia, *1*) to examine the relationship among concern, fear, and active worry; *2*) to determine whether there are differences in perceived efficacy in relation to one's ability to help prevent nuclear war, depending on the level of intervention (i.e., group or personal); *3*) to investigate some of the factors that may be associated with perceived self-efficacy; and *4*) to compare these findings with overseas research. Evidence from both informal conversations and pilot interviews with children and teenagers had suggested that young people, while they saw adults and groups of people as being able to have some influence in relation to a wide range of social issues, typically saw themselves, *as children*, as having little or no ability to change things.

METHOD

Subjects

As one part of a study in 1987–88 which used both interviews and questionnaires to examine a wide range of reactions—beliefs, attitudes, and behavior, including coping strategies—of New Zealand children and teenagers to nuclear issues, 52 students participated in in-depth interviews and 1,875 completed a comprehensive questionnaire that asked questions about their perceptions of their lives and of the future in general, and then about nuclear issues specifically. The interviewees were selected randomly from school class rolls, and the questionnaires were administered to whole classes of students at primary, intermediate, and secondary schools. The schools were selected randomly from Education Department lists covering suburbs across the greater metropolitan area of Auckland (New Zealand's largest city). Both the interview and the questionnaire samples were selected evenly from the full range of socioeconomic groups, and included the three main ethnic groups in New Zealand (Samoan, Maori, and Pakeha [white]) in approximate proportion to their representation in the general population. The respondents to both interviews and questionnaires were aged 9 to 18, with approximately equal numbers of males and females.

Questions. The students were asked to rate their own efficacy and that of three other categories of people (phrased in the interviews and questionnaire as "kids as a whole," "citizens as a whole," and "New Zealand as a whole"). These ratings also took into consideration whether they had personally encountered people involved in antinuclear activity and, if so, who the particular people were. Amongst other questions, the students were asked: *1*) to list their three main fears in relation to the future and then their three main day-to-day worries; *2*) their "main feeling about the chance of a nuclear war happening;" *3*) how much they "actually worry about the chance of a nuclear war;" *4*) their personal philosophy in relation to nuclear war (prevention or survival); *5*) who is primarily responsible for preventing nuclear war; *6*) whether they or a parent had been involved in peace or antinuclear activities; and *7*) how much they thought adults were concerned about nuclear war. (As data from these additional seven questions are presented for purposes of correlation only, the full findings are not presented here.)

RESULTS AND DISCUSSION

The quotes in this section are taken from the interviews with the permission of the young people concerned, and were chosen to reflect the questionnaire findings which are represented in the quantified data. Age and gender differences are discussed, but ethnic and socioeconomic differences are omitted as these were in general not statistically significant.

Fear and Worry About Nuclear War

In tandem questions, the students were asked to list the three things they were most afraid of about the future, and then to list the three things they "actually worry about from day to day." (It was made clear to them that they could list the same or different things in these two questions.) Relative to other concerns, issues related to peace, war, and nuclear war were not major fears or worries for these young people. Only 15.8% of all listed fears were to do with peace (5.5%) or war (10.3%). Peace and war categories combined ranked as the most commonly named fear, although only marginally ahead of fears for one's own life and health (14.8%) or for the general welfare of one's friends and family (11.3%), while as a separate category war and nuclear fears ranked only third. As a source of actual worry, however, even when combined into one category, peace (2.8%) and war (3.7%) issues constituted less than 7% of all listed worries, and ranked only fifth after several other personal and family concerns. As a separate category, war and nuclear worries ranked tenth, well behind worries about education (19.8%), others' welfare (14.3), one's own life and health (11.9%), and a wide range of worries about personal relationships, happiness and prosperity, and personal adequacy and acceptability. It appears that nuclear issues are not a major source of either fear or worry affecting more than a small proportion of these young people. The evident distinction between fear and active worry was reflected as well in responses to subsequent questions which asked specifically about reactions to the possibility of a nuclear war.

Emotional Reactions

Questionnaire respondents were asked to choose (from a list of response options generated by interviewees) the "main feeling" they had when they thought about the chance of nuclear war. Only half said they felt "scared" (see TABLE 1), and these were more likely to be younger children ($\chi^2 = 153.27$, $df = 36$, $p < .001$) and females ($\chi^2 = 58.31$, $df = 4$, $p < .001$). A response of anger was most common amongst those aged 14 and over, and sadness was a more common reaction amongst older teenagers. Responses of "sad" and "angry" were equally common to both genders.

While these responses demonstrate that young people are, almost without exception, concerned about nuclear war, fear is not necessarily their major reaction to

TABLE 1
Primary Emotional Reactions and Frequency of Worry with Regard to Nuclear War

REACTIONS	AGES:			
	9–13	14–15	16–18	ALL
Scared	62%	47%	35%	51%
Angry	20	30	30	25
Sad	12	13	19	14
Other	6	10	16	10
WORRY				
A Lot	12%	6%	5%	9%
Quite Often	13	11	12	13
Sometimes	35	35	31	34
Not Much/At All	40	48	52	44

the so-called nuclear "threat;" if fear is not presumed by researchers it is likely that this will be their subjects' primary reaction to the possibility of a nuclear war (*Barnhart-Thompson & Stacey, 1987*).

Frequency of Worry

TABLE 1 also shows that only a very small minority of these people (9%) reported that they actually worried frequently, even fewer than the 13% frequent worriers in the only other study (*Taylor & Patten, 1987*) that has asked about frequency of worry, as distinct from intensity of fear. This is not to discount the need to recognise that, in real numbers, a lot of young people may worry often about nuclear war and probably need help in trying to cope positively with these feelings if they are not to feel depressed or helpless. However it is apparent that, in New Zealand at least, the vast majority of young people do not appear to worry about a nuclear threat, but hold a very pragmatic attitude (*Oliver, 1989a*), as is evident in their interview responses:

> I just think about it, and what could happen. But not really worry about it. But sometimes it just makes me shiver. (*Carol, 12*)
>
> Not much. No point. (*Chris, 14*)
>
> Because I think that worrying about it wouldn't do any good, and that would make it worse really, worrying about it. *Daniel, 11*)
>
> I suppose I do worry, but I try to shut it out. You just say, "I don't care. I'll go on with my life," whenever you think about it. (*Maria, 16*)
>
> . . . not a lot, because I keep it to myself. But I'm pretty worried about it. But I know that there's not much that I can do about it, so you don't want to worry about it, because I've got a whole lot of things that I have to think about, with school and that. (*Vince, 13*)

This last response shows how worry is distinct from *being worried*, and also how fear, worry, and perceived self-efficacy are linked. Although these attitudes and the pragmatic behavior that accompanies them may be indeed functional in the short term, by allowing young people to "cut off" from worry through a variety of more or less complex defense mechanisms (*Oliver, 1989a*), this strategy may actually exacerbate a sense of disempowerment and helplessness in the long run. It is clear also that some are more at risk of worrying frequently than others, particularly younger children ($\chi^2 = 123.66$, $df = 36$, $p < .001$; see TABLE 1). This reaction is readily understandable for younger children, since they are more confused and less knowledgeable than teenagers about nuclear issues (*Fernando, 1989*), and therefore more likely to exaggerate the potential threat and impact on themselves. However, it is also possible that they feel less able to have any kind of influence in relation to nuclear issues.

Efficacy

In response to a question asking how much respondents thought that they, or other categories of people, could "do to help prevent a nuclear war," the efficacy ratings showed striking variation, depending on the category of respondent. TABLE 2 shows a progressive and dramatic decrease in perceived antinuclear effectiveness as respondents considered their own ability to exert influence, in comparison to that of adults or of New Zealand as a nation.

Citizen and national efficacy. Consistent with findings in earlier New Zealand studies, a majority of respondents believed that there was a lot that the nation as a whole (72%), and to a lesser extent ordinary citizens (58%), could do to help prevent nuclear war. Moreover, many actually considered that New Zealand, as a nuclear-free nation, now has a responsibility to persuade others to follow suit. This was often conceived in terms of showing others how to resist the influence of the "superpowers," as was evident in interview responses:

> Well, it showed them that people don't agree with it . . . and that a little country can stand up for what they believe. (*Nicola, 16*)
> . . . so we could set one of the biggest examples of nuclear freedom. So that helps, because it shows that a little country can stand up to a big superpower. I feel proud of that. (*Ferron, 12*)
> We can still help, because we're one of the nuclear-free places, so we *have* to show the other countries how. (*Katrina, 12*)
> . . . [We] have made a stand, and with some luck other countries will follow . . . . [We] can't back down now, because it's going to look like they have won with their nuclear weapons. (*Adam, 17*)

TABLE 2

Youngsters' Sense of Efficacy for Self, Youth, Citizens, and the Nation as a Whole

CATEGORY	MEAN SCORE[a]	HIGH EFFICACY	LOW EFFICACY
Self	3.7	16%	66%
Kids	3.0	37	33
Citizens	2.4	58	15
New Zealand	2.0	72	10

[a] Ratings were on a five-point scale; high efficacy ratings include points 1–2 on the scale, low efficacy were points 4–5.

These responses also demonstrate the confidence that young people have in the ability of citizens or nations with relatively little power to exert a strong positive influence; they seem clearly to endorse the need for appropriate and effective modeling, this time on an international basis! National efficacy ratings were higher for primary school children ($\chi^2 = 90.13$, $df = 36$, $p < .001$), whose views about the New Zealand government's ability to influence other nations tended to be much more idealistic; for example:

> They can show other countries how not to have nuclear bombs and ships—like here. (*Paul, 10*)
> We're already a nuclear-free country, so we could ask the other countries to do that and if [they did so] one by one, every country might become nuclear-free. (*Heidi, 10*)

This sense of collective and national efficacy was associated strongly with a preventionist attitude toward nuclear war ($\chi^2 = 110.19$, $df = 8$, $p < .001$), that is, a belief that it was better to try personally to work toward preventing a nuclear war. In contrast, those low on efficacy were more likely to take either a survivalist or passivist approach, believing that it was better to plan for how to survive a nuclear war, or simply to leave it up to others to sort out. Those reporting high efficacy were also more likely to have a parent who was at some time involved in antinuclear activity ($\chi^2 = 51.86$, $df = 8$, $p < .001$)—evidence of the importance of adult models. However, as the efficacy ratings in TABLE 2 show, this strong sense of group efficacy does not appear to filter down to the individual level, nor to apply as much when young people consider their ability to have some influence as a generational cohort.

Self-efficacy and youth efficacy. While ratings of national and citizen efficacy were very high, a majority of the students (66%) still felt virtually powerless personally to have any effective impact on the antinuclear process. This was especially so for 9–10-year-olds, but also for middle teenagers ($\chi^2 = 51.94$, $df = 36$, $p < .05$), which probably represents a realistic assessment by young people of their status and influence vis-a-vis adults in our society. These ratings are borne out by interview responses in which young people express the view that their ideas and feelings are not taken seriously by adults, and by their perception of the injustice in this double standard:

> I'm too young, and I'm not very important to them. They should give the children a chance . . . it's not fair. They've lived their life but we're just starting ours, and they're going to destroy everything. (*Mark, 9*)
> To them I'm just a 15-year-old kid "mouthing off." I'd like to do something but I'm just another brick in the wall. (*Wiremu, 15*)

> It makes me feel like just giving up sometimes. You want to do some-
> thing but you can't. (*Helen, 15*)

These findings are consistent with an earlier New Zealand study by Gray and Valentine (*1984*), who found that less than half their sample thought that they could do anything at all to help prevent a nuclear war and were very equivocal about the effectiveness of the limited activities, such as protests, which they did think they could be part of. Even at a collective level of efficacy, most students (63%) did not believe that young people could do a great deal to help prevent nuclear war. However, twice as many (37%) believed that "kids as a whole" could do something than the mere 16% who felt efficacious personally. The irony is that it is at this stage in their lives that people are probably most strongly motivated to social action. New Zealand studies in the past few years have shown repeatedly that young people are overwhelmingly opposed to nuclear weapons (*Oliver, 1989b*), and that banning them totally would be the first action of most if they "ran the world" (*Sides, 1987*).

Self-efficacy was also related significantly to other beliefs and attitudes about nuclear war. For example, those with the highest self-efficacy ratings were much more likely to think that a nuclear war would never happen ($\chi = 37.47$, $df = 16$, $p = .002$); to know a parent, other adult, or age-peer who was actively involved in peace or antinuclear activity ($\chi^2 = 61.99$, $df = 4$, $p < .001$); and to espouse a preventionist approach ($\chi^2 = 74.25$, $df = 8$, $p < .001$). Those with a parent who had been involved in antinuclear activity reported significantly higher efficacy for themselves ($\chi^2 = 43.77$, $df = 8$, $p < .001$) and for youth in general ($\chi^2 = 35.38$, $df = 8$, $p < .001$). and were more likely to see nuclear war prevention as the responsibility of everyone, rather than merely the responsibility of politicians and governments ($\chi^2 = 40.99$, $df = 18$, $p < .002$). It is significant, however, that of those who said they did know someone who was currently active in helping to prevent nuclear war, half of the people named turned out to be either the respondent or an age-peer, rather than an adult.

While it is difficult to be sure about the causal direction amongst these various factors, it appears that believing in one's own ability to have some influence may make young people more determined to help prevent a nuclear war from happening, and that having some kind of role model or personal experience in peace activity contributes substantially to such beliefs and attitudes.

Models

In response to the question, "Do you actually know any people yourself who are doing something to help prevent a nuclear war? *If* you do, please say who," only 8% of the students (150 respondents) answered affirmatively; 89% responded negatively, and the balance gave no answer. (Answers of "Yes" which then names someone apparently not known personally, such as "Greenpeace" or "the Prime Minister," were treated as negative responses.) The people named by those who apparently did know someone personally fell into five main categories: self, an age peer, parent, teacher, or other adult. As was noted above, it is striking that 13% of the 150 respondents names themselves and 37% named a friend or same-age peer as the person they knew who was taking action. Twenty-seven percent named a parent, 11% a teacher, and 12% some other adult or group of adults. Thus, only half of the youngsters who responded affirmatively—less than 4% of the *total* sample—could identify an adult whom they knew to be doing something to help prevent a nuclear war. Furthermore, the 17 students who named a teacher actually named the same three people, all women. Of the 40 who named a parent, only five named their father.

Sex and Age Differences

While studies have shown repeatedly that girls are more pessimistic than boys about the likelihood of nuclear war (*Barnhart-Thompson & Stacey, 1987; Oliver, 1989a; Patten, 1987*), the girls' sense of efficacy generally was the same as for boys or somewhat higher, a pattern also found in overseas studies (*Solantaus, Rimpela, Taipale, & Rahkonen, 1984*). Two factors that may help to explain this apparent anomaly are the empowering effects of the women's movement in general on this younger generation, and especially the very evident leading roles played by women in the peace and antinuclear movements in New Zealand and elsewhere. Both of these factors bear out the critical importance of effective role modeling by adults in children's development of social and personal action (*Bandura, 1977*); it is significant in this regard that the large majority of adult models named by students in the present study were women.

The lower efficacy ratings of younger children for themselves and for "kids" and citizens as a whole, which also mirror overseas findings (*Tizard, 1986*), would seem to reflect their particular world view as children—that it is more difficult for them to imagine ordinary people having any influence at all over something as powerful as nuclear weaponry or a "superpower" nation. However these young children were more likely than were teenagers to believe that New Zealand, at a national or governmental level could do something to prevent nuclear war ($\chi^2 = 90.14$, $df = 36$, $p < .001$). This suggests that older children and teenagers, although they have more experience of their own ability to influence because of their greater participation in peace activities, probably hold a more skeptical or realistic view of New Zealand's very limited ability to have any real influence beyond its own borders:

> [The government] can take a stand and say they don't want any part of it. . . . But I don't think there's anything else. (*Natalie, 12*)

So we're not going to let nuclear warships in here, and sure, it's a first step. But that is only here, and there probably aren't any arms aimed here. (*Earl, 15*)

CONCLUSIONS

It appears from comparisons of these findings with the generally lower efficacy perceptions of young people in other countries (*Griffin & Prior, 1990; Solantaus & Rimpela, 1984; Sommers et al., 1984*) that New Zealand's social-political ethos of opposing nuclear weapons, and particularly its international antinuclear stand in the face of sometimes aggressive opposition, have provided young New Zealanders with a strong belief in the ability of both ordinary adults and even very small nations to influence the process of nuclear weapons reduction and war prevention. However, this sense of efficacy does not generalize to a personal level for most young people, the apparent exceptions being those who do have exposure to the activities of others. These findings support the conclusions of others (*Boehnke et al., 1988; Sommers et al., 1984*) that the influence of parents and other salient adults in children's lives is vital in transmitting antinuclear attitudes and motivating social action, and that to hold any real belief in their own efficacy, young people need either very immediate demonstrations or personal experience of effective action.

These conclusions are consistent with those of Bandura (*1984*) and others, that personal mastery experiences are an important part of developing and maintaining a sense of control and resourcefulness. McMurray and Prior (*1987*) have noted also that there is a distinction between efficacy expectations per se (e.g., "I can do something") and positive *outcome* expectations (e.g., "What I do will have an effect"). Their study showed that although Australian teenagers felt equally *able* to engage in antinuclear activities, they also felt that adult engagement in the same behavior would have a greater impact. This relative lack of perceived self-efficacy is ironic considering the substantial impact that some direct appeals by children have had on the "superpower" leaders. It is unlikely that children, or adults, will maintain a sense of self-efficacy unless they continue to see some positive outcomes from their own actions or those of fairly immediate others. If they are to develop a sense of optimism, a trust in adults, a belief in their own ability to help shape the future, and a sense of social responsibility in general, it seems that young people need to see effective modeling by adults close to them. For the most part, it seems, this does not happen. In the present study a majority of the students (62%) felt that adults care little or not at all about the possibility of a nuclear war. However, those who reported an active parent were, not surprisingly, much more likely to believe that adults do care a great deal ($\chi^2 = 50.61$, $df = 8$, $p < .001$).

It also appears that in order to hold any belief in efficacy generally, young people need to believe that adults genuinely care both about the future of the world and about what young people can contribute to it. Knowing that one's nation is nuclear-free and that this has come about through citizen action, and even feeling that nuclear freedom is a part of one's national identity, does not necessarily translate into a sense of personal influence. Research on people's reactions to other environmental problems has shown repeatedly that a sense of concern, or even fear, and a desire to do something are not in themselves sufficient impetus for people to engage in social action (*Braithwaite & Law, 1977; Fiske, 1987; Terry, 1971*). This is all the more likely for young people, who are very aware of their limited influence in a world controlled by adults. In order to feel that they can do something to prevent their own futures from being cut short by a nuclear war, young people evidently need to see the adults close to them involved.

> . . . because we are the future. So we should have more say than anyone else really. Some of us are pretty young to try to understand this nuclear thing, but . . . it's our world, and we're only just growing up, and it's all going to be wasted otherwise. (*Moses, 17*)

REFERENCES

Bachman, J. (1983). How American high school seniors view the military. *Armed Forces and Society, 10*, 86–104.

Bandura, A. (1977). Self-efficacy: Toward a unifying theory of behavior change. *Psychological Review, 84*, 191–215.

Bandura, A. (1984). Recycling misconceptions of perceived self-efficacy. *Cognitive Therapy and Research, 8*, 231–256.

Bandura, A. (1986). *Social foundations of thought and action: A social cognitive theory.* Englewood Cliffs, NJ: Prentice-Hall.

Barnhart-Thompson, G., & Stacey, B. (1987). Nuclear war issues: reaction of New Zealand adolescents. *New Zealand Physician, 14*, 60–63.

Beardslee, W. R., & Mack, J. E. (1982). The impact on children and adolescents of nuclear developments. In R. Rogers (Ed.), *Psychosocial aspects of nuclear developments* (Task Force Report No. 20). Washington, DC: American Psychiatric Association.

Boehnke, K., Macpherson, M., Meador, M., & Petri, H. (1988). How West German adolescents experience the nuclear threat. *Political Psychology, 10*, 419–443.

Braithwaite, V.A., & Law, H. G. (1977). The structure of attitudes to doomsday issues. *Australian Psychologist, 12*, 167–174.

Clements, K. (1989). *Back from the brink.* Wellington: Allen & Unwin.

College declared nuclear free. (1983, September 29). *Wairarapa Times-Age.*

Deutsch, M. (1984). Some methodological considerations in studies of children and the threat of nuclear war. In T. Solantaus, E. Chivian, M. Varanyan, & S. Chivian (Eds.), *Impact of the threat of nuclear war on children and adolescents*. Proceedings of an International Symposium, 4th Congress of International Physicians for the Prevention of Nuclear War, Helsinki-Espoo, Finland.

Escalona, S. (1982, February). *Growing up with the threat of nuclear war: Some indirect effects on personality development*. Paper presented at a symposium on "Preparing for nuclear war: The psychological effects," Yeshiva University, New York.

Falconer, B. A. (1988). *Children and the threat of nuclear war*. Unpublished masters thesis, La Trobe University, Melbourne, Australia.

Fernando, K. (1989). *Young people's knowledge about nuclear issues*. Unpublished masters thesis, Psychology Department, University of Auckland.

Fernando, K., & Oliver, P. (1988). *What do we tell the children?* Auckland: Psychologists for Peace.

Fiske, S. (1987). People's reaction to nuclear war. *American Psychologist, 42*, 207–217.

Gray, B., & Valentine, J. (1984). Nuclear war: The knowledge and attitudes of New Zealand secondary school children. *New Zealand Family Physician, 11*, 121–122.

Griffin, M., & Prior, M. (1990). Young people and the nuclear threat. *Journal of Youth Studies, 7*, 40–43.

Hamilton, S. B., van Mouwerik, S., Oetting, E. R., Beauvais, F., & Keilin, W. G. (1987). *Storm, stress, and the threat of nuclear war: An examination of adolescent worries and their mental health implications*. Manuscript submitted for publication.

Hesse, P., Goodman, L., Mack, J., & Beardslee, W. (1987, July). *Politically active adolescents in the nuclear age*. Manuscript submitted for publication.

Hesse, P., Goodman, L., Mack, J., & Beardslee, W. (1987, July). *Politically active adolescents in the nuclear age*. Paper presented at the International Society for Political Psychology, San Francisco.

Ingleby, D. (1986, August). Limitations of the psychological approach to war and peace. In *Proceedings of the Congress of European Psychologists For Peace*. Finnish Psychological Society, San Francisco.

McMurray, N., & Prior, M. (1987). *Adolescents' cognitive appraisals, efficacy expectations, and level of involvement in nuclear issues*. Unpublished manuscript, Melbourne and La Trobe Universities.

McSweeney, K. (1985). Children's views on nuclear issues. *Set: Research information for Teachers, 1*, item 14. Wellington: New Zealand Council for Educational Research.

Oliver, P. (1989a). Reactions of young New Zealanders to nuclear issues. *Community Mental Health in New Zealand, 4*, 23–40.

Oliver, P. (1989b, August). *Young people's concepts and beliefs about peace and war: Cultural and political influences*. Paper presented at the New Zealand Psychological Society Annual Conference, Auckland.

Patten, M. D. (1987, May/June). *The psychological impact of the threat of nuclear war on adolescents in New Zealand*. Paper presented at the International Physicians for the Prevention of Nuclear War (IPPNW) 7th World Congress, Moscow.

Ponzo, E. (1986, August). Italian adolescents' concern about the threat of nuclear war. In *Proceedings of the Congress of European Psychologists For Peace*. Finnish Psychological Society, Helsinki.

School nuclear free. (1983, November 24). *Taranki Herald*, p. 12.

Schuman, H., Ludwig, J., & Krosnick, J. A. (1986). The perceived threat of nuclear war, salience, and open questions. *Public Opinion Quarterly, 60*, 519–536.

Shallcrass, J., & Gavriel, V. (1983). *Images of the year 2000*. Unpublished manuscript, Victoria University of Wellington, New Zealand.

Sides, C. (1987, December). *Adolescent views of the contemporary world*. Paper presented at the Australian Association of Research in Education/New Zealand Association of Research in Education Conference, Christchurch.

Solantaus, T., Rimpela, M., Taipale, V., & Rahkonen, O. (1984). Young people and the threat of war: Overview of a national survey in Finland. In T. Solantaus, E. Chivian, M. Vartanyan, & S. Chivian (Eds.), *Impact of the threat of nuclear war on children and adolescents*. Proceedings of an International Symposium, 4th Congress of International Physicians for the Prevention of Nuclear War, Helsinki-Espoo, Finland.

Sommers, F., Goldberg, S., Levinson, D., Ross, C., & LaCombe, S. (1984). Children's mental health and the threat of nuclear war: A Canadian pilot study. In T. Solantaus, E. Chivian, M. Vartanyan, & S. Chivian (Eds.), *Impact of the threat of nuclear war on children and adolescents*. Proceedings of an International Symposium, 4th Congress of International Physicians for the Prevention of Nuclear War, Helsinki-Espoo, Finland.

Taylor, A. J. W., & Patten, M. D. (1987). The attitudes and responses of Wellington adolescents to nuclear war and other nuclear issues. *New Zealand Journal of Psychology, 17*, 36–40.

Terry, M. (1971). *Teaching for survival*. New York: Ballantine.

Threat of the bomb has children under pressure. (1984, September 30). *New Zealand Times*.

Tizard, B. (1985). Problematic aspects of nuclear education. *Set: Research information for teachers, 1*, item 9. Wellington: New Zealand Council for Educational Research.

Tizard, B. (1986). The impact of the nuclear threat on children's development. In M. Richards & P. Light (Eds.), *Children of social worlds: Developmental in a social context*. Cambridge: Polity Press.

Wahlstrom, R. (1984). Fear of war, conceptions of war, and peace activities: Their relation to self-esteem in young people. In T. Solantaus, E. Chivian, M. Vartanyan, & S. Chivian (Eds.), *Impact of the threat of nuclear war on children and adolescents*. Proceedings of an International Symposium, 4th Congress of International Physicians for the Prevention of Nuclear War, Helsinki-Espoo, Finland.

Zeitlin, S. (1984). What do we tell Mom and Dad? *Family Therapy Networker, 8*, 28, 39.

PART VII: PSYCHOSOCIAL ISSUES

29

Are Head Start Effects Sustained? A Longitudinal Follow-up Comparison of Disadvantaged Children Attending Head Start, No Preschool, and Other Preschool Programs

Valerie E. Lee

University of Michigan, Ann Arbor

J. Brooks-Gunn

Educational Testing Service and Russell Sage Foundation

Elizabeth Schnur

Harlem Hospital Center, New York

Fong-Ruey Liaw

University of Michigan, Ann Arbor

This study investigates the sustained effects into kindergarten and grade 1 of Project Head Start for disadvantaged black children. Participation in generic Head Start programs was compared to both no preschool and other preschool experience for disadvantaged children in two American cities in 1969–1970. Incorporating both pretest/posttest and compar-

Reprinted with permission from *Child Development*, 1990, Vol. 61, 495–507. Copyright © 1990 by the Society for Research in Child Development, Inc.

We wish to express our continuing gratitude to Virginia Shipman, without whom the Educational Testing Service Head Start Longitudinal Study would not exist. Her care and dedication in conceptualization and data collection for the study were extreme and her commitment to the field of early childhood education enduring. We also gratefully acknowledge the support of the Center for Research in Mental Retardation of the Little City Foundation, Chicago, for secondary data analysis for this phase of the study. The original study was supported by the Administration for Children, Youth, and Families, Department of Health and Human Services, Washington, DC. Many people at the Educational Testing Service contributed to the study, most recently James Rosso and Norma Norris with data retrieval and Sam Messick with general support. We are also grateful for the editorial assistance of Helen M. Marks.

ison group information, the study has advantaged over other Head Start impact studies. Both preprogram background and cognitive differences were controlled in a covariance analysis design, using dependent measures in the cognitive, verbal, and social domains. Children who attended Head Start maintained educationally substantive gains in general cognitive/analytic ability, especially when compared to children without preschool experience. These effects were not as large as those found immediately following the Head Start intervention. Findings suggest an effect of preschool rather than of Head Start per se. Initial findings of greater effectiveness of Head Start for children of below average initial ability were reduced but not reversed. The diminution of effects over time, especially for low-ability children, may reflect differences in quality of subsequent schooling or home environment.

Head Start generally is perceived as one of the few enduring successes of the Johnson administration's "war on poverty" (Conger, 1988). The creators of the program had hopes that the early intervention would help disadvantaged children to break the "cycle of poverty by enabling them to start school on an equal footing with their more privileged peers" (Zigler & Valentine, 1979). But, despite the benefits that have been demonstrated to accrue to disadvantaged children in Head Start and other early intervention programs (Barnett, 1985; Lazar & Darlington, 1982; McKey et al., 1985; Schweinhart & Weikart, 1980), the distance between children who have been in Head Start and their more advantaged peers remains considerable (Hebbeler, 1985; Lee, Brooks-Gunn, & Schnur, 1988).

In addition, recent attention has been directed to the question of whether early interventions—Head Start and other programs—yield long-term effects (Barnett, Frede, Mobasher, & Mohr, 1987; Evans, 1985; Hebbeler, 1985; Meyer, 1984; Schweinhart & Weikart, 1980, 1983; Seitz, Rosenbaum, & Apfel, 1985). If effects "wash out" with time, as some have suggested (McKey et al., 1985), we need to address the question of when, to what degree, and why the effect diminishes. Moreover, when dealing with an experience as multifaceted as schooling, it is essential to examine effects in terms of multiple indicators, rather than a single measure such as IQ (Bronfenbrenner, 1975; Rutter, 1983). Thus the question becomes, how do the various aspects of the Head Start experience affect young children, and how do those various effects change over time?

Head Start studies. Since its inception, Head Start had been the subject of a vast array of studies, varying in quality, design, and focus. Summarizing all extant literature and unpublished studies in a focused and coherent form, the Head Start Evaluation, Synthesis, and Utilization Project (McKey et al., 1985) reported immediate positive and educationally meaningful effects of Head Start. These effects were followed, however, by variously declining performance in subsequent years and few meaningful differences between Head Start and control groups on any measure by the second year after the end of Head Start attendance (i.e., by grade 1). Effects were evaluated in terms of educational (as well as statistical) significance, defined as an effect size (ES) or difference in standard deviation (SD) units of at least .25. Many of these studies may have underestimated the efficacy of Head Start, however, given the paucity of statistical controls for initial differences in cognitive *and* demographic characteristics of those who did and did not attend Head Start (Hebbeler, 1985; Lee et al., 1988; Woodhead, 1988).

A handful of studies included in the Synthesis Project, which have looked at longer-term consequences on more "socially relevant" educational comes, have found Head Start "graduates" more likely to complete high school and less likely to repeat a grade or to be placed in special education classes. McKey et al. (1985) have concluded that, despite the loss over time of the Head Start advantage on specific cognitive measures, children who attended Head Start were at a more global advantage in school by virtue of having gained an important measure of social competence that enabled them to ". . . progress in school, stay in the mainstream, and satisfy teachers' requirements better than their peers who did not attend" (p. III-21). With effects near or above the educationally meaningful level at the end of the Head Start year, but fading thereafter, factors such as self-esteem, social behavior, and achievement motivation mirror patterns observed with cognitive measures.

Studies on the impact of demographic factors on cognitive outcomes report contradictory results. While children from classes with initially higher average IQ or SES demonstrated greater immediate effects of Head Start (an advantage that disappeared by grade 3—McKey et al., 1985; Schweinhart & Weikart, 1980), studies focusing on individual rather than classroom measures of ability found larger Head Start benefits accruing to children initially more cognitively disadvantaged (Lee et al., 1988; Miller & Bizzell, 1983).

Other preschool programs for disadvantaged children. Besides the Synthesis Project, several notable studies have examined the longitudinal effects of preschool interventions on disadvantaged children on a range of socioemotional and cognitive measures. These studies include the Consortium for Longitudinal Studies (Lazar & Darlington, 1982), Head Start in Maryland (Hebbeler, 1985), and the Educational Testing Service (ETS) Head Start Longitudinal Study (HSLS)—Lee et al., 1988). The Consortium studies, however, do not examine ordinary Head Start preschools. Moreover, some studies that did include Head Start had other goals and were not involved in evaluating Head Start per se. For example, the Louisville Experiment (part of the consortium) was designed to evaluate program variation in the context of carefully designed Head Start classroom settings, rather than comparing Head Start to no preschool experience (the major comparison in the Synthesis Project studies). While consortium findings have clear relevance for Head Start, they are not representative of the general Head Start experience. Their selection for the consortium depended on their being especially high-quality preschool ". . . research and demonstration programs . . . [whose] curricula were carefully designed and implemented" (Lazar & Darlington, 1982, p. 65).

The consortium examined preschool effects on four outcomes: school competence, ability, children's attitudes and values, and impact on the family. While significant effects were found in all four areas, the most striking was the reduced likelihood of program children being placed in special education classes during their school careers. The findings are interpreted as showing clear benefits of intervention both to individuals (in terms of allowing them to achieve school success, and, presumably, the concomitant benefits) and society (in terms of the relative cost of special education).

Two studies included in the consortium, the Louisville (Miller & Bizzell, 1983, 1984; Miller & Dyer, 1975) and High/Scope–Perry Preschool (Schweinhart & Weikart, 1980; Schweinhart, Weikart, & Larner, 1986), continued to collect extensive data on their subjects after participation in that collaboration. Both projects, concerned primarily with the effects of specific preschool curricula on disadvantaged children, followed a design including random assignment. Despite a strong design and longitudinal data collections, the Louisville results are tempered by high attrition rates at later follow-ups. High/Scope researchers, while finding the most positive long-term results of any study of preschool for disadvantaged children, also encountered high attrition. Moreover, others have questioned these findings for placing evaluation and program development in the same hands (Bereiter, 1986). Even more than the Louisville study, the Perry Preschool Project was not a generic Head Start program but an experimental, well-articulated, intensive, and multiyear program.

Project Follow Through was designed to examine whether a continuing program would produce more sustained effects. While results are equivocal, since a large proportion of children in Follow Through never attended Head Start, and a large number of children used for comparison purposes did in fact attend Head Start, early studies indicated that 2 years after preschool, Head Start effects were sustained only for those also in Follow Through (Abelson, 1974; Kennedy, 1978).

One-year study of Head Start using the HSLS data. The present article builds upon a recent study examining children's 1-year gains in Head Start (Lee et al., 1988) using data collected in the ETS Head Start Longitudinal Study (HSLS—Educational Testing Service, 1971; Shipman, 1972). In that study, children in Head Start centers in two cities in school year 1969–1970 were compared to two comparison groups: (*a*) disadvantaged children not in preschool that year (the traditional control group) and (*b*) children in non-Head Start preschools for disadvantaged children. Although all subjects lived in disadvantaged neighborhoods and were thus presumed eligible for Head Start, children in the two comparison groups (especially in other preschool programs) were initially advantaged on social background (mother's education, household crowding, single-parent family, and maternal reading habits) and in cognitive, socioemotional, and motor control status. Moreover, Head Start children were considerably more likely to be black, with black children lower on all social and cognitive measures at program entry.

The study evaluated all measures after the preschool year, presenting results with and without statistical adjustment for demographic differences. Unadjusted cognitive gains favored Head Start over both comparison groups for three of the four outcomes (ES = .21 to .40). Because of significant program-by-background interactions that would otherwise obviate use of an analysis of covariance (ANCOVA) design, adjusted gains were presented separately by race. Adjusted results showed significant Head Start effects for blacks only. Head Start was significantly more effective for blacks than either comparison group on a measure of impulsivity (ES = .27, .32) and significantly more effective than no preschool on a measure of sociocognitive development (ES = .32). Head Start effects significantly favored black students who ranked below average in initial cognitive status. Thus, Head Start appeared to work best for students who needed it most (i.e., those initially the most socially and cognitively disadvantaged).

The study's strengths resulted mostly from the careful initial design of the HSLS. While the Synthesis Project summarized studies either by comparison group or pretest/posttest design, this study incorporated both comparison features. Unlike the majority of evaluation studies that examine either single centers or specific educational models, the HSLS includes data from Head Start centers in multiple sites, and considerable efforts were made to canvas all children in designated disadvantaged neighborhoods in those cities in the study. The study's design included two comparison groups, a wide range of dependent measures, examination of results separately by race, as well as measures of initial status on cognitive *and* family/child characteristics, allowing statistical adjustment for potential bias due to the acknowledged nonequivalence of comparison groups.

The present study is a follow-up of the Lee et al. study, with our inquiry restricted to the black HSLS sample. Using an array of measures of cognitive and social competence, we have examined the impact of Head Start relative to both comparison groups 1 and 2 years after the preschool experience (i.e., at the end of kindergarten and grade 1). An issue of interest for the study is the change over time that accrues to children of differing cognitive ability levels, given the earlier findings.

METHOD

Original sample. This study is a longitudinal follow-up of a study described above using data from the HSLS (ETS, 1971; Lee et al., 1988; Shipman, 1972). Subjects in the earlier study included 969 disadvantaged children aged 4 to 5 years in Trenton, NJ, and Portland, OR, 696 (or 72%) of whom were black. Selection procedures used in a neighborhood canvassing procedure in elementary school districts with a substantial proportion of the population eligible for Head Start, so that a large proportion of all age-appropriate and possibly eligible children in the two communities were included in the study. Children from families speaking a foreign language and those with severe handicaps were excluded (Shipman, 1970). At the outset, children were tested and then enrolled in Head Start (46%), other preschool programs for disadvantaged children (22%), or were not in preschool (33%) in 1969–1970. Group assignment was subject to family choice and was not under experimental control.

Present sample. Children from the original sample who remained in their communities and who attended half-day public school kindergartens in 1970–1971 and grade 1 in 1971–1972 were eligible for the follow-up.[1] All black children in the original sample who had available data in 1969, 1970, 1971, and 1972 (hereafter referred to as Times 1–4, respectively) comprised the present sample. Although the original sample contained 173 white children, we restricted the present study to black children since nonrandom attrition 1 and 2 years past intervention (Times 3 and 4) was significantly more likely for whites and was larger for the No Preschool and Other Preschool than for the Head Start group, obviating the possibility of separate-by-race analyses due to unacceptably small white samples in comparison groups. The 1-year study, moreover, found significant positive effects for Head Start only for black children, though it was impossible to determine whether the lack of effects for whites resulted from race differences or low statistical power. We believe that lack of concern about ethnicity is a serious shortcoming of the preschool efficacy literature (Ogbu, 1985; Washington, 1985), and we regret that cross-race comparisons were not possible here.

Subjects are 646 black children with some data in the three follow-ups (1970, 1971, 1972) and family background and test data at the base year (1969). This represents 93% of the original sample of black children (see Table 1). The small number of missing cases were statistically similar (in terms of family background and ability) to the analytic sample. Slightly over half (54%) of the children were from Trenton. Half (51%) of the children had spent the preschool year in Head Start, 32% did not attend preschool, and 17% attended other preschools. Both Head Start and non-Head Start programs were standard preschools (not day-care) and were at least 8 to 9 months in duration. Other preschool programs existed under the sponsorship of universities, churches, and private organizations. Details on the preschool programs and on the elementary schools attended by most of the study children

---

[1]Eligibility data were obtained as part of the interview with the mother in the spring of the Head Start year (Year 2). In 1969, the Head Start poverty guidelines were $3,000 for a family of three, with an increment of $600 for each additional person (Shipman, 1972).

TABLE 1
Sample Sizes for Head Start, No Preschool, and Other Preschool Groups for Two Sites

Site	Head Start	No Preschool	Other Preschool	Total
Trenton, NJ	142	106	47	295
	(48.1%)	(35.9%)	(15.9%)	
Portland, OR	191	98	62	351
	(54.4%)	(27.9%)	(17.7%)	
Subtotal	333	204	109	646
	(51.5%)	(31.6%)	(16.9%)	

(particularly those having 50% or more of study children in at least one class) are available in Lindstrom and Shipman (1973).[2]

Outcome measures. Dependent measures tapped aspects of cognitive functioning other than verbal production and included variables designed to examine other aspects of school readiness, such as social competence. The subset used here was selected from a larger set measured at Times 3 and 4 (Shipman, 1972), based on their diversity from one another, on reasonably low proportions of missing data, and on reasonable proportions of explained variance. These measures tap three domains: verbal achievement (Cooperative Primary Test), perceptual reasoning (Children's Embedded Figures Test and the Raven's Colored Progressive Matrices), and social competence (California Preschool Competency Scale and the Schaefer Classroom Behavior Inventory). The first two domains are primarily cognitive.[3]

The Cooperative Primary Test (1965–1967), a nationally normed achievement test for grades 1.5 to 2.5, assessed *verbal achievement* at Time 4, with scores derived for listening skills, word analyses, and reading (50 to 60 items each).[4] Z score forms of subtests were summed (alpha reliability .80). The test was group administered by classroom teachers to target classrooms (i.e., those containing at least 50% children who had been previously tested—Bridgeman & Shipman, 1975). Two tests measured the second cognitive domain, *perceptual reasoning*. Given at Times 3 and 4, the Children's Embedded Figures Test, a modification of the same

---

[2]Some comparisons with current Head Start programs are in order. Our sample contained more blacks (and no Hispanics) compared to current figures (i.e., in 1970 the Trenton sample was 94% black; in 1986, 66% black and 17% Hispanic; in 1970, the Portland sample was 82% black, but 31% black and 16% Asian in 1986—Administration for Children, Youth, and Families, 1987). In addition, even though more mothers of young children are in the work force today than in the early 1970s, the availability of day-care services is still an issue, especially in disadvantaged communities (Schweinhart, 1985). Head Start is still one of the few child-care options available for 4-year-olds.

[3]The Matching Familiar Figures Test was given at Times 3 and 4 (Kagan, Rusman, Day, Albert, & Phillips, 1964). Positive but nonsignificant effects were found for Head Start compared to the two comparison groups.

[4]The Cooperative Primary Test—Math was also given, but since we found very few effects in either direction, we have not included it here.

test for 5–10-year-olds, measured differentiation and perceptual functioning (Dreyer, Nebelkopf, & Dreyer, 1969; Witkin, Oltman, Raskin, & Karp, 1971). At Time 4, the Raven's Colored Progressive Matrices Test (Raven, 1965) presented a perceptual reasoning task not relying on verbal performance (Sets A, AB, and B). The task required selecting the piece that would complete a partially formed pattern from a set of six alternative graphics for 36 items (Bridgeman & Shipman). Test/retest reliabilities range from .85 to .92; interitem consistency is above .95. The test exhibits moderate correlations with intelligence tests relying more heavily on verbal performance.

Measures of *social competence* used teacher ratings. On the California Preschool Social Competency Scale (LeVine, Elzey, & Lewis, 1969), kindergarten teachers used 30 items to rate "a child's successful integration into a preschool program" (Lytton, 1978, p. 510) at Time 3. Items tap work habits, communication, interpersonal relations, frustration, and help seeking. Interrater reliability ranges from .75 to .86, with split-half reliabilities above .90 (LeVine et al., 1969). While the test has clear face validity, no information on predictive validity exists, as there is no recognized standard of social competence with which it could be compared (Lytton, 1978). At Time 4, teachers completed a version of the Schaefer Classroom Behavior Inventory (CBI—Schaefer & Aaronson, 1967). Our analyses employed the task orientation scale.[5] The two inventories measure somewhat different competencies, as evidenced by their modest correlation ($r = .299$).

Family background, demographic, and site measures. Independent measures included a variety of familial and demographic measures obtained through interviews with mothers at the base year. The subset used includes: sex (1 = female, 0 = male), father's presence in the household (1 = yes, 0 = no), the proportion of children to adults in the household, and social class (SES).[6] The two sites were dummy coded (1 = Trenton, 0 = Portland). As children's age, family crowding, and the amount the mother reported reading to the child showed no significant differences between the program groups, these measures were not included as covariates. The general ability factor[7] controlled for cognitive functioning differences at the outset of the preschool year.

---

[5]The revised Schaefer Classroom Behavior Inventory (Schaefer & Edgerton, 1983) includes features of the earlier test as well as others (specifically, task orientation). The newer scale has adequate internal consistency, factor structure, and predictive validity to measures developed in the late 1960s (Anderson & Messick, 1974; Zigler & Trickett, 1978).

[6]Since eligibility data were collected *after* the preschool/Head Start decision was made, and since a large proportion of mothers were either unable or unwilling to provide income information, we constructed an SES factor to account for possible initial familial differences. The factor was constructed as the mean of standardized versions of nonmissing values of (*a*) mother's education, (*b*) occupation of household head on the Hollingshead scale, and (*c*) family income at Time 2. Alpha reliability: .58.

[7]Factor weights of tests given at Time 1 (Lee et al., 1988) for a general ability control were: Peabody Picture Vocabulary Test, .64; Caldwell Preschool Inventory, .73; Motor Inhibition Test, .33; Eight-Block Sorting Task, .52. Factor explained 56% of the combined variance, with alpha reliability of .72.

Subgroup background differences. Because group membership was not under experimental control, and because acceptance into Head Start was dependent in part on family circumstances, it is not surprising that children in the three program groups differed on demographic and family characteristics. Since, unfortunately, it is not unusual to find social background related to cognitive functioning, it is also not surprising that cognitive ability is related to group membership (Schnur & Brooks-Gunn, 1989).

A comparison of initial background differences (at Time 1) across program groups showed that black children enrolled in Head Start were the least advantaged, in terms of demographic, family, and general ability characteristics. While there were no sex differences in program enrollment, students in Head Start came from families of significantly lower SES, were significantly less likely to have a father in the house, and had fewer adults per child in the household. The children who initially attended other preschools were relatively the most advantaged of this generally disadvantaged group of preschoolers, which is not surprising since modest fees are often associated with such preschools. On every demographic and ability measure (except gender), these children were significantly more advantaged than those in Head Start. Head Start children were similar to those who did not attend preschool in general ability level, with both groups differing from the Other Preschool group on this measure.

Differences in both SES and general ability at program entry were particularly marked, with Head Start children considerably below their Other Preschool counterparts (.67 and .43 SD, respectively). Given these significant differences among the program groups, statistical adjustment for such variation was required to properly evaluate the effects of Head Start participation on cognitive and social functioning in the early primary grades. Indeed, given our findings and those of other evaluations, adjustment for such initial differences should be considered mandatory in studies without random assignment.

Subgroup outcome differences. Since children initially enrolled in Head Start and No Preschool scored almost one-half SD below their Other Preschool counterparts in general ability at program entry, it would be reasonable to find a similar pattern of cognitive and social functioning 2 or 3 years later. Group mean scores are found in Table 2, with mean differences as well as proportions and distribution of missing data on each measure tested for statistical significance. While the proportions of missing data were not trivial (between 24% and 45%), only two of the dependent measures had nonrandom missing data, judged by either SES or ability. In every case, subjects missing data on the dependent measure were more advantaged than those with data. This means that statistical adjustment for background and general ability might *underadjust*, but never overadjust, for preexisting differences.[8]

---

[8]This pattern of missing data is unusual. Commonly in educational research, students with missing

TABLE 2

Means and Standard Deviations of Dependent Measures for Three Program Groups

Measure	Head Start	No Preschool	Other Preschool	Missing Data (Proportion)
Perceptual reasoning:				
Embedded Figures Test (Time 4):				30.3[a]
Mean	7.32	6.59	6.90	
SD	(3.75)	(3.77)	(3.16)	
Raven's Progressive Matrices (Time 4):				23.7[a]
Mean	15.27	15.45	16.09	
SD	(3.47)	(3.27)	(3.96)	
Verbal achievement:[b]				
Cooperative Primary Test (Time 4):				45.4[a]
Mean	−.02	−.15	−.01	
SD	(.95)	(.74)	(.92)	
Social competence:[b]				
California Preschool Competency Test (Time 3):				37.3[c,d]
Mean[e]	79.20	72.46	83.60	
SD	(19.68)	(21.19)	(21.77)	
Schaefer Classroom Behavior Inventory (Time 4):				42.1[d]
Mean[e]	16.64	18.23	18.33	
SD	(5.81)	(5.35)	(5.63)	

[a] Mean difference on demographic and ability measures between retained and missing subjects not statistically significant, measured with *t* tests.

[b] Missing data for these measures are due, in large part, to the fact that data were collected only in classrooms with high proportions of sample subjects.

[c] Mean difference on social class between retained and missing subjects favors missing cases, $p < .05$.

[d] Mean differences on general ability between retained and missing subjects favor missing cases, $p < .05$.

[e] Mean difference between Head Start and No Preschool groups significant, $p < .05$.

In most cases, unadjusted differences in dependent measures were minor. Only on the two measures of social competence were differences between Head Start and comparison groups significant (in opposite directions). As the three groups differed on many demographic and cognitive background measures, such initial differences have to be taken into account to appropriately evaluate program effects. While comparison of the unadjusted program means at Times 3 and 4 indicates the actual cognitive and social competence levels of disadvantaged black children within the three experimental preschool conditions at the end of kindergarten or grade 1, substantive conclusions about program efficacy should not be drawn from these comparisons.

Analytic procedures. The aim of an impact study of this type is to make inferences that attempt to attribute students' cognitive performance levels uniquely to their preschool experiences. Because students with different backgrounds may

---

data are less socially and academically advantaged. This unusual pattern is likely to reflect the HSLS focus on Head Start and on testing in schools in poor neighborhoods.

"grow" at different rates in the absence of treatment, initial background and cognitive group differences must be controlled in multivariate analyses. As before, we employed an ANCOVA research design with ordinary least squares regression.[9] The use of ANCOVA is restricted to situations where significant interactions between background factors and program participation are not present (Anderson et al., 1980; Cohen & Cohen, 1983). In no case were program-by-initial-status interactions significant.

The three program variations were captured by two effects-coded variables, representing contrasts of Head Start with No Preschool or Other Preschool conditions. Covariates included initial cognitive status and the set of demographic variables described above. Dependent measures were the test scores presented in Table 2. Possible sex differences and program-by-gender interactions received careful attention. Although no sex effects were found in the original study, the possibility of emerging gender differences in primary school could not be discounted. Separate-by-gender analyses were run on those measures where significant sex differences were found.

RESULTS

Results of the covariance analyses are presented (in Fig. 1) as adjusted differences in outcome scores between Head Start and comparison groups in standard deviation (ES) units.[10] Positive coefficients favor Head Start; negative coefficients favor the comparison group. Analytic models generally explained between 10% and 25% of the variance in the dependent measures.[11] At the end of kindergarten, children who had Head Start preschool experience scored significantly higher on the California Preschool Competency Test than those who did not attend preschool (ES = .34). Other effects, while not statistically significant, are mostly positive (i.e., favorable to Head Start).

While standard statistical testing is the most common method to determine the "significance" of effects, consideration of the "substantive significance" of effects has been suggested by well-respected researchers (Cohen, 1977; Rosenthal & Rosnow, 1984) and followed by the Synthesis Project. Rosenthal and Cohen have both concluded that effects should be considered "small" if less than .2 SD,

---

[9]While we believe ANCOVA is the best technique to create statistically equivalent comparison groups, such "equivalence" is of course limited by the appropriateness and reliability of control variables included.

[10]Effect sizes are computed by first doubling the unstandardized regression coefficient for the particular contrast, then summing it with the coefficient of the other contrast. This sum is divided by the SD of the dependent measure for the entire sample (Draper & Smith, 1981).

[11]In general, the proportion of variance explained is highest for measures of social competence (.23 for California Preschool Competency, .16 for Schaefer) and lower for the cognitive tests (.10 for Raven's, .16 for Cooperative Primary Test, .07 for Embedded Figures Test).

"medium" if between .2 and .5 SD, and "large" if greater than .5 SD. Effects less than .1 SD are trivial. Looked at in this way, the substantive educational significance of effects is determined by their absolute magnitudes and direction (i.e., ≥ .2 SD). Figure 1 thus shows several medium "educationally significant" effects favoring Head Start. For example, Head Start is favored on the Cooperative Primary Test (ES = .28) compared to No Preschool and compared to both groups on the Embedded Figures Test (ES = .24 and .27 for the No Preschool and Other Preschool comparisons, respectively). While Head Start effects are lowest on the Schaefer Inventory, they do not reach educational significance. All educationally significant effects (4 out of 10) favor Head Start.

Because of earlier findings of 1-year Head Start gains favoring low-ability black children, we divided the sample into below- and above-average groups on general ability and used identical ANCOVA designs. While the same pattern was not characteristic of longer-term follow-up results, effects were generally larger when investigated separately for children of differing initial ability. Of the nine effects that met the criterion of educational significance, six were positive for Head Start. In terms of sex differences, there were significant effects in social competence favoring girls ($p \leq .001$ for California Competency Test, $p \leq .01$ for the Schaefer)— noteworthy but not surprising. We thus examined Head Start effects separately for male and female children, finding one significant ($p \leq .01$) and substantial (ES = .49) Head Start effect (compared to No Preschool) favoring males on the California Preschool Competency measure, and effect also significantly different from that for females (ES = .23).

DISCUSSION

Summary of findings. Participation in Head Start has enduring effects for disadvantaged black children through Grade 1 on some measures of school success, particularly compared to no preschool attendance. Five tests measured skills in two domains: cognitive ability and social competence. Educationally substantive effects favoring Head Start appeared in the cognitive domain (specifically the Embedded Figures and Cooperative Primary Tests, but not the Raven's), and these effects were larger than those reported in the Synthesis Project for grade 1. Thus, we have evidence of continuation of an effect demonstrated immediately after the Head Start experience (Lee et al., 1988). These effects were found when initial social and cognitive differences between those who did and did not have a Head Start experience were controlled.

Taking the findings of the two studies together, it is clear that strong effects favoring Head Start relative to both comparison groups at the end of the preschool year have been attenuated but not dissipated by the end of grade 1, supporting the Synthesis Project results. The particularly strong Head Start effects for black chil-

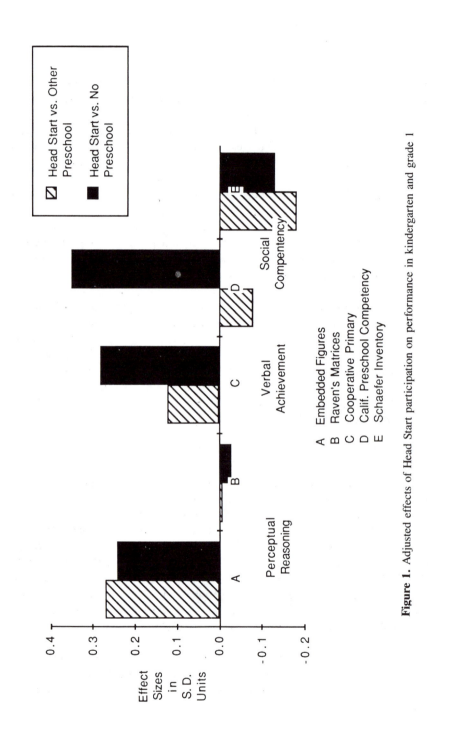

Figure 1. Adjusted effects of Head Start participation on performance in kindergarten and grade 1

dren of lower ability found at the end of the preschool year, however, have not been sustained through the early primary years. Moreover, whereas 1-year Head Start gains were favorable to both comparison groups, sustained effects are more prevalent in comparison to children without preschool experience than compared to those who attended other preschools for disadvantaged children. We interpret this as indicating that disadvantaged black children benefit from any preschool experience compared to none at all. In fact, Head Start serves the least advantaged of children in poor neighborhoods and is likely to have been the major preschool option available to poor families in 1970. While this may be changing, given the increase in state- and city-sponsored programs for disadvantaged preschool children and the expected increases in child care programs for mothers in AFDA-sponsored workfare initiatives, Head Start is still the focus of discussions on preschool for disadvantaged children.[12]

Possible explanations. Two logical (and not mutually exclusive) explanations might account for our findings of a diminution of effects over time. Both explanations are related to the fact that black Head Start enrollees enter preschool and elementary school at a particular cognitive and social disadvantage. In 1970 as well as today, Head Start serves less than a third of all eligible children. Available evidence suggests that the most disadvantaged (i.e., the poorest of the poor) are being enrolled today, as before (Hebbeler, 1985).

The first explanation is associated with the subsequent school experiences of these disadvantaged children. We know that social background is related to *what school* students attend, with residential location the determining factor. Particularly poor children are likely to be concentrated in low-SES schools, and this relation is exacerbated for minority children in urban areas (Ogbu, 1986; Spencer, Brookins, & Allen, 1985; Wilson, 1987). Particularly poor (and minority) children are also likely to receive less favorable treatment in such schools, resulting in reduced learning opportunities (Alexander & Entwisle, 1989; Rist, 1970; Sorensen, 1987). Such social disadvantages are compounded by differential treatment in school based on lower cognitive status (Barr & Dreeben, 1983; Rist, 1970). Thus, these children's elementary school experiences, relative to their more socially and cognitively advantaged counterparts, could very likely "undo" the advantages accrued as a result of a year in Head Start. It is unrealistic to expect a 9-month intervention—either Head Start or any preschool program—to overcome the past or future accumulated effects of disadvantage. As Zigler has stated repeatedly, "We simply cannot inoculate children in 1 year against the ravages of a life of deprivation" (1987, p. 258).

Another explanation relates to family environment. Children with less educated parents, with fathers less likely to be present, whose family incomes are especially

---

[12]It has been suggested that contemporary intervention programs for disadvantaged preschoolers are better designed and potentially more efficacious than those of almost 2 decades ago. Under this view, these results may be seen as representing a lower bound for effectiveness of the Head Start program.

low, are likely to experience some academic deprivation associated with such environmental conditions (Lee, 1985; White, 1982). The less advantaged home backgrounds of Head Start children relative to the comparison groups considered here could also contribute to "undoing" the immediate advantages from the Head Start experience, and such conditions are likely to be confounded with the unfavorable school and classroom experiences discussed above.

Policy implications. There are three policy implications we draw from this study, the first two of which relate to the results themselves, while the third concerns what is *not* in this article. First, the fact that Head Start (and other preschool programs) has some effects that are sustained through the early primary years argues in favor of continuing (and possibly increasing) federal support for preschool programs for disadvantaged youngsters. The second implication—one we would like to highlight—relates to the amelioration of the particularly strong effects found after a year of the program for the most cognitively disadvantaged students. If 1 year of an intense educational experience targeted for such children can show strong effects, the more abbreviated compensatory programs perhaps available to such children are unlikely to overcome what are likely to be especially poor school experiences. Chapter 1, for example, is a pull-out program for cognitively disadvantaged children in low-SES schools of only 2 to 3 hours/week. Such findings suggest that a more intense program "works," while a less intense one probably does not. This argues for widespread expansion of stimulating educational experiences targeted at cognitively and socially disadvantaged young children in the elementary years.

The third policy implication is drawn from the nature of the HSLS itself. Renewed interest in preschool children for disadvantaged children forces us to look at data collected nearly 2 decades ago. We have chosen to analyze the HSLS data because of their strong design: large samples, generic Head Start programs, two comparison groups, two diverse sites, carefully collected baseline and longitudinal measures. However, we are forced to *impute* the effectiveness of current Head Start programs from a rather dated study. Why? There are literally no studies of such quality currently available. The HSLS was a federally funded effort begun during the War on Poverty. Such studies are intense and expensive. Without federal support for careful program evaluation, as well as support for the programs themselves, the concerned and interested public is in no position to judge whether such programs are *worth* supporting. We believe that the results presented here argue for an intensification of support for compensatory preschool and early elementary programs. We argue that such program support must be accompanied by federally financed and carefully designed evaluation efforts.

While it is gratifying to find sustained effects of Head Start participation for black children, it is also unfortunate that we are unable to provide evidence of the program's efficacy for nonblack children (including whites). We do not believe that the effects are restricted to blacks—not that Head Start is a "black" program.

Indeed, only 40% of Head Start enrollees in 1985–1986 were black (ACYF, 1987). This and other evaluations of Head Start (e.g., Lazar & Darlington, 1982; McKey et al., 1985) at present provide better and more complete data on blacks, but such results say nothing about Head Start's applicability to other ethnic groups.

Clearly, if we wish to "close the gap" between advantaged and disadvantaged children, educational services need to go beyond the provision of short-term interventions. Policy decisions that support the expansion of preschool programs without addressing the more fundamental question of trying to alter what happens to disadvantaged children in our nation's public schools are shortsighted. Research such as this, which provides evidence of some success of preschool education for disadvantaged children, could be used to support arguments for what might be politically expedient and even short-sighted "solutions" to a pervasive problem (Woodhead, 1988). Inducing sustained and successful academic experiences for children of poverty *throughout* their educational careers, rather than focusing on efforts to "fix" the problem with 1-year preschool programs (however successful they may be), is absolutely essential.

REFERENCES

Abelson, W. (1974). Head Start graduates in school: Studies in New Haven, Connecticut. In S. Ryan (Ed.), *A report on longitudinal evaluations of preschool programs: Vol. 1. Longitudinal evaluations* (pp. 1–4). Washington, DC: Department of Health, Education, and Welfare.

Administration for Children, Youth, and Families (ACYF). (1987, January). *Project Head Start statistical fact sheet.* Washington, DC: Department of Health and Human Services, Office of Human Development Services.

Alexander, K. L., & Entwisle, D. R. (1989). Achievement in the first 2 years of school: Patterns and processes. *Monographs of the Society for Research in Child Development, 53*(2, Serial No. 218).

Anderson, S., Auquier, A., Hauck, W. W., Oakes, D., Vandaele, W., & Weisberg, H. I. (1980). *Statistical methods for comparative studies: Techniques for bias reduction.* New York: Wiley.

Anderson, S., & Messick, S. (1974). Social competency in young children. *Developmental Psychology, 10,* 282–293.

Barnett, W. S. (1985) Benefit-cost analysis of the Perry Preschool Program and its long-term effects. *Educational Evaluation and Policy Analysis, 7,* 333–342.

Barnett, W. S., Frede, E., Mobasher, H., & Mohr, P. (1987). The efficacy of public preschool programs and the relationship of program quality to efficacy. *Educational Evaluation and Policy Analysis, 10,* 37–49.

Barr, R., & Dreeben, R. (1983). *How schools work.* Chicago: University of Chicago Press.

Bereiter, C. (1986). Does direct instruction cause delinquency? *Early Childhood Research Quarterly, 1,* 289–292.

Bridgeman, B., & Shipman, V. C. (1975). *Predictive value of measures of self-esteem and achievement motivation in 4- to 9-year-old low-income children* (ETS Technical Report Series PR-75-241). Princeton, NJ: Educational Testing Service.

Bronfenbrenner, U. (1975). Is early intervention effective? In M. Guttentag & E. Streuning (Eds.), *Handbook of evaluation research* (Vol. 2, pp. 519–603. Beverly Hills, CA: Sage.

Cohen, J. (1977). *Statistical power analysis for the behavioral sciences.* New York: Academic Press.

Cohen, J., & Cohen, P. (1983). *Applied multiple regression/correlation analysis for the behavioral sciences*, 2d ed. Hillsdale, NJ: Erlbaum.

Conger, J. (1988). Hostages to fortune: Youth, values, and the public interest. *American Psychologist*, **43**, 291–300.

Cooperative Primary Test. (1965–1967). Consulting tests and services. Educational Testing Service, Princeton, NJ.

Draper, N. R., & Smith, H. (1981). *Applied regression analysis, 2d ed.* New York: Wiley.

Dreyer, E. S., Nebelkopf, F., & Dreyer, C. A. (1969). Note concerning stability of cognitive style measures in young children. *Perceptual and Motor Skills*, **28**, 933–934.

Educational Testing Service. (1971, July). *Disadvantaged children and their first school experiences: Preliminary description of the initial sample prior to school enrollment.* Princeton, NJ: Educational Testing Service.

Evans, E. (1985). Longitudinal follow-up assessment of differential preschool experience for low income minority group children. *Journal of Educational Research*, **78**, 197–202.

Hebbeler, K. (1985). An old and a new question on the effects of early education for children from low income families. *Educational Evaluation and Policy Analysis*, **7**, 207–216.

Kagan, J., Rusman, B. L., Day, D., Albert, J., & Phillips, W. (1964). Information processing in the child: Significance of analytic and reflective attitudes. *Psychological Monographs*, **78**, 598.

Kennedy, M. M. (1978). Findings from the Follow Through Planned Variation Study. *Educational Researcher*, **7**, 3–11.

Lazar, I., & Darlington, R. (1982). Lasting effects of early education: A report from the consortium for longitudinal studies. *Monographs of the Society for Research in Child Development*, **47**(2/3, Serial No. 195).

Lee, V. E. (1985). *Investigating the relationship between social class and academic achievement in public and Catholic schools.* Unpublished doctoral dissertation, Harvard University.

Lee, V. E., Brooks-Gunn, J., & Schnur, E. (1988). Does Head Start work? A 1-year follow-up comparison of disadvantaged children attending Head Start, no preschool, and other preschool programs. *Developmental Psychology*, **24**, 210–222.

LeVine, S., Elzey, S. S., & Lewis, M. (1969). *California Preschool Social Competency Scale.* Palo Alto, CA: Consulting Psychologists Press.

Lindstrom, D. R., & Shipman, V. C. (1973, June). *Disadvantaged children and their first school experience: Characteristics of urban preschool centers: Analysis of the preschool center inventory* (ETS Tech. Rep. Series, PR-72-21). Princeton, NJ: Educational Testing Service.

Lytton, H. (1978). Commentary on the California Preschool Social Competency Scale. In *The eighth mental measurements yearbook* (pp. 512–513). Highland Park, NJ: Gryphon.

McKey, R. H., Condelli, L., Granson, H., Barrett, B., McConkey, C., & Plantz, M. (1985, June). *The impact of Head Start on children, families and communities* (final report of the Head Start Evaluation, Synthesis and Utilization Project). Washington, DC: CSR.

Meyer, L. (1984). Long-term academic effects of the direct instruction Project Follow Through. *Elementary School Journal,* **84,** 380–394.

Miller, L. B., & Bizzell, R. P. (1983). Long-term effects of four preschool programs: Sixth, seventh, and eighth grades. *Child Development,* **54,** 727–741.

Miller, L. B., & Bizzell, R. P. (1984). Long-term effects of four preschool programs: Ninth- and tenth-grade results. *Child Development,* **55,** 1570–1587.

Miller, L. B., & Dyer, J. (1975). Four preschool programs: Their dimensions and effects. *Monographs of the Society for Research in Child Development,* **40**(5/6, Serial No. 162).

Ogbu, J. U. (1985). A cultural ecology of competence among inner-city blacks. In M. B. Spencer, G. K. Brookins, & W. R. Allen (Eds.), *Beginnings: The social and affective development of black children* (pp. 45–66). Hillsdale, NJ: Erlbaum.

Ogbu, J. U. (1986). The consequences of the American caste system. In U. Neisser (Ed.), *The school achievement of minority children* (pp. 19–56). Hillsdale, NJ: Erlbaum.

Raven, J. C. (1965). *Guide to using the Coloured Progressive Matrices: Sets A, AB, & B.* London: H. K. Lewis.

Rist, R. C. (1970). Student social class and teacher expectations: The self-fulfilling prophesy in ghetto education. *Harvard Educational Review,* **40,** 411–451.

Rosenthal, R., & Rosnow, R. L. (1984). *Essentials of behavioral analysis: Methods and data analysis.* New York: McGraw-Hill.

Rutter, M. (1983). School effects on pupils' progress: Research findings and policy implications. *Child Development,* **54,** 1–29.

Schaefer, E. S., & Aaronson, M. R. (1967). *Classroom Behavior Inventory.* Unpublished form, University of North Carolina.

Schaefer, E. S., & Edgerton, M. (1983, August). *Unified model for academic competence, social adjustment, and psychopathology.* Paper presented at the American Psychological Association meeting, Anaheim, CA.

Schnur, E., & Brooks-Gunn, J. (1989). *Who attends Head Start? A comparison of Head Start attendees and nonattendees from three sites in 1969–1970.* Princeton, NJ: Educational Testing Service.

Schweinhart, L. J. (1985). *Early childhood development programs in the eighties: The national picture.* High/Scope Early Childhood Policy Papers, no. 1. Ypsilanti, MI: High/Scope Press.

Schweinhart, L. J., & Weikart, D. (1980). Young children grow up: The effects of the Perry Preschool Program on youths through age 16. *Monographs of the High/Scope Educational Research Foundation,* vol. **7.** Ypsilanti, MI: High/Scope Press.

Schweinhart, L. J., & Weikart, D. (1983). The effects of the Perry Preschool Program on youths through age 15—a summary. In Consortium for Longitudinal Studies (Ed.),

As the twig is bent . . . Lasting effects of preschool programs (pp. 71–101). Hillsdale, NJ: Erlbaum.

Schweinhart, L., Weikart, D., & Larner, M. (1986). Consequences of three preschool curriculum models through age 15. *Early Childhood Research Quarterly, 1,* 15–45.

Seitz, V., Rosenbaum, L. K., & Apfel, N. H. (1985). Effects of family support intervention: A ten-year follow-up. *Child Development, 56,* 376–391.

Shipman, V. C. (1970). *Preliminary description of the initial sample prior to school enrollment* (ETS Tech. Rep. Series, PR-70-20). Princeton, NJ: Educational Testing Service.

Shipman, V. C. (Ed.) (1972). *Disadvantaged children and their first school experience* (ETS Tech. Rep. Series, PR-72-27). Princeton, NJ: Educational Testing Service.

Sorensen, A. B. (1987). The organizational differentiation of students in schools as an opportunity structure. In M. T. Hallinan (Ed.), *The social organization of schools* (pp. 103–156). New York: Plenum.

Spencer, M. B., Brookins, G. K., & Allen, W. R. (Eds.). (1985). *Beginnings: The social and affective development of black children.* Hillsdale, NJ: Erlbaum.

Washington, V. (1985). Head Start: Now appropriate for minority families in the 1980s? *American Journal of Orthopsychiatry, 55,* 577–590.

Washington-Smith, V., with assistance of Oyemade, U. J. (1987). *Project Head Start: Past, present, and future trends in the context of family needs: A source book.* New York: Garland.

White, K. R. (1982). The relationship between socioeconomic status and academic achievement. *Psychological Bulletin, 91,* 461–481.

Wilson, W. J. (1987). *The truly disadvantaged: The inner city, the underclass, and public policy.* Chicago: University of Chicago Press.

Witkin, H. A., Oltman, P. K., Raskin, E., & Karp, F. A. (1971). *Manual for the Children's Embedded Figures Test.* Palo Alto: CA: Consulting Psychologists Press.

Woodhead, M. (1988). When psychology informs public policy: The case of early childhood intervention. *American Psychologist, 43,* 443–454.

Zigler, E. F. (1987). Formal schooling for four-year-olds? No. *American Psychologist, 42,* 254–260.

Zigler, E. F., & Trickett, P. K. (1978). IQ, social competence, and evaluation of early childhood intervention programs. *American Psychologist, 33,* 789–798.

Zigler, E. F., & Valentine, J. (Eds.). (1979). *Project Head Start: A legacy of the war on poverty.* New York: Free Press.

30

The Seventh Jack Tizard Memorial Lecture: Aspects of Adoption

Lionel Hersov

University of Massachusetts Medical Center, Worcester

Adoption has a long history and there has been a change in traditional assumptions and practice. It is now seen as a form of child care, one of a spectrum of resources for children in need. Adopted children generally show a good outcome but are over-represented in clinical populations. This trend is likely to continue as older children with histories of severe deprivation, neglect, abuse and institutionalization are placed. New light has been thrown on "telling" in adoption by developmental studies. Adoption disruption increases with age and other factors at placement, requiring further research into its origins and management.

INTRODUCTION

In September 1973, Professor Jack Tizard gave the Second Emanuel Miller Lecture to the Association for Child Psychology and Psychiatry; the title was *The upbringing of other people's children: implications of research and for research* (Tizard, 1974). In it he outlined the opportunities which a residential care setting provided for studying the effects of the environment upon children's development, saying that "one can sidestep the otherwise almost insurmountable problems of heredity and environment which confound the interpretation of findings obtained from studies of children living in their own homes" (p. 161).

In a different way, adoption also involves the upbringing of other people's children and adoption studies have helped to clarify some of the relative influences of heredity and environment on development and psychopathology. A basic research question has become an applied question for mental health professionals, pediatricians,

Reprinted with permission from *Journal of Child Psychology and Psychiatry*, 1990, Vol. 31, No. 4, 493–510. Copyright © 1990 by the Association for Child Psychology and Psychiatry.
Delivered at the ACPP Annual Conference, Friday 30 June 1989.

developmental psychologists, adoption workers, and adoptive and perhaps biological parents (Plomin & DeFries, 1985).

I like to think that Jack Tizard would have been intrigued by data coming from recent adoption practice and research, although he would probably have remained unconvinced by some of the claims made in what remains a complex area.

The practice of adoption has its origin in the beginnings of human society. The Babylonian code of Hammurabi, the oldest written set of laws, includes a section on adoption dealing with some of the legal issues that still concern us today (Benet, 1976). Such ancient civilizations as the Egyptians, Chinese, Indians and Romans practiced adoption, as it was among several possible ways of providing an heir, safeguarding the succession of wealthy families by property inheritance, as well as ensuring the continuity of ancestral worship. In many of these societies, adoption met the needs of wealthy man who lacked heirs, so adult males were often adopted (Benet, 1976).

In India, among Hindus, adoption was a way of providing a male child for the demands of religious ceremonies. The adopting father declares "I accept thee for fulfillment of religion. I take thee for the continuation of lineage" (Hastings, 1908, p. 110).

There were other ways of bringing children into a family other than adoption. Under Islamic law, the rescue of abandoned children was allowed without permitting adoption (Tizard, 1977). Another man's son will have his father's name if taken into another family, where he will be called a brother. The obligation to be charitable to those less fortunate can thus lead to taking other children into a family (Benet, 1976).

Adoption has only recently become a recognized practice in Western Society and it was in the United States of America, with its egalitarian ideas, that modern adoption practice developed. Historians and legal scholars concur that the American law on adoption emerged in the middle of the 19th century with the passage in 1851 of the Massachusetts statute "An Act to Provide for the Adoption of Children" (Kawashima, 1981/1982). The Act is agreed to be the first general law of adoption in the United States and Britain. It was aimed at the *welfare* of children in contrast to the traditional adoption systems which existed in different societies outside the common law. These traditional systems were to benefit adoptors, whereas the Massachusetts law saw adoption as a charitable act, a way of giving a homeless child a more humane upbringing than life in an institution. There are great differences, obviously, between the 1851 law and current adoption laws, but in both, the child's welfare and adopting parents' rights are safeguarded (Presser, 1972). More children are legally adopted in the U.S.A. than any other country.

The adoption arrangement, traditional or modern, is a *triangular* relationship between the natural parents, the child and the adopting parents, serving these parties, through different functions (Sorosky, Baran & Pannor, 1984). The interests of each may differ widely. The child's welfare is enhanced through a better material upbringing and superior education than the natural parents can often provide. Parental burdens may be eased and their hopes for their child realized in a more congenial family environment with better stimulation, wider experience and vocational choice. The reasons and motives of the adopting parents are more varied, a desire to perpetuate their family and pass on the family tradition in tangible form, the satisfaction of rearing a child often in addition to their own, or to make the lives of an infertile couple more lively and meaningful by including a child (Kawashima, 1981/1982).

Each year many thousands of children are adopted. The majority are illegitimate births, but increasing numbers result from legal termination of biological parents' rights because of abuse or neglect. Other children become available for adoption because of parental death, abandonment, or voluntary relinquishment by parents. Also, an increasing number of foreign-born children are being adopted. Accurate figures on adoption in the U.S.A. are not easily available because only a small number of states publish their statistics, and the last federal effort to collect national data ceased in 1975 (Adoption Factbook, 1985). A recent national health survey suggests that there are approximately 1.3 million adopted children under 18 years of age (or roughly 2% of the child population) (Zill, 1985). Nearly two-thirds of all adoptions are related or intrafamilial and the remainder are adopted extrafamilially, i.e., by unrelated adults. It is these that have received major research attention. Since legislation was enacted in the U.S.A. in 1980 in order to provide permanence for children in their own homes and adoptive families, more older children and those with special needs are entering adoptive placements. In California the percentage of older-child adoptions rose from 4.6% in 1970 to 44.1% in 1980 (Barth, Berry, Carson, Goodfield & Feinberg, 1986).

CHANGING TRENDS IN ADOPTION PRACTICE

Since the 1920s, until fairly recently, adoption was seen primarily as a service for childless couples, to provide them with a child of their own to cement the marriage, and meet the adults' emotional needs. The concept of adoption currently in vogue requires a different professional approach and poses different problems. As Barbara Tizard has pointed out (Tizard, 1977), adoption is now seen as *a form of child care*, one of several ways of bringing up children whose parents are unable to do so, or simply will not look after them. As a result, different criteria now exist for placement. Earlier on, proof of infertility was required, the racial origins and health of the child were closely examined, and attempts were made to match infant and couple. At present, any child in need can be considered for adoption, whatever his color, family history, state of health or handicap, and level of intelligence.

Placement today does not necessarily reproduce the pattern of family life that was attempted by earlier adoptions. Adoption is seen as one way of purposefully influencing the circumstances of a child's life by removing children from adverse environments and placing them in families likely to advance their intelligence and social development.

Adoptive parenting is different today and possibly more demanding and difficult. Nowadays, older couples will be accepted because they appear very suitable for a particular child, whereas in earlier times, they might have been turned down on the grounds of age. There is also increasing discussion about so-called "open" or "inclusive" adoption, where birth parents retain contact with their child after adoption, particularly when older children are adopted, while the adoptive parents have permanent responsibility for care, custody and control (Borgman, 1982).

Pediatricians and mental health professionals working with children and families can become interested in many aspects of adoption. There is curiosity about the *effects* of terminating the relationship between a child and his natural parents or foster-parents, in the light of modern attachment theory. For example, it is believed by some that this experience places the child at greater risk for psychological disturbance and academic failure than his or her non-adopted peers. Others believe that the move to a more nurturing environment confers benefits for later development, which outweigh theoretical objections to this course of action.

There are several other reasons for interest: (1) the understanding of how this unusual family pattern affects the interaction of nature and nurture during development adds to knowledge about development in general; (2) a knowledge of the interplay of factors, which may make for increased vulnerability to psychiatric disorder, could perhaps lead to effective methods of prevention, intervention and treatment; (3) there is much interest in how adopted infants and children fare as they grow older, i.e. the study of the outcome of adoption. It has been suggested that when one is making judgments on the outcome, one should look at adopted children and families in comparison with non-adopted children without parents since infancy, as well as children who have been living with natural parents since birth, as some of the better studies have done (Tizard, 1977); (4) it is obviously helpful for a clinician to be able to form an opinion about possible psychiatric disorder in the children, as well as to be able to assist adopted children and their families when problems arise. Accurate prediction is obviously very difficult but some assessment of risk factors in adoption is possible (Barth & Berry, 1988); and (5) there is also growing research literature on the characteristics of adopted children, when compared with their biological and adoptive parents. This is a specialized topic involving the inheritance of various factors and adding to the previously sparse information on adopted children as adults, and on the outcome in adult life of children adopted in different circumstances into differing family contexts. This has thrown light on the inheritance of alcoholism, criminality and some of the major psychiatric disorders, and adoption studies have been done by those working in the new inter-discipline of developmental behavioral genetics (Plomin, 1986).

ADOPTION STATISTICS AND TRENDS
IN GREAT BRITAIN AND U.S.A.

The *current pattern* of adoption is very different from that twenty-five years ago. The number of legal adoptions in Great Britain rose steadily over the 10 years from 14,500 in 1958 to a peak of nearly 27,000 in 1968 (Home Office, 1972). The figures then declined and have continued to, so that the number of orders in 1982 was just under 7900, a drop of over 50% since 1976 [Office of Population Censuses and Surveys (O.P.C.S.), 1987]. The number of adoptions by natural parents and step-parents has risen considerably, probably reflecting higher rates of divorce and remarriage. Over the last decade or so the main changes in age distribution have been a general decline in the proportion of children adopted under 2 years of age and an increase for children aged 10 and over with a particularly sharp increase for children aged 15–17 years. In 1981 50% of adoptions in Britain were of children ages 5–14 years. There were 7.2 thousand adopted in England and Wales in 1987, 9% less than in 1986 (O.P.C.S., 1989).

The data on adoption in the U.S.A. is similar in many respects. A peak of 175,000 adoptions was reached in 1970, and this fell to under 142,000 in 1982 (Adoption Factbook, 1985). The proportion of adoptions by related individuals also steadily increased until they made up 64.2% of all adoptions in 1982 and 55% in Canada. Between 1951 and 1975 the percentage of independent adoptions declined substantially in the U.S.A., while those by public and private agencies more than doubled, reflecting changes in state regulations about adoptions (Barth *et al.*, 1986). There was also a steady increase in foreign adoptions from 1979 to 1984. The Adoption Assistance and Child Welfare Act of 1980 in the U.S.A. (P. L. 96-272) embodies principles of permanency planning. It also instituted adoption subsidies for children with special needs. As a result of this law and other welfare changes, more older and special-needs children are being adopted (Barth *et al.*, 1986).

Several factors have contributed to a situation where fewer babies are being offered for adoption in both the U.K. and the U.S.A. Greater use of contraception and an increasing number of legal abortions is one. The changing attitude to ille-gitimacy and unmarried parenthood, day-care provision and other support systems, have led to many more unmarried mothers keeping their babies, as they are more able to bring up their illegitimate children on their own. The reasons for these changes are complex and not well understood, and there may yet be a swing back to the greater acceptance of adoption in the future, if conditions should alter.

Attitudes to the adoption of children of mixed race and of older children are also changing. The situation is steadily improving and it is becoming easier to place black and mixed race children. The outcome of such adoptions is apparently successful in terms of social and personal adjustment in the great majority of children, where white families adopted black children, according to several studies (Grow & Shapiro, 1974).

A WORD ABOUT ADOPTION AND RACE

There are still issues not yet settled about transracial adoption, since in many countries, concern has been expressed about the ethics and politics of transracial adoption, with charges that non-white families and children were being exploited by the white majority, with detrimental effects on the development of children.

Gill and Jackson (1983), in Britain, examined the lives and experiences of 36 transracially adopted children, who had reached adolescence, focusing on how the issue of racial background had been defined or dealt with in the families. Using criteria of family relationships, peer-group relationships, level of self-esteem and behavior disorder, they concluded that only a small number of the adoptions could be regarded as problematic, namely six children (17%) of the group, and in only one case were there indications of breakdown in the adoption. The remainder would be regarded as definitely successful, in keeping with earlier findings. On balance the outcome was as good, if not better, than a similar-aged group of white children growing up with their natural parents.

The reasons for this successful outcome were regarded as arising from the parents' commitment to caring for the child, and making him/her part of *their* family, the early age of placement so that the child grew up entirely in a white world with consistent messages and definition about their racial background. The social class of the families (mainly I and II) was a potent factor. This meant that the majority were able to live far removed from the racially mixed areas of large cities, in communities where racial tension was unlikely to be a factor, and were able to provide good schooling for their children. This in turn leads to good qualifications and power in the job market, so avoiding some of the problems normally associated with ethnic minority status.

In spite of these findings, the authors comment that the large majority of families made little attempt to give their adopted children a sense of racial pride or awareness of their racial origin. The children saw themselves as "white," in all but skin color, and had little knowledge or experience of their counterparts growing up in a black community. Their coping mechanisms appeared to depend on a denial, up till then, of their racial background.

From their experience, Gill and Jackson (1983) believe that it is vitally important for every effort to be made to find black homes for black children, whenever possible, and that more black families be encouraged to adopt. Otherwise there will be problems for a black child to develop a sense of racial identity in a white family, tensions will arise between making a child fully part of the family, while highlighting the differences. Finally, the social class influences will mean that the children will be unlikely to have significant contacts with the black community. We will have to wait to see what effect these findings will have on future adoption practice in this field. I understand that in Britain it appears that the conclusions of the study have been influencing adoption practice to some extent, and more black families are adopting black children, but with so many black children in need, transracial adoption will no doubt continue.

AGE AT ADOPTION

Another issue in adoption theory and practice has been the age of adoption. Late adoption has long been thought of as second best, or to be avoided, for several reasons, but partly because there has been a strongly held belief that early rearing experiences are critically important for later development. It has also been said that adoption placements are best made before the age of 6 months, i.e. before the infant develops focused attachments (Yarrow & Klein, 1980).

However, recent studies by Tizard (1977) and others have shown that older children can be successfully adopted. Triseliotis' and Russell's (1984) follow-up study of late adopted children, i.e. settled into their adoptive families between the ages of 2 and 8 years, also showed that the majority had a good outcome and that the rate of psychosocial problems, both in child and adult life, was below that of institution-reared children, but above that in the general population. These and other data may increase the temptation to use adoption as an outlet for the children of the most disadvantaged. However, this must be thought about most carefully. Mental health professionals, pediatricians and others experienced in child development and family pathology can play their part in weighing clinical and research data, in advising on policy and coming to individual decisions.

THE CLINICIAN'S ROLE IN ADOPTION
AND FOSTERING

What has been said so far shows how modern adoption practice today has widened in scope, and increased in complexity, requiring more knowledge, as well as access to specialist opinion, in certain instances. The wider range of older children now being considered for adoption includes those with existing psychiatric disorders and/or mental and physical handicaps. Many have earlier experienced the pressures of parental mental disorder and repeated family breakdown, meaning that some of these children are more vulnerable and sometimes more difficult to integrate into a new family. This is where knowledge of developmental psychopathology is valuable.

It is also true that hard-to-place and handicapped children are being found homes and families in greater numbers than before, but a great deal more preparation for the adoption of older children is needed than is often provided. Some children have strong ties with their families in spite of the way they have been treated and do not wish to be adopted. Others need unhurried preparation and a graded introduction to their prospective families. These obviously should be chosen with care, as well as being given adequate preparation for dealing with an older child with a past experience of failed fostering. In a situation like this, love is not enough, for the children may have many problems with authority, are often grossly insecure, with poor impulse control, as well as sometimes having a diagnosable psychiatric disorder.

Some authorities have emphasized the potential difficulties if adoption is used as a panacea in permanency planning, because foster home and group care have come in for criticism in many countries in recent years (Powers, 1984). The temptation to use adoption as a means of dealing with the children of very disadvantaged parents is hard to resist. Social workers are naturally keen to find new and permanent homes for children and these developments have brought social workers into sharp conflict with natural parents. Many of the parents still appear to retain positive feelings for their children and vice versa, in spite of the sometimes appalling histories of abuse and neglect experienced by the children. What may appear to be a clear-cut case for placement in another family often has undercurrents of emotion and prejudice which eventually undermine all but the most carefully thought out and planned placements (Kadushin & Martin, 1988).

OUTCOME OF ADOPTION

Any service dealing with children and adolescents, whether in a hospital or in the community, is bound to have adopted children referred. Questions have arisen whether adopted children are over-represented in clinical populations, whether there are distinctive social and psychological factors which differentiate adopted children and their families from natural families, and whether it is these differences which are responsible for the apparent increase in referral of adopted children for inpatient and outpatient treatment. Two different approaches have been used to assess the outcome of adoption. The first looks at the frequency of adoptees in the clinical population. The earlier clinical studies in the 1950s reported an over-presentation of adoptees in clinical populations, with adoptees likely to show aggressive and antisocial problems and learning disabilities (Hersov, 1985). Conduct disorder was more often found than emotional disorder, and boys were more often affected than girls. A study from the U.S.A. reported a high frequency of attention deficit disorders in adoptees and suggested that the diagnosis could be made in approximately 17% of adopted children (Deutsch *et al.*, 1982; Nichols & Chen, 1981). Obviously, referral bias must be taken into account, as well as the fact that attention deficit disorder has been diagnosed much more often in the U.S.A. than in Britain.

The general conclusion that emerges from these and other clinical studies is that adoptees are at greater risk. But this contrasts sharply with results of studies of non-clinical samples of adopted and non-adopted children. The discrepancy is hard to explain, but one possible difference is that clinical studies do not always specify the age of circumstances of adoption and whether the adoption is intrafamilial or extrafamilial. Studies comparing adopted and non-adopted children usually involve early placements, whereas clinical studies can include later placements with children coming from broken homes, having experienced lengthy or changing foster placements prior to adoption and being generally more exposed to stressful circumstances. In other words, they are extreme groups which differ from the rest of the distribution, whereas the comparison studies of adopted and non-adopted children consider the entire distribution, and is possible that the two groups truly differ from each other (Plomin & DeFries, 1985).

Until recently, there were more speculations about these issues than empirical facts, but recent research has provided much clearer data which can be applied in clinical practice. Adoptive families vary greatly in parental personality and family structure, and there is *not* a "standard" adoptive family. Although an adoptive family resembles an ordinary family, some maintain that it is set apart partly because of society's attitudes to illegitimacy and blood ties, so that in certain respects, adoptive parents are a minority or deviant group (Kirk, 1981). Others maintain that those who are fortunate enough to adopt an infant will still miss the experience of pregnancy and childbirth and sometimes the first few months with the infant, with later possible problems in forming secure social and emotional relationships (Reeves, 1971). A recent study bears on this issue and brings to mind T. H. Huxley's aphorism: "The great tragedy of science—the slaying of a beautiful hypothesis by an ugly fact" (p. 260, Auden & Kronenberger, 1970).

The Colorado Adoption Project, a longitudinal prospective study directed by Robert Plomin and John DeFries (1985), looked at matched adoptive and control families, adoptive and control infants, their adoptive, biological and control parents, and adoptive and control home environments. Comparisons were reported of infants at 12 and 24 months of age, on mental and motor development, temperament and behavioral problems. The sample was of 182 adopted infants and 165 non-adopted (control) infants matched on various factors, and infants were adopted between 3 and 172 days after birth (under 6 months).

The results at about 2 years after the beginning of the study showed that there were *few* differences detected on a variety of measures between the three groups of biological, adoptive and non-adoptive parents, so parental characteristics are unlikely to lead to differences between adopted and non-adopted children in the sample. Home characteristics were very similar in adoptive and control families.

Perinatal factors were not different among adopted and non-adopted infants. There were few differences in outcome measures between the two groups of infants at 12 and 24 months of age on measures of mental and motor development, temperament and behavioral problems. Age at placement was not a factor and selective placement was of no importance. Genetic factors were obviously significant, not solely influential, but point to a need to respect the genetic uniqueness of all children, adopted and non-adopted.

There were some minor differences between adopted and control infants and toddlers in terms of adjustment. For those few differences that did emerge, the adoptees generally displayed more favorable adjustment.

The overall conclusions were that there were no important differences between adopted and control infants and their families at this early age and that prediction of individual outcomes of early adoption cannot be made with sufficient certainty to be useful in predicting success or forecasting problems.

There are other broader and separate issues about the possible effects on adopted children of the characteristics of their adoptive parents and the circumstances in which they live. There is the general finding that as a group, older adopted children have I.Q. scores and scholastic attainments as good as those in the general population and substantially better than might have been expected on the basis of their biological background (Lambert & Streather, 1980; Scarr, 1981). It seems clear that this is due to the fact that, in general, adoptive parents tend to be rather better educated and of higher socio-economic status than average for the population. It appears that adoptive children's cognitive performance is responsive to their rearing environment, which tends to be above average, and adoptees perform well because they have benefited from the environment in which they were reared.

It should be noted that this also applies to transracial adoptions. One study (Scarr & Weinberg, 1976, 1978) found that black children adopted by white parents had a mean I.Q. of 110, some 20 points above comparable children reared in the black community (although some six points below the natural children in the white adopting families).

Other workers (Lambert & Streather, 1980), discussing comparable findings in their own outcome study of illegitimate and adopted children, remark that it may be that it is not adoption *per se* which is good for the children, but rather the combination of factors associated with it: (1) social class and materially comfortable homes; (2) older adopting parents who are more likely to be settled in homes and jobs; (3) family size—since adopting families tend to be smaller and the majority are two-child families, but a large number are one-child families.

One can also ask whether the same pattern of effects applies to personality differences and to psychiatric outcome. The evidence on this is more limited than with intellectual development, and the findings are dissimilar. Adoptees have a rate of psychiatric disorder which is *above that* in the general population (Von Knorring,

1983). It is certainly not as great as was originally claimed in the 1950s and 1960s, based on studies of selected clinical populations. The facts are such that several studies show that in the U.K., U.S.A. and Canada adopted children are referred to social and psychiatric services with about twice the frequency of the general population: this difference may reflect patterns of *referral* as well as increased rates of disturbance (Hersov, 1985; Jerome, 1986; Kotsopoulos *et al.*, 1988). On the other hand, it is also clear that a minority of children show significant clinical symptoms, and most adopted children are well within the normal range with respect to behavioral, emotional and academic adjustment. Two studies of psychological and academic adjustment in adopted children, using matched control groups and valid and reliable measures, showed that adopted children were rated as more poorly adjusted compared to non-adopted children, but were still well within the normal range of behavior (Brodzinsky, Schechter, Braff & Singer, 1984a; Brodzinsky, Singer & Braff, 1984b; Brodzinsky, 1987). Adoptive children in this study were doing very well, considering the background from which they came and their exposure to earlier stresses.

The Colorado Adoption Project findings (Plomin & DeFries, 1985) show scant evidence of psychological disturbance in the pre-school period, and it appears from other studies that adoptees who begin to show problems may do so in the school years, in middle childhood and adolescence.

STUDIES FROM HOSPITAL POPULATIONS

A number of studies have been published in the U.S.A. and elsewhere on adopted adolescents undergoing hospital or residential care for psychiatric disorders, which look at frequency of adoption in hospitalized adolescents, psychiatric diagnostic categories and other clinically important associations (Fullerton, Goodrich & Berman, 1986; Piersma, 1987; Rogeness, Hoppe, Macedo, Fischer & Harris, 1988; Wun Jung Kim, Davenport, Joseph, Zrull & Woolford, 1988; Hajal, Catenaccio & Hyler, 1988).

These studies all show that a higher percentage of adopted adolescents are found in hospital populations than are found in outpatient samples. The frequency of adoptees in hospitals has ranged from 2.9 to 21.2% of consecutive admissions, as against estimates of 2.2 and 3.5% of adoptees under 18 years of age in the general population (Mech, 1973). There are many possible reasons for the excess of admissions, such as hospital admission policies, socio-economic status of families, whether it is a public or private hospital, the rate in the population of adopted adolescents in the catchment area, differences in diagnostic practice, and treatment planning. Generally, the studies are weak in terms of control groups, data about age at adoption, reasons for adoption, family size and presence of other adopted or non-adopted children in the family, and whether the adoptions were extrafamilial or intrafamilial, i.e. by a related family member or not.

The studies show that adoptees display a wide range of psychiatric disorders which differ in some respects from those found in other groups of non-adopted patients. In a few studies the groups were matched on several factors.

Adoptees show more "externalizing" disorders (Achenbach & Edelbrock, 1983) with behavior directed outward to the environment such as adjustment, conduct, oppositional and antisocial disorders. Where the diagnosis of personality disorder was made, there was a higher frequency in adopted adolescents due to an increased frequency of this diagnosis in girls (Rogeness *et al.*, 1988). Some studies reported an excess of runaway behavior in adopted adolescents, with themes of abandonment and heightened depressive affect emerging during observation and treatment (Fullerton *et al.*, 1986). Sometimes the adoption broke down during hospital admission and the youngsters did not return to their adoptive families at the completion of treatment.

One study in the U.S.A. predicted that there would be higher rates of extrafamilial adoptions among children and adolescents admitted to psychiatric hospitals, as well as among juvenile offenders attending court (Wun Jung Kim *et al.*, 1988). The prediction was correct for hospital admissions, but a significant under-representation of adopted adolescents was found among the juvenile offenders. The same socio-economic factors which influence rate of admission to psychiatric hospitals may be operating, in that middle and upper middle class families were over-represented in the samples. They may be more likely to seek psychiatric help earlier, so that their children may be possibly protected from contact with the juvenile court system by referral to outpatient and inpatient hospital services first (Wun Jung Kim *et al.*, 1988).

Although it seems true that the majority of adoptions turn out well and that cognitive abilities of adopted and non-adopted do not differ, it is a little premature to assume that adoptees have no more adjustment problems than non-adopted children. Studies in the U.S.A., France, Sweden and England (Hersov, 1985) suggest that adoptees have greater problems of adjustment. Both the National Child Development Study (Seglow, Pringle, Kellmer & Wedge, 1972), and Bohman's study from Sweden (Bohman, 1970), showed behavioral problems as rated by teachers to be more common in adopted boys. In the Swedish studies the differences noted at 11 years decreased by age 15 and late adolescence (Bohman, 1978).

REASONS FOR THE EXCESS OF REFERRALS
TO CLINICS AND HOSPITALS

Several factors have been put forward to explain this excess of disturbance in adopted children, generally. These include: (1) biological and social factors related to pregnancy and perinatal experience in children coming from disadvantaged homes, such as inadequate prenatal care, poor nutrition, drug and alcohol abuse and mental illness in the parents (Seglow *et al.*, 1972; Crellin, Pringle, Kellmer & West, 1971); (2) experiences prior to final placement in an adoptive family, including the transition from foster care to adoptive home, after attachments have been made (Yarrow & Klein, 1980); (3) interference with the formation of normal attachments in early life, with later effects on personality and relationships; (4) adoption after an early infancy and childhood spent in an institution, with problems in adapting to family life; (5) the social stigma surrounding adoption (Kirk, 1981); (6) problems over identity in adolescence arising from confusion or uncertainty over unknown origins (Sants, 1964; Humphrey & Humphrey, 1986); (7) there is also the suggestion that adoptees are at higher risk for genetic factors leading to increased psychopathology. Genetic influences have been implicated in antisocial behavior, criminality, alcoholism and some psychiatric disorders (Bohman & Sigvardsson, 1985; Mednick *et al.*, 1983). There is a high rate of unmarried mothers among the biological mothers of non-relative adoptees (Seglow *et al.*, 1972). With pregnancy effects controlled, these mothers score highly on measures of psychopathology and there is possible genetic transmission of psychopathology to the children (Bohman, 1978; Loehlin, Willerman & Horn, 1982); and (8) difficulties arising from the "telling" process, affecting family relationships.

"TELLING" IN ADOPTION

One of the more difficult problems facing adoptive parents has to do with the adoption–revelation process, i.e. when, what and how to tell children initially about their being adopted, and how to manage the subsequent and often persistent questions that the child asks, with increasing age and cognitive and emotional development. It has been suggested that the vulnerability of some adopted children to psychological, emotional and academic problems has to do with issues arising from inappropriate or clumsy telling.

Professional workers in adoption practice regard family communication as a crucial issue, for it has been said that it is the "telling" that *proves* the adoption (Raynor, 1980). It is also a test of the parents' security in their role, their sensitivity to the child's questions and need for information or reassurance, and their own capacity to accept and understand the child's background.

Most professionals are quite insistent about the necessity of "telling" early in the child's life, i.e. between 2 and 4 years, starting with the simplest facts and providing increasing information as the child develops and comes to understand and adjust to their unique family situation (Mech, 1973).

Apart from this ground rule, there seems little agreement as to method and timing of "telling" and until recently, very little empirical data on children's understanding of adoption. Some clinicians working in the psychoanalytic framework maintain that repeated early telling of how the child was "chosen" can lead to feelings of mistrust and being unloved and unwanted, which may persist into adolescence and early adulthood, because the child perceives the information as a rejection and desertion by the natural parents (Peller, 1961). On the other hand, it is argued that the risks of attempted secrecy and denial are much greater because the risks of "finding out" later, possibly from someone outside the family, may shake the child's trust in their parents.

Tizard (1977) noted that young children often show mixed feelings in response to statements that they are different, were specially chosen, or that their biological parents had not brought them up. Holbrook (1984), in her study of 10–13-year old adopted and fostered children, found there were marked individual differences in the kind of information the children wanted. It was striking that parents wishing to shield their children from potentially hurtful truths, sometimes shied away from discussion, when children would welcome it. Many parents waited for the child to take the initiative, whereas these same children said they would prefer their parents to take the lead. It is clear that false explanations about adoption or about the biological parents are resented by adoptees, who find out the truth when they are older, but there is no clear association between parents' willingness to communicate the facts and adoption outcome (Triseliotis, 1973).

Schwartz (1975), in a commonsense article on guidelines to pediatricians involved in potential early intervention in problems arising in adopting families, makes several useful observations. He found in 44 adoptive families, that pre-school children, because of their egocentric thinking and self-centered view of the world, find statements about being "chosen" very positive and only rarely react with concern, negative responses or questions about this information. During middle childhood, latency, or the stage of concrete operational thinking, the earliest level of information is no longer sufficient, for the child can now think more logically and appraise information more realistically. The child also develops new and different perceptions about being adopted and therefore different from other children, within or outside his family. They have many new unanswered questions in spite of having been told earlier, but parents may not appreciate the need for additional information in keeping with this new developmental level. The older school child may want to know what their parents look like, but not their names. When adolescent, they want to know their parents level of education as well as their work, their abilities and what sort of person they are. In late adolescence and adulthood they can be interested in the medical history of their natural parents, especially when their own marriage is likely.

More recently in the U.S., Brodzinsky, Schechter and Brodzinsky (1986) interviewed 200 adopted and non-adopted children, aged 4–13 years, about their understanding of adoption.

They found that most pre-school children are unlikely to understand much about adoption, even when told about it by their parents and referring to themselves as "adopted." By 6 years of age, most children *do* differentiate between birth and adoption as alternative paths to parenthood. They also appreciate the *permanence* of adoptive family relationships. Between 8 and 11 years, their conception of adoption broadens in terms of appreciation of the uniqueness of the family and what this entails.

For some children between 8 and 11 years, this increase in knowledge gives rise to anxiety about the permanence of their status in the family. The data showed that much of the child's fantasy life is focused on the biological parents' potential for reclaiming the child and so disrupting adoptive family life. These findings are of particular interest, because the period of 8–11 years is the time when many adoptive children are referred for psychiatric assessment, and is also a period of increased disturbance in some longitudinal studies of adopted children (Bohman, 1970; Lambert & Streather, 1980). It may be a vulnerable period in which anxiety, insecurity and associated problems become manifest. As the children grow older, their uncertainty diminishes and they come to recognize the legal process of transfer of parental rights to adoptive parents.

The study also has important implications for adoption practice, particularly the advice given to parents about "telling." It questions a central assumption underlying the recommendation that early "telling," i.e. before 5 years of age, gives a child a basic understanding of their unique position in a family, as well as establishing a trusting relationship and facilitating a sense of confidence and positive self-image. The study questions whether pre-school-age children are really capable of understanding their adoptive status.

Others have also found that parents far too often overestimate the child's knowledge and unrealistically assume that there is no further need for disclosure and discussion as the child grows older (Raynor, 1980; Holbrook, 1984). The developmental aspect should be stressed in advice to parents, for if this issue is handled effectively, it may well forestall some of the problems of behavior and relationships which arise during late childhood and early adolescence. It is also at these later stages that adopted children show a less positive view of adoption as they grow older, possibly from exposure to negative comment from their peers and from their own awareness of the problems that can arise in being adopted (Brodzinsky *et al.*, 1984a, b).

ADOPTION DISRUPTION

I have spoken earlier about the finding that more older children and those with special needs are being placed for adoption. Many studies have shown that "adoption disruption" increases with age at adoption. "Disruption" is the preferred term to "failed adoption" and is defined as all placements which ended with the return of the child to the agency (Barth, 1988).

Barth and Berry (1988) carried out a prediction study on children aged 4 years or older who were placed in adoption in 13 California counties from January 1980 to June 1984. Slightly more than half of the children were male and most children were placed alone, rather than with siblings, in a family of their own race with adoptive parents not of the same religion as birth parents. Over two-thirds were adopted by foster parents rather than new adoptive parents. The mean age at placement was 7.2 years and more than 60% of the children were white. The average time in foster care prior to adoption placement was 35 months.

Only 10% of the placements disrupted and the average time to disruption was 18 months. The figures were lower than feared and, in general, the disruption rate is decreasing rather than increasing, possibly because selection of children and families is improving in quality.

Disruption rates were higher for children *not* adopted by foster parents, so the increase in foster parent adoption during the preceding years may account for the downward trend in disruption. The difference in stability of foster adoptions holds only for non-minority children. Foster adoptions were no more successful for children who had been previously placed for adoption or for children over 12 years of age.

FACTORS ASSOCIATED WITH DISRUPTION

The outcome in adoption results from a complex number of factors, and no single characteristic of a child, family or adoption practice is a reliable guide to predicting the outcome of placement. Certain features suggest a risk of disruption. Children with a previous adoptive placement, older children, children with problems of behavior or relationships, children adopted without subsidy, and adoptive mothers with higher education were found significantly more often in disrupted placements (Barth, 1988). Sibling adoptive placements in homes with no other children are unusually unlikely to disrupt.

The findings from the prediction study strongly support the conclusions of earlier studies that the amount and type of information and pre-placement preparation is crucial to a successful outcome. The views of families and social workers differ widely about the amount and quality of information given to a family. When not informed in advance, families had particular difficulty adjusting to children who had been sexually abused or who had serious behavior problems.

Families that adopted children who differed considerably from what they had hoped for had more difficult placements, but the difficulties could be ameliorated by providing more and accurate information. Families with the highest-risk placements reported receiving the least accurate information. Families who reported receiving realistic information were over-represented in the group with placements who were predicted to disrupt but did not (Barth *et al.*, 1986).

Fewer than half of the families reported getting adequate information about their child's psychological, dental, medical, educational and neurological background, birth history and early childhood development, and few post-placement services were offered and these were generally insufficient to prevent disruption.

A child is an active partner in the adoption process, as his or her behavior strongly influences the success or otherwise of the placement. Data on behavior were collected 3 months after placement using the Child Behavior Checklist (Achenbach & Edelbrock, 1983), a valid and reliable measure much used in the U.S.A. and other countries. For all adoptive children, the most common behavior problems noted by parents were inability to concentrate, excessive demands for attention, immaturity, impulsiveness, stubbornness, temper tantrums, poor school work and no apparent guilt after misbehavior. Children in placements which disrupted were significantly more likely to display high levels of interpersonal or externalizing problem behaviors, including meanness, cruelty, fighting, threatening behavior and vandalism. They also showed less increase in parent–child reciprocity over time, such as curiosity, showing affection, caring about parental approval and satisfaction of need for attention, unlike those children where placement was successful.

CONCLUSIONS

With the change in traditional assumptions and concepts in adoption practice, we should think of a spectrum of resources for children in need which includes adoption, fostering with a view to adoption, long- and short-term fostering, and residential care. There will always be a demand for these resources, even though one may hope that improvements in family welfare policy will reduce the need for substitute family care.

Transracial adoption and finding families for "hard to place" children has developed apace. Successful outcome using the usual criteria may not necessarily leave black or colored children with the appropriate sense of identity, but only further studies will clarify this.

There is no single reason why adopted children are over-represented in clinical populations and knowing what we do about the multifactorial causation of child and adolescent psychiatric disorder, this should not come as a surprise. The data from adoption studies show the importance of genetic factors in the major disorders, but the common-or-garden problems are still the result of the interaction of nature and nurture, and the intervention should focus on the latter. Recent empirical research is showing the importance of some developmental issues, while providing a more balanced view of some traditional beliefs about telling.

As older children and those with special needs are increasingly placed for adoption, they will take a central place in permanency planning. It is also this population who are more prone to adoption disruption and psychiatric disorder, given some of the circumstances mentioned earlier. The types of disturbed behavior they display mean that both they and their adoptive parents may require clinical intervention. Further research is needed to better understand factors leading to disruption as well as the provision of better adoption programs and practice, including post-placement support, and this is clearly where the challenges lie in the future.

REFERENCES

Achenbach, T. M. & Edelbrock, C. (1983). *Manual for the child behavior checklist and revised child behavior profile*. Burlington: Burlington University Associates in Psychiatry.

Adoption Factbook (1985). *United States data, issues, regulations and resources*. Washington, DC: National Committee for Adoption, Inc.

Auden, W. H. & Kronenberger, L. (1970). *The Faber book of aphorisms*. London: Faber and Faber.

Barth, R. P. (1988). Disruption in older child adoptions. *Public Welfare, 6,* 23–44.

Barth, R. P. & Berry, M. (1988). *Adoption and disruption rates, risks and responses*. New York: Aldine de Gruyter.

Barth, R. P., Berry, M., Carson, M. L., Goodfield, R. & Feinberg, B. (1986). Contributions to disruption and dissolution of older-child adoptions. *Child Welfare, 65,* 359–371.

Benet, M. K. (1976). *The politics of adoption*. New York: The Free Press.

Bohman, M. (1970). *Adopted children and their families*. Stockholm: Proprius.

Bohman, M. (1978). An eighteen-year prospective longitudinal study of adopted boys. In E. J. Anthony & C. Chiland (Eds), *The child in his family: Vulnerable children* (pp. 473–486). New York: Wiley.

Bohman, M. & Sigvardsson, S. (1985). A prospective longitudinal study of adoption. In A. R. Nicol (Ed.), *Longitudinal studies in child psychology and psychiatry* (pp. 137–155). Chicester: Wiley.

Borgman, R. (1982). The consequences of open and closed adoption for older children. *Child Welfare, 61,* 217–226.

Brodzinsky, D. M. (1987). Adjustment to adoption: a psychosocial perspective. *Clinical Psychology Review, 7,* 25–47.

Brodzinsky, D. M., Radice, C., Huffman, L. & Merkler, K. (1987). Prevalence of clinically significant symptomatology in a nonclinical sample of adopted and nonadopted children. *Journal of Clinical Child Psychology, 16,* 350–356.

Brodzinsky, D. M., Schechter, D. E., Braff, A. M. & Singer, L. M. (1984a). Psychological and academic adjustment in adopted children. *Journal of Consulting and Clinical Psychology, 52,* 582–590.

Brodzinsky, D. M., Schechter, D. E. & Brodzinsky, A. B. (1986). Children's knowledge of adoption. Developmental changes and implications for adjustment. In R. D. Ashmore

& D. M. Brodzinsky (Eds), *Thinking about the family: Views of parents and children* (pp. 205–232). Hillsdale, NJ: Lawrence Erlbaum.

Brodzinsky, D. M., Singer, L. M. & Braff, A. M. (1984b). Childrens' understanding of adoption. *Child Development, 55,* 869–878.

Crellin, E., Pringle, M. L., Kellmer, D. & West, P. (1971). *Born illegitimate: Social and educational implications.* Windsor: National Foundation for Educational Research.

Deutsch, C. K., Swanson, J. M., Bruell, J. H., Cantwell, D. P., Weinberg, F. & Baren, M. (1982). Overrepresentation of adoptees in children with attention deficit disorder. *Behavioral Genetics, 12,* 231–237.

Fullerton, C. S., Goodrich, W. & Berman, L. B. (1986). Adoption predicts psychiatric treatment resistances in hospitalized adolescents. *Journal of the American Academy of Child Psychiatry, 25,* 542–551.

Gill, O. & Jackson, B. (1983). *Adoption and race.* London: Batsford.

Grow, L. J. & Shapiro, O. (1974). *Black children, white parents: A study of transracial adoption.* New York: Child Welfare League of America, Inc.

Hajal, F., Catenaccio, R. & Hyler, I. (1988). Adopted adolescents in the psychiatric hospital and their families. Paper presented at the Annual Meeting of The American Academy of Child and Adolescent Psychiatry, Seattle, WA, October 1988.

Hastings, J. (Ed.) (1908). *Encyclopedia of religion and ethics.* New York: Charles Scribner and Sons.

Hersov, L. (1985). Adoption and fostering. In M. Rutter & L. Hersov (Eds), *Child and adolescent psychiatry: Modern approaches* (2nd edn, pp. 101–117). Oxford: Blackwell.

Holbrook, D. (1984). Knowledge of origins, self-esteem and family ties of long-term fostered and adopted children. Report to the Holden Trust.

Home Office (1972). *Report of the Departmental Committee on the Adoption of Children.* Chairmen: His Honor, Judge F. A. Stockdale and Sir William Houghton. Home Office: Scottish Education Department Cmnd 5107; London: Her Majesty's Stationery Office.

Humphrey, M. & Humphrey, H. (1986). A fresh look at genealogical bewilderment. *British Journal of Medical Psychology, 59,* 133–140.

Jerome, L. (1986). Overrepresentation of adopted children attending a children's mental health center. *Canadian Journal of Psychiatry, 31,* 526–531.

Kadushin, A. & Martin, J. A. (1988). *Child Welfare Services* (4th edn). New York: Macmillan.

Kawashima, Y. (1981/1982). Adoption in early America. *Journal of Family Law, 20,* 677–696.

Kirk, H. D. (1981). *Adoptive kinship.* Toronto: Butterworths.

Kotsopoulos, S., Cote, A., Joseph, L., Pentland, N., Stavrakaki, C., Sheahan, P. & Oke, L. (1988). Psychiatric disorders in adopted children: a controlled study. *American Journal of Orthopsychiatry, 58,* 608–612.

Lambert, L. & Streather, J. (1980). *Children in changing families: A study of adoption and illegitimacy.* London: Macmillan.

Loehlin, J. C., Willerman, L. & Horn, J. M. (1982). Personality resemblances between unwed mothers and their adopted-away offspring. *Journal of Personality and Social Psychology,* **42,** 1089–1099.

Mech, E. V. (1973). Adoption: a policy perspective. In B. Caldwell & H. Ricciuti (Eds), *Review of child development research,* Vol. 3 (pp. 467–508). Chicago: University of Chicago Press.

Mednick, S. A., Moffitt, T. E., Pollock, V., Talovic, S., Gabrielli, W. F. & Van Dusen, K. T. (1983). The inheritance of human deviance. In D. Magnusson & V. Allen (Eds), *Human development: An interactional perspective* (pp. 221–242). New York: Academic Press.

Nichols, P. L. & Chen, T. C. (1981). *Minimal brain dysfunction: A prospective study.* Hillsdale, NJ: Erlbaum.

Office of Population Censuses and Surveys (1987). *Adoptions in England and Wales, notified during 1985 and 1986.* Reference FM3 87/1, London: H.M.S.O.

Office of Population Censuses and Surveys (1989). *Marriage and divorce statistics* (Series FM2, No. 14). London: H.M.S.O.

Peller, L. E. (1961). About "telling the child" about his adoption. *Bulletin of the Philadelphia Association for Psychoanalysis,* **11,** 145–154.

Piersma, H. L. (1987). Adopted children and inpatient psychiatric treatment: a retrospective study. *The Psychiatric Hospital,* **18,** 153–158.

Plomin, R. (1986). *Development, genetics and psychology.* Hillsdale, NJ: Erlbaum.

Plomin, R. & DeFries, J. C. (1985). *Origins of individual differences in infancy. The Colorado adoption project.* New York: Academic Press.

Powers, D. (1984). The hurried adoption of older children. Lessons from the American experience. *Association for Child Psychology and Psychiatry Newsletter,* **6,** 11–13.

Presser, S. B. (1972). The historical background of the American law of adoption. *Journal of Family Law,* **11,** 443–516.

Raynor, L. (1980). *The adopted child comes of age.* London: George Allen and Unwin.

Reeves, A. C. (1971). Children with surrogate parents: cases seen in analytic therapy and an aetiological hypothesis. *British Journal of Medical Psychology,* **44,** 155–171.

Rogeness, G. A., Hoppe, S. K., Macedo, C. A., Fischer, C. & Harris, W. A. (1988). Psychopathology in hospitalized, adopted children. *Journal of the American Academy of Child and Adolescent Psychiatry,* **27,** 628–631.

Sants, H. J. (1964). Genealogical bewilderment in children with substitute parents. *British Journal of Medical Psychology,* **37,** 133–141.

Scarr, S. (1981). *Race, social class, and individual differences: New studies of old problems.* Hillsdale, NJ: Lawrence Erlbaum.

Scarr, S. & Weinberg, R. A. (1976). I.Q. Test performance of black children adopted by white families. *American Psychologist,* **31,** 726–739.

Scarr, S. & Weinberg, R. A. (1978). The influence of "family background" on intellectual attainment. *American Sociological Review,* **43,** 674–692.

Schwartz, E. M. (1975). Problems after adoption: some guidelines for pediatrician involvement. *The Journal of Pediatrics,* **87,** 991–994.

Seglow, J., Pringle, M. L., Kellmer, D. & Wedge, P. (1972). *Growing up adopted*. Windsor: National Foundation for Educational Research.

Sorosky, A. D., Baran, A. & Pannor, R. (1984). *The adoption triangle*. New York: Anchor Books.

Tizard, B. (1977). *Adoption: A second chance*. London: Open Books.

Tizard, J. (1974). The upbringing of other people's children: implications of research and for research. *Journal of Child Psychology and Psychiatry,* **15,** 161–173.

Triseliotis, J. (1973). *In search of origins: The experiences of adopted people*. London: Routledge and Keegan Paul.

Triseliotis, J. & Russell, J. (1984). *Hard to place: The outcome of late adoptions and residential care*. London: Heinemann.

Von Knorring, A. L. (1983). *Adoption studies on psychiatric illness: Epidemiological, environmental and genetic aspects*. Sweden: Umeå University Medical Dissertations (New Series), No. 101.

Wun Jung Kim, Davenport, C., Joseph, J., Zrull, J. & Woolford, E. (1988). Psychiatric disorder and juvenile delinquency in adopted children and adolescents. *Journal of the American Academy of Child and Adolescent Psychiatry,* **27,** 111–115.

Yarrow, L. J. & Klein, R. P. (1980). Environmental discontinuity associated with transition from foster to adoptive homes. *International Journal of Behavior and Development,* **3,** 311–322.

Zill, N. (1985). Behavior and learning problems among adopted children: findings from a U.S. national survey of child health. Paper presented at the biannual meeting of the Society for Research in Child Development, Toronto, Canada.